Acute and Emergency Care in Athletic Training

Michelle A. Cleary, PhD, ATC

Chapman University

Katie Walsh Flanagan, EdD, LAT, ATC

East Carolina University

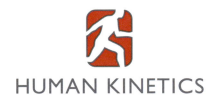

HUMAN KINETICS

Library of Congress Cataloging-in-Publication Data

Names: Cleary, Michelle A., 1970- author. | Flanagan, Katie Walsh, author.
Title: Acute and emergency care in athletic training / Michelle A. Cleary,
  Katie Walsh Flanagan.
Description: Champaign, IL : Human Kinetics, [2020] | Includes
  bibliographical references and index.
Identifiers: LCCN 2018028441 (print) | LCCN 2018028936 (ebook) | ISBN
  9781492587163 (e-book) | ISBN 9781492536536 (print)
Subjects: | MESH: Athletic Injuries--therapy | Emergency Treatment |
  Emergency Medical Services | Sports Medicine--methods
Classification: LCC RD97 (ebook) | LCC RD97 (print) | NLM WA 292 | DDC
  617.1/027--dc23
LC record available at https://lccn.loc.gov/2018028441

ISBN: 978-1-4925-3653-6 (print)

The web addresses cited in this text were current as of September 2018, unless otherwise noted.

Senior Acquisitions Editor: Joshua J. Stone
Developmental and Managing Editor: Amanda S. Ewing
Copyeditor: Joanna Hatzopoulos Portman
Proofreader: Chernow Editorial Services, Inc.
Indexer: Rebecca L. McCorkle
Permissions Manager: Dalene Reeder
Senior Graphic Designer: Nancy Rasmus
Cover Designer: Keri Evans
Cover Design Associate: Susan Rothermel Allen
Photograph (cover): Patrick S. Blood/Icon Sportswire
Photographer (interior): Gregg Henness, unless otherwise noted
Photographs (interior): © Human Kinetics, unless otherwise noted
Photo Asset Manager: Laura Fitch
Photo Production Coordinator: Amy M. Rose
Photo Production Manager: Jason Allen
Senior Art Manager: Kelly Hendren
Illustrations: © Human Kinetics, unless otherwise noted
Printer: Walsworth

We thank East Carolina University in Greenville, North Carolina, for assistance in providing the location for the photo shoot for this book.

Printed in the United States of America   10 9 8 7 6 5 4

The paper in this book was manufactured using responsible forestry methods.

Human Kinetics
1607 N. Market Street
Champaign, IL 61820
USA

United States and International
Website: **US.HumanKinetics.com**
Email: info@hkusa.com
Phone: 1-800-747-4457

Canada
Website: **Canada.HumanKinetics.com**
Email: info@hkcanada.com

E6893

Tell us what you think!
Human Kinetics would love to hear what we can do to improve the customer experience. Use this QR code to take our brief survey.

CONTENTS

Preface   vii

Acknowledgments   ix

CAATE Standards   xi

PART I — Introduction to Acute and Emergency Care in Athletic Training

Chapter 1   The Interprofessional Health Care Team   3

Characteristics of a Good Team 4 • Sports Medicine Setting 6 • Breakdowns in Teamwork 15 • Effective Practices in Teamwork 18 • Professional Attributes of Effective Health Care Providers 18 • Therapeutic Behaviors 19 • Summary 25

Chapter 2   Prevention and Risk Management Strategies   27

Risk Management 27 • Infectious Diseases 28 • Standard Precautions 34 • Exposure Control Plans 43 • Legal Responsibility 43 • Summary 52

Chapter 3   Planning for Emergencies   53

Epidemiology of Medical Emergencies in Sports 54 • Emergency Planning in Sports 54 • Developing an Emergency Action Plan for Each Venue 56 • Developing Acute Care and Emergency Protocols for Major Trauma and Medical Emergencies 57 • Consulting With Institutional Authorities and Working With Local EMS Providers 58 • Obtaining and Maintaining Emergency Equipment and Supplies 62 • Reviewing the EAP and Training Personnel 62 • Communicating During an Emergency 68 • Mass Care and Catastrophic Incidents 71 • Post-Catastrophic Injury or Post-Critical Incident Plan 72 • Evidence for Best Practices in Emergency Preparedness 74 • Summary 75

Chapter 4   The Emergency Examination   77

Scene Size-Up 79 • Initial Assessment 82 • Identify the Chief Complaint or Concern 89 • Focused Assessment 91 • Monitor the Critically Injured or Ill Patient 93 • Reassessment 100 • Patient Hand-Off 100 • Evidence for Injury Scoring Systems 101 • Summary 103

Chapter 5   Emergency Medications and Administration   105

Medical Direction and Oversight 105 • Best Practices for Safe Administration of Medication 107 • Medication Administration 108 • Oral Medication Administration 110 • Sublingual Medication Administration 110 • Metered-Dose Inhaler Administration 111 • Oxygen Administration 112 • Nebulized Medication Administration 115 • Emergency Medication Injection 116 • Intravenous Access 120 • Summary 131

PART II   Immediate Management of Acute Injuries and Illnesses

Chapter 6   Immediate Management of Bleeding, Shock, and Immunologic Emergencies   135

Overview of the Circulatory System 136 • Hemorrhage 136 • Shock 152 • Anaphylactic Reactions and Immunologic Emergencies 160 • Evidence 177 • Summary 177

Chapter 7   Immediate Management of Musculoskeletal Injuries   179

Overview of the Structures 179 • Classification of Injuries 183 • Shoulder Dislocation 187 • Elbow Dislocation 191 • Finger Dislocation 193 • Hip Dislocation 194 • Knee Dislocation 195 • Ankle Dislocation 197 • Humeral Fractures 200 • Colles' Fracture 202 • Pelvis Fracture 203 • Femur Fracture 205 • Tibia-Fibula Fractures 207 • Ankle Fractures 208 • Management of Lower-Leg Fractures 209 • Compartment Syndrome 214 • Ring Avulsion 215 • Summary 216

Chapter 8   Traumatic Injuries to the Head and Face   217

Overview of the Head and Face 217 • Overview of Head Injuries 220 • Scalp Lacerations 220 • Skull Fracture 221 • Concussion 221 • Chronic Traumatic Encephalopathy 225 • Intracranial Pressure 226 • Intracerebral Contusion 226 • Epidural Hematoma 226 • Subdural Hematoma 227 • Headaches 228 • Stroke 231 • Seizures 233 • Altered Mental Status 236 • Overview of Facial Injuries 236 • Corneal Abrasion and Foreign Objects in the Eye 238 • Retinal Detachment 239 • Hyphema 240 • Tympanic Membrane Rupture 240 • Facial Fractures 241 • Temporomandibular Joint Dislocation 242 • Dental Injuries 242 • Laryngeal Injuries 242 • Summary 245

Chapter 9   Traumatic Injuries to the Spine   247

Anatomy and Physiology of the Spine 247 • Pathophysiology 252 • Emergency Medical Care of Injuries to the Spine 254 • Equipment Removal 269 • Summary 279

Chapter 10   Injuries of the Thorax and Lungs   281

Overview of Anatomical Structures in the Thorax 281 • Respiratory Assessment 286 • Using Supplemental Oxygen 286 • Airway Maintenance 288 • Rib Fracture 291 • Sternoclavicular Joint Injury 293 • Pulmonary Embolism 295 • Pneumothorax, Hemothorax, and Hemopneumothorax 297 • Asthma 299 • Summary 302

Chapter 11   Life-Threatening Cardiac Conditions   303

Overview of the Cardiovascular System 303 • Epidemiology of Sudden Cardiac Death 307 • Etiology and Pathophysiology of Acute Cardiac Conditions 308 • Field Assessment Techniques for Emergent Cardiac Conditions 315 • Immediate Management of Sudden Cardiac Arrest 315 • Emergency Preparedness for Sudden Cardiac Arrest 321 • Clinical Decision Making 323 • Evidence: Cardiovascular Screening 323 • Evidence: Factors Affecting Survival After Sudden Cardiac Arrest 325 • Summary 325

Chapter 12   Injuries and Illnesses of the Abdominopelvic Region   327

Overview of Anatomical Structures in the Abdomen and Pelvis 327 •
Trauma to Abdominal Organs 332 • Injuries to the Liver and
Spleen 332 • Injury to the Kidneys 335 • Appendicitis 337 • Acute
Abdominopelvic Concerns for Female Athletes 339 • Acute Trauma to
Male Genitals 340 • Summary 342

Chapter 13   Life-Threatening Metabolic Emergencies   343

Overview of the Anatomical Structures in Metabolic Emergencies 343 •
Diabetes 344 • Hypoglycemia and Hyperglycemia 348 • Summary 351

Chapter 14   Exertional Sickling and Rhabdomyolysis   353

Exertional Rhabdomyolysis 353 • Sickle Cell Trait 358 • Evidence:
Factors That Increase Risk of Exertional Rhabdomyolysis 362 •
Summary 362

Chapter 15   Environmental Emergencies   365

Lightning Emergencies 365 • Heat-Related Emergencies 368 •
Cold-Related Emergencies 372 • Altitude-Related Emergencies 375 •
Summary 377

Appendix A: Model Exposure Control Plan   379
Appendix B: SCAT-5   383
Glossary   393
References   405
Index   435
About the Authors   448
Contributors and External Reviewers   449

PREFACE

Acute and Emergency Care in Athletic Training is an essential text on prehospital care of the acutely injured or ill patient. It is written for the professional-level health care student. Athletic training programs of all levels can benefit from the content that addresses the National Athletic Trainers' Association (NATA) educational competencies relating to immediate management of acute injuries and illnesses to physically active people. While athletic training curricula include examination of musculoskeletal and medical conditions, this text specifically addresses the patient care that is provided between the field and the emergency department. These areas of prehospital health care have been previously addressed in the literature in the form of position statements, consensus statements, and interassociation proclamations. However, until now, they have not been available in a comprehensive text for the prehospital care of the patient who is injured or ill.

This text is a significant addition to the literature as an interprofessional resource describing the most up-to-date information available in the medical literature. In the spirit of interprofessional collaborative practice, evidence from a variety of health care professions was consulted in the writing of each chapter. Drawing from the literature in the emergency response system, paramedic training, and emergency medicine resources, this text is the first to comprehensively review the literature for the most current evidence to support clinical practice. In addition to position and consensus statements from the NATA and other professional organizations, this text provides more review of the literature and application to practice. This text specifically focuses on the competencies identified in the CAATE 2020 standards and the new skills and techniques ATs must be prepared to use in an emergency situation. This is one of the first texts directed at masters-level professional programs that includes the definitive knowledge and skills needed for clinical decision-making during a medical emergency. This book and its online ancillaries aim to benefit the graduate athletic training student and educators in preparing the next generation of prehospital health care teams.

Organization

This text provides the essential knowledge and skills that a competent entry-level health care professional should be able to provide in the prehospital setting. The reader will find a systematic approach to acute and emergency care in the athletic training setting.

Part I of this text provides a comprehensive understanding of how current AT practice fits into the overall health care system. Athletic trainers have always been primary care providers who work interprofessionally with other HCPs. However, this section of the text demonstrates how the interprofessional health care team must communicate, cooperate, and collaborate in the management of medical emergencies. The evolution of health care services is described as well as how appropriate precautions can minimize risk and prevent medical errors. Further described is a collaborative approach to emergency planning and the steps necessary to effectively manage an emergency response and implement an effective post-catastrophic or critical incident plan. The emergency examination is detailed to allow the student to focus on each step in a systematic, consistent manner that allows a successful hand-off to the next level care provider. Throughout the first 5 chapters, the new CAATE standards as well as evidence-based practice are interwoven into providing readiness for the AT to provide emergency services, administer emergency medicines, and provide patients with the best possible care when faced with an emergency.

Part II of this text takes a body systems approach to describing how to examine, treat, and manage common acute injuries and illnesses of the immune, musculoskeletal, nervous, respiratory, cardiac, metabolic, and thermoregulatory systems. It is assumed the graduate AT student has a basic understanding the underlying anatomy and physiology of the body, and detailed coverage of this content is not included. However, a deep understanding of the etiology and pathophysiology of common conditions as well as how to respond are included in each chapter as important aspects of clinical decision-making during an emergency.

Unless otherwise noted, the chapters in part II are organized in a linear fashion, beginning with a brief overview of the relevant anatomy and physiology of the body system. (A basic knowledge of human anatomy, physiology, health, and wellness is assumed, and foundational information is therefore not included.) Next, the text provides an in-depth description of the epidemiology and etiology of each condition as well as how to recognize the signs and symptoms during the emergency examination. In addition, it includes field assessment techniques (e.g., diagnostic accuracy and clinical prediction rules) and immediate management techniques (e.g., indication, contraindications, and transportation techniques).

Special Features

To aid in the learning process, this text includes the following special elements:

- Red Flag boxes assist the reader in rapidly identifying potentially limb- or life-threatening conditions.
- Clinical Skills boxes detail in a step-by-step fashion how to complete a specific skill.
- Decision-making algorithms and decision trees assist the learner in recognizing important steps that depend on the individual patient scenario.
- Glossary terms are set in bold type and defined in the end-of-book glossary.

In addition, students will benefit from the full-color illustrations detailing anatomy, various conditions, spine boarding, equipment removal, and more.

Web Study Guide

The accompanying web study guide provides two case studies per chapter. The case studies highlight the specific application of examination, management, and return-to-participation considerations of specific acute or emergent medical conditions. The case studies help athletic trainers make clinical decisions, determine appropriate techniques, and apply prevention strategies taught in this text. Access the web study guide at www. HumanKinetics.com/AcuteAndEmergencyCareIn AthleticTraining.

Instructor Ancillaries

Instructors have access to a full array of ancillaries.

- The **presentation package** has more than 700 slides that cover the content of each chapter. Select figures and tables are also included.
- The **image bank** contains most of the figures and tables from the text. Instructors can use these individual files to supplement lecture notes and create student handouts.
- The **text package** contains more than 380 questions that instructors can use to build tests and quizzes.
- The **instructor guide** includes chapter summaries, ideas for activities, and suggested websites to consult for more information. The instructor guide also provides answers to the case studies in the web study guide, allowing instructors to easily grade students' answers.

Access the ancillaries at www.HumanKinetics.com/ AcuteAndEmergencyCareInAthleticTraining.

ACKNOWLEDGMENTS

This text would not be possible without the clinical athletic trainers who have tirelessly provided health care to innumerable athletes over the past half century. Their contributions have propelled the profession forward into the modern health care system of today. I am proud to be part of the evolution of the athletic training profession, and I look forward to seeing how the future unfolds. As for my part in writing this book, I would not have had the time or energy needed without the support of my best friend and partner in life—my husband, Geoff Maloney. I am eternally grateful to him and to other family and friends who have supported me over the years. My mom, Roberta McCaw, has always encouraged me to push the limits of what seems possible so that I could achieve my goals. My dad, Jack Cleary, has been a driving force for knowing how to succeed and believing that I deserved to lead a fabulous life full of hard work, fun, and adventure. Chris Long (my other best friend) and his better half, Lety Pulido, have inspired and motivated me to be the best version of myself and to strive to lead a long and healthy life. My gratitude goes to all these people and all the others who have encouraged, supported, and mentored me and who have toiled, sweated, and succeeded with me. Thank you.

—Michelle Cleary

This textbook is dedicated to the athletic training students, faculty, and fellow athletic trainers who made my life better and challenged me to become a better athletic trainer and instructor. A special thank-you for Dr. Sharon Rogers Moore, who taught me how to make off-field learning an art and how to be a wonderful friend, and who let me bounce every idea I had off her. Together with my AT faculty and staff, she makes coming to work fun. Thank you to my youthful, energetic parents, Phyllis Walsh Kelly and Gerald Kelly, who by their actions and words remind me to always keep learning, to be inquisitive, to be thankful for everything, and to be kind—always. And thank you to Sean Bryce Flanagan, my wonderful and patient husband who keeps me laughing, keeps me grounded, and makes my world brighter.

—Katie Walsh Flanagan

Thank you to the wonderful staff at Human Kinetics! Without the inspiration of Josh Stone to create this textbook and the careful and tenacious work of Amanda Ewing to make our words better, this project would never have happened. We have to point out the extraordinary work of Amanda, who was persistent, patient, and encouraging every step of the way. We have a special thank you to HK photographer Gregg Henness, who rescheduled the photo shoot around Hurricane Florence to get the perfect images we needed for the text; to Dalene Reeder, who worked hard behind the scenes to secure the permissions; and to Nancy Rasmus, who designed the book to make it enjoyable reading.

We were lucky enough to work with dedicated and brilliant authors who researched their respective content areas and brought forth cutting-edge and evidence-based information to each chapter. Thank you for the generosity of Ron Courson and the University of Georgia. Mr. Courson unselfishly gave us full access to his images for the management of an acute spinal injury (featured in chapter 9), and we could not be more grateful. Thank you also to Battalion Chief Sparrow of the Fire/Rescue/EMS Department in Greenville, North Carolina, for her generosity in loaning us medical equipment for the photo shoot.

—Michelle and Katie

CAATE STANDARDS

The following Commission of Accreditation of Athletic Training Education (CAATE) 2020 standards are covered in this text:

Standard 56: Advocate for the health needs of clients, patients, communities, and populations.

- Annotation: Advocacy encompasses activities that promote health and access to health care for individuals, communities, and the larger public.

Standard 59: Communicate effectively and appropriately with clients/patients, family members, coaches, administrators, other health care professionals, consumers, payors, policy makers, and others.

Standard 61: Practice in collaboration with other health care and wellness professionals.

Standard 62: Provide athletic training services in a manner that uses the best evidence to inform practice.

Standard 63: Use systems of quality assurance and quality improvement to enhance client/patient care.

Standard 64: Apply contemporary principles and practices of health informatics to the administration and delivery of patient care, including (but not limited to) the ability to do the following:

- Use data to drive informed decisions
- Maintain data privacy, protection, and data security
- Use medical classification systems (including International Classification of Disease codes) and terminology (including Current Procedural Terminology)
- Use an electronic health record to document, communicate, and manage health-related information; mitigate error; and support decision making

Standard 65: Practice in a manner that is congruent with the ethical standards of the profession.

Standard 66: Practice health care in a manner that is compliant with the BOC Standards of Professional Practice and applicable institutional/organizational, local, state, and federal laws, regulations, rules, and guidelines. Applicable laws and regulations include (but are not limited to) the following:

- Requirements for physician direction and collaboration
- Mandatory reporting obligations
- Health Insurance Portability and Accountability Act (HIPAA)
- Family Education Rights and Privacy Act (FERPA)
- Universal Precautions/OSHA Bloodborne Pathogen Standards
- Regulations pertaining to over-the-counter and prescription medications

Standard 69: Develop a care plan for each patient. The care plan includes (but is not limited to) the following:

- Assessment of the patient on an ongoing basis and adjustment of care accordingly
- Collection, analysis, and use of patient-reported and clinician-rated outcome measures to improve patient care
- Consideration of the patient's goals and level of function in treatment decisions
- Discharge of the patient when goals are met or the patient is no longer making progress
- Referral when warranted

Standard 70: Evaluate and manage patients with acute conditions, including triaging conditions that are life threatening or otherwise emergent. These include (but are not limited to) the following conditions:

- Cardiac compromise (including emergency cardiac care, supplemental oxygen, suction, adjunct airways, nitroglycerin, and low-dose aspirin)
- Respiratory compromise (including use of pulse oximetry, adjunct airways, supplemental oxygen, spirometry, meter-dosed inhalers, nebulizers, and bronchodilators)
- Conditions related to the environment: lightning, cold, heat (including use of rectal thermometry)
- Cervical spine compromise
- Traumatic brain injury
- Internal and external hemorrhage (including use of a tourniquet and hemostatic agents)
- Fractures and dislocations (including reduction of dislocation)
- Anaphylaxis (including administering epinephrine using automated injection device)
- Exertional sickling, rhabdomyolysis, and hyponatremia
- Diabetes (including use of glucometer, administering glucagon, insulin)
- Drug overdose (including administration of rescue medications such as naloxone)
- Wounds (including care and closure)
- Testicular injury
- Other musculoskeletal injuries

Standard 71: Perform an examination to formulate a diagnosis and plan of care for patients with health conditions commonly seen in athletic training practice. This exam includes the following:

- Obtaining a medical history from the patient or other individual
- Identifying comorbidities and patients with complex medical conditions
- Assessing function (including gait)
- Selecting and using tests and measures that assess the following, as relevant to the patient's clinical presentation:
  - Cardiovascular system (including auscultation)
  - Endocrine system
  - Eyes, ears, nose, throat, mouth, and teeth
  - Gastrointestinal system
  - Genitourinary system
  - Integumentary system
  - Mental status
  - Musculoskeletal system
  - Neurological system
  - Pain level
  - Reproductive system
  - Respiratory system (including auscultation)
  - Specific functional tasks
  - Evaluating all results to determine a plan of care, including referral to the appropriate provider when indicated

Standard 72: Perform or obtain the necessary and appropriate diagnostic or laboratory tests—including (but not limited to) imaging, blood work, urinalysis—to facilitate diagnosis, referral, and treatment planning.

Standard 74: Educate patients regarding appropriate pharmacological agents for the management of their condition, including indications, contraindications, dosing, interactions, and adverse reactions.

Standard 75: Administer medications or other therapeutic agents by the appropriate route of administration upon the order of a physician or other provider with legal prescribing authority

Standard 76: Evaluate and treat a patient who has sustained a concussion or other brain injury, with consideration of established guidelines:

- Performance of a comprehensive examination designed to recognize concussion or other brain injury, including (but not limited to) neurocognitive evaluation, assessment of the vestibular and vision systems, cervical spine involvement, mental health status, sleep assessment, exertional testing, nutritional status, and clinical interview
- Re-examination of the patient on an ongoing basis
- Recognition of an atypical response to brain injury
- Implementation of a plan of care (addressing vestibular and oculomotor disturbances, cervical spine pain, headache, vision, psychological needs, nutrition, sleep disturbance, exercise, academic and behavioral accommodations, and risk reduction)
- Return of the patient to activity/participation
- Referral to the appropriate provider when indicated

Standard 78: Select, fabricate, and/or customize prophylactic, assistive, and restrictive devices, materials, and techniques for incorporation into the plan of care, including the following:

- Durable medical equipment
- Orthotic devices
- Taping, splinting, protective padding, and casting

Standard 80: Develop, implement, and assess the effectiveness of programs to reduce injury risk.

Standard 81: Plan and implement a comprehensive pre-participation examination process to affect health outcomes.

Standard 82: Develop, implement, and supervise comprehensive programs to maximize sport performance that are safe and specific to the client's activity.

Standard 83: Educate and make recommendations to clients/patients on fluids and nutrients to ingest prior to activity, during activity, and during recovery for a variety of activities and environmental conditions

Standard 85: Monitor and evaluate environmental conditions to make appropriate recommendations to start, stop, or modify activity in order to prevent environmental illness or injury.

Standard 86: Select, fit, and remove protective equipment to minimize the risk of injury or re-injury.

Standard 88: Perform administrative duties related to the management of physical, human, and financial resources in the delivery of health care services. These include (but are not limited to) the following duties:

- Strategic planning and assessment
- Managing a physical facility that is compliant with current standards and regulations
- Managing budgetary and fiscal processes
- Identifying and mitigating sources of risk to the individual, the organization, and the community
- Navigating multipayor insurance systems and classifications
- Implementing a model of delivery (for example, value-based care model)

Standard 89: Use a comprehensive patient-file management system (including diagnostic and procedural codes) for documentation of patient care and health insurance management.

Standard 90: Establish a working relationship with a directing or collaborating physician.

- Annotation: This standard is specific to preparing an athletic trainer to fulfill the Board of Certification Standards of Professional Practice, specifically Standard 1, "The Athletic Trainer renders service or treatment under the direction of, or in collaboration with a physician, in accordance with their training and the state's statutes, rules and regulations."[1]

Standard 91: Develop, implement, and revise policies and procedures to guide the daily operation of athletic training services.

- Annotation: Examples of daily operation policies include pharmaceutical management, physician referrals, and inventory management.

Standard 92: Develop, implement, and revise policies that pertain to prevention, preparedness, and response to medical emergencies and other critical incidents.

Standard 93: Develop and implement specific policies and procedures for individuals who have sustained concussions or other brain injuries, including the following:

- Education of all stakeholders
- Recognition, appraisal, and mitigation of risk factors
- Selection and interpretation of baseline testing
- Agreement on protocols to be followed, including immediate management, referral, and progressive return to activities of daily living, including school, sport, occupation, and recreation

PART I

Introduction to Acute and Emergency Care in Athletic Training

Although not all emergencies are preventable, being prepared as a health care team is essential in responding effectively to an emergency. When an emergency arises, all individuals involved must come together and perform as a team that functions in a planned, practiced, and effective manner. Health care professionals (HCPs) must understand the roles and responsibilities of all team members, treat others with respect, and provide seamless health care in stressful situations. To do so, the team must communicate effectively, practice legally and ethically, and plan for emergencies. Developing an emergency action plan, having it approved, reviewing and training staff, and other important steps are necessary to effectively manage an emergency response and implement an effective post-catastrophic or critical incident plan. Once the athletic trainer (AT) is confident in planning and preparedness, the emergency examination becomes a natural and efficient process that focuses on the patient. Chapter 1 describes how effective teamwork involves using best practices, and chapter 2 explains how to take appropriate precautions to minimize risk and prevent medical errors. Preparing and planning for an emergency response are essential to providing the best possible care as the patient transitions through the health care system. Chapter 3 describes how the AT should plan to provide acute or emergency care and transfer care of the patient to emergency medical services (EMS) or next-level provider should a life-threatening injury or illness occur. Planning for emergencies is essential to maximizing patient outcomes and avoiding errors or mistakes. With thorough and detailed planning, the AT is able to coordinate the response to an emergency or other critical incident with skill and professionalism.

Chapter 4 describes the keys to an effective emergency examination including following a routine, systematic approach that allows for a consistent and appropriate decision-making process. It is essential that the AT has a practiced, effective approach to providing emergency care and hand-off to the next-level HCP. Chapter 5 provides clear guidelines on emergency medication administration methods and techniques for use by the AT in the prehospital setting. Using current techniques, educational standards, and skills training ensures that ATs are prepared to provide patients with the best evidence-based care available when faced with an emergency.

CHAPTER 1

The Interprofessional Health Care Team

OBJECTIVES

After reading this chapter, you will be able to do the following:

- Summarize how interprofessional health care teams work collaboratively to improve patient care.

- Distinguish the roles and responsibilities of members of the sports medicine health care team.

- Explain factors that lead to medical errors.

- Examine how effective teamwork practices and professional behaviors reflect core values and ethics.

Since the turn of the 21st century, health care has changed enormously, and the rapidity of change continues to accelerate. Health care providers (HCPs) are integrating new information and technology into management of injuries and illnesses in the physically active population. The modern health care system is complex and rapidly evolving with new evidence, practice guidelines, position statements, and predication rules; no single clinician can absorb and use all this information. To provide optimal health care, the specific knowledge and skills require specialized providers, diagnosticians, pharmacists, emergency care personnel, and a variety of other health care services. Examples of health care teams include the following:

- Disaster response teams
- Teams that perform emergency procedures
- Hospital teams caring for acutely ill patients
- Home health care teams caring for home-bound patients
- Office- or clinic-based care teams
- Geographically disparate teams that provide **ambulatory care**
- Teams limited to one clinician and patient
- Teams that include the patient and family as well as a number of supporting health professionals

In the health care system, the clinician operating in isolation is now seen as undesirable. This lone ranger works long and hard to provide the care needed, but the dependence on solitary resources and perspective may put the patient at risk.[1] **Team-based health care** is the provision of health services to individuals, families, and their

3

communities by at least two health providers who work collaboratively with patients and their caregivers—to the extent preferred by each patient—to accomplish shared goals within and across settings to achieve coordinated, high-quality care. The overall **health care system** is the diverse people who collaborate in order to direct their specialized capabilities toward common goals for the patient. Health care teams are coordinated by design, and each clinician must cultivate certain interpersonal and team-based skills that are uncommon in practice and not often taught.[2]

An effective team has team members, including the patient, who communicate with one another and share observations, expertise, and decision-making responsibilities to optimize patient care. Good teamwork has the ability to reduce errors and improve care for patients. In the context of a complex health care system, effective teamwork is essential for minimizing adverse events. Mistakes are often caused by miscommunication with other providers caring for the patient or misunderstandings of roles and responsibilities of each team member. Good communication between patients and their HCPs is essential, and patients must be fully informed and educated about their treatment and medication. A common reason for patients taking legal action against HCPs is poor communication between health care professionals, patients, and their caregivers.[3]

Characteristics of a Good Team

An effective team is two or more people who interact dynamically, interdependently, and adaptively toward a common and valued goal, who have been assigned specific roles or functions to perform, and who have a limited life span of membership. Examples of teams include sporting teams, military units, aircraft crews, and emergency response teams. According to the Agency for Healthcare Research and Quality,[4] members of a health care team interact dynamically and have the common goal of delivering health services to patients. Regardless of their nature, all teams share these characteristics:

- They possess specialized and complementary knowledge and skills.
- They know their role and the roles of other team members.
- They interact with one another to achieve a common goal.
- They make decisions.
- They possess specialized knowledge and skills and often function under high-workload conditions.

- They act as a collective unit because of the interdependency of the tasks performed by team members.

A driving force behind the transition of the HCP from being cowboy lone ranger to a member of a pit crew is the complexity of modern health care.[1] For example, in a Formula One pit crew, each member of the crew has a specific task, role, or responsibility; knows the roles of others on the crew; and communicates well with other members of the crew. The pit crew has a common goal of achieving a 9-second pit stop and winning the race. To accomplish a successful pit stop, members of the crew must act as a unit and trust one another with shared values and ethics. Similarly, effective teams throughout health care—regardless of the specific tasks, patients, and settings—are guided by these basic principles, which guide the functioning of the interprofessional **collaborative health care** team:[2]

- *Shared goals*: The team—including the patient and, as appropriate, family members, or other support people—works to establish shared goals that reflect patient and family priorities and can be clearly articulated, understood, and supported by all team members.
- *Clear roles*: Expectations are clear for each team member's functions, responsibilities, and accountabilities, which optimize the team's efficiency and often make it possible for the team to take advantage of division of labor, thereby accomplishing more than the sum of its parts.
- *Mutual trust*: Team members earn each other's trust, creating strong norms of reciprocity and greater opportunities for shared achievement.
- *Effective communication*: The team prioritizes and continuously refines its communication skills. It has consistent channels for candid and complete communication, which are accessed and used by all team members across all settings.
- *Measurable processes and outcomes:* The team agrees on and implements reliable and timely feedback on successes and failures in both the functioning of the team and achievement of the team's goals. These measures are used to track and improve performance immediately and over time.

As multiple clinicians provide care to the same patient, clinicians become a team—a group working toward one common aim, namely, the best possible patient care. Because each clinician relies on information and action from other members of the team, there is an obligation to strive for perfection in the science and practice of interprofessional team-based health care.[2] Although these concepts of interprofessional collaborative practice were developed for use in **primary care** for chronically ill adults, the core principles or competencies are easily adapted to apply to the work of health care teams in ambulatory care and sports medicine settings.

Teams are everywhere in health care—the surgeon, operating-room technician, operating-room nurse, and anesthesiologist in the operating suite; the oncologist, radiologist, and surgeon treating a cancer patient; the physician, medical assistant, and receptionist in a small family practice office;[5] or athletic trainer (AT), athletic training students, physical therapists, sports nutritionist, and strength and conditioning specialist all working together to provide high-level health care services. **Interprofessional practice** (or **collaborative practice**) is key to the safe, high-quality, accessible, patient-centered care desired by all. Interprofessional collaborative health care is the practice of approaching patient care from a team-based perspective according to these core competencies:[6]

- *Values/ethics for interprofessional practice*: Work with individuals of other professions to maintain a climate of mutual respect and shared values.
- *Roles/responsibilities:* Use the knowledge of one's own role and those of other professions to appropriately assess and address the health care needs of patients and to promote and advance the health of populations.
- *Interprofessional communication*: Communicate with patients, families, communities, and professionals in health and other fields in a responsive and responsible manner that supports a team approach to the promotion and maintenance of health and the prevention and treatment of disease.
- *Teams and teamwork*: Apply relationship-building values and the principles of team dynamics to perform effectively in different team roles to plan, deliver, and evaluate patient/population-centered care and population health programs and policies that are safe, timely, efficient, effective, and equitable.

Interprofessional health care teams understand how to do the following:[2]

- Strengthen the health care system.
- Optimize the skills of team members.
- Share patient management.
- Provide high-quality health care to patients.
- Improve patient outcomes.

According to the World Health Organization (WHO), collaborative practice happens when multiple HCPs from different professional backgrounds work together with patients, families, caregivers, and communities to deliver the highest quality of care. It allows HCPs from a variety of professions to engage any individual whose skills can help achieve local health goals.[3] Quality health care is dependent on people from various professions working together to address patient needs. When disciplines work together toward a shared goal that focuses on the patient (**patient-centered** or **participatory care**), health care is optimized. Collaborating as an interprofessional team reflects the changes in the health system that focus on the **Triple Aim**[6] to simultaneously improve these 3 dimensions of health care:

- Patient outcomes
- Quality of care
- Cost of care delivery

The incorporation of multiple perspectives in health care offers the benefit of diverse knowledge, skills, and experiences. However, in real-life clinical practice, the shared responsibility of a patient is challenging and requires collaboration while striving to improve systems and skills and adhere to best practices in interdisciplinary team-based care.[7] The high-functioning interprofessional team is now widely recognized and accepted as an essential tool for constructing a more patient-centered, coordinated, and effective health care delivery system.[2]

The national conversation about the need for interprofessional collaboration began when the **Institute of Medicine** (**IOM**, now recognized as the Health and Medicine Division of the National Academies) emphasized the importance of interprofessional practice within the health care environment. Now most health care education accrediting bodies, including the **Commission on Accreditation of Athletic Training Education (CAATE)**, require students to experience interprofessional teamwork in their clinical settings. Interprofessionalism is increasingly an important part of health care professional education, especially in athletic training, which has always been interprofessional by necessity. HCPs must identify themselves as an integral part of a larger health care team rather than simply learn their discipline-specific role, so that patients can receive the best care, which is the ultimate goal of each specialty. The focus is on the patient as a whole rather than a specific diagnosis or treatment provided by a specific HCP.[8] The athletic trainer (AT) has long been an advocate for injured athletes who are patients in the health care system. ATs have always viewed the patient as a whole and excel at viewing individual patients within the context of their setting or sport. ATs are HCPs who collaborate with physicians and a variety of other HCPs. The AT is a specialist in providing primary care services comprised of prevention, emergency care, clinical diagnosis, therapeutic intervention, and rehabilitation of injuries and medical conditions. Therefore, it is essential that ATs play a role in the health care team in order to offer their unique and vital perspective to the patient's needs.

Sports Medicine Setting

Patient-centered, multidisciplinary health care occurs routinely in the AT clinical setting (e.g., when a patient requires surgery and rehabilitation). In this context, interprofessional teamwork from the injury on the field, to the operating room, to the pharmacy, to the rehabilitation clinic, and back to the playing field all require interdisciplinary practice. One of the most prominent examples of current interprofessional patient care is multidisciplinary rounds, when an interprofessional team meets to discuss and develop a patient care plan together.[8] However, the sports medicine setting is different from any other in health care. Somewhat similar to an ambulatory care clinic, a busy AT clinic serves a large patient population with difficulty routinizing what happens each day. One complex patient—such as a patient with a cervical spine injury, a patient with an acute asthma attack, or a patient with an acute diabetic emergency—can disorganize an AT clinic for a whole day. With hundreds of patients and

the need to provide acute, chronic, and preventive care services, organizing and administering an AT clinic is a major challenge. Further complicating services, HCPs rarely talk to one another, usually communicating through written notes, reports, and prescriptions.[8]

As the delivery of health care evolves to become more interconnected, coordinating care between ATs, physical therapists, physician assistants, orthopedic technologists, nurse practitioners, pharmacists, physicians, and other health care professionals has become increasingly important (figure 1.1). For ATs who would like to be more involved in the entire patient care process or increase interprofessionalism in their practice, they must start by embracing the identity of the AT as part of a patient's health care team. When caring for a patient, the AT should make an effort to talk to the professionals in other disciplines involved in the patient's care. Talking about a patient to other HCPs helps to identify common goals and pave the way for collaborative efforts to reach these goals. Many hospital grand rounds involve multiple disciplines, and ATs can join these meetings in person or through conference call. The best way to learn more—and change the way health care is provided—is to be the change and become involved in the process.[8]

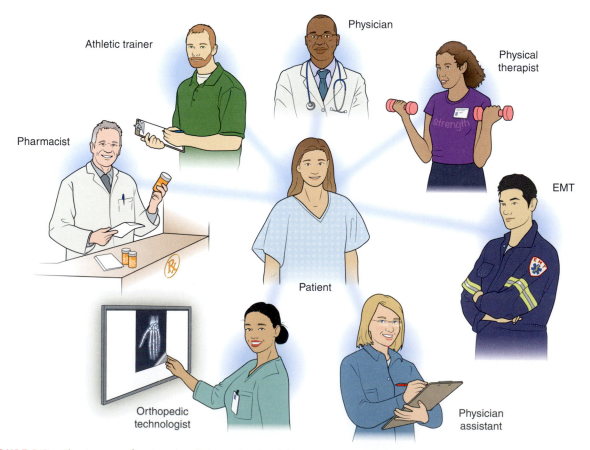

FIGURE 1.1   The interprofessional collaborative health care team.

Role of the Athletic Trainer

The AT is a HCP who collaborates with physicians to optimize activity and quality of life for patients of both the physically active and the sedentary population. The AT provides care procedures used in acute and emergency situations, independent of setting. Clinical practice in accordance with the AT's level of training and within the state's statutes, rules, and **regulations** is required in most states and ensures that a person has achieved basic knowledge and skill to be a competent HCP. ATs must be licensed or registered in states that have regulated **practice acts** before practicing athletic training. Additionally, each AT renders service or treatment under the direction of or in collaboration with a physician. ATs and physicians collaborate to optimize activity and participation of patients by providing acute and emergency care for injuries or medical conditions involving impairment, functional limitations, and disabilities.[9] To provide the best possible care, ATs collaborate with a physician or medical director in a relationship of mutual trust and confidence. ATs need to develop a close working relationship with physicians so that competent decision making occurs through a collaborative process. This relationship facilitates open communication and shared understanding of expectations, and it allows the AT to truly be an extension of the physician, operating under standing orders and following written policies and procedures. The physician should be willing to communicate with the AT at any time and make patient evaluation and follow-up care a priority.[10] Additional responsibilities of the AT include the following:

- Developing and implementing a comprehensive emergency action plan (EAP)
- Evaluating, recognizing, diagnosing, referring, and treating injuries
- Providing acute and emergency care
- Developing and implementing rehabilitation programs for injured athletes
- Establishing criteria for safe **return to participation** or **return to play (RTP)** and implementing the RTP process
- Planning and implementing comprehensive programs to prevent injury and illness among clients
- Maintaining and operating treatment facilities for both practice and game situations that follow national and local standards
- Determining which venues and activity settings require the on-site presence of the athletic trainer and physician and which require that they be available
- Maintaining accurate medical records for each client

Athletic Training Settings

ATs practice in a variety of settings. They practice in traditional settings, such as secondary school, college, or university; and nontraditional places, such as the physician's office, physical therapy clinic, performing arts center, industrial setting, and military base, among others. A variety of administrative models exist for the sports medicine clinic, chains of command, and selection and evaluation of the sports medicine team. Further, different athletic training settings vary widely in staffing, resources, and budgets. Regardless of the setting or administrative model used, staff responsibilities should be clearly defined to include the supervisory relationship. In addition, the institution must establish a clear line of unchallengeable authority for the physician and AT.[10]

In traditional school athletic departments, the AT is often supervised and evaluated by an athletic director who is unaware of best practices. Situations in which the athletic director is also a coach may present an inherent **conflict of interest**. Sports medicine physicians and ATs are often presented with an ethical dilemma when an individual athlete's best medical interests conflict with the performance expectations of authority figures (e.g., coaches, parents). The legal responsibility for the decision to allow an injured athlete to return to sports participation must belong to a licensed physician.[10] In this setting, often a coach determines the AT's work hours, report times, and duties.

In a medical model of health care, administrative alignment of the athletic health care unit exists within a larger health care system. Often university health services or another health care organization or clinic is aligned with a medical director who serves as the director of athletic medicine, often the physician. Another HCP supervises and evaluates the AT's performance and medical competence. Student-athlete medical records are stored in a database on campus and shared by the health center nurses, physicians, and ATs. At the beginning of the year or season, a written plan for provision of medical service (as opposed to sport *coverage*) is developed, approved by administration, and communicated to all coaches, staff, and personnel. The plan includes the following:[11,12]

- Predetermined high-risk sports or events occur when the AT is present.
- Coaches of high-risk sports do not hold practice unless an AT is present.
- Predetermined AT clinic hours are communicated to coaches before the season begins.
- Low-risk practices or events take place when an AT is available in the clinic.
- Low-risk sports have coaches versed in the EAP specific for the facility.

- First aid and CPR certification are required for all coaches.[11,12]

Aligning the athletic training clinic with the medical model may allow the AT to do the following:[11-13]

- Have access to a greater variety of HCPs and a supportive infrastructure for care coordination (i.e., electronic medical record system).
- Share patient care duties as a collaborative team, which improves patient care, decreases work hours, and improves quality of life for the HCP.
- Work around 40 hours per week with hours documented, just as in a clinic.
- Not cover low-risk sport practices or events; rather, medical care is provided during high-risk sports or events.
- Have access to additional professional development opportunities.
- Have job performance evaluations conducted by another HCP.
- Have more staff hired and with higher salary.[12]

Role of the Patient, Parent, and Family

Once a client is injured and receives care by an AT, he becomes a patient who must be an active participant in medical decisions. Parents or guardians may be involved if the patient is a minor. Sports medicine providers develop and maintain a relationship of trust and confidence with the patient and the parent or guardian. The AT must communicate effectively and truthfully with the patient and other people involved in the patient's care.[9] The patient must understand the short- and long-term risks associated with continued athletic participation. The collaborative participatory decision-making process involves a discussion between the patient and the AT in simple language so that the patient understands any potential adverse consequences, including catastrophic consequences. Sports medicine HCPs should determine the patient's capacity to make the necessary decision and ensure that the patient is free of coercion or manipulation. Collaborative decision making may include the following:

- Informing the patient, parent or guardian, or other person involved in the patient's care of any risks involved in the treatment plan
- Operative and nonoperative treatment options, with outcomes described so that the patient understands the advantages and disadvantages of each
- Treatment options that may delay RTP but further the patient's best medical interests

- Treatment options that may hasten RTP but are not in the patient's best medical interests[10]

Role of the Physician or Medical Director

Like all HCPs, the physician's first obligation is the well-being of patients under the care of the health care team. The physician's judgment should be governed only by medical considerations and not be influenced by coaches or parents. The physician must have the ultimate authority for making medical decisions regarding an athlete's safe participation.[10,13] The physician shares her medical expertise in a collaborative relationship with the patient, family, ATs, and other members of the health care team to make decisions about treatment and clearance for RTP. However, to manage ethical and medicolegal issues it is essential that the physician have the authority to do the following:

- Establish an organizational hierarchy with a chain of command to manage injuries and illnesses.
- Coordinate the assessment and management of injuries and medical problems.
- Decide on clearance to participate, same-day RTP, and post–game-day RTP.
- Conduct an effective preparticipation examination.
- Integrate medical expertise with the athletic care network.
- Perform best practices according to evidence.
- Provide documentation and keep medical records.[10,13]

Role of Emergency Medical Services

Emergency medical services (EMS) is a local government (or contracted) emergency medical safety net of community-based HCPs that is fully integrated with the overall health care system. EMS includes the following:

- Emergency medical responder (EMR)
- Emergency medical technician (EMT)
- Advanced EMT (AEMT)
- Paramedic

In most U.S. communities, when people need emergency medical care they call 9-1-1. Appropriate EMS resources are dispatched, EMS personnel respond, and they provide care to the patient in the setting where the injury or illness occurred (e.g., home, field, work, industrial and recreational settings). In the case of emergency calls, EMS personnel are unique in that they typically have a duty to act (see chapter 2). In some cases, such as sporting events or other mass participation events (e.g., a marathon), EMS personnel stand by in an ambulance. Increasingly, EMS personnel are working in traditional health care settings such as hospital emergency departments (EDs), urgent care centers, physicians' offices, and long-term care facilities. EMS personnel's **scope of practice** includes skills and knowledge that represent a continuum of complexity and risk that have **medical oversight** from a medical director. The medical director is a physician who is legally responsible for all patient care aspects of the EMS system. Prehospital care providers are the medical director's designated agents or are delegated by the medical director.

As the licensure level increases from EMR to paramedic, the knowledge required to practice safely, the skill complexity (the difficulty in acquiring and maintaining skill competency), and the potential for harm increase.[14]

Emergency Medical (or First) Responder

The EMR's primary role is to initiate immediate lifesaving care to **critical** patients who require the services of EMS. This level of training requires 24 to 60 hours of instruction beyond basic first aid. EMRs work alongside other EMS and HCPs as an integral part of the emergency care team to provide simple, noninvasive interventions to reduce the morbidity and mortality associated with acute medical and traumatic emergencies. Typically, the EMR is the first to arrive on the scene while awaiting additional EMS response and provides limited skills that are effective and safe to perform with medical oversight. This professional also comforts the patient and family while awaiting additional EMS personnel to arrive, then transfers care to a higher level of care. Under medical oversight, EMRs perform basic interventions with minimal equipment.[14]

Basic Skills of the EMR

- Airway and breathing:
  - Inserting oropharyngeal airway adjuncts
  - Using positive pressure ventilation devices such as the bag-valve mask
  - Suctioning upper airway
  - Providing supplemental oxygen therapy
- Pharmacological interventions:
  - Administering unit dose auto-injectors for lifesaving medications intended for self- or peer rescue
- Medical or cardiac care:
  - Using an automated external defibrillator (AED)
  - Trauma care

- Manual stabilization of suspected cervical spine injuries
  - Manual stabilization of extremity fractures
- Bleeding control
- Emergency moves, such as extrication from a car accident

Emergency Medical Technician

The EMT is part of the EMS response and provides a progressive increase in the level of assessment and care. The EMT is a mid-level provider of prehospital emergency medical services that augments prehospital critical care and provides rapid on-scene treatment. Education requirements for an EMT include completion of a state-approved course that exceeds educational standards and basic life support for the HCP. The primary role of the EMT is to provide basic emergency medical care and transportation for critical and **emergent** patients who require EMS. With medical oversight, EMTs perform interventions with the basic equipment typically found on an ambulance. The EMT's scope of practice includes basic, noninvasive interventions to reduce the morbidity and mortality associated with acute out-of-hospital medical and traumatic emergencies.[14] The EMT transports all emergency patients to an appropriate medical facility but is not prepared to make decisions independently regarding the appropriate disposition of patients.

Basic Skills of the EMT

- Airway and breathing:
  - Inserting of oropharyngeal or nasopharyngeal or supraglottic airway adjuncts
  - Airway suctioning
  - Pulse oximetry
  - Using positive pressure ventilation devices, such as manually triggered ventilators and automatic transport ventilators
- Pharmacological interventions:
  - Assisting patients in taking their own prescribed medications, including supplemental oxygen, inhaled bronchodilators, epinephrine, and nitroglycerin
- Administering over-the-counter medications with appropriate medical oversight:
  - Oral glucose for suspected hypoglycemia
  - Aspirin for chest pain of suspected ischemic origin
- Trauma care:
  - Application and inflation of the **pneumatic antishock garment** (PASG) for fracture stabilization

Advanced Emergency Medical Technician

The primary role of the AEMT is to provide basic and limited **advanced-level emergency medical care** and transportation for critical and emergent patients who require EMS. Education requirements for an AEMT include completion of a state-approved course that exceeds educational standards. Usually employed in ambulance services, AEMTs often work in conjunction with EMTs and paramedics; however, these professionals are also commonly found in fire departments as nontransporting first responders. Under medical oversight, AEMTs perform interventions with the basic and advanced equipment typically found on an ambulance.[14]

Basic Skills of the AEMT

- Airway and breathing:
  - Inserting airways that are *not* intended to be placed into the trachea
  - Tracheobronchial suctioning of an already intubated patient
- Patient assessment:
  - Pharmacological interventions
  - Establishing and maintaining peripheral intravenous access
  - Establishing and maintaining intraosseous access in a pediatric patient
  - Administering (nonmedicated) intravenous fluid therapy
  - Administering the following:
    - Sublingual nitroglycerin to a patient experiencing chest pain of suspected ischemic origin
    - Subcutaneous or intramuscular epinephrine to a patient in anaphylaxis
    - Glucagon to a hypoglycemic patient
    - Intravenous dextrose to a hypoglycemic patient
    - Inhaled beta-agonists to a patient experiencing wheezing or difficulty breathing
    - A narcotic antagonist (e.g., naloxone), which is especially effective with morphine to a patient suspected of narcotic overdose
    - Nitrous oxide for pain relief

Paramedic

The paramedic is a HCP, predominantly in the prehospital and out-of-hospital environment, who works mainly as part of EMS, such as on an ambulance. The scope of practice of a paramedic includes autonomous decision making around the emergency care of patients. The paramedic's scope of practice includes invasive and pharmacological interventions to reduce the morbidity and mortality associated with acute out-of-hospital medical and traumatic emergencies. The paramedic has the knowledge associated with, and is expected to be competent in, all of the skills of the EMT and AEMT. The major difference between the paramedic and the AEMT is the ability to perform a broader range of advanced skills. These skills carry a greater risk for the patient if improperly or inappropriately performed, are more difficult to attain and maintain competency in, and require significant background knowledge in basic and applied sciences.[14]

Basic Skills of the Paramedic

- Airway and breathing:
  - Performing endotracheal intubation
  - Performing **percutaneous** cricothyrotomy
  - Decompressing the pleural space
  - Performing gastric decompression
- Pharmacological interventions:
  - Inserting an intraosseous cannula
  - Enteral and parenteral administration of approved prescription medications
  - Accessing indwelling catheters and implanted central IV ports for fluid and medication administration
  - Administering medications by IV infusion
  - Maintaining blood or blood products infusion
- Medical/cardiac care:
  - Performing cardioversion, manual defibrillation, and transcutaneous pacing

Role of the Emergency Department

Emergency medicine is a **medical specialty** that involves acute care of internal medical and surgical conditions. Emergency medicine encompasses planning, oversight, and medical direction for community emergency medical response, medical control, and disaster preparedness.[15] Emergency departments (EDs, formerly known as emergency rooms) are staffed with **emergency physicians** who treat many patients and either admit the patient to the hospital or release the patient after treatment. ED personnel have a broad range of knowledge and advanced procedural skills that often include surgical procedures, trauma resuscitation, advanced cardiac life support, and advanced airway management. Many specialists with the ability to provide a variety of skills are involved in the ED (see Roles and Responsibilities of Emergency Medicine Specialists).

Scope of Practice for Emergency Medical Service Personnel

Airway and Breathing Minimum Skills

Emergency Medical Responder

- Oral airway
- Bag-valve-mask maneuver
- **Cricoid pressure** (Sellick's maneuver)
- Head-tilt–chin-lift
- Jaw-thrust
- Modified chin lift
- Airway obstruction, manual removal
- Oxygen therapy
- Nasal cannula (NC)
- Non-rebreather face mask
- Upper airway suctioning
- Manual blood pressure (BP)

Emergency Medical Technician

- Humidifiers
- Partial rebreathers
- Venturi mask
- Manually triggered ventilator (MTV)
- Automatic transport ventilator (ATV)
- Oral and nasal airways
- Pulse oximetry
- Manual and automated BP

Advanced EMT

- Esophageal-tracheal multilumen (Combitube) airways
- Blood glucose monitor

Paramedic

- Bilevel positive airway pressure (BiPAP) and continuous positive airway pressure (CPAP)
- Needle chest decompression
- Chest tube monitoring
- Percutaneous cricothyrotomy
- End-tidal carbon dioxide (ETCO$_2$) capnography
- Nasogastric or orogastric (NG/OG) tube
- Nasal and oral endotracheal intubation
- Airway obstruction removal by direct laryngoscopy
- Positive end-expiratory pressure (PEEP)
- Electrocardiogram (ECG) interpretation
- Interpretive 12-lead blood chemistry analysis

Pharmacological Intervention Minimum Skills

Emergency Medical Responders

- Technique of medication administration
  - Unit dose auto-injectors for self- or peer care

Emergency Medical Technician

- Assisted medications
- Assisting a patient in administering personal prescribed medications, including auto-injection
- Technique of medication administration:
  - Buccal
  - Oral
- Administered medications:
  - Physician-approved over-the-counter medications (e.g., oral glucose, aspirin for chest pain of suspected ischemic origin)

> continued

Advanced Emergency Medical Technician

- Technique of medication administration
  - Aerosolized
  - Subcutaneous (SQ)
  - Intramuscular (IM)
  - Intraosseous (IO)
  - Intravascular (IV)
  - Nebulized
  - Sublingual (SL)
  - Intranasal
- Peripheral IV insertion
- IV fluid infusion

- Pediatric IO
- IV push of D50 and narcotic antagonist only
- Administered medications:
  - SL nitroglycerin for chest pain of suspected ischemic origin
  - SQ or IM epinephrine for anaphylaxis
  - Glucagon IV and D50 for hypoglycemia
  - Inhaled beta-agonist for dyspnea and wheezing
  - Narcotic antagonist
  - Nitrous oxide for pain relief

Paramedic

- Technique of medication administration:
  - Endotracheal
  - IV (push and infusion)
  - NG
  - Rectal
  - IO
  - Topical
- Central line monitoring

- IO insertion
- Venous blood sampling
- Accessing implanted central IV port
- Administered meds—physician-approved medications
- Maintain blood administration
  - Thrombolytics initiation

Minimum Skills for Emergency Trauma Care

Emergency Medical Responder

- Manual cervical stabilization
- Manual extremity stabilization
- Eye irrigation

- Direct pressure
- Hemorrhage control
- Emergency moves for endangered patients

Emergency Medical Technician

- Spinal immobilization
- Seated spinal immobilization—long board
- Extremity splinting
- Traction splinting

- Mechanical patient restraint
- Tourniquet
- PASG
- Cervical collar
- Rapid extrication

Advanced Emergency Medical Technician

- Same as skills for EMT

Paramedic

- Morgan lens for eye irrigation

Minimum Skills for Medical/Cardiac Care

Emergency Medical Responder

- CPR
- AED
- Assisted normal delivery

Emergency Medical Technician

- Mechanical CPR
- Assisted complicated delivery

Advanced Emergency Medical Technician

- Same as skills for EMT

Paramedic

- Cardioversion
- Carotid massage

- Manual defibrillation
- Transcutaneous heart pacing

Emergency medicine professionals provide valuable clinical, administrative, and leadership services to the ED and other sectors of the health care delivery system.[15] ED personnel also provide episodic primary care to patients during off hours and for those who do not have primary care providers. Emergency medicine is distinct from urgent care, which refers to immediate health care for less emergent medical conditions.[15]

Examples of Emergency Medical Equipment and Skills

Equipment

- Bag-valve mask
- Chest tube
- Defibrillator (AED/ICD)
- Electrocardiogram (ECG) machine
- Intraosseous infusion (IO)
- Intravenous therapy (IV)

- Tracheal intubation
- Laryngeal tube or Combitube
- Nasopharyngeal airway (NPA)
- Oropharyngeal airway (OPA)
- Pocket mask

Emergency Pharmacology

- Atropine
- Amiodarone
- Epinephrine/adrenaline

- Magnesium sulfate
- Sodium bicarbonate
- Naloxone

Life Support

- First aid
- Cardiopulmonary resuscitation (CPR)
- Basic life support (BLS)
- Advanced cardiac life support (ACLS)
- Advanced trauma life support (ATLS)

- Care of the critically ill surgical patient (CCrISP)
- Neonatal resuscitation program (NRP)
- Pediatric advanced life support (PALS)
- Acute care of at-risk newborns (ACoRN)

Scoring System

- Injury Severity Score (ISS)

Roles and Responsibilities of Emergency Medicine Specialists

- *Anesthesiology:* Manage a difficult airway, relieve pain, and care for the patient before, during, and after surgery.
- *Cardiology:* Treat a heart attack; insert stents, pacemakers, and valves.
- *Cardiothoracic surgery:* Place a chest tube; provide surgery for trauma to heart, lungs, and great vessels.
- *Critical or intensive care medicine:* Diagnosis and management of life-threatening conditions requiring resuscitation, sophisticated organ support, and invasive monitoring.
- *Emergency nursing:* **Triage** patients, perform rapid, accurate physical examination, complete early recognition of life-threatening conditions.
- *Emergency psychiatry (MD):* Identify and treat attempted suicide, drug dependence, alcohol intoxication, and acute depression.
- *Neurology:* Manage traumatic brain injury (TBI), strokes, epilepsy, and pain.
- *Obstetrics and gynecology (OB/GYN):* Diagnose a pregnant patient with vaginal bleeding.
- *Otorhinolaryngology/ear, nose, and throat (ENT):* Multiple subspecialties involved with trauma and reconstructive surgery of the head, face, and neck; severe or recurrent epistaxis (nosebleeds); dizziness; and hearing loss.
- *Ophthalmology (MD):* Treat immediate threats to the visual system that can lead to permanent loss of visual function if left untreated.
- *Orthopedics and orthopedic surgery:* Perform surgical and nonsurgical treatment of musculoskeletal trauma and sports injuries; reduce (set) a fractured bone or dislocated joint.
- *Pediatric emergency medicine:* Diagnose and care for undifferentiated acute illnesses or injuries in children.
- *Plastic surgery:* Suture a complex laceration; perform reconstructive surgery, craniofacial surgery, hand surgery, microsurgery; treat burns.
- *Radiology:* Conduct and interpret imaging such as x-ray radiography, ultrasound, computed tomography (CT), and magnetic resonance imaging (MRI).
- *Trauma surgery:* Perform initial resuscitation and stabilization of traumatic injuries; lead the trauma team, including nurses and support staff.

Role of Additional Members of an Interprofessional Collaborative Health Care Team

The interprofessional collaborative health care team involves participation and input from multiple HCPs including athletic trainers, physicians, nurses, pharmacists, physical therapists, occupational therapists, speech and language pathologists, social workers, psychologists, and potentially administrative staff. From the patient's point of view, coordination and provision of emergency care should be seamless. This coordination of emergency medicine services requires a full range of health care professionals, such as 9-1-1 and ambulance dispatch, EMS, ED care, operating room or **intensive care unit (ICU)**, and the involvement of additional specialists. In addition, it must be tightly linked by interoperable communications, transmission of patient information, and consensus clinical protocols.[16,17] The role these health care professionals play varies between health care teams and with different patients:

- *Physician assistant (PA):* With a supervising physician, conducts physical exams, orders and interprets tests, diagnoses illnesses, performs procedures, prescribes medications, and assists in surgery.
- *Pharmacist (PharmD):* Often first point of contact for patients with health inquiries with a significant role assessing medication management and referring patients to a physician.
- *Occupational therapist (OT):* Treats patients with disabling conditions to develop, recover, or maintain daily living and work skills.

- *Orthopedic technologist, certified (OTC):* Extension of a physician and assists in the treatment of the orthopedic patient in casting, splinting, wound closure, and more.
- *Physical therapist (PT):* Uses specially designed exercises and equipment to help patients regain or improve their physical abilities.
- *Social worker:* Assesses the psychosocial functioning of patients and families and intervenes as necessary, such as connecting patients and families to necessary resources, providing psychotherapy, counseling, or strengthening their network of social supports.
- *Speech and language pathologist (SLP) or speech therapist:* Evaluates, diagnoses, and treats communication, cognition, voice, and swallowing disorders.
- *Marriage and family therapist (MFT):* Provides psychotherapy to families and couples in intimate relationships to nurture change and development.
- *Psychologist (PsyD):* Diagnoses, treats, and studies mental processes; performs counseling and psychotherapy.
- *Psychiatrist (MD):* Medical doctor specializing in diagnosis, prevention, study, and treatment of mental disorders.

Roles of professionals on the health care team are often flexible and opportunistic in that leadership changes depending on the required expertise or the professional that has the most patient contact; in many cases the AT serves this role. In patient-centered care, the patient and their family or caregivers are engaged as a valuable part of the health care team.[18]

Role of Athletic Training Students

The role of the AT student is to learn to be a good health care professional by studying an accredited program; observing respected, experienced HCPs; and gaining practical clinical experience involving patients. The role of the AT student is not to act as a licensed HCP or as substitute staff in an understaffed AT clinic. Being an AT student is a privilege with the opportunity to learn by examining and treating real patients under the supervision of a licensed AT (in states where AT practice is regulated). Most patients understand that students have to learn and that the future of health care depends on training. The student's opportunity to interview, examine, and treat patients is a privilege granted by each of those patients. In most situations, a student cannot examine a patient unless the patient has given consent. Students and clinicians should always ask permission from each patient before they physically touch or seek personal information from them. They should also be aware that patients may withdraw this privilege at any time and request that the student stop what he is doing.[18] AT students should be considered part of the collaborative health care team. With this responsibility, students are important in providing optimal patient-centered care and preventing medical errors.

Breakdowns in Teamwork

Breakdowns in teamwork happen when human factors lead to violations of evidence-informed rules, guidelines, and principles. Occasionally health professionals break professional rules, such as using incorrect hand hygiene techniques or allowing junior or inexperienced providers to work without proper supervision. Occasionally, students may observe health care professionals on duty who may use shortcuts in procedures without understanding the correct technique. Such behaviors are not acceptable and are considered a **violation**, or deliberate deviation from an operating procedure, standard, or rule.[18] **Systems thinking** is a process of understanding organizations and how events are interdependent. Using systems thinking to understand errors and failures ensures that when such an event occurs, one performs an examination to learn from the error rather than automatically placing blame. Paying careful attention to the multiple factors associated with an incident provides insight as to where or how the system breakdown occurred in order to learn from the experience and prevent it in the future.

To ensure quality of coordination of continuous care for all patients, follow these guidelines:

- Provide information to the right people at the right time to ensure that patients receive continuous care and treatment.
- Accurately transfer information about a patient's status and care plan to another team member or health care team.
- Record information clearly and legibly.
- Document patient records to show patient progress.
- Communicate clinical findings clearly to other members of the health care team.
- Effectively manage medications.

Using evidence-informed guidelines and principles can allow the health care team to safely and efficiently complete tasks such as the following:

- Administering medications
- Handing off (handing over) information
- Moving patients

- Documenting treatment, medications, and other orders electronically[18]

Situations Associated With Increased Risk of Error

A great deal of health care depends on the professionals providing the care, and human factors can result in errors in procedures, practices, communication, and breakdowns in the health care team. Basic tasks have become quite complicated because of the increasing complexity of health care systems. Addressing human factors can reduce errors by focusing on how HCPs function and interact within the workplace. Types of errors are defined as follows:

- *Errors* occur because of one of two main types of system failures. Either actions do not go as intended (slip or lapse) or the intended action is wrong (mistake).
- *Slip* is an error of execution that is observable.
- *Lapse* is an error of execution that is not observable.
- *Mistake* is a failure that occurs when the intended action is actually incorrect.

For example, a slip is accidentally pushing the wrong button on a piece of equipment whereas a lapse is a memory failure, such as forgetting to ask about drug allergies before administering a medication. A mistake is a failure of planning (i.e., the plan is wrong). A rule-based mistake occurs when the wrong rule is applied, and a knowledge-based mistake occurs when a clinician does not take the correct course of action. An example of a rule-based mistake would be making an incorrect diagnosis and embarking on an inappropriate treatment plan. Knowledge-based mistakes tend to occur when HCPs are confronted with unfamiliar clinical situations.[3,18-21]

Here are some other situations associated with increased risk of error:

- *Students or novice clinicians*: Students and novice clinicians are particularly vulnerable to errors under certain circumstances. In the case of students, it is essential that a student not perform a procedure on a patient or administer a treatment for the first time without appropriate preparation and supervision. Students must first understand the correct procedure, why it is correct, and when to apply it; and practice on a mannequin or other simulated environment. The first time a student performs a procedure or administers a treatment, the student should be properly supervised and provided correction. Students are in a privileged position. Patients do not expect students to know much, and they appreciate that they are learning. Therefore, students should not pretend or let others present them as having more experience than they do.

- *Time shortage*: Time pressures encourage people to cut corners and take shortcuts when they should not, such as not properly cleansing hands, a pharmacist not taking the time to properly counsel a patient receiving medication, or a midwife not properly informing a woman about the stages of delivery.

- *Inadequate checking*: The simple act of checking can prevent medical errors in many situations. Routinely checking drugs allows all members of the health care team to ensure each patient receives the correct dosage of the correct drug by the correct route. Providers should observe good working relationships in a health care team that has habitual checking routines built into their professional routines. Checking is a simple thing that students can start practicing as soon as they are placed into a clinical environment or **community care** setting.

- *Poor procedures:* Factors contributing to poor procedures include inadequate preparation, inadequate staffing, and inadequate attention to the particular patient. Providers may be asked to use a piece of equipment without fully understanding its function or how to use it. Before using any piece of equipment for the first time, providers should familiarize themselves with it. Watching someone use a piece of equipment and then talking with that person about the procedure for which it is used is very instructive.

- *Inadequate information:* Providing consistent quality health care and treatment depends on each health care professional recording the patient details accurately, in a timely way, and in legible handwriting in the patient record (medical record, drug chart, or other method used for storing patient information). It is crucial that students and clinicians habitually check the information being recorded and ensure that the information they write is legible, accurate, and up to date. Misinformation, incorrect information, and inadequate information often contribute to adverse events. Accurate verbal transmission of information is also crucial. Because multiple health care professionals are involved in caring for a patient, it is essential that verbal and written communications are checked and accurate.

Here are some system-wide ways to prevent medical errors:

- *Standardize common processes and procedures.* Even students who work in only one clinic or facility may observe each health care professional doing certain things differently. Providers may have to relearn how to perform procedures when moving from one person or clinic to the next. Health care facilities that have standardized procedures, as appropriate, help staff by reducing reliance on memory, which also improves efficiency and saves time. Discharge forms, prescribing conventions, and types of equipment can all be standardized within a clinic or among several clinics at an institution.

• *Routinely use checklists.* The use of checklists has been successfully applied in many areas of human endeavor, such as studying for examinations, traveling, and shopping. For example, using Safe Surgery checklists has increased the use of checklists in many health care activities. Students and clinicians should develop a habit of using checklists in their clinical practice, particularly when an evidence-based way of selecting or implementing treatment exists.[18,22]

Individual Factors That Predispose to Errors

These individual factors can predispose a clinician to making errors:

• *Reluctance or unwillingness to ask for help*: Asking for help is an essential skill for HCPs. Having confidence and willingness to ask for help often depends on a person's self-perception as a health care professional or perception of workplace hierarchy. Especially for students, asking for help is expected. However, many providers find asking questions challenging, which limits their ability to recognize their limitations and learn from experience. Lack of confidence can affect whether providers ask for help in mastering a new skill. Providers must have the confidence and be willing to ask for help, even with simple tasks, so they can ask for help when it is really needed.

• *Transition to autonomous practice*: The transition to practice as an autonomous HCP is often a time of inadequate competence and stress. Even some graduating medical students have deficiencies in basic clinical skills in their first years of practice. This situation may be a result of a reluctance to ask for help as students or inadequate knowledge and skill. For example, understanding the crucial signs of acute illness, airway obstruction, or basic life support are specific areas in which novice clinicians have inadequate knowledge and skills.

• *Dependence on memory*: Many students and novice clinicians think that if they can regurgitate the technical information stored in textbooks, they will be good HCPs. However, the amount of information that many HCPs are required to know is far beyond that which can be memorized. The human brain is only capable of

CLINICAL SKILLS

Strategies to Reduce Medical Errors

Reducing medical errors involves a variety of individual strategies. To ensure that the best care is provided to the patient, use the following self-monitoring skills:[18]

- Take care of your own health (e.g., eat well and sleep well).
- Be aware of your fatigue.
- Avoid reliance on memory.
- Routinely use checklists.
- Simplify processes.
- Standardize common processes and procedures.
- Decrease reliance on perseverance.
- Know the personnel, environment, and task(s).
- Prepare and plan (What if _____ happens?).
- If you do not know something, ask questions.
- Use mnemonic devices to help monitor yourself. For example, using the mnemonic I'M SAFE helps you self-monitor for the following:

  Illness

  Medication (prescription and others)

  Stress

  Alcohol

  Fatigue

  Emotion

remembering a finite amount of information. Students should not rely on memory, particularly when several steps are involved. Guidelines and protocols have been developed to help health care professionals provide care and service following the best available evidence. Students should get into the habit of using checklists and not rely on memory.

• *Fatigue*: Memory is affected by fatigue. Fatigue is a known factor in errors involving HCPs, often the result of the excessive hours that doctors and nurses work. Long hours and sleep deprivation disrupt circadian rhythms and general well-being. Working long hours, mandatory overtime, and inadequate rest time can lead to increased errors.

• *Stress, hunger, and illness*: When clinicians feel stressed, hungry, or ill, they do not function as well as when these issues are addressed. Therefore, students and HCPs must monitor their own status and well-being. Students and clinicians should be mindful of the fact that if they are feeling unwell or stressed, they are more likely to make errors. Burnout in novice clinicians has led to errors and even to ATs leaving the profession. Stress and burnout are related.[3,18-22]

Effective Practices in Teamwork

Being an effective member of a health care team involves a variety of skills that are learned and practiced early in life and at the outset of an academic program. To promote good teamwork, every health care student should learn, practice, and use the following strategies:[3,6,18]

• *Always introduce yourself.* Let everyone on the team know your name and profession, even if you are only working with them for a few minutes.

• *Learn and use people's names.* Some professionals do not take the time to learn the names of the HCPs they are working with. It is worth the effort to learn names; when you use people's names rather than refer to them by their profession, such as "Nurse" or "Doctor," you create better relationships with them.

• *Be assertive when required.* This skill is universally difficult, but if a patient is at risk of serious injury then the HCPs, including students, must speak up. Senior clinicians will be grateful in the longer term if one of their patients avoids a serious adverse event.

• *Ask for clarification.* If something does not make sense, ask for clarification or find out the other person's perspective.

• *Conduct a pre-brief and debrief.* Whenever possible, conduct a briefing before and after a team activity. This meeting encourages every member of the team to contribute to discussions about how it went and what can be done differently or better next time. When conflict occurs, concentrate on *what* is right for the patient instead of *who* is right or wrong.

• *Delegate tasks to a specific person.* When assigning or delegating a task, look directly at the person and confirm the person has the information needed to complete task. Talking into the air is an unsafe practice because a person may think the responsibility of the task is for someone else.

• *Use effective team communication skills.* Read back and close the communication loop in relation to patient care information. State the obvious to avoid confusion, such as in this example:

> • Sarah (AT): "James, please take Jameel to have an X-ray."

> • James (AT student): "OK, Sarah. I will take Jameel to have an X-ray now."

Professional Attributes of Effective Health Care Providers

The NATA has developed the Code of Ethics while the Board of Certification has created the Standards of Professional Practice and Code of Responsibility. These principles define specific abilities and behaviors that a graduate of an accredited athletic training education program should demonstrate, including the following:[9,23]

• *Honesty and integrity*: Represents one's own and others' abilities honestly; is truthful and sincere; accepts responsibility for one's actions; is able to reflect on one's personal reactions to encounters with others. Most settings involve confidential medical records and other patient information. It is important to be trusted with such information on a need-to-know basis and not share inappropriate information with others.

• *Respect*: Adheres to confidentiality and professional boundaries; works toward conflict resolution in a collegial way; demonstrates consideration for the opinions and values of others; shows regard for diversity.

• *Responsible*: Is present and punctual for all learning experiences; is able to cope with challenges, conflicts, and uncertainty; recognize one's limits and seeks help; recognizes the needs of others and responds appropriately; demonstrates willingness to discuss and confront problematic behavior of self and others.

• *Dependable:* Must be reliable—shows up to work when scheduled and does assigned work (and hopefully pitches in to help others with theirs). A dependable person can be trusted in many situations.

• *Competent:* Takes responsibility for one's own learning; participates equally and collegially in groups; demonstrates self-reflection and accurate self-assessment; is able to identify personal barriers to learning; works with colleagues to manage difficult situations.

• *Mature:* Demonstrates emotional stability; is appropriately confident yet humble; demonstrates appropriate professional dress, demeanor, and language; accepts constructive criticism and applies it in a useful way; inspires confidence in others; displays appropriate emotions; is not hostile, disruptive, confrontational, aggressive, or isolated; does not engage in behavior that endangers or threatens self or others.

• *Empathetic:* A HCP must develop the ability to relate to another person's situation (putting yourself in someone else's shoes) without feeling sorry for them (detachment). Having empathy allows the AT to gain trust and insight, which helps the AT provide better care for the patient.

• *Effective communicator:* Is able to communicate effectively with others; demonstrates courteous and respectful communication, even in difficult situations; uses active listening; communicates with empathy and compassion.

• *Lifelong learner:* Lifelong learning is a commitment to continue to learn throughout the career. It is not sufficient to learn information only to pass the tests and obtain a degree, the AT must always be learning new information, skills, and technology to provide the best possible care to patients.[9,23]

Therapeutic Behaviors

Therapeutic behaviors are interpersonal communication skills that are consciously applied by the HCP in both verbal and nonverbal ways. The HCP can help patients feel valued and important to the participatory decision-making process when using therapeutic behavior skills such as the following:

• Being respectful, polite, and punctual

• Encouraging the patient to continue treatment or a rehabilitation program

• Reducing distance between the patient and the HCP to demonstrate desire to be involved while

---

Core Values and Professional Behaviors of an Athletic Trainer

Core Values
• Accountability
• Altruism
• Compassion
• Caring
• Excellence
• Integrity
• Professional duty
• Social responsibility

Professional Behaviors
• Commitment to learning
• Interpersonal skills
• Communication skills
• Effective use of time and resources
• Use of constructive feedback
• Problem solving
• Professionalism
• Responsibility
• Critical thinking
• Stress management

Based on National Athletic Trainers Association (2016); Commission on Accreditation of Athletic Training Education (2015).

maintaining appropriate interpersonal distance (details follow)

- Actively listening by restating and reflecting to validate the HCP's interpretation of the patient's message
- Remaining silent at times to display acceptance
- Incorporating open-ended questions to allow the patient control of the conversation
- Directing the conversation toward important topics
- Seeking clarification to demonstrate the desire to understand
- Summarizing to help the patient focus on relevant information

Every patient interaction is unique to the setting, roles, and circumstances during that interaction. However, in any setting, successful patient interaction requires having self-awareness, following intuition, and ensuring sensitivity to the patient's needs.[25] The following therapeutic behaviors are described next:

- Interpersonal distance
- Interpersonal communication
- Appropriate touch
- Professional boundaries
- Confidentiality
- Emotional intelligence
- Cultural competence
- Collaborative practice
- Ethical practice

Interpersonal Distance

When interviewing or talking to a patient, maintaining appropriate interpersonal distance involves an awareness of personal space and how distance between people affects communication (figure 1.2). The degree to which people feel comfortable depends on with whom they are communicating. As trust is established between two people, a smaller distance between the two people becomes comfortable. A high sense of trust is necessary to be within a patient's intimate space. Additionally, appropriate interpersonal distance depends heavily on culture. In most cultures when interviewing a patient, use social distance by remaining between 4 and 10 feet (~1-3 m) from the patient.[25]

Interpersonal Communication

An important aspect of the therapeutic relationship is understanding how interpersonal communication can help a patient feel confident that he will be treated cour-

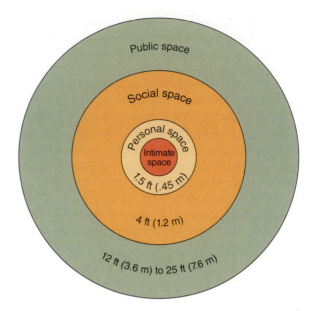

FIGURE 1.2   Interpersonal distances.

teously and that the HCP has genuine concern for his well-being.[25] Many practice settings are located in diverse areas with cultures that are different from that of the HCP. Verbal communication with patients and families from different cultures requires sensitivity to respond appropriately and withhold judgment. A language barrier between the HCP and the patient or family may require an interpreter or forms written in another language. Cultural sensitivity (see Cultural Competence) is a key factor in communicating with someone who speaks a different language, or who has different beliefs or values. Being sensitive to another person's culture requires interpersonal skills with verbal and nonverbal communication. In addition, effective interpersonal communication techniques are essential for obtaining informed consent for procedures and open disclosure (details in chapter 2). Practicing effective interpersonal communication involves the following:

- Actively encouraging patients and caregivers to share information
- Actively sharing information with patients and caregivers
- Showing empathy, honesty, and respect for patients and caregivers
- Appropriately informing patients and obtaining informed consent for treatments and interventions, and supporting patients in making informed choices
- Showing respect for each patient's religious, cultural, and personal beliefs and individual needs
- Describing and understanding the basic steps in an open-disclosure process

- Meeting patients' complaints with respect and openness
- Applying patient-engagement thinking in all clinical activities
- Demonstrating the ability to recognize the importance of patient and caregiver engagement for good clinical management[8,18]

Patient and caregiver engagement involves interpersonal communication skills with the patient and family, bystanders, and the rest of the health care team as an essential part of high-quality patient care. In a traditional athletic setting, the AT must be able to effectively coordinate the variety of people often present at a game or competition and transfer the patient's care to EMTs, nurses, and physicians in the emergency department. Actively listening is necessary in order to fully understand the nature of the patient's problem, quickly organize thoughts, and accurately verbalize instructions to the patient, bystanders, and other HCPs.[26]

Nonverbal Communication

Nonverbal communication (body language) is extremely important when engaging patients, family, and caregivers. In stressful situations, patients may misinterpret your gestures and movements as threatening. To reduce stress and anxiety, sit or kneel at the same level or at a lower level than the patient whenever practical. In a calm, professional manner, speak slowly, clearly, and distinctly with close attention to your tone of voice. Maintain a calm, confident manner while making the patient physically comfortable and relaxed. Demonstrate caring and sensitivity by determining what the patient needs in order to be comfortable (e.g., sitting or lying down, covered with a blanket, having a friend or relative nearby).[27] The SURETY model (table 1.1) is an acronym for nonverbal communication techniques used to create an effective therapeutic space, emphasizing appropriate touch and intuition.

Closed- and Open-Ended Questions

When interviewing the patient to obtain a history of the injury or illness, open- and closed-ended questions may be used for different reasons, depending on the patient's level of consciousness, intensity of pain, difficulty breathing, or the urgency of the situation. When the patient is unable to provide long or complete answers to questions, **closed-ended questions** are appropriate. These questions are answered in short or single-word (yes or no) responses:

- Are you having trouble breathing?
- Do you take medications for asthma?

TABLE 1.1　Using the SURETY Model to Create an Effective Therapeutic Space

Sit at an angle.	Sit at a slight angle to create a nonconfrontational comfort zone or personal space. Sitting directly opposite a patient may be interpreted as confrontational or make the patient feel vulnerable or unwilling to discuss her concerns.
Uncross legs and arms.	Uncross your legs and arms to communicate an open and receptive body position. Crossed arms or legs communicate defensiveness, disinterest, or superiority.
Relax.	A relaxed body position allows the patient to relax and feel more comfortable. Leaning in demonstrates active listening but may be uncomfortable or impractical to maintain.
Use **E**ye contact.	Use appropriate eye contact to communicate respect and attention. Wandering eyes (e.g., looking at the window or clock) indicate loss of interest or inattention.
Touch respectfully.	Respectful use of touch communicates compassion, empathy, and understanding. Sensitive use of touch is often appropriate. However, the use of touch is not universal, and cultural sensitivity is essential. Gushing hugs or kisses are not appropriate in the health care setting. Appropriate touch in safe zones such as the hand, lower arm, or shoulder may communicate warmth, caring, and understanding. Generally avoid all other areas of the body, which require the consent (or implied consent; see chapter 2) of the patient during a physical examination.
Your intuition matters.	Deliberate use of intuition in clinical practice has no universal guidelines. However, as the HCP gains experience and confidence, intuition becomes important. In clinical practice, you often need to follow your gut.

Be mindful that personal space is influenced by culture, upbringing, and individual preference. Use intuition to respond to signs of discomfort or stress.

Based on College of Nurses of Ontario (2006); Stickley (2011).

Closed-ended questions are often limited in that the information provided usually has less detail and is uninformative. **Open-ended questions** allow a free flow of conversation and provide the patient time and space to respond.[27] Open-ended questions require a level of detail from the patient to provide an answer. In situations with less urgency, the initial interview with the patient should use open-ended questions, as appropriate, such as "Hi. My name is Michelle, and I am an athletic trainer here to help you. What seems to be bothering you today?" Open-ended questions to understand the patient's concerns include the following:

- What seems to be the problem?
- How can I help?
- What helped you feel better?

When communicating with patients, it is best to ask a single question, wait for an answer, and then ask another question. Consider how the patient will feel with a coach or authority figure nearby. When talking to a patient about an injury or illness, you should ask coaches and other authority figures to leave. Patients often conceal an injury in order to continue playing in a game or competition. Patients may be afraid that they will be restricted from participation and be unwilling to communicate their concern or provide information about the injury. On the other hand, a severely ill or injured patient without his or her loved ones nearby may be difficult and stressful. The presence of family, friends, or teammates during the patient interview can be helpful in reducing anxiety. Often additional or unnecessary people surrounding the patient may hinder the interview process and create a violation of patient privacy. Whenever possible, interview the patient in a private area or office, or ask others to step outside during the interview with the patient. However, when in a private area, it is prudent to have a neutral adult such as an administrator or other staff or personnel present to avoid any **appearance of impropriety**.[27]

Appropriate Touch

When interviewing the patient, consider using appropriate touch to communicate caring and compassion. However, be mindful that touch is a powerful tool that should be used consciously and sparingly. Appropriate touch varies with culture, and many people are uncomfortable being suddenly touched by a stranger. Avoid touching the patient's torso, chest, or face simply as a means of communication, because these areas are often considered intimate. When it is necessary to touch these areas, ask permission to touch the patient (for more details on consent, see chapter 2), slowly move closer to the patient, and avoid invading the patient's personal space. Ultimately every patient is different, and it is essential to assess each

situation to determine when touch is appropriate for the patient. To appropriately touch a patient, approach slowly and touch the patient's shoulder or arm with your right hand, if possible. Holding the patient's hand allows you to do the following:

- Reassure the patient
- Show care and compassion
- Actively listen to what the patient is saying
- Allow a slight distance for communication[25,26]

Professional Boundaries

An integral part of the HCP–patient relationship, boundaries are based on respect and **primacy of the patient**. Professional boundaries represent legal, ethical, and professional standards of practice. Establishing boundaries of a relationship between the professional and patient is the HCP's responsibility. The boundaries must have a specific purpose and health goal. The professional relationship terminates when the identified goal is met. It is never acceptable for the HCP to put his job first or act in any manner that does not advocate for the patient's best interests and well-being. The Board of Certification (BOC) Code of Professional Responsibility (Code 1.2)[9] requires ATs to do the following:

- Protect the patient from undue harm.
- Always act in the patient's best interests.
- Advocate for the patient's welfare.
- Take appropriate action to protect patients from HCPs or athletic training students who are impaired or engaged in illegal or unethical practice.

The BOC Code of Professional Responsibility requires that the AT develop patient care relationships that maintain trust and confidence with the patient (or the parent or guardian of a minor patient) and does not exploit the relationship for personal or financial gain (Code 1.5). Violation of the patient's boundaries occurs when personal benefit to the HCP exists at the expense of the patient. A sports medicine example would be when an AT or physician makes RTP decisions that benefit her own position or job at the risk of the patient. Another example might be engaging in a romantic or sexual relationship with a current patient or having knowledge of abuse or misconduct to a patient by a physician and failing to report the incident to supervisors. Code 1.6 specifically requires the AT to not engage in intimate or sexual activity with a patient or with the parent or guardian of a minor patient.[23] It is the HCP's responsibility to be self-aware of warning signs of boundary crossing such as the following:

- Frequently thinking of a patient in a personal way.
- Keeping secrets with a specific patient.
- Favoring one patient's care at the expense of another's.
- Sharing personal details with a patient to make an impression.[25]

Boundary violations are never acceptable, and it is the AT's responsibility to manage any situation professionally and therapeutically regardless of who initiated it. Anything that could compromise the patient's well-being if the relationship with an AT is continued or discontinued should be considered a warning sign requiring assessment of the situation in an objective manner.[25] Remember, the patient's best interests must be maintained, and the AT must act responsibly and stop the inappropriate behavior or report (in writing) the violation to a higher authority (more on mandatory reporting in chapter 2). It is important to follow up on the report to ensure the violation has been reported to the proper authorities.

Confidentiality

For a patient to feel safe and trust the HCP, the professional relationship requires confidentiality. During all interactions, the patient should feel comfortable reporting injuries or illnesses. Further, the patient should feel that the HCP will only share information with other HCPs or medical staff that need to know about the patient's condition. The HCP must obtain the patient's written permission to share information with anyone outside of the health care team, including employers, supervisors, coaches, or administrators. Whenever possible, use appropriate terms to communicate injury status to anyone outside the health care team, including the media. For example, when communicating with others outside the health care team, use language or estimation (educated guess) for level of activity or participation, such as the following:

- Providing health status for games, performances, or other physical activity:
  - *Questionable*—Patient is "uncertain" to participate, or there is a 50% likelihood of participating.
  - *Doubtful*—Patient is "unlikely" to participate, or there is a 75% likelihood of not participating.
  - *Out*—Patient will not participate.
- Confirming the extent of participation:
  - *Did not participate*—Patient did not participate at all.
  - *Limited participation*—Patient participated in less than 100% of normal activity.

- *Full participation*—Participated in 100% of normal activities.

The BOC's Code of Professional Responsibility (Code 1.4)[9] requires the AT to communicate effectively and truthfully with patients while maintaining privacy and confidentiality of patient information in accordance with applicable law.

Emotional Intelligence

Emotional intelligence is recognizing one's own and other people's emotions and using this information to guide thinking and behavior and adjust emotions based on the situation or physical setting. Self-awareness requires examination of your emotional reactions. It involves knowledge of how attitudes, perceptions, past and present experiences, and relationships create a lens through which you see the world and the people in it. Emotional intelligence and **self-awareness** allow the HCP to know when to step in and when to stand back. An example of emotional intelligence involves understanding that during halftime at a football game, a head coach might feel anger or frustration. Adapting the AT's behavior to this situation might involve waiting until the coach has calmed down or discussing the status of a player with an assistant coach who will communicate the patient's status (see previous section, Confidentiality) with the head coach at the appropriate time or place. Recognizing that situations or people with emotions exist outside of your control requires emotional intelligence. Further, having self-awareness means you are able to be fully present and engage with a patient in the moment rather than be distracted by the situation or other people's behavior.[29]

Cultural Competence

HCPs care for patients from many different cultural and ethnic backgrounds that affect people's perceptions of life and health. **Cultural competence** is an attitude of respect and awareness for patients from cultures different from the HCP's own and is essential for successful provision of health care to a diverse patient population. Delivering health care in a culturally competent manner is necessary in order to provide adequate and appropriate health care services to all people in a way that respects and honors their particular culturally based understandings and approaches to health and illness.[18]

Cultural competence in providing health care services requires the HCP to do the following:[18]

- Be aware of and accept cultural differences.
- Be aware of her own cultural values.
- Recognize that people from different cultural backgrounds have different ways of communicating,

behaving, interpreting information, and solving problems.

- Recognize that cultural beliefs affect how patients perceive their health, how they seek help, how they interact with health practitioners, and how they adhere to the treatments or care plans.
- Be aware of the patient's health literacy.
- Be able and willing to change the way he works to fit in with the patient's cultural or ethnic background in order to provide the patient with optimal care.
- Be aware that cultural competence includes people from low socioeconomic backgrounds. Marginalized citizens tend to be more passive. They are often reluctant to voice their opinions or preferences and may be less willing to trust their own judgment.

Cultural competence is a core value that enhances communication between the HCP and patient and facilitates better intervention, treatment, and patient outcomes. Having an open mind and accepting attitude is essential for the HCP to understand another person's perspective and provide culture-specific care. Attitudes and interpersonal skills that are culturally sensitive are necessary to successfully establish an effective HCP–patient therapeutic relationship. Highly skilled HCPs have experiences and attitudes toward patients and families that are genuine, warm, and respectful with an ability to convey support, interest, sympathy, and understanding of each patient's condition and situation. The BOC's Code of Professional Responsibility (Code 1.1) fosters nondiscrimination by mandating that the AT render quality patient care regardless of the patient's age, gender, race, religion, disability, sexual orientation, or any other characteristic protected by law. Additionally, the BOC's Code of Professional Responsibility (Code 1.4.1)[9] requires the AT to do the following:

- Demonstrate respect for cultural diversity.
- Understand the impact of cultural and religious values.
- Accept all patients by overcoming negative or biased attitudes.
- Offer consistent, nonjudgmental care to all patients regardless of background, circumstance, morals, or beliefs.
- Consider the internal perception of the patient to understand how the patient experiences the situation.

Obtaining a medical history and communicating with a patient who uses English as a second language is challenging, particularly in many large urban areas where major segments of the population do not speak English. Patients who have difficulty communicating are at greater risk of medical errors and poor outcomes. Contributing factors that perpetuate ineffective communication between a patient and HCP include a lack of the following:

- Systematic method for assessing a patient's communication needs
- Practices for effective patient communication in routine care
- Standardized training of HCPs

Effective patient–provider communication is an essential component of patient care. Improving patient–provider communication is a patient safety and quality of care concern. For communication to be effective, the information must be complete, accurate, timely, unambiguous, and understood by the patient.[30] Effectively communicating with patients who use English as a second language may involve the following:

- Using short, simple questions and simple words
- Avoiding difficult medical terms by using layperson or more common language
- Learning common words and phrases in the other language, especially common medical terms
- Using pocket cards that show pronunciation
- Finding a family member or friend to act as an interpreter
- Researching cultural differences and similarities[27]

Ethical Practice

Therapeutic relationships require the HCP to interact, communicate, and behave ethically. The NATA Code of Ethics[23] requires that the AT not engage in conduct that could be construed as a conflict of interest, reflects negatively on the athletic training profession, or jeopardizes a patient's health and well-being. It is the HCP's responsibility to report abuse and protect the patient from undue harm. Occasionally, the ATs must intervene and report an abusive situation that might be violent, threatening, or intended to inflict harm. Mandated reporting of suspected abuse is further described in chapter 2.

Ethical practice also includes documenting all procedures and services in accordance with local, state, and federal laws, rules, and guidelines (BOC Practice Standard 7). In addition, the AT should conduct research activities intended to improve knowledge, practice, education, outcomes, and policy related to health care delivery (Code 4.3).[9] An essential aspect of documentation is using **health care informatics** such as patient databases, electronic medical records, or other tracking systems. Injury **epidemiology** is using large data sets or databases to characterize the occurrence of sports injuries by identifying risk factors in order to develop injury prevention strategies and programs. Sports injuries can occur in every athlete, in every setting, at any age. Standardizing the collection of information (data) depends on valid and reliable definitions of sports injury, injury severity, and sports participation. Using standard definitions is crucial for comparing and interpreting data.

Injury surveillance is the ongoing collection of data describing the occurrence of, and factors associated with, sports injury. Injury surveillance systems (table 1.2) rely on standard definitions of injury, exposure, severity, and other elements to determine incidence, relative risk, and athlete exposures. These factors provide validity of data and useful outcomes in epidemiological research activities. Many injury prevention interventions have been established, including rules and regulations such as wearing a helmet, eliminating spearing (initial contact with the top of the head), and using a heads-up technique. These regulations are essential in reduction of injury. Several sports injury surveillance systems use data supplied by ATs as data recorders. These data are essential to describe rates, patterns, and trends of sports-related injuries. Epidemiologic analysis of these data is necessary to develop, implement, and evaluate evidence-based, targeted prevention programs to reduce the number and severity of injuries among athletes of all levels.

Summary

Emergency medicine is an important part of the clinical care provided by ATs and other HCPs who are primary care or first-line providers of immediate care to acute or emergent injuries and medical conditions. The interprofessional health care team can be found in a variety of prehospital, emergency department, urgent care clinic, and other health care settings. The AT and other prehospital HCPs are responsible for diagnosing traumatic injuries or illnesses in the acute phase, initiating resuscitation and stabilization of the patient, starting interventions and field management, coordinating care with specialists, and determining disposition regarding patients' need for referral to physicians, physician assistants, nurse practitioners, and other next-level HCPs. This group of clinicians becomes an interprofessional health care team—a group working toward one common aim, namely, the best possible patient care. Interprofessional collaborative practice is key to the safe, high-quality, accessible, patient-centered care desired by all.[3,8]

TABLE 1.2 **Sports Injury Surveillance Systems**

System	Purpose	Outcome measures
High school reporting injuries online (RIO)	Internet-based data collection tool studies all time-loss injuries in a sample of U.S. high school athletes. Weekly data are collected by ATs as data reporters.	Athletic exposure (number of athlete practices and number of athlete competitions per week) Injury (body site, diagnosis, severity, etc.) Injury event (mechanism, activity, position/event, field/court location, etc.)
National Center for Catastrophic Sport Injury Research (NCCSIR)	Conduct surveillance of catastrophic injuries and illnesses related to participation in organized U.S. sports at the collegiate, high school, and youth levels of play.	Systematic data reporting system Cases of catastrophic injuries and illnesses
High School National Athletic Treatment, Injury and Outcomes Network (NATION)	Integrates injury surveillance, treatment and patient outcomes. Uses data gathered by ATs in public high schools.	Time-loss and non-time-loss injuries Frequency and value of health care provided by ATs in the high school setting Patient-reported outcomes for patients who receive care by ATs in the high school setting

Based on information from High School RIO; National Center for Catastrophic Sport Injury Research; DatalysCenter.

 Go to the web study guide to complete the case studies for this chapter.

CHAPTER 2

Prevention and Risk Management Strategies

OBJECTIVES

After reading this chapter, you will be able to do the following:

- Define infectious disease and communicable disease.

- Describe the routes of disease transmission.

- Identify the standard precautions that are used in treating patients to prevent infection.

- Describe a risk management approach to infection prevention and control.

- Explain the concept of consent before delivery of health care.

- Determine measures to implement for preventing litigation.

Before providing care to an injured patient, best practices in the prevention of disease transmission or infection must be established. These best practices allow medical care to be administered by trained and licensed health care providers (HCPs) in order to minimize risk or significant liability exposure. Medical teams that include an athletic trainer (AT) sustain a lower incidence of injuries (both acute and recurring) than athletes at schools without ATs.[1] Therefore, strategies to minimize risk to the HCP and patient should follow standard precautions, protect health information, obtain consent, be practiced in an ethical manner, and follow state laws governing health care practice. Additionally, the AT is responsible for reporting and documenting patient care and emergency response. The AT is an expert at prehospital care and is usually the primary care provider during an emergency for sporting or athletic events, practices, and other settings. It is essential that the AT take appropriate precautions to minimize risk and prevent medical errors. This chapter describes how to manage risk, reduce the spread of infectious disease, minimize infections associated with health care, avoid medicolegal issues related to obtaining consent, maintain confidentially, and document patient care.

Risk Management

Risk management is the identification, assessment, and prioritization of risk (an uncertain possibility of a threat that leads to loss, catastrophe, or other undesirable outcome). The process of managing risk involves coordinating resources to minimize, monitor, and control the probability and impact of unfortunate events.[2] Safety is an all-encompassing strategy for reducing risk.

Developing and implementing policies and procedures for the safety of patients and employees, as well as the safe operation of the AT facility, is essential to lessen or mitigate risk. One of the most important aspects of safety and minimizing risk is employee education on the many safety and health hazards while on the job. To protect the employee and patients, it is important to follow the regulations for the operation of an athletic health care program. Regulations require a facility or organization to be in compliance with **standard precautions** and to demonstrate that compliance.

Although AT facilities are not specifically required to obtain accreditation as a health care facility, standards are detailed by the Athletic Training Board of Certification (BOC)[3] and should be followed. Facilities similar to AT clinics are generally accredited as ambulatory care clinics that provide outpatient care in facilities where patients do not remain overnight. Examples of ambulatory care facilities include the following:

- Hospital- and non–hospital-based outpatient clinics
- Physician offices
- Urgent care centers
- Outpatient surgical centers
- Imaging centers
- Physical therapy and rehabilitation centers

Large organizations, such as schools, universities, clinics, and hospitals, have insurance, legal professionals, and risk management professionals who can be helpful in identifying the regulations that apply to each program. Although many sports medicine settings or athletic health care facilities were not originally designed as health care facilities, it is important to follow the regulations and standards of health care facilities. Athletic health care services are not commonly delivered in a traditional health care facility. The BOC Facility Principles are available to ensure the quality of facilities where health care services are delivered.[3] To be compliant with regulations and standards, employers are required to do the following:

- Educate employees regarding safety and protection against accidental transmission of blood-borne pathogens.
- Provide daily maintenance and upkeep of the facility, such as housekeeping and laundry.
- Document employee education about blood-borne pathogens.
- Communicate to employees on a regular basis.
- Provide evidence that compliance is documented.[3]

Health care facilities that employ HCPs must provide a safe work environment and follow regulations and stan-dards. Additionally, facilities must ensure that the AT and other HCPs providing care to patients are highly skilled professionals with extensive knowledge that includes university-level study, appropriate certifications, and state regulations or licensure. Anyone who is working (paid or unpaid) or volunteering (including AT students) in an outpatient setting has the potential for exposure to patients and to infectious materials, including the following:

- Body substances
- Contaminated medical supplies and devices
- Contaminated environmental surfaces
- Contaminated air

Following standard precautions and protocols, including people not directly involved in patient care (e.g., AT students, clerical, housekeeping, and volunteers), will prevent potential exposure to infectious agents that can be transmitted to and from HCPs and patients.[4]

Infectious Diseases

Infectious diseases resulted in 9.2 million deaths globally in 2013 (about 17% of all deaths).[5] HCPs in the prehospital or ambulatory care setting treat patients who may have a variety of communicable or infectious diseases.

- A **communicable disease** is a disease that can be spread from one person or species to another. An example of a communicable disease is the influenza virus that spreads through air droplets when someone coughs or sneezes.
- An **infectious disease** is a medical condition caused by the growth and spread of small, harmful organisms within the body (**pathogens**). An example of an infectious disease is a *Staphylococcus aureus* bacterial infection in a wound from contact with an infected object.

Infectious agents are biological agents (pathogens) that cause disease or illness to their **host**. Many infectious agents are **microbes** present in health care settings. Patients and HCPs are the most likely sources of infectious agents and are also the most common susceptible hosts. People visiting and working in health care may be at risk of both infection and transmission. Therefore, hygiene is critical for the prevention of infection by pathogens. Several classes of pathogens can cause infection, including bacteria, viruses, fungi, parasites, and prions. Treatment of infection is primarily by **antimicrobials** that destroy disease-causing microbes. The most commonly known antimicrobials are **antibiotics**, which target bacteria. Other forms of antimicrobials are antivirals, antifungals, and antiparasitics.[6]

HCPs are at risk for exposure to serious, and sometimes deadly, diseases. Providing care to patients or handling material may spread infection from the patient to the provider or from provider to patient. While the risk for exposure varies with setting, role, and responsibility, HCPs should have appropriate **vaccines** to reduce the chances of contracting or spreading vaccine-preventable diseases to coworkers, patients, and family members. Table 2.1 provides the Centers for Disease Control and Prevention (CDC)-recommended vaccines for all workers in health care settings.

Further, hospitals, clinics, and other health care facilities require HCPs and volunteers to be screened for tuberculosis (TB), which is caused by *Mycobacterium tuberculosis*. The bacteria usually attack the lungs, but TB bacteria can attack any part of the body, such as the kidney, spine, and brain. The TB bacteria can lie dormant or be a **latent infection**; however, an **active infection** can be fatal if not treated properly.[7] These 2 types of screening tests are available for TB in HCPs:[7]

- *Initial baseline testing upon hire:* Two-step testing with a TB skin test or a TB blood test
- *Annual or serial screening:* Determined by state regulations or risk assessment outcomes

The TB vaccine should be considered for only select people who meet specific criteria, such as the following:

- HCPs in contact with a high percentage of TB
- HCPs exposed to transmission of drug-resistant TB strains and subsequent infection is likely
- HCPs exposed to settings in which TB infection-control precautions have not been implemented or have not been successful

HCPs considering the TB vaccination should be counseled regarding the risks and benefits associated with both the vaccine and treatment of latent TB infection.[7]

Routes of Disease Transmission in Health Care Settings

While all infections result from an invasion of body spaces and tissues by pathogens, different pathogens use different routes of **transmission** to spread the infectious agent. The modes of transmission vary by type of organism. Some infectious agents may be transmitted by more than one route, including the following:

TABLE 2.1 **CDC-Recommended Vaccines for Health Care Workers**

Name of vaccine	Vaccination recommendations
For all listed	Provide documented evidence of vaccine dose or complete vaccine series, or Provide current blood test indicating immunity (i.e., serologic evidence of immunity from prior vaccination); Otherwise obtain the following:
Hepatitis B (HepB or HB)	3-dose series (first dose now, second dose in 1 month, third dose approximately 5 months after second dose) with anti-HBs serologic tested 1-2 months after third dose
Influenza (Flu)	1 dose of influenza vaccine annually
Measles, mumps, and rubella (MMR)	1-2 doses of MMR (1 dose now and the second dose at least 28 days later)
Varicella (Chickenpox)	Those who have not had chickenpox (varicella), obtain 2 doses of varicella vaccine, 4 weeks apart.
Tetanus, diphtheria, pertussis (Tdap)	One-time dose of Tdap as soon as possible if you have not received Tdap previously (regardless of when previous dose of Tdap was received) Td boosters are for tetanus and diphtheria (not pertussis) and should be administered every 10 years thereafter. Pregnant HCPs must have a dose of Tdap during each pregnancy.
Meningococcal	People routinely exposed to *N. meningitidis* should obtain 1 dose.
Tuberculosis (TB)	Health care providers who have been tested and meet specific criteria for the vaccine (details in the table footnote)

State immunization laws for health care providers vary. Visit the CDC website to search for information on vaccine administration, assessment, and reporting.

Based on Centers for Disease Control and Prevention (2017); Centers for Disease Control and Prevention (2016).

- *Direct contact:* Physically touching an infected person, including sexual contact (e.g., herpes simplex virus)
- *Indirect physical contact:* Touching a contaminated **fomite**, such as a surface, including soil (e.g., *S. aureus* bacteria)
- *Airborne transmission:* Microorganism transmitted through the air (e.g., *M. tuberculosis*)
- *Droplet contact:* Coughing or sneezing on another person (e.g., influenza virus, *B. pertussis*)

Other infectious agents, such as blood-borne viruses (e.g., hepatitis B and C viruses, human immunodeficiency virus), are transmitted rarely in health care settings through percutaneous or mucous membrane exposure. Importantly, not all infectious agents are transmitted from person to person.[8]

Direct Contact Transmission

The most important and frequent mode of transmission of hospital-acquired (**nosocomial**) infections is by direct contact. Direct contact transmission involves a direct contact from body surface to body surface and physical transfer of microorganisms between a susceptible host and an infected or **colonized** person. Direct contact transmission also can occur between 2 patients; one serves as the source of the infectious microorganisms and the other as a susceptible host. Opportunities for direct contact transmission between patients and health care personnel include the following:

- Blood or other blood-containing body fluids from a patient directly enter the HCP's body through contact with a mucous membrane or non-intact skin (e.g., cuts, abrasions). For example, a HCP develops an infection from an open cut on a finger after contact with a patient without using gloves.
- A HCP with contaminated hands touches a vulnerable site, such as an open wound, causing infection in the patient.

Indirect Contact Transmission

Indirect contact transmission involves the transfer of an infectious agent through a contaminated intermediate person or object that transmits the infection to a susceptible host. Contaminated hands of HCPs are important contributors to indirect contact transmission if proper **hand hygiene** (details follow) is not performed before touching another patient. Patient-care devices may transmit pathogens if devices contaminated with blood or body fluids are shared between patients without cleaning and disinfecting between patients. Examples of opportunities for indirect contact transmission include the following:

- During routine patient care, blood is dropped onto the basketball court. If the court surface is not properly cleaned, the pathogen can be transmitted to another player days later.
- Needlesticks can allow a pathogen to move from the patient to the needle to the HCP. This route of transmission is less common with use of safety equipment such as needleless intravenous (IV) medication systems.
- Instruments that are inadequately cleaned between patients before disinfection or sterilization (e.g., scalpel, rectal thermometer, non-rebreather mask, airways) may transmit bacterial and viral pathogens.
- Disease transmission can occur by sharing a towel that has been vigorously rubbed or items of clothing in close contact with the body (i.e., socks) that have not been thoroughly washed between uses. For this reason, contagious diseases often break out on teams where towels are shared and personal items of clothing are accidentally swapped in locker rooms.
- Clothing, uniforms, laboratory coats, or isolation gowns used as personal protective equipment (PPE) may become contaminated with potential pathogens after care of a patient colonized or infected with an infectious agent.

Airborne Transmission

Airborne transmission occurs by dissemination of either airborne droplet nuclei or small particles in the respirable size range containing infectious agents that remain infective over time and distance (e.g., spores of *M. tuberculosis*). Microorganisms carried in this manner may be dispersed over long distances by air currents containing the infectious agent that is inhaled by susceptible individuals who have not had face-to-face contact with (or been in the same room with) the infectious person.[9] Airborne transmission dispersed from the source to the patient depends on environmental factors; therefore, special air handling and ventilation are important in preventing airborne transmission. An example of disease transmitted by airborne transmission is when breathing air from an infected person transmits the common cold or influenza from person to person.

Droplet Transmission

Droplet transmission occurs when respiratory droplets carrying an infectious pathogen transmit infection by traveling directly from the respiratory tract of the infectious person to susceptible mucosal surfaces of the recipient. Facial protection is required to prevent this type of transmission. Examples of respiratory droplets generated from an infected person include the following:

- Coughing, sneezing, or talking during procedures such as suctioning, endotracheal intubation, or cardiopulmonary resuscitation
- Soiled garments that have not been properly sanitized[8,10,11]

Health Care–Associated and Nosocomial Infections

The Occupational Safety and Health Administration (OSHA) has developed, published, and enforced guidelines concerning reducing risk in the workplace.[12] Additionally, the CDC[13] developed a set of protective practices for HCPs to use when providing patient care designed to prevent workers from coming in direct contact with pathogens or pathogens carried by patients (described next). Because every person is potentially infected or can spread an organism that could be transmitted in the health care setting, infection control procedures must be applied to reduce infection in patients and health care personnel.

Without the use of appropriate standard precautions, HCPs can inadvertently spread infection or become infected themselves. Pathogens can be found on contaminated equipment, bed linens, or in air droplets that are breathed into the lungs. Infection can originate from the outside environment, another infected patient, or staff that may be infected; or in some cases, the source of the infection cannot be determined. Microorganisms often originate from the patient's own skin and become opportunistic after surgery or other procedures that compromise the protective skin barrier. Infection acquired by patients during health care delivery in any setting (e.g., athletic training clinics, physical therapy clinics, ambulatory or outpatient settings) is considered a **health care–associated infection (HAI)**; while infections acquired specifically in hospitals are nosocomial infections. HAIs can cause severe pneumonia and infections of the urinary tract, bloodstream, and other parts of the body (table 2.2).

TABLE 2.2   **Common Pathogens Transmitted in the Health Care Setting**

Pathogen	Description/Transmission	Health care settings
Acinetobacter	• Group of bacteria commonly found in soil and water. • Outbreaks typically occur in intensive care units and health care settings housing very ill patients.	• Accounts for 80% of reported infections in all health care settings. • *Acinetobacter* infections rarely occur outside of health care settings.
Burkholderia cepacia	• Complex of bacteria found in soil and water. • Often resistant to common antibiotics.	• Poses little medical risk to healthy people; however, causes infections in hospitalized patients who may be more susceptible to infections.
Clostridium difficile	• Spores are easily transmitted to individuals by hands that have touched a contaminated surface or item. • Bacterium causes an inflammation of the colon (colitis). • Diarrhea and fever are the most common symptoms of infection.	• Overuse of antibiotics is the most important risk for getting *C. difficile* infection.
Clostridium sordellii	• Bacterium that causes pneumonia, endocarditis, arthritis, peritonitis, and myonecrosis • **Bacteremia** and **sepsis**, a serious bodywide response, occur rarely.	• Most cases of sepsis from *C. sordellii* occur in patients with other serious health conditions or comorbidities.
Enterobacteriaceae	• Large family of gram-negative bacteria; examples are *Klebsiella* species and *E. coli*. • Difficult to treat because of high levels of resistance to antibiotics. • Normal part of the human gut bacteria that can become **carbapenem** resistant (details follow).	• Infections are most common in patients who require devices such as ventilators, urinary **catheters**, or IV therapy, and who are taking long courses of certain antibiotics.

> continued

Table 2.2 > continued

Pathogen	Description/Transmission	Health care settings
Enterococcus	• Anaerobic bacterium normally present in human intestines, female genital tract, and outside environment. • Has a high level of intrinsic antibiotic resistance.	• Most infections occur in hospitals.
Hepatitis Common types: hepatitis A, hepatitis B, and hepatitis C	• Causes inflammation of the liver. • Group of viruses; most common types are hepatitis A, hepatitis B, and hepatitis C. • Transmitted primarily by unsafe injection practices; reuse of needles, fingerstick devices, and syringes; and other lapses in infection control.	• Delivery of health care has the potential to transmit hepatitis to both health care workers and patients. Outbreaks have occurred in outpatient settings, hemodialysis units, long-term care facilities, and hospitals.
Human immunodeficiency virus (HIV)	• Virus that destroys CD4 and T blood cells, crucial to **immunity** (helping the body fight disease). • Leads to acquired immunodeficiency syndrome (AIDS).	• Transmission of HIV to patients while in health care settings is rare. Weakened immune system is at risk for many of infections. Most exposures do not result in infection.
Influenza	• Community-based viral infection transmitted in households and community settings. • HAI prevention measures for influenza should be implemented in all health care settings.	• 5%-20% of U.S. residents acquire an influenza virus infection each year. • Many seek medical care in ambulatory health care settings; 200,000 people are hospitalized each year.
Mycobacterium abscessus	• Bacterium found in water, soil, and dust. • Contaminates medications and medical devices.	• HAIs of *M. abscessus* are usually in skin and the soft tissues under the skin. Can also cause lung infections in people with various chronic lung diseases.
Norovirus	• Group of viruses that cause **gastroenteritis**, causing an acute onset of severe vomiting and diarrhea. • Like all viral infections, noroviruses are not affected by treatment with antibiotics.	• Usually brief in healthy people. Young children, the elderly, and people with other medical illnesses are at risk for severe or prolonged infection.
Pseudomonas aeruginosa	• Strains of bacteria found widely in the environment. • Most common type causes infections in humans.	• Infections usually occur in people who are hospitalized or who have weakened immune systems.
Staphylococcus aureus (staph)	• Bacterium found on the skin and in the nose of about 30% of people and usually does not cause harm.	• Infections look like pimples, boils, or spider bites. • Most are treatable; however, strains have become antibiotic resistant.
Tuberculosis (TB)	• Infection caused by bacterium that spreads through air and can travel long distances. • Transmission in health care is from close contact with people with active infectious TB, particularly during cough-inducing procedures such as bronchoscopy and sputum induction.	• Poses recognized risk to patients and health care personnel. • Cases of multidrug-resistant tuberculosis (MDR-TB) are recognized and difficult to treat.

Based on Centers for Disease Control and Prevention (2014); OSHA (2007).

Many types of HAIs are difficult to treat with antibiotics and other medications; treatment is further complicated by **antibiotic resistance**.[11,12]

Multidrug-Resistant Organisms

Bacteria and other microorganisms that have developed resistance to antimicrobial drugs are considered **mul-tidrug-resistant organisms (MDROs)**; they are also called *superbugs*. Although the names of certain MDROs (table 2.3) describe resistance to only one agent (e.g., MRSA, VRE), these pathogens are frequently resistant to most available antimicrobial agents (table 2.4) and require special attention in health care facilities. Increasing experience with these organisms in health care is

TABLE 2.3   Common Multidrug-Resistant Organisms

Pathogen	Drug resistance	Health care settings
Methicillin/oxacillin -resistant *Staphylococcus aureus* (MRSA)	Staph bacteria resistant to certain **beta-lactam** antibiotics. Community-acquired MRSA infections are skin infections.	Infections in open wounds, invasive devices, and weakened immune systems are potentially life-threatening.
Penicillin-resistant *Streptococcus pneumoniae* (PRSP)	Strain resistant to penicillin, second-generation cephalosporins, macrolides, tetracyclines, and trimethoprim/sulfamethoxazole.	Susceptibility depends on the site of infection (e.g., meningitis, otitis media).
Vancomycin-intermediate *Staphylococcus aureus* (VISA) and Vancomycin-resistant *Staphylococcus aureus* (VRSA)	Specific staph bacteria that have developed resistance to the antimicrobial agent **vancomycin**.	More common in people with: underlying health conditions (diabetes, kidney disease), devices going into the body (catheters), previous infection, and recent exposure to antimicrobial agents.
Vancomycin-resistant enterococci (VRE)	Specific types of antimicrobial-resistant bacteria that are resistant to vancomycin.	Most infections occur in hospitals. Cephalosporin use is a risk factor for VRE colonization, infection, and transmission.
Klebsiella pneumoniae carbapenemase (KPC)	Gram-negative bacteria that have developed antimicrobial resistance, most recently to carbapenems.	Cause HAIs including pneumonia, bloodstream infections, wound or surgical site infections, and meningitis.

Based on National Health and Medical Research Council (2010); Siegel et al. (2006); Centers for Disease Control and Prevention (2016).

TABLE 2.4   Common Antibiotics Used to Treat Infection

Antibiotic class	Examples
beta-lactams penicillins	methicillin, dicloxacillin, nafcillin, oxacillin
cephems cephamycins cephalosporins	Cefoxitin, Cefotetan, Cefmetazole Ceftobiprole, Ceftaroline, Ceftolozane
carbapenems	Imipenem, Meropenem, Ertapenem
glycopeptide antibiotic	vancomycin
monobactams	aztreonam
macrolide	erythromycin
synthetic derivatives	azithromycin
protein synthesis inhibitors	tetracycline, oxytetracycline, chlortetracycline, demeclocycline, doxycycline
enzyme inhibitor	trimethoprim
sulfonamides	sulfamethoxazole

Generic drug names are in lower case; brand names are in upper case.

Based on Centers for Disease Control and Prevention (2017); Siegel et al. (2006); Occupational Safety and Health Administration (2002).

improving the understanding of the routes of transmission and effective preventive measures for MDROs. Although transmission of MDROs is most frequently documented in acute care facilities, all health care settings are affected by the emergence and transmission of antimicrobial-resistant microbes.[10] Transmission by HCPs may occur by colonization of a disease-causing organism that is present in or on the body but is not causing illness. Any HCP can become colonized with a microbe, then carry and spread infection to other health care personnel and patients.[6,10,15]

Avoiding the spread of infections reduces the necessity for antibiotics and reduces the likelihood that drug resistance will develop during therapy. Preventing infections also prevents the spread of resistant bacteria. The appropriate and safe use of antibiotics—only when needed to treat disease, when selecting the right antibiotic, and when administering the drug correctly—minimizes the development of MDROs.[6] The most relevant recommendations for prevention and control of MDRO transmissions for all health care settings are as follows:[10]

• *Infection control precautions*: Follow standard precautions during all patient encounters in all settings in which health care is delivered. Use masks according to standard precautions when performing splash generating procedures (e.g., wound irrigation, suctioning, intubation); masks are not otherwise recommended during routine care (e.g., upon room entry). Use standard precautions for patients known to be infected or colonized with MDRO.

• *Environmental measures*: Clean and disinfect surfaces and equipment that may be contaminated with pathogens more frequently, including those that are in close proximity to the patient (e.g., tables) and frequently touched surfaces in the patient care environment (e.g., doorknobs, surfaces in and surrounding showers or locker rooms).

Standard Precautions

Athletic trainers and other HCPs often work under unpredictable, adverse conditions where a patient may have exposure to pathogens while being treated for medical or trauma conditions. Any HCP can be exposed to blood while treating trauma victims, performing life support procedures, or using needles and other sharp instruments. Exposure to blood can occur from a sharps injury, such as a needlestick after use on a patient or a cut from a contaminated sharp object. Exposure can also occur from a splash to the eyes, nose, or mouth; contact on non-intact (broken or cracked) skin; or a human bite. Appropriate precautions are required when reasonable anticipation of **occupational exposure** to skin, eye, mucous membrane, or **parenteral** contact with blood or **other potentially**

infectious materials (OPIM) exists. The risk of contracting a communicable or infectious disease during patient care is a possibility; however, the potential for exposure can be minimized by using standard precautions.[16]

Standard precautions are a group of infection prevention practices that apply to all HCPs and patients, regardless of suspected or confirmed infection status, in any setting in which health care is delivered. The application of standard precautions during patient care is determined by the nature of the HCP–patient interaction and the extent of anticipated blood, body fluid, or pathogen exposure. For some interactions (e.g., performing point-of-care blood glucose testing), only gloves may be needed; however, during other interactions (e.g., intubation), use of gloves, face shield or mask, and goggles is necessary.[9] Assume that every person is potentially infected or colonized with an organism that could be transmitted in the health care setting, and apply the proper infection control practices during the delivery of health care.

Similarly, equipment or items in the patient environment likely to have been contaminated with infectious body fluids must be handled in a manner to prevent transmission of infectious agents. For each facility, the standard precautions must be detailed in a written **exposure control plan (ECP)** (details follow; see appendix A for a sample plan). These practices are designed to both protect HCPs and prevent HCPs from spreading infections among patients.

The BOC and OSHA require the following standard precautions for health care providers:[3,11,12,3,16]

• Proper hand hygiene

• Personal protective equipment (e.g., gloves, gowns, masks)

• Safe injection practices

• Safe handling of potentially contaminated equipment or surfaces

• Respiratory hygiene and cough etiquette

The following sections describe each of these elements.

Proper Hand Hygiene

Hand hygiene is the single most important practice to reduce the transmission of infectious agents in health care settings and is an essential element of standard precautions. When properly implemented, hand hygiene alone can significantly reduce the risk of cross-transmission of infection in health care facilities.[9,17]

Hand hygiene includes both handwashing with either plain or antiseptic-containing soap and water, and the use of alcohol-based products that do not require the use of water. Alcohol-based hand sanitizers (gels, rinses, foams) are the most effective products for reducing the number of pathogens on the hands of HCPs. In the absence of visibly soiled hands, approved alcohol-based products for hand disinfection are preferred over antimicrobial or plain soap and water because of their superior microbicidal activity, reduced drying of the skin, and convenience. Antiseptic soaps and detergents are the next most effective, and non-antimicrobial soaps are the least effective.[9,17] During the delivery of health care, avoid unnecessary touching of surfaces in close proximity to the patient to prevent both contamination of clean hands from environmental surfaces and transmission of pathogens from contaminated hands to surfaces (cross-contamination).[9,18]

For routinely decontaminating hands, it is recommended that HCPs use alcohol-based hand sanitizers in these situations:[9,17]

- When hands are not visibly soiled
- Before having direct contact with patients
- After contact with a patient's intact skin (e.g., when taking a pulse or blood pressure or touching a patient)
- After contact with body fluids or excretions, mucous membranes, non-intact skin, and wound dressings if hands are not visibly soiled
- After contact with inanimate objects (including medical equipment) in the immediate vicinity of the patient
- After removing gloves
- If moving from a contaminated body site to a clean body site during patient care

Alternatively, the HCP should use soap and water to wash in these situations:[9,18]

- When hands are visibly dirty or contaminated with proteinaceous material, blood, or other body fluids
- After using a restroom
- Before and after having food
- Before and after glove use
- Before and after contact with a patient, regardless of whether gloves were worn

Cleanliness of HCPs working in a health care facility, as well as the facility itself, is an important part of safe and effective treatment. Adequate facilities for handwashing or hand sanitation should be available throughout the AT facility. Not all facilities have access to sinks; however, a facility can improve sanitary conditions with the addition of hand sanitizing units. Anyone providing services in a health care facility should be educated about handwashing and personal sanitation. It is also important to develop an organizational policy for the HCPs who have direct contact with patients wearing nonnatural nails that can harbor infectious agents. The administration should regularly communicate these policies to everyone in the health care facility as well as keep records of this communication and related training.[3]

Personal Protective Equipment

To protect HCPs, staff, and the patient from infectious agents, the use of personal protective equipment (PPE) is essential. A variety of barriers (e.g., gloves, gowns, masks) used alone or in combination can protect mucous membranes, airways, skin, and clothing from contact with infectious agents.

Hand Hygiene Using an Alcohol-Based Hand Sanitizer

- Put product on hands and rub hands together.
- Cover all surfaces (dorsal and palmar) and rub until hands feel dry.
- This procedure should take around 20 seconds.

CDC Guideline for Hand Hygiene Using Soap and Water

1. Use soap and warm water.
2. Rub hands together for 10-15 seconds to work up a lather.
3. Rinse hands, then dry them with a paper towel.
4. Use a paper towel to turn off the faucet.

Based on Siegel et al. (2007). http://www.cdc.gov/ncidod/dhqp/pdf/isolation2007.pdf; Boyce (2002).

Standards for the Use of PPE

- Use PPE when the nature of the anticipated patient interaction indicates that contact with blood or body fluids may occur.
- Prevent contamination of clothing and skin during the process of removing PPE.
- Before leaving the patient's table or area, remove and discard PPE in designated (red biohazard) containers.

Based on Board of Certification Inc. (2013). www.bocatc.org/; Siegel et al. (2007). www.cdc.gov/ncidod/dhqp/pdf/isolation2007.pdf; Centers for Disease Control and Prevention (2016). www.cdc.gov/HAI/prevent/prevent_pubs.html.

Here are some recommendations for use of PPE in health care settings:[3,9,11]

- Facilities should ensure that sufficient and appropriate PPE is available and readily accessible to HCPs.
- Instruct all HCPs on the use of PPE and ensure employee compliance with governing agencies.
- Document evidence of training, education, and communication about the required use of PPE.
- Educate all HCPs on proper selection and use of PPE.
  - Post materials in a publicly available way.
  - Remove and discard PPE (other than respirators for airborne pathogens) before leaving the patient's room or care area.
  - Perform hand hygiene immediately after removal of PPE.
- Wear gloves when potential for contact with blood, body fluids, mucous membranes, non-intact skin, or contaminated equipment exists.
  - Do not wear the same pair of gloves for the care of more than one patient.
  - Do not wash gloves for the purpose of reuse.
- Wear a gown to protect skin and clothing during procedures or activities where contact with blood or body fluids is anticipated.
  - Do not wear the same gown for the care of more than one patient.
  - Wear mouth, nose, and eye protection during procedures that are likely to generate splashes or sprays of blood or other body fluids.

In the sports medicine or athletic health care setting, gloves are the most common PPE and must be routinely used. Gloves can protect both patients and HCPs from exposure to infectious materials that may be transmitted by direct or indirect contact. Gloves protect HCPs from transmission of blood-borne pathogens as long as the gloves are intact; a needlestick or other puncture that penetrates the glove barrier increases risk of transmission. Gloves manufactured for health care purposes are available in nonsterile and sterile forms. Nonsterile disposable medical gloves made of a variety of materials (e.g., latex, vinyl, nitrile) are ideal for routine, nonsurgical patient care. For contact with blood and body fluids during nonsurgical patient care, a single pair of gloves generally provides adequate barrier protection. Latex or nitrile gloves are preferable to vinyl gloves for clinical procedures that require manual dexterity or will involve more than brief patient contact. Gloves should be used to prevent contamination of the HCP's hands in these situations:

- When providing direct patient care when potential exists for direct contact with blood or body fluids, mucous membranes, non-intact skin, and other potentially infectious material
- When having direct contact with patients who are colonized or infected with pathogens transmitted by the contact route (e.g., MRSA)
- When handling, touching, or cleaning visibly or potentially contaminated patient care equipment and environmental surfaces

During patient care, HCPs can reduce transmission of infectious organisms by adhering to the principles of *working from clean to dirty* and confining or limiting contamination to surfaces that are directly needed for patient care.

Gloves must not be washed for subsequent reuse, because microorganisms cannot be removed reliably from glove surfaces and continued glove integrity cannot be ensured. Furthermore, glove reuse has been associated with transmission of MRSA and gram-negative bacteria. It is necessary to change gloves in these situations:

- During the care of a single patient to prevent cross-contamination of body sites
- If the patient interaction also involves touching portable computer keyboards or other mobile equipment

Wearing and Removing Gloves

Wearing Gloves

1. Choose the right size and type of gloves appropriate to the task.
2. Put on gloves before touching a patient's non-intact skin, open wounds, or mucous membranes, such as the mouth, nose, and eyes.
3. Change gloves during patient care if the hands will move from a contaminated body site (e.g., perineal area) to a clean body site (e.g., face).
4. Remove gloves after contact with a patient or the surrounding environment (including medical equipment) using proper technique to prevent hand contamination.

Removing Gloves

1. With both hands gloved, grasp near the cuff of one glove (a) and pull the glove from the wrist toward your fingertips until the glove folds over (b). Be careful not to touch bare skin when reaching inside of the glove.
2. Carefully grasp the fold of the glove and pull the glove away from your body until it is pulled off of your fingertips turning the glove inside out (c). Be careful not to flip any particles from the glove as it is removed.
3. Place and hold the removed glove in the palm of your gloved hand (d). Keep it wadded up as much as possible so as to more easily complete steps 4 and 5.
4. Using the ungloved hand, carefully insert 2 fingers into the cuff of the gloved hand (e). Slide your fingers down toward your fingertips until the glove folds over, turning the glove inside out while also encasing the other contaminated glove (f). Avoid touching the outside of the glove.
5. Grasp the fold of the glove, and fully remove it from your hand (g). Be careful not to flip any particles that may contaminate the area. Many germs are spread when personal protective equipment is removed.
6. Properly dispose of the gloves. Do not contaminate trash areas, especially when handling harmful substances or chemicals.
7. Thoroughly wash your hands with soap and water to ensure that any contamination from the glove removal is eliminated.

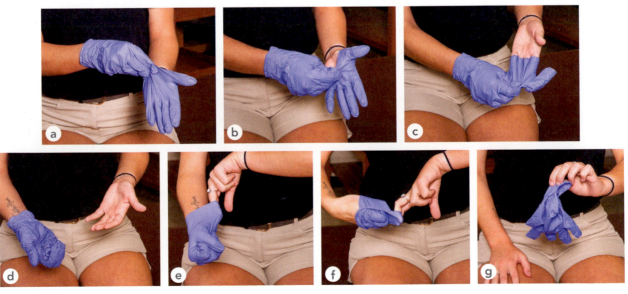

FIGURE 2.1

- Between patients to prevent transmission of infectious material

Hand hygiene following glove removal further ensures that the hands will not carry potentially infectious material that might have penetrated through unrecognized tears or that could contaminate the hands during glove removal.[9,18] Failure to remove gloves after caring for a patient may lead to the spread of potentially deadly pathogens from one patient to another.

Safe Injection Practices

ATs and other HCPs often prepare a patient for or assist in administering injections. Safe injection and other basic infection control practices during patient care are central to patient safety and standard precautions. If infection control protocols are not followed, hepatitis C virus, hepatitis B virus, and HIV can spread. Injection safety includes practices intended to prevent transmission of infectious diseases between one patient and another or between a patient and HCP, and prevent harms such as needlestick injuries (discussed later in this section). To prevent microbial contamination, all medication injections should follow **aseptic technique** (additional details in chapter 5) when handling, preparing, and storing medications and injection equipment or supplies (e.g., syringes, needles, and IV tubing).[19] Although not all prehospital care providers use injections, all ATs should be able to prepare the patient for or provide administration of medication by injection and therefore use these safe practices:

- Follow proper infection control practices and maintain aseptic technique during the preparation and administration of injected medications (e.g., perform hand hygiene).
- Never administer medications from the same syringe to more than one patient, even if the needle is changed.
- Never enter a vial with a used syringe or needle.
- Do not use medications packaged as single dose or single use for more than one patient.
- Do not use bags of intravenous solution as a common source of supply for more than one patient.
- Limit the use of multidose vials and dedicate them to a single patient whenever possible.
- Always use face masks when injecting material or inserting a catheter into the epidural or subdural space.[9,18-20]

HCPs who use or may be exposed to needles or other sharps are at increased risk of **percutaneous exposure incident**, also called a percutaneous injury or **needlestick injury**. Needlestick injury is the percutaneous penetration of skin by a needle or other sharp object, which was in contact with blood, tissue, or other body fluid before the exposure. Injuries resulting from needles and other sharps have been associated with transmission of hepatitis C virus, hepatitis B virus, and HIV to health care personnel. Prevention of sharps injuries has always been an essential element of standard precautions. These measures, used during routine patient care, include handling needles and other sharp devices in a manner that will prevent injury to the user and to others who may encounter the device during or after a procedure. Although nurses sustain the highest number of percutaneous injuries, other patient care providers (e.g., physicians, athletic trainers), laboratory staff, and support personnel (e.g., housekeeping staff) are also at risk. Needlestick injuries have been related to these unsafe health care practices:

- Recapping
- Transferring a body fluid between containers
- Failing to properly dispose of used needles in puncture-resistant sharps containers (details follow)[9,18-20]

Engineering controls are safety mechanisms built into needles and other sharps to prevent or reduce percutaneous exposure incidents. Needlestick injuries are prevented with safety needles, needle removers, retractable needles, needle shields or sheaths, needle-less IV kits, and blunt or valved ends on IV connectors (figure 2.2). HCPs using medical devices requiring manipulation or disassembly after use (e.g., needles attached to IV tubing, winged steel needles) are more likely to be injured than with a hypodermic needle or syringe. Here are some work practices that reduce the risk of needlestick injuries:

- Avoiding recapping, bending, breaking, or handing over used needles

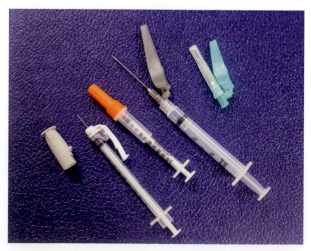

FIGURE 2.2 Safety-engineered needles and syringes.
Courtesy of Dr. Eric J. Fuchs, ATC, NRAEMT.

- Using safety features when available
- Using instruments (rather than fingers) to grasp needles, retract tissue, and load or unload needles and scalpels
- Giving verbal announcements when passing sharps
- Avoiding hand-to-hand passage of sharp instruments by using a basin or neutral zone
- Using round-tipped scalpel blades instead of pointed sharp-tipped blades
- Double gloving
- Placing used sharps in a puncture-resistant container (described next)[19,21]

Safe Handling of Potentially Contaminated Equipment or Surfaces

The prehospital HCP regularly uses medical devices with various levels of contamination with blood or body fluids. In the prehospital or ambulatory care setting, the CDC provides recommendations for safely handling contaminated medical devices in the *Guideline for Disinfection and Sterilization in Healthcare Facilities.*[22] While each setting has varying levels of use of medical devices and equipment, each facility should establish policies and procedures for containing, transporting, and handling devices.

All medical devices (table 2.5) originally labeled for use in the United States are subject to the U.S. Food and Drug Administration (FDA), which regulates manufacturing requirements and must meet strict cleaning, functionality, and sterility specifications prior to use. Medical devices are labeled by the manufacturer as either reusable

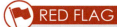

RED FLAG

If you experience a needlestick or sharps injury or are exposed to the blood or other body fluid of a patient during patient care, immediately follow these steps:[21]

1. Wash needlesticks and cuts with soap and water.
2. Flush splashes to the nose, mouth, or skin with water.
3. Irrigate eyes with clean water, saline, or sterile irrigants.
4. Report the incident to your supervisor.
5. Immediately seek medical treatment according to the exposure control plan.

or single use. All reusable medical devices must be cleaned and maintained according to the manufacturer's instructions to prevent patient-to-patient transmission of infectious agents. Single-use devices (SUDs) are labeled by the manufacturer for only a single use and do not have **reprocessing** instructions.

Contaminated objects and surfaces are possible routes to pass pathogens between patients and are associated with hospital-acquired infections. Smooth (nonporous) surfaces such as doorknobs can transmit bacteria and should be routinely cleaned. Safe environmental control practices include the following:

- Developing procedures for routine care, cleaning, and disinfection of environmental surfaces, especially frequently touched surfaces in patient-care areas

TABLE 2.5 **Classification of Medical Devices**

Classification	Description	Examples
Single-use device (SUD)	Noninvasive disposable device, intended for use on one patient during a single procedure; not intended to be reprocessed and used on another patient	Tourniquet cuffs, pulse oximeter sensors, sequential compression sleeves
Reusable medical device	Device that can be reused to diagnose and treat multiple patients	Surgical forceps, endoscopes, stethoscopes
Noncritical items	Objects that may come in contact with intact skin but not mucous membranes	Blood pressure cuffs, stethoscopes, manual ventilation bags, scissors, stethoscopes, CPR manikins
Semicritical items	Objects that contact mucous membranes or non-intact skin	Oropharyngeal or nasopharyngeal airways, oral or rectal thermometers
Critical items	Objects that enter a sterile body cavity, tissue, or vascular space	Surgical instruments; suture needles, scalpels, hemostats

Based on U.S. Food and Drug Administration (2005); U.S. Food and Drug Administration (2017).

- Handling textiles and laundry in a manner that prevents transfer of microorganisms to others and to the environment
- Using safe needles and other sharps practices (described previously)

Levels of Disinfection in Health Care Settings

Cleaning wounds and handling medical devices or equipment (table 2.6) require the use of chemical antimicrobials or **germicides** to prevent or control infection. **Antiseptics** are antimicrobial substances applied to living tissue to reduce the possibility of infection. Antiseptics are different from antibiotics that are transported through the lymphatic system to destroy bacteria within the body.[25] Disinfectants destroy microorganisms found on nonliving objects, but they do not kill bacterial spores, which requires **sterilization**. Some antibiotics are true germicides, capable of destroying bacteria (bacteriocidal), while others are bacteriostatic; they only prevent or inhibit bacterial growth. Antibacterials are antiseptics that have the proven ability to act against bacteria. Micro-

bicides destroy virus particles; they are called viricides or antivirals.[9]

Determining the level of disinfection or sterilization required for reusable medical devices and surfaces is based on the degree of risk for transmitting infections if the device is contaminated at the time of use. It is important to follow all product label instructions for cleaning and decontaminating surfaces or objects soiled with blood or body fluids. These instructions require the following:

- Personal protective equipment must be provided for and worn by the worker performing the task.
- All blood must be thoroughly removed before applying the disinfectant.
- Infectious waste disposal must be in accordance with federal, state, or local regulations.
- Disinfectant should be left on the surface for 30 seconds for HIV-1 and for 10 minutes for hepatitis B virus.[12]

Chemical germicides formulated as antiseptics, disinfectants, or sterilants (table 2.7) are regulated in the

TABLE 2.6 Products for Disinfecting and Sterilizing Reusable Medical Devices

Disinfection and sterilization products	Description
Autoclaves	Sterilization that eliminates, removes, kills, or deactivates all forms of life and other biological agents. Use steam-heated chamber under pressure until a time and temperature set point is reached.
Glutaraldehydes, such as • MetriCide • Pro Advantage • Protectop • Coecide	High-level chemical sterilant that kills all organisms except high levels of bacterial spores
Chemical germicides such as • Oxonia Active • Tek-Phene* • Ultra Clorox 6.15% Bleach	Intermediate-level disinfection which kills mycobacteria, most viruses, and bacteria
Chemical or hospital disinfectant, such as • 70% isopropyl alcohol • UltraCruz • Techspray • Isopropyl rubbing alcohol	Low-level disinfection which kills some viruses and bacteria
General decontamination cleansers, such as • Cavicide* • Sani-Cloth Plus Germicidal Disposable Cloth*	Cleaning contaminated objects or surfaces, which is general removal of debris such as dirt, food, feces, blood, saliva, and other body secretions
Skin antiseptics, such as • Betadine, povidone-iodine • iso-Betadine	Antimicrobial substances applied to skin to reduce possibility of infection

*Also effective against MRSA and VRE, according to the U.S. Environmental Protection Agency.[27]

Generic product names are in lower case; brand names are in upper case.

Based on U.S. Food and Drug Administration (2005); U.S. Food and Drug Administration (2017); World Health Organization (2016).

TABLE 2.7   **Common Disinfectants Used in Health Care Settings**

Classification	Description	Examples
Phenolic detergent germicides	Disinfectant for use on environmental surfaces of patient care tables, bed rails, laboratory surfaces, and noncritical medical devices	CiDecon LopHene STERIS Lph Se Pdi 160 Germicidal Disinfecting Wipes
Quaternary ammonium compounds	Used for environmental sanitation of noncritical surfaces, such as floors, furniture, and walls; can be used for disinfecting noncritical medical equipment	TexQ Disinfectant Microban Germicidal Cleaner Clorox Pro All-Purpose Disinfectant Cleaner
Chlorine disinfectant 5.25%-6.15% sodium hypochlorite	Broad spectrum of antimicrobial activity; widely used in health care facilities in a variety of settings	Household bleach 1:100 dilution used for spot-disinfection of countertops and floors 1:10 dilution for decontaminating blood spills
Hydrogen peroxide 3%	Active against a wide range of microorganisms; stable and effective disinfectant when used on inanimate surfaces	Hydrogen peroxide, 3% solution

Based on McDonnell and Russell (1999); Beam et al. (2016).

United States and must be registered before sale or distribution. The safety and effectiveness of each product must be disclosed on the label with the microbicidal activity, stability, and toxicity to animals and humans.

Potentially Hazardous, Contaminated Materials, or Biohazardous Materials Disposal

In the pre-hospital health care setting, biohazardous waste must be properly handled and disposed of as quickly as possible. **Biohazardous materials** are any solid or liquid waste that poses serious threat of transmitting infection to humans, including towels, gloves, and bandages. Separate containers or receptacles (figure 2.3) for the disposal

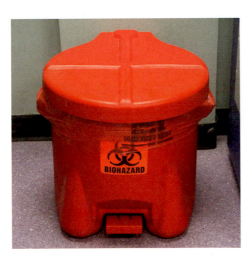

FIGURE 2.3   Biohazardous waste container with biohazard symbol.

of biohazardous materials must be available within the health care facility as well as in the medical bag. All volunteers and employees must have training and education for disposal of biohazardous waste (including **sharps**). This training must be provided on a regular, planned basis with evidence of the communication documented.[3,29,30]

Sharps Disposal

Sharps waste is a form of biomedical waste composed of used sharps, which includes any device or object used to puncture or lacerate the skin. Sharps waste must be carefully handled. Common medical materials treated as sharps waste include the following:

- Hypodermic needles
- Disposable scalpels and blades
- Contaminated glass and some plastics

Sharps waste is collected in a sharps container (figure 2.4), which is a hard plastic container used to safely dispose of hypodermic needles and other sharp medical instruments. HCPs must take extreme care in managing and disposing of sharps waste in the prehospital setting. Sharps waste must be safely handled until the hazardous materials can be properly disposed of. HCPs may use individual vials or a small, portable sharps container to dispose of sharps. Needles are dropped into the container through an opening in the top. A needle should never be pushed or forced into the container, because damage to the container or needlestick injuries may result. Sharps containers should not be filled above the indicated line, usually two-thirds full. The ideal sharps container is self-locking and sealable to prevent the sharps from easily

Recommendations for Cleaning and Disinfection or Sterilization of Medical Devices in Outpatient Settings

- Facilities should ensure that reusable medical devices (e.g., blood glucose meters and other point-of-care devices, surgical instruments) are cleaned and reprocessed appropriately prior to use on another patient.

- Reusable medical devices must be cleaned and reprocessed (disinfection or sterilization) and maintained according to the manufacturer's instructions. If the manufacturer does not provide such instructions, the device may not be suitable for multipatient use.

- Outsource responsibilities for reprocessing of medical devices to people with appropriate training.

- Maintain copies of the manufacturer's instructions for reprocessing of devices in use at the facility; post instructions at locations where reprocessing is performed.

- Annually conduct hands-on training on proper selection and use of PPE and recommended steps for reprocessing assigned devices should be provided upon hire (prior to being allowed to reprocess devices), and when new devices are introduced or policies/procedures change.

- HCPs should be required to demonstrate competency with reprocessing procedures (e.g., correct technique is observed by trainer) following each training.

- Assure HCPs have access to and wear appropriate PPE when handling and reprocessing contaminated medical devices.

Adapted from Occupational Safety and Health Administration, *Quick Reference Guide to the Bloodborne Pathogens Standard 2010*; www.osha.gov/SLTC/bloodbornepathogens/bloodborne_quickref.html.

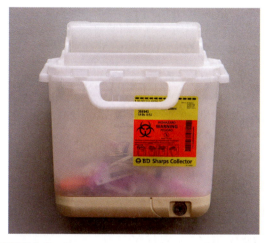

FIGURE 2.4 Sharps container for needles and other sharp instruments.

penetrating through the sides. Such units are designed so that the whole container can be disposed of with other biohazardous waste.[31]

Practice Respiratory Hygiene and Cough Etiquette

Respiratory hygiene and cough etiquette is an element of standard precautions that highlights the need for prompt implementation of infection prevention measures at the first point of encounter with the patient or in the AT facility. People with undiagnosed transmissible respiratory infections or anyone with signs of illness including cough, congestion, rhinorrhea, or increased production of respiratory secretions should practice respiratory hygiene. Cough etiquette is especially important for infection control measures in health care settings, such as emergency departments, physician's offices, and athletic training clinics.

The following precautions can help stop the spread of pathogens in the health care facility:

- Implement measures to contain respiratory secretions in patients and accompanying individuals who have signs and symptoms of a respiratory infection, beginning at the initial point of care and continuing throughout the patient encounter.

- Post signs at entrances with instructions to patients with symptoms of respiratory infection to inform HCPs of symptoms of a respiratory infection.

- Avoid touching objects after contaminating your hands.

- Avoid touching your face after touching contaminated objects.

- Cover your mouth and nose when coughing or sneezing,
- Use and dispose of tissues.
- If you don't have a tissue, cough or sneeze into your upper sleeve, not your hands.
- Wash your hands after coughing or sneezing.
- Perform hand hygiene after your hands have been in contact with respiratory secretions.
- Provide tissues and no-touch receptacles for disposal of tissues.
- Provide resources for performing hand hygiene in or near waiting areas.
- Offer masks to coughing patients and other symptomatic people upon entry to the facility, at a minimum during periods of increased respiratory infection activity in the community.
- Provide adequate personal space and encourage people with symptoms of respiratory infections to sit as far away from others as possible. If available, facilities may wish to place these patients in a separate area while waiting for care.
- Educate HCPs on the importance of infection prevention measures to contain respiratory secretions to prevent the spread of respiratory pathogens.[11]

Exposure Control Plans

Facilities with the potential for occupational exposure to blood or OPIM must develop an exposure control plan (ECP), which is a written plan (approved by experts or a legal department) to minimize potential exposure and procedures to follow in the event of exposure to blood or OPIM. The ECP applies to non–health care as well as health care settings, and it must be detailed and periodically updated. To meet minimum requirements of OSHA blood-borne pathogen standards, it is helpful to use a model document as a template to individualize the workplace ECP and tailor it to the specific requirements of the institution or organization. Elements required by the blood-borne pathogens standards should be included; minimally, the ECP should include the following:

- Policy for blood-borne pathogens
- Name and contact information of program administrator
- Determination of employee exposure
- Methods of implementation and control
- Employer or institutional requirements for hepatitis B vaccination and hepatitis B vaccine declination
- Administration of post-exposure evaluation and follow-up

- Procedures for evaluating the circumstances surrounding an exposure incident
- Employee training schedule
- Records of exposure incidents

Appendix A provides a model ECP.

The written plan must be accessible to all ATs, students, and staff either online or in a physical area available for review at all times. While preparing written plans, refer to OSHA blood-borne pathogens and hazard communication standards for specific compliance requirements.[12,30]

The ECP should describe the level of exposure for each job classification including tasks and procedures where occupational exposure exists. The procedures for evaluating the circumstances surrounding exposure incidents should be included. The ECP should also include a schedule of how other provisions of the standard are implemented, including methods of compliance, hepatitis B vaccination requirements, post-exposure evaluation and follow-up, communication of hazards to employees, and record keeping.

Legal Responsibility

Every AT should be aware that laws related to patient care exist at the federal and state levels and practice acts differ from state to state. When a state practice act or its associated rules and regulations specifically addresses clinical practice guidelines, such guidelines become the standard of care and subsequent legal expectation. ATs are responsible for practicing consistently with federal and state practice acts and with rules and regulations governing the practice of athletic training for the state in which they practice. A policy regarding who needs to know what information, and what is necessary to communicate, should be created with input from each stakeholder to clearly delineate appropriate and inappropriate sharing of information. The primary issues relating to acute and emergency care in the pre-hospital setting are as follows:

- Obtaining patient consent
- Maintaining patient confidentiality
- Reporting suspected abuse
- Documenting records and reports

Obtaining Patient Consent

Under most circumstances, consent is required from every conscious, mentally competent adult before care can be started. A person receiving care must give permission (consent) for treatment. If a person is alert, rational, and capable of making informed decisions, he has a legal right to refuse care even if he is ill or injured. A patient may also consent to some aspects of care and deny consent to others. If a patient refuses care, you cannot care for the patient; in fact, providing care may be grounds for criminal and civil action (see Refusal of Care or Against Medical Advice). A patient might agree to certain emergency medical care but not to other care. For example, a patient might agree to receive oxygen and transport but refuse insertion of an IV line. An injured person might agree to emergency care at home but refuse to be transported to a medical facility.[32]

HCPs need to be aware of these 3 types of consent:

1. Informed consent
2. Expressed consent
3. Implied consent

Informed Consent

Although ATs and other HCPs have the training and experience to make diagnoses and recommend treatment, it is accepted that the patient is most capable of deciding whether the proposed interventions are compatible with her value system and goals. Many emergency procedures, such as IV lines and blood drawing, are considered routine, and they are performed after general consent to treatment, agreed orally or in writing. Other more invasive procedures should be performed following a discussion with the patient regarding the procedure, purpose, risks, benefits, and alternatives to the proposed procedure or intervention.[33]

For treatment or transport of a minor, the law requires that a parent or legal guardian give consent. A child does not have the wisdom, maturity, or judgment to give valid consent; therefore, the law requires that a parent or legal guardian give consent for treatment or transport. In some states, depending on age and level of maturity, a minor can give valid consent to receive medical care. Obtain consent from a parent or legal guardian whenever possible; however, if a true emergency exists and the parent or legal guardian is not available, the consent to treat the minor is implied, just as with an adult. Similarly, appropriate medical care for the pediatric patient with an urgent or emergent condition should never be withheld or delayed because of problems obtaining parental consent.[32-34]

The legal basis for informed consent rests on the assumption that the patient has a right to determine what is to be done with his or her body. Informed consent is a fundamental right of patient autonomy in medical decision making. The process of informed consent requires the following:

- Disclosure of information to the patient before the patient agrees to the proposed intervention
- Voluntariness on the part of the patient to consent who is not under any influential pressures to receive the care[32-34]
- The type of care or intervention to be rendered
- The likely benefits and potential risks associated with the care or intervention
- All available options as possible alternatives to the proposed care or intervention[34]

Informed consent is valid if given orally; however, it may be difficult to prove. Having the patient sign a consent form does not eliminate the responsibility to fully inform the patient.[32] A succinct but legally defensible statement should be documented in the patient's record when consent is given. For example, "Patient has the capacity to understand. [Insert procedure] was discussed, and questions were answered. Patient chooses to [proceed/decline]."[35]

Expressed Consent

When a serious threat to life exists and the patient is unresponsive or otherwise unable to give consent, the law assumes that the patient would give consent to care and transport to the hospital. Expressed consent (or actual consent) is a type of informed consent that occurs when the patient does something, either by telling you or by taking some sort of action that demonstrates giving you permission to provide care. This may be done verbally, or by such actions such as rolling up a sleeve so that you can take his or her blood pressure or inspect an injury.[32] Most states have also adopted specific laws granting special privileges to HCPs authorizing them to perform certain medical procedures. Many states grant partial immunity to some HCPs, physicians, and nurses who give emergency instructions to HCP personnel via radio or other forms of communication.[32] The key principle to follow is that the HCP should able to affirmatively answer these 2 questions:

1. Would a reasonable patient expect a discussion of this?
2. Have I provided the patient with an understanding of what he would want to know?[35]

While documenting expressed consent will not obviate a lawsuit, it does allow for a discussion during deposition or court proceedings to explain what topics were discussed. It is optimal for the HCP to explain her experience with a procedure, as well as to ensure patients are informed of alternate treat-

---

🚩 **RED FLAG**

Be sure you know the legal age in your state as it relates to minors being able to give valid consent to receive medical care.

ment plans to avoid some of the pitfalls of informed consent.[35]

Implied Consent

When a person is unresponsive or otherwise unable to make a rational, informed decision about care, the law assumes that the patient would consent to care and transport to a medical facility. Implied consent is necessary to perform a procedure in situations that do not allow time to obtain informed consent or the patient is incapable of giving it. State laws support the right of a HCP in an emergency to act without the expressed consent of the patient, relying instead on implied consent (If the patient could give consent, they would likely do so). Implied consent applies in these conditions:

1. If the patient is unable to communicate his wishes
2. If the situation demands immediate action

In this case, the HCP should assume that the patient would want the most appropriate medical treatment, and she would assume risks of necessary procedures. Whenever possible, it is preferable to communicate with family members for consent; if time is limited, the HCP should proceed with treatment.[35]

Good Samaritan Laws

When a HCP is off duty, providing care in an emergency situation presents a variety of legal or moral obligations to act. In most U.S. states, no law exists that requires a person to assist another in an emergency while off duty. However, a HCP may be held liable if there is a *special relationship*. For example, if someone causes an accident, that person then has the duty to rescue, if able. That person must at least call 9-1-1 (or other appropriate emergency number) to obtain help.[36] U.S. state laws enacted to protect HCPs and other emergency personnel from being sued because of providing help to a victim during an emergency situation are **Good Samaritan laws** or volunteer protection laws. Good Samaritan laws are based on the principle that a HCP who reasonably helps someone should not be liable for errors or omissions while providing good-faith emergency care.[6] These statutes provide immunity from liability in emergency situations where no remuneration (compensation) exists and the actions of the HCP are not grossly negligent. For example, an off-duty AT that stops to help someone on the side of the road is provided immunity from liability as long as reasonable care is provided using the resources or equipment available at the time. The HCP cannot be sued for injuries to the patient during the incident.[37] In order for the Good Samaritan law to be applicable, these 5 elements must be satisfied:

1. The incident must be an emergency.
2. The act of rendering care must be voluntary.
3. The victim receiving care must be accepting of it (expressed or implied consent).
4. The care provided must be a good faith effort to help.
5. The provider must not receive reimbursement for any of the care provided.

Furthermore, to avoid litigation, the care rendered must not be considered grossly negligent.[36]

However, Good Samaritan laws do not extend to HCPs who provide medical care or treatment in the course of their employment or if remuneration is expected. While most state Good Samaritan laws protect all people who give assistance in an emergency, some state Good Samaritan laws protect only certain people, such as trained emergency personnel.[38] All HCPs should know the Good Samaritan law where they are practicing and be mindful of how the law applies in an emergency situation, including the following:

- The HCP who volunteers to provide emergency assistance should limit care to those functions that are within the scope of practice, education, training, and experience. For example, if the AT has not been adequately trained to perform intubation, it is not advisable to try to administer one at the scene of an accident. Rather, maintaining an airway and instituting CPR, if needed, would be a better course of action.

- Once the AT or other HCP begins rescue efforts, those efforts must be continued until the provider becomes exhausted (and therefore unable to continue) or until other qualified personnel (e.g., paramedics, physicians) assume the care of the patient.

- ATs and other rescuers should never take compensation for the care they render at the scene of an emergency. Good Samaritan laws were enacted to protect those who voluntarily assist. Accepting compensation affects the voluntariness of the care and may result in loss of protection. Rather than a victim having to establish that the care given was grossly negligent (intentionally harmful, willful, and wanton), he or she may have a lower burden of just proving the actions were unreasonable under the circumstances.[37]

Mandated Reporting

In some states, mandatory reporting laws require that people in health care professions report suspected child abuse or neglect to a proper authority, such as a law enforcement agency or child protective services. In other states, the mandatory reporting laws require that any person who suspects child abuse or neglect report any such instance. ATs working in the school setting are considered mandated reporters and must report suspected child abuse or neglect. Similarly, ATs providing care to adults must report suspected or witnessed abuse of victims of sexual (or other) misconduct by anyone in the organization including coaches and physicians. Mandated reporters are encouraged to report their suspicions immediately and not to investigate or wait for absolute proof, which can lead to further harm directed at the suspected victim. Mandatory reporters are required to report the facts and circumstances that led them to suspect that a person has been abused or mistreated. The reporter does not have the burden of providing proof that abuse or mistreatment has occurred.[55]

According to the US Department of Health and Human Services, institutional reporting is required for the HCP to be a mandated reporter while working (or volunteering, such as a student) as a staff member of an institution, such as a school or hospital, at the time he or she gains the knowledge that leads him or her to suspect that abuse or neglect has occurred. Many institutions have internal policies and procedures for handling reports of abuse, and these usually require the person who suspects abuse to notify the head of the institution that abuse has been discovered or is suspected and needs to be reported to child protective services or other appropriate authorities. Regardless of any policies within the organization, the mandatory reporter is not relieved of his or her responsibility to report to the appropriate authority first and then notify the institution that a report has been made. An employer is expressly prohibited from taking any action to prevent or discourage an employee from making a report.[55]

Maintaining Patient Confidentiality

Ensuring that a person's health information is properly protected is a major responsibility of all HCPs. It is a challenge to provide confidentially while allowing the flow of health information needed to provide and promote high-quality health care. U.S. federal laws and rules allow important uses of information while protecting the privacy of patients or clients. **Protected health information (PHI)** is individually identifiable health information as protected by federal law. Most PHI is protected and should not be released without the patient's permission. These regulations apply to all forms of communication, written and verbal. To ensure protection of the patient's right to confidentiality, information cannot be provided to anyone other than those directly involved in the care of the patient. It is essential that all personnel and staff are aware of all policies and procedures relating to patient confidentiality.[39]

HIPAA Statutes, HITECH, and the Privacy and Security Rules

All confidential health information is protected by the U.S. **Health Insurance Portability and Accountability Act (HIPAA)** of 1996. This federal law established mandatory patient privacy rules and regulations to safeguard patient confidentiality. The act provides guidance on the types of information that are protected, the responsibility of health care providers regarding that protection, and penalties for breaching that protection. The **Privacy Rule** applies to any health care provider who transmits health information in electronic form. Hospitals, clinics, other outpatient services, and HCPs are considered **covered entities**.[40] The Privacy Rule (2000) establishes national standards for the protection of certain health information, while the Security Rule (2003) establishes a national set of security standards for protecting certain health information that is held or transferred in electronic form. The Security Rule operationalizes the protections contained in the Privacy Rule by addressing the safeguards that covered entities must put in place to secure individuals' electronic protected health information (ePHI).[39] The HIPAA Privacy Rule requires covered entities to develop and distribute a **notice of privacy practices** that provides a clear, user-friendly explanation of people's rights with respect to their personal health information and the privacy practices of health care providers. A model notice of privacy practices should be provided by the employer or developed for the AT setting following models found online.[41]

The Health Information Technology for Economic and Clinical Health (HITECH) Act, which was enacted as part of the American Recovery and Reinvestment Act of 2009, significantly increases the penalty for violations of the HIPAA rules and encourages prompt corrective action.[42] This act also provides incentives related to creation of a national health care infrastructure and adoption of **electronic health record (EHR)** systems among providers. Because this legislation anticipates a massive expansion in the exchange of ePHI, the HITECH Act also widens the scope of privacy and security protections available under HIPAA; it increases the potential legal liability for noncompliance; and it provides for more enforcement. The primary aspects of HITECH related to HCPs in the prehospital setting include the following:

- *Enforcement*—Mandatory penalties are imposed for **willful neglect**.
- *Notification of breach*—Unauthorized use and disclosure of **unsecured PHI** (unencrypted PHI). The covered entity must provide notification of the breach to affected people.[43]
- *Electronic health record access*—Provides people with a right to obtain their PHI in an electronic

format (ePHI). A person can also designate that a third party be the recipient of the ePHI.

- *Business associates and business associate agreements*—Contractual agreements are required of business associates who are required to comply with the safeguards contained in the HIPAA Security Rule.[44]

Other statutes protect all individually identifiable health information that is created, received, maintained, or transmitted in electronic form. Although many AT clinics in schools, universities, and other non-traditional settings may not be considered a covered entity, health care providers in these settings should follow all privacy laws.

Confidentiality Policies

Although many AT clinics may not be considered covered entities, these settings may still be required to follow other federal statutes or institutional requirements. Specifically relating to school is the **Family Educational Rights and Privacy Act (FERPA)**. Often confusion exists on the part of school administrators, HCPs, and others as to how these laws apply to records maintained on students. FERPA protects the privacy of student education records and gives parents certain rights to their children's education records until they reach 18 years of age. Certain disclosures are allowed without consent or authorization under both FERPA and HIPAA laws, especially those related to health and safety emergency situations.[45] An AT facility housed in a school or other institution must educate all personnel about record storage and managing confidential patient information (e.g., FERPA and HIPAA). A clear policy must be documented and communicated to all staff and students about record storage and managing of confidential patient information. It should include the following:

- Evidence of the communication of relevant or applicable laws (e.g., HIPAA, FERPA, HITECH) or notice of privacy practices is documented.
- All interactions between patients and ATs or other health care providers are documented in the health records of each patient and securely maintained.
- The facility has a locked file cabinet for all patient medical or health files.
- Electronic and paper copies of health information are protected and accessible or transferred only to authorized people (i.e., FERPA, HIPAA, HITECH).
- A physical space exists for private conversations with patients and their parents.
- A private place exists for conducting evaluation or treatments when necessary.

- Communication occurs with employees about their responsibility for ensuring the confidentiality of health care information.[3]

Protecting Patient Information

Any communication between the AT and the patient is considered confidential and generally cannot be disclosed without written permission from the patient (or parent, if patient is a minor). Confidential information includes the patient history, assessment findings, and treatment provided. Each school, facility, institution, or clinic must have and enforce rules and regulations for managing sensitive information, including the documentation, storage, and dissemination of medical records, as well as the use of **electronic medical records (EMRs)**.[40] Examples of sensitive information include the following:

- Pre-participation exams
- AT medical records
- Physician visits and follow-ups
- Diagnostic reports
- Phone calls, emails, and text messages

It is important for AT facilities to document patient care and the information must be properly stored and secured (including EMRs). Having confidential information that is not properly secured puts the facility at risk of potential lawsuits in the event that data are stolen.[3]

Documenting Records and Reports

The purpose of complete and accurate patient record documentation is to facilitate patient care and continuity of care. Records and reports provide a means of communication between HCPs about medical status, treatment, planning, and delivery of care. Standards of competence require that the AT be familiar with **health informatics** in the administration and delivery of patient care. ATs and other HCPs use EMRs to search, retrieve, and use information derived from online databases and internal databases for clinical decision support. Patient care must be documented using a legally compliant method (digital or paper) that maintains patient data privacy, protection, and security. Whenever possible, medical classification systems (including International Classification of Diseases; ICD codes) and terminology (including Current Procedural Terminology; CPT) should be used. Advantages of using an EMR include communicating and managing health care–related information, mitigating errors, and supporting clinical decision making.[46]

Regardless of institutional or organizational requirements, it is essential to document and save a complete and accurate record of all incidents that require acute or emergency care. Most institutions require submitting a written report to supervisors any time an ambulance is summoned or a patient is transferred to the emergency department. Medicolegal experts consider a complete and accurate record of any emergency trauma or medical incident as an important safeguard against legal action. Absence or a substantially incomplete record may require remembering the events, exam findings, actions, and interventions during a legal case. Should a legal case arise, the person who completed the report is usually the person who will be summoned to provide testimony with the written record as evidence. Providing testimony should not be based on memory or an inadequate report. The written report reflects that a professional image and a concise, well-written document—including correct spelling and grammar—will reflect good patient care.[32]

It is essential to accurately and thoroughly compile and maintain reports and records of all events and patients receiving care. Having a comprehensive system of documenting patient care reports also helps the HCP evaluate health care services provided over time. Additionally, medical records or reports are an integral part of **continuous quality improvement** efforts.[32]

Patient Care Report

The **patient care report (PCR)** or **prehospital care report** is the legal document used to record all aspects of care provided to the patient, from initial assessment to arrival at the hospital. The report is used as a record of events, actions, and interventions provided to the patient as well as documenting transfer of care to the next-level HCP. All information collected during patient care becomes part of the patient's medical record.[32] Gathering patient information begins upon approaching the patient and continues during assessment, treatment, and transfer to the hospital. The PCR facilitates efficient continuity of patient care by describing the nature of the patient's injuries or illness at the scene and the treatment provided. Although the report might not immediately be used at the hospital, the information will be an important part of the patient's overall health care record. The report serves the following 6 functions:

1. Continuity of care
2. Legal documentation
3. Education
4. Administrative information
5. Essential research record
6. Chart review by clinician for evaluation and continuous quality improvement[32]

The narrative of the PCR is an important section where the facts related to the care provided to the patient are described. This section must be written objectively and with concise, clear language. It is important to document all positive findings as well as pertinent negative findings. Pertinent negative findings generally warrant no medical care or intervention but show evidence of the thoroughness of the examination and history of the complaint.[32] Abbreviations and acronyms are common in medical documentation. It is vital that people minimize use of abbreviations; and when they do use them, they should do so in a consistent manner to prevent errors and miscommunication.[34] The report should contain only approved abbreviations (see table 2.8). Unfamiliar or seldom-used abbreviations can confuse other HCPs and potentially lead to an adverse outcome.[47]

In the prehospital setting, common methods of documentation include the following:[32,47]

- *SOAPM:* Subjective objective assessment plan, and medical necessity (figure 2.5)
- *ICHART:* Incident, chief complaint, history, assessment, treatment (Rx), transportation, and (optional) exceptions (table 2.9)

Reporting Errors

When documenting patient care, accuracy, objectivity, and completeness are essential. It is important to record observations, actions, and interventions while keeping opinions, assumptions, and adjectives to a minimum. Likewise, when documenting the chief complaint, use the patient's exact words in quotation marks. All data relating to all aspects of patient care and the treatment process should be included. Each PCR should be signed with the HCP's first name or initial, last name, and professional status (AT). When documentation errors are made, correct the error promptly. For inaccuracies, errors, or mistakes, draw a single line through the incorrect information and write "mistaken entry" next to it. Add the correct information and an explanation on the next available line, then initial the changes. Never erase or scribble over an erroneous entry, which could appear like an improper cover-up if the case were involved in a lawsuit.[47]

Refusal of Care or Against Medical Advice

A responsible HCP communicates effectively and truthfully with patients and other people involved in the patient's treatment or care.[3] Occasionally, a patient may want to disregard the HCP's medical decision or terminate treatment of the illness or injury. **Against medical advice (AMA)** occurs when a patient refuses treatment or transportation, or leaves a health care facility against the recommendation of a HCP. A clear conversation with the patient about these questions, followed by clear documentation of the answers in the medical record, ensures the best care possible for the patient and may reduce liability.[50] A formal decisional capacity evaluation includes the following:

TABLE 2.8 Common Medical Abbreviations Used in Prehospital Care Reports

$\bar{p}$	After	IV	Intravenous
$\bar{a}$	Before	JVD	Jugular venous distention
Δ	Change	KVO	Keep vein open
↓	Decrease	LOC	Loss of consciousness
$\bar{q}$	Every	LS	Lung sounds
↑	Increase	MI	Myocardial infraction
$\bar{c}$	With	MOE	Moves all extremities
$\bar{s}$	Without	MOI	Mechanism of injury
AAA	Abdominal aortic aneurysm	N/G	Nasogastric
ABC	Airway, breathing, circulation	N/V	Nausea/vomiting
ABD	Abdomen	N/V/D	Nausea/vomiting/diarrhea
ACLS	Advanced cardiac life support	NAD	No apparent distress
ALOC	Altered level of consciousness	NG	Nasogastric
ALS	Advanced life support	NPO	Nothing by mouth
AMA	Against medical advice	OD	Overdose
AMI	Acute myocardial infarction	OPA	Oropharyngeal airway
APAP	Acetaminophen	P	Pulse
ASA	Aspirin	PC	After eating
AVPU	Alert, verbal, painful, unresponsive	PERL	Pupils equal and reactive
BID	Twice a day	PID	Pelvic inflammatory disease
BP	Blood pressure	PMH	Previous medical history
BS	Blood sugar	PO	By mouth
c/c	Chief complaint	PRN	Whenever necessary
C/O or c/o	Complains of	Pt	Patient
CA	Cancer	PTA	Prior to arrival
CAD	Coronary artery disease	QID	4 times/day
Cx	Chief complaint	QXh	Every X hours
CHF	Congestive heart failure	R/O	Rule out
Clr	Clear	resp	Respirations
CNS	Central nervous system	Rx	Treatment/prescription
CP	Chest pain	s/s	Signs/Symptoms
CSF	Cerebral spinal fluid	SL	Sublingual
CSM	Circulation/Sensory/Motor	SNT	Soft, nontender
CVA	Cerebral vascular accident	SOB	Short of breath
cx	Chest	SPO2	Pulse oximeter oxygen saturation
D/C	Discontinue	Sx	Symptoms
Dx	Diagnosis	Sz	Seizure
EMS	Emergency medical system	TIA	Transient ischemic attack
ETOH	Alcohol	TID	3 times/day
FROM	Full range of motion	TKO	To keep open
fx	Fracture	U/A	Upon arrival
HA	Headache	UTI	Urinary tract infection
HTN	Hypertension	V-Fib	Ventricular fibrillation
Hx	History	V-Tac	Ventricular tachycardia
IM	Intramuscular	WNL	Within normal limits
IO	Intraosseous		

Subjective
- Patient's age, gender, and chief complaint
- Events that transpired prior to EMS arrival
- History of present illness (e.g., HPI, SAMPLE, or OPQRST; see chapter 4)

Objective
- How the patient was found in terms of location and position
- Level of consciousness (LOC or AVPU; see chapter 4)
- Vital signs

Assessment
- Overall impression of the patient

Plan
- List of treatment in chronological order
- Important findings and results of physical exam
- Where the patient was transported and if any changes were noted en route

Medical Necessity (Optional)
- Why, when, and where the patient was transported by ambulance[48]

FIGURE 2.5 SOAPM method of documenting patient care.

TABLE 2.9 **ICHART Technique Used for Patient Care Documentation**

Incident	Brief details of the incident including location and reason for assistance Time on site/venue and location of patient How the patient was found
Chief complaint (CC or Cx)	Patient's age, gender and chief complaint Documentation of information from family members, friends, or bystanders using quotation marks Reason AT was called
History (Hx)	Brief history of events leading to incident Mechanism of injury (MOI) or nature of illness (NOI) Symptom assessment
Assessment (Ax)	Level of consciousness (LOC) and pain assessment Important findings and results of physical exam Vital signs
Treatment (Rx)	List of treatment in chronological order
Transportation (Tx)	If the patient was transported by ambulance, when, where the patient was transported, and if any changes were noted en route

See chapter 4 for additional assessment details. See table 2.8 for common medical abbreviations used in writing reports.
Based on Pollack and Beck (2012); EMTResource.com (2014).

- Does the patient understand and appreciate the diagnosis, prognosis, likelihood of risks and benefits, and treatment alternatives?
- Can the patient make and communicate a choice?
- Is the patient being coerced by an authority figure such as a teammate, coach, or parent?
- Can the patient articulate a reason for the refusal that is consistent with her values?[51]

If it is determined that the patient has capacity, is adequately informed of the risks, and still insists on refusing treatment against medical advice, the AT should document the discussion or action. Proper documentation

This is to certify that I, _____, a patient at _____ (name of health care facility), am refusing at my own insistence and without the authority of and against the advice of my _____ (athletic trainer/physician's name), request to _____ (terminate treatment, return to participation) against medical advice.

The medical risks and benefits have been explained to me by a member of the medical staff, and I understand those risks and benefits.

I hereby release the health care facility, its administration, personnel, and my athletic trainers/physician from any responsibility for all consequences, which may result by my leaving under these circumstances.

Medical Risks

The risks have been explained to the patient, including the following:

_____ Death

_____ Worsening illness, chronic pain

_____ Additional pain and/or suffering

_____ Permanent disability/disfigurement

Other: _____

_____

_____

Medical Benefits

_____ History/physical examination, further additional testing and treatment as indicated

_____ Radiological imaging, such as the following:

_____ CAT scan

_____ X-rays

_____ Ultrasound (sonogram)

_____ Laboratory testing

_____ Potential admission and/or follow-up

_____ Medications as indicated for infection, pain, blood pressure, etc.

Other: _____

_____

_____

Please return at any time for further testing or treatment.

Patient signature _____ Date _____

Physician signature _____ Date _____

Witness _____ Date _____

FIGURE 2.6 Sample AMA form. This form should be approved by risk management or legal counsel before use.[50,54]

must be recorded in the patient's chart and should include these specific elements:[52,53]

- Formalities:
  - Signature of HCP and patient
  - Date and time of AMA discussion and signature on form
- Personalized to patient:
  - Medical condition(s)
  - Specific risks and benefits of proposed treatment and alternatives
  - Specific consequences of leaving AMA
- Report of results of mental capacity assessment:
  - Patient's mental status and capacity to make medical decisions
  - Patient understanding of proposed treatment
  - Patient understanding of consequences of refusing treatment
  - Patient's reason for refusal of admission or treatment ("The patient has decided to leave against medical advice because _____.")
- Lists of follow-up instructions:
  - Self-care and when to seek medical attention
  - Arrangements with relatives ("Follow-up has been discussed and arranged with Dr. _____.").

Although AMA forms and procedures do not completely insulate emergency personnel from liability in a medical malpractice action, properly executed AMA forms (figure 2.6) and procedures can confer important legal protections. Any form used for AMA should be reviewed and approved by risk management or legal counsel.

Summary

ATs, team physicians, and other HCPs must be familiar with strategies for prevention and managing risk relating to patient care in the prehospital setting. All facilities should be compliant with relevant health care accreditation requirements or follow the BOC Facilities Principles. These principles provide accountability to patients, parents, administrators, and stakeholders that supplies, equipment, and facilities are high quality and in good working order. Additionally, HCPs should be current on vaccinations and practice standard precautions necessary to prevent the spread of infection—both health care–associated and nosocomial infections. These practices and responsible use of antibiotics will prevent drug-resistant infections in the health care setting. All personnel should undergo training on standard precautions and other OSHA requirements and should have access to the ECP for each facility. Additionally, state and federal regulations should be followed to ensure that protected health information is handled in compliance with applicable laws such as HIPAA and FERPA. Institutions should have their policies and procedures reviewed by legal counsel or risk management officers to ensure legal compliance. Protected health information should be disclosed only on the advice of legal counsel, by written authorization, or for a public health risk. Every attempt should be made to limit information to only what is necessary and eliminate identifying documentation.

 Go to the web study guide to complete the case studies for this chapter.

CHAPTER 3

Planning for Emergencies

OBJECTIVES

After reading this chapter, you will be able to do the following:

- Recognize the illnesses and injuries most commonly associated with medical emergencies.

- Develop, coordinate, and implement an emergency action plan (EAP).

- Identify and obtain the emergency equipment and supplies that should be available during an emergency.

- Justify approval of an EAP from institutional authority and coordinate with emergency medical services (EMS).

- Create a plan for training personnel, practicing, and revising the EAP at least annually.

- Implement best practices in communication with other health care providers.

- Summarize the essential components of a post-catastrophic injury or critical incident plan.

Sports-related injuries can have a substantial detrimental effect on the long-term health of athletes and physically active people. Each year in the United States, more than 2.6 million youth sport participants are treated in an emergency department (ED) for sport- and recreation-related injuries.[1] Although most sport-related injuries are considered minor emergencies, life-threatening illnesses or injuries do occur with relative frequency. Severe injuries are generally considered third-degree joint or tissue damage in which gross instability and complete tear or rupture of the involved tissues occurs. Medically disqualifying (MDQ) injuries are severe enough to be season or career ending. These severe injuries are concerning because they often result in time lost from sport participation and school, social costs, and economic costs of medical care.[2,3] Health care providers (HCPs) must be prepared to manage life- and limb-threatening emergencies associated with athletics and physical activity, such as the following:

- Abdominal injuries
- Anaphylaxis (severe allergic reaction)
- Bleeding (severe)
- Blunt chest trauma or severe breathing problems
- Burns
- Catastrophic brain injuries
- Cervical spine injuries
- Chest pain and sudden cardiac arrest
- Choking
- Concussion and other head injuries
- Diabetes and hypoglycemia
- Exercise-induced asthma

- Exertional heatstroke and other environmental injuries and illnesses
- Exertional hyponatremia
- Exertional sickling
- Extremity fractures resulting in compartment syndrome
- Fractured femur or pelvis
- Open fractures
- Poisoning or drug overdose
- Stroke
- Seizure
- Shock

When proper steps are taken to prevent, recognize, and treat major medical conditions that athletes and other physically active people may experience, nearly all deaths and serious injuries that have long-term complications can be avoided. Particular concern is for school-based athletics, especially during practices and competitions.[4] Boden[5] reported that 4 conditions account for more than 90% of **catastrophic injuries** in high school athletes. These 4 conditions—cardiac injuries, exertional heatstroke, head and spinal cord injuries, and exertional sickling—as well as other medical conditions (e.g., asthma, lightning injuries, hyponatremia) can have serious consequences. Being prepared for the 4 most common catastrophic conditions provides an appropriate starting point for implementing emergency guidelines. Each of these and other serious injuries and illnesses is addressed in future chapters. This chapter describes the personnel and infrastructure planning that is necessary in any setting and can be particularly challenging in a school-based athletic setting. These factors must be considered as the athletic trainer (AT) prepares for EAPs, coaching education, safety of strength and conditioning sessions, and access to on-site AT services. When sound policies are in place, all athletes will have the best opportunity for proper prevention, recognition, and treatment of the myriad medical conditions they may experience.[4,6]

Epidemiology of Medical Emergencies in Sports

Medical emergencies occur relatively frequently in sports, and HCPs must be prepared to implement and manage an emergency response. For example, in U.S. high schools, ATs reported MDQ injuries using the High School Reporting Information Online (RIO) system.[2] In a 5-year period, ATs reported 59,862 total injuries including 3,599 MDQ injuries (6.0% of all injuries). Most MDQ injuries (60.4%) occurred in competition, and 39.5% occurred in practice. Football had the highest MDQ injury rate of 26.5 per 100,000 athlete exposures (AEs) and the highest competition rate of MDQ injuries (93.1 per 100,000 competition AEs). The next-highest MDQ injury rates were in gymnastics (18.6 per 100,000 AEs) and wrestling (17.9 per 100,000 AEs). MDQ injuries varied by sport, sex, and type of athletic activity and occurred most frequently as a result of player–player contact.

The National Collegiate Athletic Association (NCAA) monitors injuries among college student-athletes at member schools.[7] In all NCAA sports during a 5-year period, an estimated 1,053,370 injuries occurred, representing an average of 210,674 total injuries per year; among them, 134,498 (63.8%) occurred during practices. An annual average of 46,231 (21.9%) were time-loss injuries that required at least 7 days before the athlete could return to full participation; 18.1% required surgery; and 4.1% required emergency transport.[7] Of practice-related injuries requiring emergency transport, 29.4% were sprains and strains; however, during competition, the largest proportions of injuries requiring emergency transport were fractures, stress fractures, dislocations, subluxations (25.8%), and concussions (22.0%). Football teams were estimated to have the highest competition injury rate (39.9 injuries per 1,000 AEs), and the third-highest overall injury rate (9.2 per 1,000 AEs) after men's wrestling (13.1) and women's gymnastics (10.4). Overall, football accounted for the largest proportions of all time-loss injuries (26.2%), surgery (40.2%), and emergency transport (31.9%).[7]

Similarly, documentation of injuries to collegiate athletes at a Canadian university over a 4-year period[3] revealed that men sustained 1,155 injuries, with 13.3% of them being severe; while women sustained 502 injuries, 17.7% of which were severe.[3] Although men generally incur more injuries, women tend to have a significantly higher proportion of severe injuries. Furthermore, women reported a significantly higher proportion of concussions.[3]

Emergency Planning in Sports

These findings in collegiate and secondary school sports emphasize the need for development, implementation, and evaluation of emergency planning and providing medical services for high-risk sports. Sport health professionals, school nurses, and primary care physicians who care for the physically active must ensure that all athletic programs are in compliance with national guidelines for emergency preparedness. The AT must set expectations and communicate levels of medical services provided based on level of risk for each sport. Further, epidemiological data should be used to determine the presence of ATs during specific sporting events and at different venues. Emergency planning is essential for preparedness to respond to a variety of incidents defined as follows:

- *Emergencies* are unplanned or imminent events that affect or threaten the health, safety, or welfare of people and require a planned and coordinated response.
- *Catastrophic injuries* result in severe functional disability, surgery, medical disqualification, and possibly sudden death.
- *Critical incidents* are unexpected traumatic events involving personal or professional threat that evokes extreme stress, fear, or injury.
- *Traumatic events* are incidents people experience, witness, or are confronted by and that involve actual, threatened, or perceived death or serious injury or threat to their own or others' physical and emotional integrity.

Emergencies, catastrophic injuries, and **critical incidents** do occur in sports, and sport health professionals must be prepared to prevent, recognize, and manage these medical emergencies and traumatic injuries[8] when they occur. Proper planning and management of these events is essential to reduce the immediate physical and emotional trauma, economic costs, and the potential risk of long-term sequelae.[2] Emergency preparedness in athletics involves the following:

- Planning for medical services
- Identifying life- or limb-threatening injuries and illnesses
- Providing for the safety of the patient
- Limiting further injury by proper management
- Providing medical care at the site of practice or competition
- Transferring care to the next HCP

Athletic organizations have a duty to develop an emergency plan that can be implemented immediately when necessary and to provide appropriate standards of health care to all sports participants.[9] An **emergency action plan (EAP)** is a written document that follows guidelines or standards of a professional or federal organization. For example, the Occupational Safety and Health Administration (OSHA) provides standards for safety in the workplace; similarly, an EAP provides **protocols** and procedures to follow in the event of a sport-related emergency in a school, field, arena, stadium, or other venue. In general, the purpose of an EAP is to facilitate and organize actions during emergencies of all kinds. A well-developed plan must include proper training so that all medical and other staff or personnel understand their roles and responsibilities within the plan. On the other hand, a poorly prepared plan is more likely to lead to a disorganized emergency response, resulting in confusion, injury, and possibly death.[10] Comprehensive emergency planning must be in place for all venues to ensure an efficient and structured response to an emergency. Core elements of a comprehensive written EAP include the following:[8,10-12]

- All medical personnel or other staff involved in the planning process
- Specifications about what each staff member should do during an emergency
- Proper training of likely responders for emergencies
- Providing access to early defibrillation through on-site automated external defibrillator (AED)
- Establishing an effective and efficient communication system
- Practicing and reviewing the response plan with potential first responders at least annually

An effective emergency response requires development, implementation, and coordination of a planned and

Potential Emergencies and Critical Incidents

- Bomb threat
- Campus violence (e.g., armed intruder, active shooter, hostage)
- Earthquake
- Evacuation
- Extreme weather (e.g., heat, cold, lightning)
- Fire (inside or outside)
- Flood
- **Hazardous material (HAZMAT)**/waste spill
- Infectious disease (e.g., pandemic influenza)
- Shelter in place
- Utility failure (e.g., power, water)

practiced response, risk reduction, training, and equipment.[13] The focus should not be only possible trauma or medical emergencies; the entire health care team may be called to respond to other emergency situations involving terrorism, natural disasters, or another catastrophe. While local police and fire rescue teams are generally responsible for management and investigation of many catastrophic events, often the AT is the first HCP on the scene. For example, the medical staff for the Boston Marathon is one of the most comprehensive medical teams in the world. Coordinating the medical care for a race of this scope—more than 27,000 runners—is a massive undertaking and includes more than 130 ATs, AT students, nurses, emergency medical technicians (EMTs), and physicians. The medical team coordinates with hospitals along the route to orient them on common running injuries and cold-water immersion techniques, and it includes ambulance services and fire departments for every town along the route. This level of preparation and coordination prepared the medical team for the 2013 Boston Marathon bombings.[14] ATs and physicians were the first on the scene and were immediately available to respond to blast trauma, fractures, and amputations. Although these injuries are not common and most practitioners have not been specifically trained in treating these injuries, the AT skills learned and practiced can be translated to a broad range of trauma or medical conditions.

It is essential to collaborate with responsible people likely to be available during an emergency, such as AT students, coaches, managers, or other staff. Similarly, local emergency service personnel must be involved in the development and implementation process. As appropriate, include responsible, trained personnel that can supervise and coordinate emergency response activities. All people with a role in the EAP must understand how their responsibilities relate to others in the plan. Practicing the EAP annually or when new personnel are introduced to the team is essential in order for all involved to know their role and responsibility as well as those of others.

An EAP is useful for ensuring a safe and successful response only when content is current, accurate, and clear; and all medical personnel and other staff are sufficiently educated and trained before an actual emergency. Successful development and implementation of an EAP should follow the steps shown in figure 3.1.[10,15]

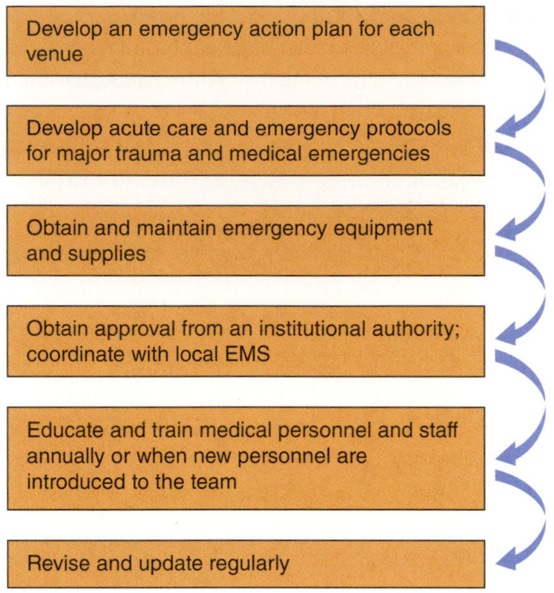

Developing an Emergency Action Plan for Each Venue

Emergency situations or life-threatening conditions can arise at any time during athletic events. Therefore, expeditious action is necessary to provide the best possible care to participants. Organizations and institutions have a duty to develop an EAP that can be implemented

FIGURE 3.1 Steps for successful development and implementation of an EAP.

immediately when necessary and to provide appropriate standards of health care to all sports participants.[9] Any organization or institution sponsoring athletic activities or events must develop and implement a written EAP that is venue specific and is written, posted, and practiced by all who have responsibility for the acute management of athletes' injuries and illnesses.

A well-planned emergency response requires much more than simply drafting an EAP. Although all safety precautions have been followed, emergencies can still occur. It is useful to identify conditions or situations that may place athletes, students, faculty, staff, or event attendees at risk for developing a life-threatening condition, then train and equip personnel to provide the appropriate response for those conditions.[13] The medical personnel and staff must be prepared for a variety of emergency scenarios. Before drafting the EAP, think of the worst-case scenario for each venue. Imagine how an emergency response would unfold, including EMS using a stretcher and an ambulance arriving. Consider people's professional positions and roles as well as specific or necessary skills. Ask yourself the following questions:

- Who is likely to be available to help in an emergency situation? Is this person responsible, able to follow directions, and willing to train for and practice an emergency response? What skills does each person have?

- What is the best way for an ambulance to enter the campus/stadium/arena? Are the gates locked? Who has keys? Is this person always available?

- How would EMS bring a **gurney** to the field/court/gymnasium/pool? Do they have to use stairs? Does the doorway have double doors? What other obstacles might EMS encounter on the way to the patient?

- What is the role of campus security or police? What is the role of the physician or medical director? When are they available on-site?

- How far away is the nearest level I trauma center?

Each venue or site requires a separate plan that involves emergency communication, personnel, equipment, and transportation. Core elements to an effective EAP include the following:[16,17]

- Identifying roles and responsibilities of personnel involved

- Acquiring necessary emergency equipment

- Ensuring access to early defibrillation

- Specifying emergency supplies and equipment needed

  - Dates and signatures of maintenance of emergency equipment

- Establishing a communication system to mobilize the emergency care response

  - Determining the mode of emergency transportation

  - Providing explicit directions to the venue or activity location

- Training likely first responders in cardiopulmonary resuscitation (CPR) and AED use

- Delineating those responsible for documenting details relating to the emergency

- Debriefing and evaluating the emergency response

- Post-event or post-catastrophic incident guidelines

- Practicing, reviewing, and rehearsing the response plan with potential first responders at least annually

- Specific dates and attendees of regular, planned, rehearsal of the EAP

Developing Acute Care and Emergency Protocols for Major Trauma and Medical Emergencies

The goal of an acute care or emergency protocol for specific trauma or medical emergencies is to establish the correct conduct and procedures to be followed in an emergency. A well-thought-out, established, and approved protocol should effectively reduce the life-threatening nature of some emergencies and maximize the chances of survival from a catastrophic emergency. Such a protocol has the potential to save the greatest number of lives with the most efficient use of equipment and personnel.[13] Guidelines have been published for emergency preparedness and acute care of many life-threatening injuries and conditions.[11] Table 3.1 lists many of the National Athletic Trainers' Association (NATA) current position statements (available at the time of printing) recommending the development of established protocols for responding to emergencies. Emergency protocols for each of these conditions are addressed in future chapters.

Knowledge and best practice in the athletic training profession are constantly changing. As new research and experience broaden people's understanding, changes in research methods, professional practices, or medical treatment may become necessary. ATs must always rely on their own experience and knowledge in evaluating and using any information, methods, techniques, or protocols. In using such information or methods they should be mindful of their own safety and the safety of others, including parties for whom they have a professional responsibility. Each situation and patient requires the provider to carefully and independently consider each of the recommendations. Variables such as institutional human resource guidelines, state or federal statutes, rules, or regulations, as well as regional environmental conditions, may affect the relevance and implementation of these recommendations. The NATA and the Inter-Association Task Force advise their members and others to carefully and independently consider each of the recommendations, including the applicability of some to any particular circumstance or person.[6]

The EAP should include medical direction and protocols with the objective of providing immediate, high-quality patient-centered care. Part of the high-quality continuity of care requires an appointed or designated team physician or medical director and an adequate number of HCPs, specifically and most appropriately ATs. The AT's role is to be an extension of the team physician, operating under standing orders and following written protocols. The team physician and AT must communicate to properly evaluate, diagnose, treat, and provide follow-up care. Legally, the AT is acting under the direction of a licensed physician; ultimately, this role is clearly defined in standing orders authorizing the athletic trainer's clinical practice decisions. The clinical responsibilities of an AT must always be performed consistent with the written or verbal instructions of a physician or standing orders and acute care protocols that have been approved by a program's designated medical director.[18]

TABLE 3.1   **NATA Position Statements on Acute Care and Emergency Management of Sport-Related Injuries and Illnesses**

Last updated	Topic	DOI or URL
2017	Best practice guidelines for athletic training documentation	https://www.nata.org/practice-patient-care/risk-liability#documentation
2017	Fluid replacement for the physically active	doi: 10.4085/1062-6050-52.9.02
2016	Management of acute skin trauma	doi: 10.4085/1062-6050-51.7.01.
2016	Cardiovascular care of college student-athletes	doi: 10.4085/j.jacc.2016.03.527.
2016	Preventing and managing sport-related dental and oral injuries	doi: 10.4085/1062-6050-51.8.01
2015	Exertional heat illnesses	doi: 10.4085/1062-6050-50.9.07
2015	Exercise-associated hyponatremia	doi: 10.1097/JSM.0000000000000221
2014	Management of sport concussion	doi: 10.4085/1062-6050-49.1.07
2013	Lightning safety for athletics and recreation	doi: 10.4085/1062-6050-48.2.25.
2013	Preventing sudden death in secondary school athletics	doi: 10.4085/1062-6050-48.4.12
2013	BOC facility principles	www.bocatc.org/public-protection#facility-principles
2012	Athletic HCP "time-outs" before athletic events	https://www.nata.org/sites/default/files/timeout.pdf
2012	Preventing sudden death in sports	doi: 10.4085/1062-6050-48.4.12
2010	Skin diseases	doi: 10.4085/1062-6050-45.4.411
2009	Acute management of the cervical spine–injured athlete	doi: 10.4085/1062-6050-44.3.306
2008	Environmental cold injuries	doi: 10.4085/1062-6050-43.6.640
2007	Emergency preparedness and management of sudden cardiac arrest	www.ncbi.nlm.nih.gov/pubmed/17597956
2007	Management of the athlete with type 1 diabetes mellitus	www.ncbi.nlm.nih.gov/pubmed/18176622
2005	Management of asthma in athletes	www.ncbi.nlm.nih.gov/pubmed/16284647
2004	Head-down contact and spearing in tackle football	www.ncbi.nlm.nih.gov/pubmed/15085218
2002	Emergency planning in athletics	www.ncbi.nlm.nih.gov/pubmed/12937447

BOC = Board of Certification for the AT

Consulting With Institutional Authorities and Working With Local EMS Providers

Communicating with an institutional administration and local EMS providers is essential to implementing an effective EAP. The EAP must be a written document that is reviewed and approved by the medical director, institutional administration, risk management or general counsel, as well as local EMS and EDs or emergency medical facilities. A signature page including the date the plan was approved, reviewed, and distributed should be the first page of the document. To provide direction, leadership, and accountability, designate an EAP coordinator—most likely the medical director, supervising AT, or other HCP associated with the institution or organization. The EAP coordinator should identify who will be responsible and trained to respond to an emergency—including but not limited to ATs, AT students, officers, facility directors, managers, nurses, and physicians.[11] All personnel must know who the coordinator is and understand that this person has the authority to make decisions during emergencies. The EAP coordinator should be responsible for the following:[10]

- Assessing the situation to determine whether an emergency exists
- Activating emergency procedures
- Overseeing emergency procedures
- Notifying and coordinating with outside emergency services
- Directing evacuation or other mass care if necessary

Assembling the Emergency Response Team

High-quality continuity of care requires an appointed or designated physician or medical director and an adequate number of HCPs, specifically and most appropriately ATs,[18] to lead the emergency response team. The emergency response team should include the school nurse, directing physicians, and ATs in development of the EAP. The EAP should specify each person's role in the emergency response as well as in documenting, evaluating, and providing post-event support of athletes, coaches, students, teachers, and staff. Whenever possible, the EAP coordinator should assign specific tasks to each team member; multitasking can cause confusion or oversight of important tasks during an emergency. Each practice or event should have an emergency response team with the following roles in an emergent situation:[9]

- *Provide immediate, on-site acute care.* In an emergent situation, acute care and management of the injury or illness must be provided by the person on the scene with the most qualifications or highest credential. In most situations, the physician or EMS will not be the first on the scene; rather the AT is most likely the best-qualified person to activate the EAP and provide immediate, on-site acute care. People with lesser credentials or without training specific to the situation should yield to those with more appropriate training.[16] Others who are most likely to be on-site and have keys to gates or can otherwise be helpful, such as administrators, managers, or groundskeepers, should be included or invited to review the EAP.

- *Retrieve equipment.* Anyone on the emergency team who is familiar with the types and location of the specific equipment needed, including AT students, managers, and coaches, can fill this role.

- *Activate EMS.* When no ambulance or emergency transportation is present, EMS must be activated as soon as possible because response time is critical during an emergent or a life-threatening situation. Any member of the emergency response team who is calm under pressure, can follow the plan, communicates well over the telephone, and is familiar with the location and address of the event or venue can fill the role of activating EMS.

- *Direct EMS to the location of the patient.* Once EMS is activated, one member of the emergency response team must be responsible for directing EMS to the scene by personally meeting the EMS personnel as they arrive and providing explicit instructions to the location of the injured or ill patient. This task is appropriate for AT students or other staff with knowledge of the facility.

In some cases, the person initiating the EAP might be a non-HCP such as a coach, official, student, teammate, teacher, school nurse, or institutional personnel associated with practice, competition, skill instruction, and strength and conditioning activities.[9,11,16] In instances where the EAP is activated by someone other than the EAP coordinator, clear instructions for reporting incidents of EAP activation should be in place. Coaches or other institutional personnel should be aware of the importance of reporting, communicating, and following up after the incident. All people most likely to be on-site should be trained in the EAP, AED use, CPR, first aid, and prevention of disease transmission. In addition, staff or personnel at each venue (e.g., announcers, media, food vendors, janitors, equipment or field managers) should have the following:[12]

- General awareness of the emergency plan
- Familiarity with the location of the AED(s) and bringing the AED to the patient
- Understanding of the emergency communication plan (detailed in the next section)

Coordinating and Integrating With EMS

The EAP coordinator should develop the plan with input from the local EMS agency and integrate the plan with the local EMS system. The local EMS agency should be encouraged to conduct an on-site pre-incident visit to identify problems, such as restrictive passages through parking lots, doors, stairs, or any areas that are inaccessible to an ambulance crew with a stretcher or gurney. To effectively coordinate and integrate with EMS, the EAP should include the following:

- Contact information for the local EMS agency and dispatchers
- Contact information for the EAP coordinator and institutional administrator(s)
- Instructions to notify parents or school district personnel of the emergency

- Location and type of emergency equipment available on-site at each venue
- Detailed floor plans and maps of the property

A copy of the final EAP should be provided to the local EMS system and dispatcher. This information can be entered into the computer-aided systems at the EMS dispatch center and linked to the venue address with the name and contact numbers for the EAP coordinator and institutional administrators.[13] As part of the annual review of the EAP, provide a current document (updated as necessary) to designated emergency facilities and EMS, and review with staff and administrators in advance of an emergency or catastrophic event.[16]

Identify Emergency Transportation and Emergency Care Facilities

High-risk or highly attended events should have an ambulance on-site, particularly when the EMS response time is potentially lengthy. Nationwide, the Fire and Emergency Services[20] (FEMS), the U.S. government department that provides emergency and fire safety services, estimates the average response time to be 4 to 7 minutes or as long as 9 minutes, which varies greatly in rural or urban areas. In a cardiac emergency, the time from collapse to AED shock must be approximately 3 minutes; therefore, on-site medical staff or personnel must be prepared to provide immediate CPR and defibrillation.[13]

Ambulances should be available on-site for high-risk events that are planned and coordinated ahead of time; however, many other venues (field, arena, assembly line, training facilities) and events (practices, conditioning, weight training) are generally not required to have an ambulance on-site. When an ambulance is available on-site, it must be at a designated location that enables rapid access and a cleared route for entering and exiting the venue, such as in the end zone near an open gate.[9]

For emergency transportation that is not on-site, the EAP must indicate the best route for an ambulance

---

Activating the EMS System

In the United States, the universal emergency telephone number is 9-1-1, and the availability of cellular phones with **global positioning systems (GPSs)** in most locations has greatly helped EMS notification and dispatch. When the emergency is detected by a law enforcement or other public vehicle, notification may occur by radio. When the 9-1-1 call is made, the EMS dispatcher follows a list of questions to gather information from the caller:[9]

- Your (the caller's) name, location address, and telephone number
- Description of the scene, such as the number of patients or special environmental hazards
- Patient's name and age
- Exact location of the patient
- Patient's condition or disposition (nature and severity of the problem)
- Initial first aid or treatment provided
- Specific directions to locate the scene of the emergency (e.g., "Use the Palm Street entrance on north side of the stadium, enter through Gate number 1 near Walnut Street.")
- Other information as requested by the dispatcher

The caller should not hang up; stay on the phone until otherwise instructed.

From this information, the EMS dispatcher's role is to determine the following:[19]

- The relative urgency of the emergency
- The nature and severity of the problem
- Anticipated response time to the scene
- Appropriate EMS response including level of training (EMR, EMT, AEMT, paramedic) needed for the EMS response
- Need for additional EMS units, fire rescue, HAZMAT team, air medical support, or law enforcement

to rapidly enter and exit each venue. Part of the EAP must identify a dedicated staff person or administrator assigned to each event with keys to all access points and who is familiar with the directions for EMS personnel arriving to the specific facility or venue. Clearly posted written directions should be available to read to the EMS response dispatcher and global positioning satellite coordinates should medical air transport be needed.[11] Once the ambulance has arrived, the EAP should include a protocol for an adult to accompany the patient to the emergency medical facility; ideally, this person is a parent or family member, but an adult representative of the institution should make every effort to ride with the patient to provide information and support. An excellent resource with a sample EAP with templates to be indi-

vidually customized can be found at the Korey Stringer Institute website.

The nearest emergency medical facility and its level of service (table 3.2) must be identified in the EAP. For cases requiring a higher level of care, the EAP should include contact information and the location of the nearest regional trauma center. Maintaining an open line of communication with emergency care facilities is essential in the unfortunate event of a catastrophic medical emergency.[16]

All trauma centers require a commitment to the following:

1. Continuous quality improvement of trauma care through a formal quality assessment program and prevention

TABLE 3.2 **Levels of Trauma Centers**

	Description	Services provided
Level I	A comprehensive regional resource that is a tertiary care facility; capable of providing total care for every aspect of injury from prevention through rehabilitation	• Provides 24-hour in-house coverage by general surgeons. • Includes availability of care in specialties such as orthopedic surgery, neurosurgery, anesthesiology, emergency medicine, radiology, internal medicine, and critical care. • May also include cardiac, hand, pediatric, and microvascular surgery and hemodialysis • Referral resource for communities in nearby regions • Provides leadership in prevention and public education to surrounding communities. • Committed to organized research to help direct new innovations in trauma care. • Provides continuing education of the trauma team members.
Level II	Ability to initiate definitive care for all injured patients	• Provides 24-hour immediate coverage by general surgeons. • Includes availability of orthopedic surgery, neurosurgery, anesthesiology, emergency medicine, radiology, and critical care. • Tertiary care needs such as cardiac surgery, hemodialysis, and microvascular surgery may be referred to a level I trauma center.
Level III	Ability to provide prompt assessment, resuscitation, and stabilization of injured patients and emergency operations	• Provides 24-hour immediate coverage by emergency medicine physicians and prompt availability of general surgeons and anesthesiologists. • Has transfer agreements for patients requiring more comprehensive care at a level I or level II trauma center. • Provides back-up care for rural and community hospitals.
Level IV	Ability to provide ATLS before transfer to a higher level trauma center	• Provides basic ED facilities to implement ATLS protocols and 24-hour laboratory coverage. • Transfer to higher-level trauma centers following formal transfer agreements.
Level V	Provides initial evaluation, stabilization, and diagnostic capabilities; and prepares patients for transfer to higher levels of care.	Includes basic ED facilities to implement the following: • ATLS protocols • Trauma nurse(s) and physicians available upon patient arrival. • Has after-hours activation protocols if facility is not open 24 hours a day.

ATLS = advanced trauma life support; ED = emergency department

Trauma center levels are verified by the American College of Surgeons (ACS), which verifies the presence of resources for optimal care of the injured patient.

Based on Pollack and Beck (2012); American College of Surgeons (2014).

2. Public education and outreach within its community

3. Continuing education of nursing and allied health personnel or the trauma team

4. Prevention efforts and an active outreach program for its referring communities (except level V)

Obtaining and Maintaining Emergency Equipment and Supplies

Equipment is an important part of any medical EAP, starting with a first aid kit and CPR barrier devices and should include access to an AED. Equipment should be carefully selected based on the types of emergencies likely to develop at each venue. For example, if football, gymnastics, or diving events take place on campus, a backboard with restraints should be available to immobilize an athlete with suspected spine injury. Epinephrine can be lifesaving for victims with **anaphylaxis** (severe allergic reaction), such as that resulting from a bee sting, a severe food allergy, or latex allergy. Some states encourage the use of **epinephrine** injection or **epinephrine auto-injectors** for emergency treatment of severe allergic reactions. If state regulations allow (see chapter 2), epinephrine should be included in the emergency equipment, and appropriate staff should be trained in its use (described in chapter 5). A physician's prescription is often required to purchase emergency medications, although each state has different regulations.[13]

The EAP must list the equipment as well as the location of the equipment required to manage the emergency. It is essential that the emergency response team be familiar with the terminology, function, and operation of each piece of emergency equipment before an emergency occurs.[9]

Equipment should be maintained in good operating condition (e.g., AED batteries are charged, the oxygen tank is full, and spine boards and other vacuum or air splinting equipment is functioning properly). Emergency equipment should be checked for good working order, and medications should be checked for expiration on a regular basis. Essential members of the emergency team are responsible for properly cleaning, storing, and maintaining emergency equipment. Storing equipment in a clean, environmentally controlled area will aid in maintaining good condition of equipment.[22] Each venue or facility must have a checklist with the EAP coordinator or other responsible team member's signature and dates of inspection recorded and maintained. Routine maintenance checklists that are documented at regular intervals (e.g., monthly, every season) should include the following:

- Checking expiration dates on medications and promptly removing and replacing expired medications

- Checking expiration date of defibrillation pads on the AED

- Checking and documenting the battery charge on the monitor and AED

Any equipment is useless unless it is readily accessible in an emergency. First aid and resuscitation equipment should be placed in a central, highly visible, and accessible location near a telephone; and all faculty, staff, and students should know where the equipment is stored. If the institution is large (e.g., large high school or university), it may be necessary to keep duplicate equipment in several areas. Because injuries are most likely to occur during athletic activities, the athletic facilities should be considered high-priority areas for placement of equipment such as the first aid kit and spine boards. Emergency equipment, including the AED, should not be stored in a locked office or cabinet, because locking it might delay emergency care.

EMS and 9-1-1 centers must know in advance where emergency equipment is kept in the venue or on school property. This knowledge can prevent failure to use available equipment (such as an AED) because responders are unaware of the existence or location of the equipment. If the 9-1-1 center knows where emergency equipment is located, the dispatcher can inform the rescuer where to find the equipment and can instruct rescuers in the use of the equipment before the arrival of EMS personnel.[13]

Reviewing the EAP and Training Personnel

Annually, when new personnel are added, or at the beginning of each sport season, the EAP must be practiced, rehearsed, and documented. When schools have an AED, they are more likely to rehearse and practice the EAP.[23] The written plans must be available to all

 RED FLAG

An AED must be kept in the venue or in a central location, such as the athletic training clinic, so that responders are aware of its existence and location. If the AED is located in a locked room, such as the school nurse's or principal's office, ATs will be unable to access the AED when needed and use it before the arrival of EMS personnel.

Suggested On-Site Medical Supplies and Medications

General

- Access to a communication device and list of important local emergency telephone numbers, including police, fire department, EMS, poison control center, and school district emergency numbers
- Alcohol swabs and povidone-iodine swabs
- Bandages (sterile and nonsterile)
- Blankets
- Cooling tub and tarp for rapid whole-body cooling
- Dextrose 50% in water (D50W; or D25 for the pediatric patient) IV solution
- Disinfectant
- Extra ice water for cooling
- Fast-acting carbohydrate (glucose tablets, honey)
- Flashlight
- Gloves, sterile and nonsterile, disposable (variety of sizes)
- Oral fluid replacement for dehydration
- Oral glucose source for hypoglycemia (sugar packet, honey, glucagon)
- Oxygen
- Paper and pens
- Rectal thermistor (e.g., DataTherm Continuous Temperature Monitor)
- Multipurpose scissors or emergency shears
- Sealed moist towelettes (hand wipes)
- Sharps box and red bag
- Tongue depressor
- Tweezers

Cardiopulmonary

- Airway equipment (oropharyngeal and nasopharyngeal airways, supraglottic airways) and bag-valve mask
- ACLS drugs and equipment (crash cart)
- AED
- Blood pressure cuff
- Cricothyrotomy kit
- Epinephrine 1:1000 in a prepackaged unit/epinephrine auto-injector
- IV fluids and administration set
- Large-bore angiocath for tension pneumothorax (14-16ga)
- Pocket mask
- Short-acting beta-agonist bronchodilator/albuterol metered-dose inhaler
- Stethoscope

Head and Neck/Neurologic

- Cervical collar
- Dental kit
- Eye kit/shield for traumatic eye injuries

> continued

Suggested On-Site Medical Supplies and Medications   *> continued*

- Face mask removal tool
- Screwdrivers
- Pen light
- Nasal packing material
- Oto-ophthalmoscope
- Pin or other sharp object for sensory testing
- Reflex hammer
- Spine board and attachments or restraints

Orthopedic/Wound Injuries

- Adhesive tape (1-2 in./2.5-5 cm wide)
- Biohazard waste bag (3.5-gallon/13-L capacity)
- Crutches
- Elastic roller bandage, 4 and 6 inches (10 cm and 15 cm) wide
- Extremity splints for musculoskeletal injuries
- Ice with bags or disposable instant-activating cold packs
- Hemostatic agents
- Local anesthetic/syringe/needles
- Scalpel
- Skin staple applicator
- Slings
- Sterile eye pads
- Sterile gauze/trauma pads and roll gauze
- Suture set/Steri-Strips
- Topical antibiotics
- Tourniquet
- Wound irrigation materials (sterile normal saline, 10-50 cc syringe)

ACLS = advanced cardiac life support; AED = automated external defibrillator; IV = intravenous
Based on Hazinski et al. (2004); Olympia et al. (2007).

personnel and kept in a prominent location in the AT clinic or facility. Best practices for reviewing the EAP include the following:

- Regularly (at least annually) schedule a review, rehearsal, training, and practice in order to ensure that all involved personnel understand their roles and responsibilities during an emergency.[16]

- When new staff members are hired, review the EAP upon initial assignment of duties, especially if new staff members have a role in the EAP.

- Review the EAP with other institutional staff such as cleaning personnel, administrators, and field managers to ensure that response efforts will be coordinated with their role during practices and events, enhancing the effectiveness of the plan.

- Review and coordinate the EAP with local emergency responders such as the fire department, local HAZMAT teams, or other outside responders, to ensure that the capabilities of these outside responders are used optimally.[10]

Unfortunately, a general lack of available personnel exists to plan for emergencies and implement an EAP in many settings, in particular the secondary school setting. According to a benchmark study,[24] only 37% of public high schools employed a full-time AT, although larger schools were much more likely to do so. Having a full-

Automated External Defibrillator

The EAP must include access to emergency and lifesaving equipment such as an AED. Secondary schools that have AEDs (86.5%) also have an established EAP, compared to 47.4% of schools without AEDs. Of the schools with an EAP, 67.8% of schools with AEDs developed the EAP in consultation with local EMS, compared with 57.6% of schools without AEDs.[23]

A response time of less than 3 minutes from collapse to delivery of electrical rescue shock is ideal. This response time includes the time it takes to do the following:

- Recognize an emergency.
- Notify designated responders.
- Access the AED.
- Reach the victim.
- Apply the electrodes.
- Deliver the first shock.

If a facility has only one AED, it should be centrally located so that it can be brought to the site of sudden cardiac arrest through activation of the EAP. All staff should know the location of the AED. Consideration should be given to the most populated areas and proximity to athletic facilities. For large schools and complexes with distant or multiple athletic facilities, duplicate equipment may be needed. The AED should be:[12]

- highly visible,
- located near a telephone or other means of activating the EMS system and on-site response team,
- easily accessible during all hours the facility is open, including any sponsored event after usual working hours,
- secured but not placed in a locked box, cabinet, or room that is inaccessible at the time of an emergency,
- routinely maintained and tested (with documentation) according to the manufacturer's directions,
- checked for equipment readiness by on-site event personnel for each athletic event, and
- distributed to medical staff along a race course or stadium. (Use bicycle, golf cart, or emergency vehicles for rescue teams.)

time AT in every U.S. high school that sponsors athletic activities should be a priority. It ensures that athletes have access to critical medical services and also that best practices for preventing sudden death are implemented.[4] Barriers to hiring ATs are primarily budgetary in nature but are also related to general misconceptions regarding the value and role of the athletic trainer, particularly in the secondary school setting.[25] In general, reasons for lack of planning and preparation for catastrophic conditions or critical incidents are multifactorial and include the following:

- Lack of funding to support the presence of ATs at all athletic events, to provide training for athletic trainers and other sport health professionals in the use of the AED, first aid, and CPR, to purchase

and stock important emergency equipment and medications, and to maintain safety of athletic fields and venues;

- Deficiency in the evidence supporting adherence of ATs and schools to guidelines for emergency preparedness; and
- Disbelief by sport health professionals and school officials that serious emergencies related to athletics, albeit rare, may occur.[8,24,25]

To address these concerns, the NATA recommends a time-out system be adopted for athletic health care. Before the start of each athletic event (practice or competition), a time-out should be held to convene the athletic HCPs who comprise the emergency response team. The purpose of the meeting is to go through a pre-event checklist reviewing the venue's EAP. The concept of a time-out is common in athletics and medicine. For example, time-outs are taken immediately before surgery when all operating-room participants stop to verify the procedure, patient identity, correct site, and side. Similarly, coaches and athletes call time-out to gather the team together and discuss game strategies or call a play. This new application of time-out is expected to save lives by ascertaining that all those involved in emergency care are properly briefed and ready before a potentially dangerous or life-threatening injury occurs.[26]

A pre-event time-out will help produce a decisive, coordinated emergency response and outcome. Typically the AT is the first person to respond to an athletic emergency situation. Others, such as physicians and EMTs, also are involved and need to be part of the pre-event briefing so that they are fully informed. To ensure the athlete receives the best care when an emergency arises, effective communication with all relevant parties is critical.[26]

Practicing, Evaluating, and Revising the Plan

Each institution or organization should practice and evaluate the EAP with participation of all relevant personnel, including the following:

- ATs
- AT students
- Facility administrators
- Coaches, managers, or administrators usually present during practices or events
- Nurse or other HCP on-site
- Directing physicians
- Local EMS system

Specifically designated rescuers should participate in unannounced practice drills on a regular basis (e.g., at the beginning of each sport season or school year and repeated during the year) to promote an efficient, organized, and timely response to life-threatening medical emergencies anywhere in the facility. These practice drills should include mock emergency situations with real-time participation by students, staff, and faculty as members of the response or communication team.

During each practice drill, an observer should record the following:[12,13]

- Critical time intervals:
  - Time from development of the emergency to 9-1-1 call
  - Time from development of the emergency to administration of first aid
  - Time from collapse to bystander initiation of CPR (if indicated)
  - Time from collapse in cardiac arrest to delivery of first shock from AED
  - Time of arrival of EMS personnel to the patient
- Availability and function of emergency equipment

More frequent practice sessions will improve the effectiveness, efficiency, and organization of the response. Any modifications to the response plan based on practice drills should be documented.[12]

After each drill, review performance of each component of the plan and revise the EAP as needed to improve performance and efficiency. Identify the strengths and weaknesses of the plan in order to improve it and to better serve the next emergency.[13] Procedures and personnel change frequently, so review the contents of the plan regularly and update it whenever staff or responsibilities change. In addition, the plan should be updated when changes occur in the layout or design of the facility or in the equipment, which may affect evacuation routes. Generally, the most common outdated item in plans is the facility and agency contact information. Consider placing this important information on a separate page in the front of the plan so that it can be readily updated.[10]

Educating and Training Personnel

Before implementing the EAP, the director of sports medicine or head AT must designate an AED coordinator and train enough personnel to assist in safe and orderly emergency response. All staff members must be informed of their roles and responsibilities in EAP. Each staff member should be initially assigned to a role in the EAP and notified when the plan changes. Staff must be educated about the function and elements of the EAP, including types of potential emergencies, reporting procedures, alarm systems, evacuation plans, and shutdown procedures. To minimize confusion, clearly communicate

 RED FLAG

The NATA recommends a time-out before the start of each athletic event, practice, or competition. The time-out involves all athletic HCPs who comprise the emergency response team. The purpose of the time-out is to go through a pre-event checklist and review the venue's EAP.

Checklist for Emergency Preparedness

Preseason Planning

- ☐ Complete a preparticipation examination of all athletes to identify medical conditions that may predispose the athlete to certain life-threatening emergencies or injuries.
- ☐ Develop a watch list for athletes with medical conditions.
- ☐ Develop a chain of command that establishes and defines the roles and responsibilities of institutional administrators, officials, and sports medicine staff.
- ☐ Establish a policy to assess environmental concerns and playing conditions to modify or suspend practice or competition.
- ☐ Identify and designate an institutional administrator to serve as public information officer (PIO).
- ☐ Establish and regularly rehearse a comprehensive, practical, and flexible written EAP developed by organizational or institutional personnel in consultation with local EMS.
- ☐ Educate and train coaches, managers, and school staff about the EAP as well as in use of the AED, CPR, and first aid.
- ☐ Establish a clear mechanism for communication to EMS, and identify the mode of transportation to designated emergency receiving facilities.
- ☐ Establish a plan to provide proper documentation and keeping of medical records.

Pre-Event Preparation

- ☐ Prepare a sideline medical bag with specific equipment and medications.
- ☐ Check and confirm communication equipment is charged and in working order.
- ☐ Maintain emergency equipment and supplies at all venues, athletic fields, or arenas for specific sport-related emergencies.
- ☐ Monitor sports equipment for safety and fit.

Event/Game Day Preparation

- ☐ Assess environmental concerns and playing conditions.
- ☐ Ensure the presence of medical personnel at the competition site.

Pre-Event Time-Out

- ☐ Meet and greet all athletic HCPs to review the EAP.
- ☐ Establish the location and role of each provider present (e.g., AT, EMT, MD).
- ☐ Establish how communication will occur (e.g., voice commands, radio, hand signals). Confirm the primary means of communication as well as the secondary or back-up method of communication. Ensure all batteries are fully charged.
- ☐ For all high-risk events, identify where the ambulance is physically located. Identify the planned route for the ambulance entrance and exit, ensuring the route is unencumbered. Determine whether the ambulance is a dedicated unit or on stand-by. If an ambulance is not on-site, confirm the mechanism for calling one.
- ☐ Designate the closest and most appropriate trauma center in the event of emergency transport. Consider the most appropriate facility for the injury or illness when selecting the hospital.
- ☐ Identify the type and location of emergency equipment; check to confirm it is in working order and fully ready for use.
- ☐ Ask whether any issues exist that could potentially impact the implementation of the EAP (e.g., construction, weather, crowd flow).[26]

> continued

Checklist for Emergency Preparedness   > *continued*

Postseason Evaluation

☐ Summarize injuries and illnesses that occurred during the season.

☐ Review performance of personnel in following the EAP and revise as necessary.

☐ Improve medical and administrative protocols.

☐ Implement strategies to improve sideline preparedness.

☐ Document checking equipment and medications for expiration dates.

AED = automated external defibrillator; CPR = cardiopulmonary resuscitation; EMS = emergency medical services
Based on Olympia et al. (2013); Drezner et al. (2007); Courson (2007); Andersen (2002); NATA (2018).

---

who will be in charge during an emergency. All staff members—including administrators, coaches, and the entire emergency response team—must feel ownership and responsibility for their roles in the planning, implementation, and documentation of the EAP. To ensure the entire staff is engaged in the EAP, all staff members should be taught the following:[11]

- Potential threats, hazards, and protective actions
- When to telephone the EMS service (phone 9-1-1)
- When to phone other facility or medical personnel
- Means for locating or contacting family members
- Where to find the emergency equipment
- How to clear crowds
- How to direct arriving EMS personnel to all sites on campus
- How to communicate with other HCPs, specifically EMS
- When events require documentation and how to write an incident report

If training is not practiced and reinforced it will be forgotten, so staff should be trained again annually, including protection against blood-borne pathogens; personal protective equipment; and restricting unauthorized access to the site of the emergency.[10] During the annual review of the EAP, all personnel involved must be considered and informed of any revisions or modifications. All changes to the document should be reviewed, with feedback requested, and approved by the institution and EMS.[16]

Communicating During an Emergency

Establishing a clear, rapid, accessible mechanism and system for communicating with the appropriate emergency care service providers is a critical element of an effective EAP. The following are keys to an effective and efficient communication system:[11,13,16]

- Establish systems ahead of time for each venue or health care facility to alert on-site responders to the emergency and location within the venue. This step is essential in order to prevent critical delays caused by a rescuer running from a distant facility or field.
- Connect all parts of the facility to the EMS system, including indoor facilities and practice fields.
- Include current emergency telephone numbers for the nearest hospital and trauma center, directing physician, university (or school) health center, and campus police or security.

Activation of the internal response team should be simultaneous with activation of the EMS system. This communication network can be developed through existing telephones, cellular telephones, walkie-talkies, alarms, or an intercom or public address system that links the rescuer directly to the EMS. The emergency communications system must be established ahead of time and should be checked before each practice or competition to ensure proper working order. Mobile phones provide a quick and easy way to activate EMS; however, the EAP coordinator must ensure that cellular phones are charged and that cellular coverage exists. A back-up communication plan must be in place in case of loss of cell phone coverage, which may result from the following:

- Power outages and lost battery charge
- Insufficient tower coverage (Many rural areas do not have cellular coverage.)
- Phone system overload
- Damaged cell towers from wind, lightning, or other natural disasters

Failure of the primary communication system requires a back-up communication plan such as a landline phone or two-way radio. Post the EAP at every venue and near telephones, including the role of the first responder, a listing of emergency contact numbers, street address, and directions to guide the EMS personnel.[11]

Interprofessional Communication With Other Health Care Providers

Effective communication is an essential component of prehospital care that links members of sports health care teams with responders from EMS, fire, and law enforcement agencies. Timely, clear communication allows team members to work together efficiently and safely. Knowing the capabilities of the team's communication system is essential for the best use of available resources.[19,27]

Verbal communication skills are vital for gathering information, effectively coordinating the response, and instructing personnel. Excellent verbal communication is also an integral part of organizing, summarizing, and transferring information about the patient's care to the EMTs, nurses, and physicians in the ED. Best practices for verbal communication within the health care team include the following:[19,27]

- Use professional language and demeanor.
- Introduce yourself to the team.
- Clarify your role.
- Read or report back; in other words, close the communication loop.
- State the obvious to avoid false assumptions.
- Ask questions, check and clarify.
- Delegate tasks to specific people.
- Use objective (e.g., specific, fact-based, measurable, observable) terms and avoid subjective (e.g., opinions, interpretations, points of view, emotions, judgment) language.
- Always echo the orders back to avoid misunderstandings.
- Repeat vital signs and other information as needed.
- Ask for clarification if an order, report, or finding is not clear or seems inappropriate.
- Remember that U.S. federal laws protect a patient's right to privacy. Do not give any health information about the patient to anyone other than those directly involved in the care of the patient.

Providing the Oral Report

Reporting responsibilities begin with the initiation of patient care and continue until the patient is transferred to the next level of care. The oral report is often provided at the same time that the paramedic, nurse, or physician is examining the patient or moving the patient from the ground or examination table to a stretcher or gurney.

Therefore, it is essential to provide information in a complete, precise way. In addition, it may be necessary to briefly explain the role of the AT in the management of the patient's care. The oral report must include the following components:[19]

1. *Opening information.* Briefly introduce yourself and your role at the facility. Include the patient's name and chief complaint, nature of illness, or mechanism of injury. For example, "Good afternoon. My name is Sandy, and I am the athletic trainer for this university. I have evaluated the patient and called for transport to the nearest trauma center. Our patient here is Damian Lewis. Damian is a 22-year-old football player complaining of neck pain of 9/10 after being tackled in a game this afternoon."

2. *Detailed information.* Include additional findings indicating the severity of the condition. For example, "He denies losing consciousness, has no history of neck injuries or concussion, and has a mechanism of injury of spinal loading."

3. *Relevant patient history.* Include information that was not already provided. For example, "Damian was unable to move his hands or feet and has paresthesia in his arms and legs. We suspect cervical spine injury and promptly immobilized him on the spine board."

4. *Pertinent findings of the physical exam.* Relay any pertinent findings of the physical exam. For example, "We noted point tenderness near C6-C7, distal muscle weakness, and diminished deep tendon reflexes of the Achilles and wrist extensors."

5. *The patient's response to treatment.* It is especially important to report any changes in the patient or the treatment provided since initiating care. Include treatments given en route. For example, "Once immobilized, his pain subsided to 7/10 and he was able to move his fingers and toes. Oxygen was initiated by non-rebreather mask at 15 minutes. Because he was lying in a nonneutral position, we used the Xcollar to immobilize him in the position found."

6. *Vital signs.* Vital signs must also be assessed initially and during transport. For example, "His initial vitals included a blood pressure of 112/84 mm Hg, a pulse of 72 bpm, respirations of 14 breaths/min. We did not assess core body temperature. His vitals were generally unchanged upon transport to the ED."

7. *Other information.* Include any other information gathered that was not important enough to report earlier, any patient medications, and any other details provided by team members or family. For example, "Teammates reported seeing Damian tackle using the top of his helmet before he collapsed to the ground. We found him prone with his head turned to his left side."

Transfer of Care

Transfer of care (also called patient hand-off or hand-over) is a crucial time during which errors in communication can result in adverse patient outcomes.[27] This important transition involves communication strategies that are purposeful, concise, and simple to reduce errors. Be mindful that not all HCPs are aware of the qualifications of the AT in the care of the patient. Transfer of care of the patient must be only to someone with your level of training or higher—usually the EMTs at the scene, physician, or ED personnel.

Once the next-level provider is ready to take responsibility for the patient, a crucial part of transferring the patient's care from one provider to another is providing a formal report of the patient's condition. The communication process during a patient transfer ensures that the information provided to the next-level care provider is received and understood correctly. Several techniques or strategies can assist timely and accurate hand-off,[27] such as this check-back or echo strategy:

- Sender initiates message.
- Receiver accepts message and provides feedback.
- Sender double-checks in order to ensure the message is understood.

Similarly, a call-out exchange is a simple communication technique for ensuring that information conveyed by the sender is understood as intended by the receiver.

For example, a call-out exchange between an AT and an EMT might be as follows:

> EMT: "Airway status?"
>   AT: "Airway clear."
> EMT: "Breath sounds?"
>   AT: "Breath sounds decreased on right."
> EMT: "Blood pressure?"
>   AT: "BP is 96/92."

Documenting and Reporting the Incident

Incident reports are an essential method of documenting, evaluating, and monitoring certain serious occurrences, as well as ensuring that the necessary people receive the information. The EAP coordinator should ensure the documenting and reporting occur and follow all institutional or organizational incident-reporting policies. Documentation is the written portion of the emergency response that becomes part of the permanent or official record. Adequate reporting and accurate records do the following:[19]

- Ensure continuity of patient care.
- Facilitate proper transfer of responsibility.
- Provide a detailed account of an incident so that appropriate follow-up action can be taken.

CLINICAL SKILLS

The Patient Hand-Off: The I PASS the BATON Strategy

I	*Introduction:* Introduce yourself, your role, and job and the name of the patient.
P	*Patient:* Provide name, identifiers, age, sex, location.
A	*Assessment:* Present chief complaint, vital signs, symptoms, and diagnosis.
S	*Situation:* Share current status or circumstances, including code status, level of (un)certainty, and recent changes and response to treatment.
S	*Safety concerns:* Share critical lab values or reports, socioeconomic factors, allergies, and alerts (falls, seizure, etc.).
the	
B	*Background:* Discuss comorbidities, previous episodes, current medications, and family history.
A	*Actions:* What actions were taken or are required? Provide brief rationale.
T	*Timing:* Discuss level of urgency and explicit timing and prioritization of actions.
O	*Ownership:* Know who is responsible (person/team), including patient/family.
N	*Next:* Discuss what will happen next. What are anticipated changes? What is the plan? Are there contingency plans?

Reprinted from *Multi-Professional Patient Safety Curriculum Guide*, World Health Organization, pg. 139, copyright 2012.

- Comply with the requirements of health departments and law enforcement agencies.
- Provide a reliable tool for evaluation of policies, procedures, performance, and patterns.
- Fulfill the organization's administrative policies.
- Fulfill regulatory agency or accrediting body requirements.
- Potentially reduce exposure and minimize vulnerability when investigated in litigation.

Any incident or event that requires activation of the EAP and summoning EMS is a critical incident that requires providing internal documents and reports to the institution or organization. To report a critical incident, the EAP coordinator should immediately do the following:[28]

- Complete a critical incident report and ensure that it contains details of the actions taken during and after the incident.
- Summarize the response to the incident with detailed explanations of any opportunities to improve the response to a similar incident in future and any systems that may have failed for quality improvement.
- Provide copies of the critical incident report with the summary for approval by the institution's risk management or general counsel.
- Save the originals of all documentation relating to the critical incident in a confidential file to be recorded in the institution's official recordkeeping system.
- Save all incident reporting and facts documentation, including details of the responses taken, copies of related emails and letters, records of significant interactions, and contact details for all people involved in the response process.
- Send copies of the final report and summary document to the institutional official (athletic director, principal, chancellor) who has the responsibility to report a critical incident.

All medical personnel must know what events require documentation and what is expected of them in terms of that documentation. Further, all medical personnel should receive training and practice in how to write an incident report. Important documentation includes a report that

- is written objectively,
- distinguishes facts from assumptions,
- avoids hearsay, and
- eliminates jargon.

To ensure completion and make it as easy as possible to write an accurate and complete report, developing a form is useful. To keep the form simple, use check boxes or fill-in-the-blank responses wherever possible (e.g., day, date, time, location of incident). A form is not necessary or applicable to every incident as long as the report includes the following items:

- Day, date, and time of the incident
- Name and title of the person writing the report
- Exact location of the incident
- Conditions (e.g., weather, lighting, wet turf)
- List of key participants and role
- Complete description of the incident in chronological order
- Events leading up to the incident
- Time EMS was called
- Preliminary or field diagnosis and treatment or interventions provided
- Resolution of the incident
- Injury, condition, or disablement as a result of the incident
- People notified of the incident (include name/title/date/time)
- People receiving a copy of the report (include name/title)
- Signature of the author and date of the report

Statements from key participants or observers directly involved in the incident may be part of a comprehensive incident report or may be attached as a supplemental report; follow institutional reporting policies.[28]

Mass Care and Catastrophic Incidents

A **mass care (or casualty) incident (MCI)** is a catastrophic incident that results in the need to provide medical care to multiple patients outside of traditional hospital settings. ATs may be called upon to provide initial medical or trauma care during a large-scale disaster at a school or workplace or mass gathering events such as sporting events or a marathon. An MCI may result from a wide range of emergencies, such as fires, floods, earthquakes, hurricanes, tornadoes, tsunami, riots, mass shootings, spilling of HAZMAT, and other natural or human-caused incidents. MCIs require advanced planning in order to do the following:[29,30]

1. Initiate the MCI response.
2. Triage or identify the most severely injured patients.

3. Move patients to a safe area to begin treatment.

4. Transport patients to arranged or staged ambulances to the nearest appropriate hospital or trauma center.

5. Facilitate the local or regional **incident command system (ICS)** for extended or long-term emergency response.

Planning for an MCI response begins long before the catastrophe. Planning should involve local EMS who usually have protocols for managing emergencies during large events. Basic MCI training may be as simple as a tabletop exercise with the EMS providers. The goal is to have all medical staff comfortable with assuming various roles during a disaster. EMS systems typically conduct regional MCI drills annually and should include the school, organization, or other safety personnel. Drills may include scenarios with varying implications for scene safety, such as a building collapse or a terrorist attack. The emergency response team should have a well-thought-out plan to respond to an MCI scenario with 5 or more patients that can be scaled up or down as needed.[30]

Incident Command System

The United States has a national system that includes a regional or local ICS. Any MCI requires a system for the command, control, and coordination of emergency response. At the incident scene, the ICS facilitates a consistent response allowing agencies to work together using common terminology and operating procedures while controlling personnel, facilities, equipment, and communications. While the ICS may provide an extended or long-term response, advance planning for an MCI is essential to maximize patient care and outcomes and minimize chaos, panic, radio traffic, and impact on area ambulance services and hospital resources.

Venue Evacuation

A comprehensive institutional or organizational MCI response plan must provide evacuation policies, procedures, and escape routes. These plans are necessary so that all personnel and guests or visitors understand who is authorized to order an evacuation, under what conditions an evacuation would be necessary, how to evacuate, and what routes to take. Exit diagrams should be used to identify the escape routes to be followed from each specific facility location. Evacuation procedures also describe actions staff should take before and while evacuating such as shutting windows, turning off equipment, and closing doors behind them.[10]

Public Information Officer

During a critical incident or MCI, the institution or organization should have a plan for communicating with the public by identifying an institutional representative as a public information officer (PIO or IO). This person serves as the conduit for information to and from internal and external stakeholders, including the media or other organizations seeking information directly from the incident or event. The PIO is also responsible for ensuring that MCI command staff is kept apprised of what is being said or reported about an incident. Managing information allows public questions to be addressed and rumors to be managed, and it ensures that other such public relations issues are not overlooked.[31] This role may be assumed by an athletic director or administrator who coordinates with the public announcer providing announcing guidelines[32] for addressing emergency situations or security situations during public events.

Post-Catastrophic Injury or Post-Critical Incident Plan

Each institution or organization should include a post-catastrophic injury or post-critical incident plan within the EAP. A catastrophic injury is a situation in which a life has been lost from any cause or a way of life has been permanently altered, such as spinal paralysis, blindness, or loss of a limb. Other possible events that might require a post-critical incident plan could be when a coach who works closely with the athletes has just sustained a fatal heart attack, an athlete has been fatally struck by a car while crossing the street, or an athlete is in intensive care with a staph infection and has lost one or more limbs to amputation. In addition, as previously mentioned, a critical incident may involve an event related to MCI, campus violence, natural disaster, or terrorism.

The post-catastrophic injury or post-critical incident plan should outline the procedures for responding to this kind of event, including the following:[11,16,33]

- A crisis management team that has a designated institutional official or PIO to call family members to notify of the incident and to release information to public or media

- Protocol for holding post-event debriefing within days of the incident for all personnel involved

- Local crisis services and mental health counselors to assist students, teammates, families, and rescuers

- List of administrative and legal personnel from the institution or organization to be contacted and informed of the incident

- Forms for documenting actions and reporting events during the incident

- Methods for data collection, reporting, and incident response evaluation and review

- Protocols for training institutional personnel
- Maintenance logs for emergency equipment

As with all established policies and procedures, it is critical that the EAP be reviewed and approved by the institution or organization's legal counsel and followed consistently.

Create the Crisis Management Team

In the case of a catastrophic injury or crisis event, the EAP should designate members of a crisis management team and outline the post-incident procedures and protocols to be followed. The team should include the PIO who will call the parents, guardians, or other family members of a student athlete, coach, or staff member. This person is designated ahead of time and may be the director of athletics, head AT, head coach, or any other appropriate person (head of security, physician) designated to make the call. Designating the PIO in advance is useful to maintain control over information gathering and dissemination to the public. This person should be available to answer any questions important to the family and ensure that families and loved ones receive accurate and timely information in a compassionate way. At this time, information can be gathered to arrange for the family to travel to campus or the hospital if appropriate.

It is important to keep the number of people providing information to a minimum. Often after a catastrophic event too many people are talking about the incident while charged with emotion, and they may provide inaccurate details. The plan should explicitly address how affected athletes, teams, or families will be supported if they prefer not to engage with the media, including strategies for keeping the media separate from families and staff who may experience unwanted media attention.[31,34] Finally, consider a plan for a catastrophic incident while traveling. It is recommended to establish a point person who will remain on-site to manage information gathering, act as an institutional representative, and meet the parents or guardians on their arrival at the remote location.[34]

Conducting a Post-Incident Evaluation

The crisis management team should conduct a post-event evaluation. It is critical both to document the details of the event and to allow system improvement. Included in the post-event plan should be a protocol requiring institutional officials or administrators to hold a post-event debriefing meeting of all involved personnel. This meeting should be scheduled to occur within 48 to 72 hours after the incident and should provide the opportunity for an open discussion of what worked, what did not work, and how to improve the response plan. This process

enables revision of the response plan to improve actions during the next emergency.

The debrief meeting also serves to decrease feelings of isolation and provide people affected by the incident with a facilitated session to assist in normalizing thoughts and feelings. Discussion is valuable in exploring differing perspectives of the incident and sharing similar thoughts and feelings.[35] Post-incident counseling should be available to athletes, coaches, and medical staff whenever a traumatic event occurs (details in the following section). Most school districts have designated counseling staff to offer mental health support services. The EAP should identify resource personnel before an emergency arises with contact numbers for use in the post-incident response.[13] Pre-established incident report forms to be completed by all responders should be included to facilitate a summary report with recommendations for site management and modifications to the existing EAP, if needed. Feedback, particularly of a positive nature, should also be provided to responders.[11]

Providing Psychological First Aid

An essential component of the post-catastrophic event plan is to arrange for counseling services for individuals as well as the team affected by the incident. The mental health providers must be established ahead of time. Teammates, coaches, ATs, and staff should be encouraged to participate in grief counseling[34] with trained personnel to talk about death and injury with clarity and compassion. A variety of support personnel who can provide acute intervention when responding to the psychosocial needs of children, adults, and families affected by catastrophic events may be identified. Use local resources such as the local children's hospital, medical center, or community mental health agency as a starting point to identify qualified people to serve in this role. Having these components in place before the need arises is an effective way to help survivors and others affected by a catastrophic incident manage post-catastrophic distress and adversities, and to identify those who may require additional services.[36]

Catastrophic events and critical incidents often lead to feelings of post-traumatic stress that affects people in the workplace and in their personal life. A catastrophic incident may lead to **post-traumatic stress disorder (PTSD)**, which can involve the following:

- Nightmares or dreams related to the events
- Intrusive thoughts
- Preoccupation with details of the incident
- Attempts to avoid trauma-related cues or triggers
- Sense of guilt that the response was inadequate or that not everyone could be saved

- Guilty feelings (i.e., survivor's guilt) for having survived when others died[37]

Psychological first aid (PFA) is an evidence-informed approach used by mental health and disaster response workers to help people of all ages in the immediate aftermath of a catastrophic incident, campus violence, natural disaster, or terrorism. This technique is designed to reduce the initial distress caused by traumatic events and to foster short- and long-term adaptive functioning and coping. Using this strategy does not assume that all survivors will develop mental health problems or long-term difficulties in recovery. Instead, it is based on an understanding that disaster survivors and others affected by such events experience a broad range of early reactions (e.g., physical, psychological, behavioral, spiritual). Some of these reactions cause enough distress to interfere with adaptive coping, and recovery may be helped by support from compassionate and caring PFA responders. These HCPs in mental health may be embedded in a variety of response units, including first-responder teams.[31]

Most responders successfully cope with the psychological aftermath of critical incidents by talking with one another informally. However, professional help may be needed. HCPs should never be ashamed if the services of a mental health professional are needed. Post-incident debriefing may be helpful to reduce post-traumatic stress, but responders experiencing serious or ongoing symptoms may need individual help from a qualified professional.[30]

As part of the ongoing commitment to the AT profession, the NATA has developed the ATs Care program, a peer-to-peer support program to assist members in the aftermath of a critical incident or catastrophic event. A study conducted by NATA found that 82% of members surveyed felt they were not prepared to deal with the psychological impact of catastrophic events.[38] The ATs Care program has created a network of ATs trained in PFA from a leading organization in crisis management training. The training enables members to enhance knowledge of crisis intervention in order to equip them to support their peers in the aftermath of a critical incident. This network of ATs provide psychological and emotional support through the following:[38]

- Phone calls
- On-scene assessment support
- Post-incident defusing
- One-on-one interaction
- Group debriefings and follow-up

The ATs Care program also provides materials to educate NATA members about the psychological impact a critical incident can have on their personal and professional lives.

Evidence for Best Practices in Emergency Preparedness

Acquiring an AED is an essential part of a comprehensive EAP. Many institutions and organizations are financially challenged; however, more effort is needed to explore options for limited budgets. School-based AED programs have demonstrated a high survival rate for people suffering sudden cardiac arrest (SCA) in U.S. high schools. A cross-sectional study of U.S. high schools from 2006 to 2009[23] examined the relationship between high schools having an AED on campus and other measures of emergency preparedness for SCA. A comprehensive survey on emergency planning for SCA was completed by principals, athletic directors, school nurses, and ATs representing 3,371 high schools with and without AEDs. The major findings of this study were as follows:

- 82.6% (2,784 of 3,371) of schools reported having 1 or more AEDs on campus, with an average of 2.8 AEDs per school.
- 17.4% (587 of 3,371) of schools had no AEDs.
- Schools more likely to have an AED were
  - large, with an enrollment of more than 500 students (relative risk [RR] = 1.12, 95% confidence interval [CI] = 1.08-1.16, $P = .01$); and
  - suburban compared to rural (RR = 1.08, 95% CI = 1.04-1.11, $P < .01$), urban (RR = 1.13, 95% CI = 1.04-1.16, $P < .01$), or inner-city schools (RR = 1.10, 95% CI = 1.04-1.23, $P < .01$).
- Schools with 1 or more AEDs were more likely to do the following:
  - Ensure access to early defibrillation (RR = 3.45, 95% CI = 2.97-3.99, $P < .01$)
  - Establish an EAP for SCA (RR = 1.83, 95% CI = 1.67-2.00, $P < .01$)
  - Review the EAP at least annually (RR = 1.99, 95% CI = 1.58-2.50, $P < .01$)
  - Consult EMS to develop the EPA (RR = 1.18, 95% CI = 1.05-1.32, $P < .01$)
  - Establish a communication system to activate emergency responders (RR = 1.06, 95% CI = 1.01-1.08, $P < .01$)

Implementing school-based AED programs is a key step associated with emergency planning for young athletes with SCA. Schools with limited resources should do the following:

- Investigate applicable state and federal grants to fund AED programs.
- Develop funding programs.
- Elicit financial support from the local community, parenting, and fundraising groups.[11]

Understanding sport- and sex-specific patterns is essential to the development of effective, targeted preventive interventions to reduce the incidence and severity of sport-related injuries. Season- or career-ending injuries in adolescents and young adults are concerning because of the limitation on the benefits of physical activity. The costs associated with severe sports injuries include the following:

- Time lost from the sport itself
- Time lost from work or school
- Social costs when removed from the team environment
- Economic costs associated with medical care
- Permanent disability

Rates and patterns of medically disqualifying (MDQ) injuries (season- or career-ending injuries) among U.S. high school athletes overall, by sport, and by sex were determined in U.S. high schools using an injury surveillance system.[2] From 2005 to 2014, participating high school ATs received weekly emails reminding them to complete weekly exposure reports capturing the number of athlete competitions and athlete practices and the number of reportable injuries for each sport in session at their school. This study defined MDQ injuries as those reported by ATs as medical disqualification for the season or career. Major findings from this investigation were as follows:

- 6.0% of all reported injuries (3,599 of 59,862 injuries) were MDQ injuries.
- 60.4% of MDQ injuries occurred during competition.
- Football had the highest injury rate (26.5 per 100,000 AEs), followed by gymnastics (18.6) and wrestling (17.9).
- MDQ injury rates were higher among girls in these sex-comparable sports:
  - Basketball (rate ratio [RR], 1.6; 95% CI, 1.3-2.0)
  - Cross country (RR = 2.6; 95% CI = 1.0-7.5)
  - Soccer (RR = 1.6; 95% CI = 1.3-1.9)
  - Track and field (RR = 2.6; 95% CI = 1.7-4.0)
- Player–player contact was most common (48.2%) MDQ injury mechanism.
- Knee (33.7%) was most commonly injured body site.

- Sprains/strains (35.9%) were most common MDQ injury diagnosis.
- Knee sprains/strains (25.4%) were most common specific MDQ injury.
- Anterior cruciate ligament (ACL) was the most commonly injured knee structure.
- Among boys, fracture was the most common diagnosis in 3 sports, and sprain/strain was the most common in 6 sports.
- Among girls, sprain/strain was the most common diagnosis in 9 sports, and fracture was the most common only in softball.

According to this data set of high school athletes, MDQ injuries vary by sport, sex, and type of athletic activity and occur most frequently as a result of player–player contact. These findings should prompt additional research into the development, implementation, and evaluation of targeted injury prevention efforts.

Summary

Most sport-related injuries are considered minor emergencies; however on occasion, a life-threatening injury or illness may occur, and the AT must be prepared to provide acute or emergency care and transfer care of the patient to EMS or next-level provider. Although catastrophic or critical incidents are not common, planning ahead is essential to maximize patient outcomes and avoid errors or mistakes. Standing orders or protocols with the directing physician as well as an EAP for each venue are necessary to appropriately manage an emergency. The plan should be developed, coordinated, and integrated with EMS; then practiced, reviewed, evaluated, and revised on at least an annual basis. All new members of the medical staff should be informed, educated, and trained for their role in the event of an emergency. The EAP coordinator should implement MCI or post-catastrophic incident plan including plans for venue evacuation. In addition, a PIO should be identified who will release current, correct information, and a crisis management team should be assembled to provide support services such as psychological first aid. All these activities involve professional communication skills that are essential during transfer of care (patient hand-off). With thorough and detailed planning, the AT is able to coordinate the response to an emergency or other critical incident with skill and professionalism.

 Go to the web study guide to complete the case studies for this chapter.

CHAPTER 4

The Emergency Examination

OBJECTIVES

After reading this chapter, you will be able to do the following:

- Identify the components of the emergency examination process.

- Distinguish the steps of the initial assessment process, including identifying and treating life threats.

- Determine appropriate equipment needed and whether immediate transport is required.

- Perform focused assessment based on patient presentation.

In the prehospital setting, performing an emergency examination of an acutely ill or injured patient is essential to appropriate patient care. This chapter serves as an overview of the emergency examination process and provides a preview of the contents of subsequent chapters that relate to specific acute and emergency care situations. The information gathered during the emergency examination process determines which emergency interventions or lifesaving measures will be required. Formulating a **differential diagnosis** and making a **field (on-site) diagnosis** provide guidance for clinical decision making and correct prehospital care. An accurate field diagnosis also determines the equipment needed, additional help required, and urgency of transportation, as well as determines the level of care needed during transport and at the hospital or trauma center. When making clinical decisions, always consider the platinum 10 minutes and the golden hour, described as follows:[1-4]

- *Platinum 10 minutes:* The critical interval during which emergency personnel assess the situation and decide to initiate treatment or transport immediately; it is also known as *stay and play or load and go.*

- *Golden hour*: The approximate time during which treatment of shock or traumatic injuries is most critical for emergency treatment to improve the patient's chances of survival.

A critical component of prehospital care is the emergency examination that begins with the initial assessment. During the initial assessment, the athletic trainer (AT) or health care provider (HCP) must be able to quickly and accurately determine whether the patient is acutely ill (medical) or injured (trauma). Each step in the emergency examination must be performed in order, but with experience, multiple steps can be performed simultaneously. Most experienced practitioners find that in medical patients, 80% of key information in making a diagnosis is from the history and 20% is from the physical exam. However, in acutely injured trauma patients, 20% of the important information comes from the history and 80% from the physical exam.[5] The availability of additional HCPs or trained assistants makes the examination process more efficient, although there must always be one (usually the most-experienced or highest-ranking) provider making final decisions on interventions, treatment, and transportation for further diagnosis and definitive care.

Having a systematic approach to the emergency examination is important to ensure that each patient is examined in a consistent and appropriate manner depending on the individual presentation. The AT or HCP should practice and become competent in conducting each assessment and performing the skills following a consistent routine (figure 4.1). Approaching the examination in an organized rather than random manner is essential so that you don't miss key signs and symptoms. With practice and experience, using a systematic approach to patient examination will become second nature. As addressed in chapter 2, patient care requires informed consent or implied consent in the case of an emergency. This chapter presents the components of the emergency examination including scene size-up, initial assessment, focused history, focused assessment, and reassessment to be conducted individually for each patient.

During the examination of the patient, the HCP gathers information relating to the condition and develops a differential diagnosis list. Essential elements in making a differential diagnosis include information from the patient (symptoms) and information found during the assessment (signs). Both signs and symptoms are abnormal findings that provide valuable information relevant to a potential medical condition. During the history section of the examination, the patient experiences and

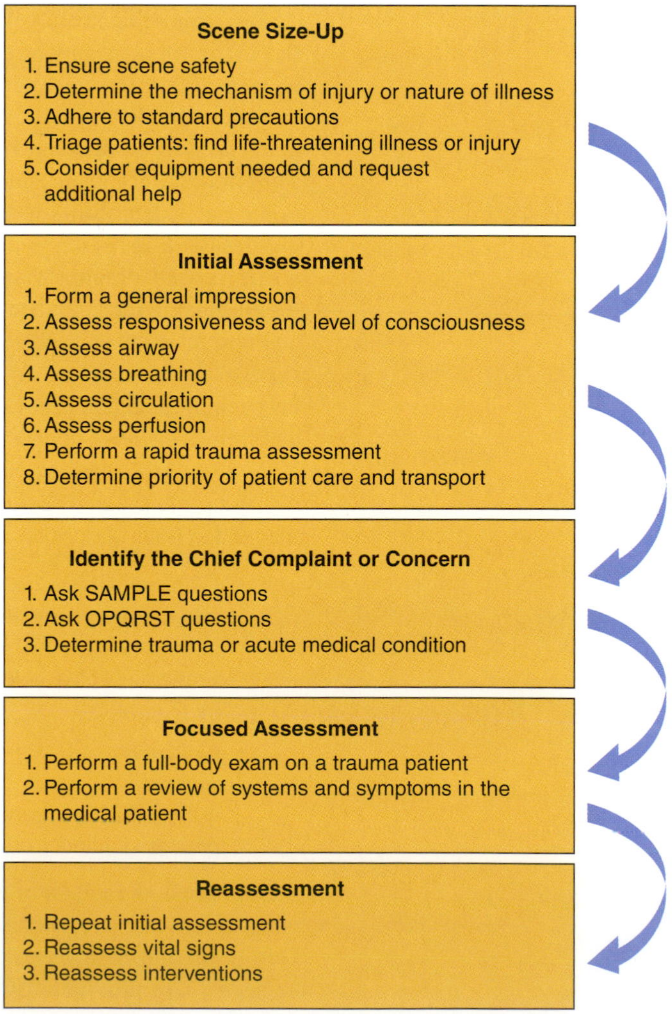

Scene Size-Up

1. Ensure scene safety
2. Determine the mechanism of injury or nature of illness
3. Adhere to standard precautions
4. Triage patients: find life-threatening illness or injury
5. Consider equipment needed and request additional help

Initial Assessment

1. Form a general impression
2. Assess responsiveness and level of consciousness
3. Assess airway
4. Assess breathing
5. Assess circulation
6. Assess perfusion
7. Perform a rapid trauma assessment
8. Determine priority of patient care and transport

Identify the Chief Complaint or Concern

1. Ask SAMPLE questions
2. Ask OPQRST questions
3. Determine trauma or acute medical condition

Focused Assessment

1. Perform a full-body exam on a trauma patient
2. Perform a review of systems and symptoms in the medical patient

Reassessment

1. Repeat initial assessment
2. Reassess vital signs
3. Reassess interventions

FIGURE 4.1   Components of the emergency examination.

reports a **symptom**, whereas the physical assessment reveals a **sign** or objective indication that an abnormal finding exists. For example, a patient reports a symptom of tingling paresthesia; only the patient experiencing the symptom can directly report the sensation. On the other hand, erythema is a sign; anyone observing the skin can identify redness. Individually, signs and symptoms may be nonspecific; but in combination, the AT can begin to suspect or at least suggest certain diagnoses, facilitating the process of developing differential diagnoses. In some cases, the signs or symptoms specifically indicate a diagnosis; however, the AT should be careful not to develop tunnel vision and neglect to rule out the other potential or concomitant conditions that may be present.

In many cases, the HCP will provide emergency care for an acute condition based on symptoms without a definitive diagnosis. For example, a 55-year-old male coach who reports to the AT clinic with chest pain may be having a heart attack, or he may be experiencing heartburn because he ate a chili dog for lunch and forgot to take his acid reduction medication. A thorough history must be performed to determine that he reports pain that is crushing, radiating down the left arm or up into the jaw; he is pale and sweaty; the episode began while he was pushing a sled on the football field; he has a history of coronary bypass surgery; and he is taking nitroglycerin for angina pectoris. Based on this information, it appears he should be treated for a myocardial infarction. Many conditions may have similar signs and symptoms, and with experience, being able to formulate a list of potential conditions or injuries a patient may be experiencing becomes easier. However, it is essential to collect all pertinent information and interpret how the signs and symptoms fit together before deciding on a course of action. Having strong assessment skills is essential in performing an effective, efficient, and thorough examination that serves as the foundation for all patient care.

Scene Size-Up

The beginning of the emergency examination begins with scene size-up. This essential component of the examination reveals information regarding the scope or magnitude of the situation, including the patient's general condition.[5-8] During the scene size-up, the AT observes the patient and her surroundings. Before entering the scene or approaching the patient, consider a general overview of the number of patients and severity of their conditions.

Ensure Scene Safety

Ensuring the safety of the provider is the first element of the scene size-up. Before entering an emergency situation, your own personal safety is a primary concern. If you or

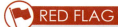

RED FLAG

Consider rapid transport if the initial assessment identifies a priority patient, including but not limited to these conditions:

- Poor general impression
- Unresponsiveness (no gag or cough reflex)
- Responsiveness but not following commands (altered mental status)
- Shock (hypoperfusion)
- Uncontrolled bleeding
- Severe pain in any location or sudden onset of the following:
  - Abdominal pain or pressure
  - Breathing that is abnormal, difficult, or painful
  - Chest pain with systolic blood pressure (BP) <100 mm Hg
  - Choking
  - Coughing up or vomiting blood
- Head injury
- Ingestion of poisonous or toxic substance
- Loss of consciousness or fainting (syncope)
- Mental status changes (unusual behavior, confusion, lethargy)
- Pain that is sudden or severe
- Shortness of breath
- Spine injury
- Vision changes or difficulty
- Vomiting that is severe or persistent

another HCP are injured in the field or other environment, it adds one more patient and potentially redirects response efforts away from the patients most in need of care. For example, an AT witnesses a severe collision of 2 players during a football game. She notices that one of the players was completely limp as he hit the ground. Before running onto the field, the AT must wait for the official to stop the play; otherwise, the AT may be tackled.

While most scenes are safe, being aware of the environment and situation before approaching the patient is an important step in ensuring your own safety. This situational awareness varies from minimal to intense based on changing facts as the response unfolds. Awareness and observation must be part of every response and are essential parts of ensuring the safety[9] of the HCP. Once the AT has determined the scene is safe to enter, the next step in the emergency assessment is to determine whether the patient has a traumatic injury or acute illness.

Determine the Mechanism of Injury or Nature of Illness

Establishing the patient's general condition begins with observing the position of the patient and the immediate environment in determining whether the patient has a traumatic or medical condition. The AT continues to gather information while approaching the patient, including witnessing the injurious incident or observing the surrounding environment. Witnessing the event or gathering information from others who did see the event provides information that may lead to a higher **index of suspicion** for certain injuries or conditions.[5-8]

Mechanism of injury (MOI) is used to establish a trauma patient and helps in the decision-making process of performing a rapid trauma exam or a slower and more focused exam. Unfortunately, MOI does not always match the severity of injury. In many cases the MOI may seem severe, yet the patient is able to stand and walk off the field. In other cases, the MOI appears to be minor, but signs and symptoms indicate a severe injury or medical condition. For example, a head-to-head collision in football may appear to be relatively minor, but the patient may fall to a knee and experience signs and symptoms of a concussion or mild traumatic brain injury (TBI). A lack of significant MOI should not be used to rule out injury, and a significant MOI does not always indicate a severe injury. An essential step in determining a field diagnosis is matching the MOI with trends in **vital signs** or other indications of trauma. As a rule, approach MOI with caution as a significant predictor of injury, because it is not necessarily an important prognostic indicator of severity of injury.[9-10]

RED FLAG

Significant MOIs include the following:[1-4]

- Vehicle collision or ejection from vehicle
- Falls greater than 20 feet (6 m) for adults or 10 feet (3 m) for infants and children
- Bicycle collision
- Blunt trauma to the chest
- Penetrating wounds of the head, chest, or abdomen
- Head trauma with intracranial lesion
- Spinal cord injury
- Exsanguination or uncontrolled hemorrhage

Nature of illness (NOI) is specific to making a correct field diagnosis of an acute medical condition. Assessments of medical conditions are largely based on history, while trauma exams are predominantly based on physical examination. The information gathered relating to the NOI is essential in forming the **general impression**. For example, patients with severe respiratory distress or altered levels of responsiveness are high priorities for acute care and transportation.[7] Because the NOI begins during the patient assessment, it is important to make an accurate determination of the type of medical problem the patient has by evaluating information from a variety of sources. This process of information gathering may begin with a coach who brings the patient to you, from teammates or family members, or from the **patient presentation**.

Adhere to Standard Precautions

Standard precautions are the infection prevention practices intended to reduce the risk of transmission of blood-borne and other pathogens from both identified and unrecognized sources of infection.[6] These minimum infection prevention practices are essential in any setting in which health care is delivered and apply to all patient care, regardless of suspected or confirmed infection status of the patient.[9] These best practices are designed to both protect the HCP and prevent the provider from spreading infections from patient to patient or from patients to healthy people. According to the Centers for Disease Control and Prevention (CDC),[10] standard precautions include hand hygiene; use of personal protective equipment such as gloves, gowns, or masks; safe injection practices; safe handling of potentially contaminated equipment and surfaces; and respiratory hygiene (cough etiquette). For more about standard precautions, see chapter 2.

Triage Patients: Find Life-Threatening Illness or Injury

Making decisions about the most appropriate care and transport for severely injured or acutely ill patients in the prehospital setting is a critical skill. **Field triage** of trauma patients is the process of rapidly and accurately evaluating patients to determine the extent of their injuries and the appropriate level of medical care required. The goal is to transport all seriously injured patients to medical facilities capable of providing appropriate care, while avoiding unnecessary transport of patients without critical injuries to trauma centers.[11] These decisions are made through the triage process, which involves an assessment of pathophysiology, MOI/NOI, and special patient considerations.[3] Triage is traditionally used in situations involving mass casualties (e.g., active shooter, terrorism) or natural disasters in which multiple casualties could stress or overwhelm local prehospital and hospital resources.[10] However, in the prehospital setting, the field triage process is designed to ensure that the appropriate decision is made to transport one or more acutely injured or ill patients and to ensure they are sent to the hospital or trauma center (discussed in chapter 3) best equipped to manage their specific injuries. According to the CDC's *Guidelines for Field Triage of Injured Patients*,[10] the decision to transport injured or acutely ill patients depends on specific criteria related to physiologic, anatomical, MOI, and special considerations. Prehospital HCPs must be skilled in recognizing individual injured patients who require transport to a specialized trauma center following standard recommendations and guidelines.

In the event of a mass casualty incident (MCI) or other catastrophic event such as a bus accident, terrorism, or active shooter, field triage decisions are primarily made during the scene size-up and initial assessment in which life-threatening injuries are recognized and initially treated. **S**imple **t**riage **a**nd **r**apid **t**reatment (START) is a triage method used by first responders and medical personnel to quickly classify victims during an MCI based on the severity of injury.[14-16] Table 4.1 organizes injury categories by color.

The START strategy evaluates the severity of injury of each victim as quickly as possible, then identifies or tags each victim in about 30 to 60 seconds. If available, triage tags or tape is placed near the patient's head so that when more help arrives, the patients are easily recognizable for the extra help to ascertain the direst cases.[11,14-16] A triage tag (figure 4.2*a*) is a card that is easy to use and understand with front and back body diagrams. The tag is color coded for patient prioritization with perforated tear-offs. The tag is placed on each patient, then the colors are torn off until the color at the bottom matches the patient's classification. The rescuer completing the initial START triage does *not* fill out the tag; she only tears off the color strip and attaches the tag to the patient. The rescuer should write the time and initial the tag. The string allows for easy attachment. The tags are sequentially numbered for recordkeeping. Tape imprinted with triage terms (figure 4.2*b*) is used to prioritize patients using color categories (see table 4.1).

As responders approach the scene, all ambulatory patients are asked to walk to a designated location for further assessment. Patients who can walk unaided and follow commands are designated "minor" (color coded green). Those in whom no respirations are present are tagged as "deceased" (color coded black). Patients who did not move are then assessed individually using the acronym RPM, described as follows:[10,11,16]

- ***Respiration:*** After manually positioning airway ≤30 breaths/min
- ***Perfusion:*** Presence of radial pulse, or capillary refill <2 sec
- ***Mental status:*** Ability to follow commands

RED FLAG

Field triage guidelines: Any of the following findings indicate that the patient should be transported to a trauma center.[2-4,10,12,13]

- *Physiologic criteria:* Glasgow Coma Scale < 14, systolic BP <90 mm Hg, or respirations < 10/min or > 29/min
- *Anatomic criteria:* Penetrating injuries to the head and torso, flailing chest, multiple long-bone fractures, or other significant injuries
- *Significant MOI criteria:* Fall from height for adult >20 feet (6 m) or child >10 feet (3 m) or 2-3 times the child's height, ejection from a vehicle, or a death in the same passenger compartment or significant intrusion of damage into the passenger compartment
- *Special patient or scene considerations:* Age of the patient, pregnancy, additional specific injuries, and the judgment of the prehospital HCP[10]

TABLE 4.1 **Triage Color Categories**

Color	Priority	Description
Red: Immediate	1	May survive with immediate medical attention; may not survive if treatment is delayed. Any compromise to respiration, hemorrhage control, or shock control could be fatal.
Yellow: Delayed	2	Should survive with medical attention. Injuries are potentially life-threatening, but can wait.
Green: Minor	3	Walking wounded. Does not require rapid medical attention but may require stabilization, monitoring, or transport.
Black: Expectant/Deceased	4	Seriously injured and unlikely to survive. Pain medication only should be provided until death.

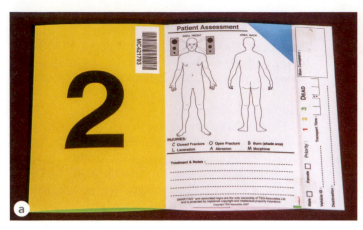 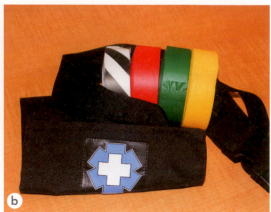

FIGURE 4.2   *(a)* Triage tag for patient prioritization. *(b)* Triage tape.

4.2b Courtesy of Dr. Eric J. Fuchs, ATC, NRAEMT.

Although it is straightforward to use, the START triage technique is limited in its rigid assignment of patients to categories based on vital signs (described in the following section) that may change rapidly, as well as human factors (inability to detect a radial pulse, difficulty in visualizing breathing, etc.).[11]

Consider Equipment Needed and Request Additional Help

A medical emergency such as a myocardial infarction in a spectator or a potential cervical spine injury in an athlete will both require specialized equipment and an ambulance with basic life support equipment and personnel (discussed in chapter 3). Patients meeting the field triage criteria of red or yellow may need advanced life support and rapid transport to the nearest level I trauma center. Depending on the location of the venue or facility, rural areas may require resources such as air medical evacuation to the nearest appropriate level trauma center. Many trauma or medical situations require equipment or other resources to properly handle the emergency, such as the following:

- Automated external defibrillator (AED) and pulse oximeter
- Supplemental oxygen, bag-valve mask
- Materials to control bleeding
- BP cuff and stethoscope
- Equipment removal supplies (e.g., shears, screwdriver, cutter)
- Portable/mobile electrocardiogram (ECG) monitor
- Spine board and accessories for c-spine stabilization

- Ambulance and emergency medical services (EMS) personnel
- Law enforcement or fire department
- Helicopter for air medical evacuation

All the components of the size-up are interrelated for the HCP's safety and rapid, efficient patient care. Cardiac and pulse oximetry monitors are not mandatory for performing an initial assessment. However, these pieces of equipment are essential in accurate recognition of some medical conditions. If equipment and additional resources are available, all should be present at the patient's side and used to facilitate the next step in the emergency examination—the initial patient assessment.

Initial Assessment

The initial assessment (also called the primary survey) involves quickly determining any life-threatening conditions and immediately treating these conditions. Approaching the patient during the scene size-up involves evaluating potential or actual scene hazards and threats, protecting yourself, identifying threats to life, and deciding on the need for additional resources. You must take these critical steps before making initial direct contact with the patient. The initial patient assessment begins with greeting the patient and introducing a sense of trust and rapport. The patient must feel that you are calm, in control, and competent. The overall goals of the initial assessment (which in an experienced HCP are often conducted simultaneously) are as follows:[3,4,17]

- Ensure scene safety.
- Determine MOI and NOI, establish whether the patient is a medical or trauma patient.

- Adhere to standard precautions.
- Form a general impression.
- Determine responsiveness or level of consciousness using the Glasgow Coma Scale (GCS) or Alert, Voice, Pain, Unresponsive (AVPU) scale.
- Stabilize the cervical spine.
- Assess airway, breathing, circulation, disability, and exposure.
- Identify and begin to treat immediate or imminent threats to life.
- Determine the priority of care.

The components of the initial assessment may be altered based on the patient presentation keeping in mind that an in-depth physical exam or assessment of vital signs (described next) is performed during the focused assessment.[7] Once you have completed these steps, then it is possible to effectively determine priorities in patient care and transport.

According to the *Advanced Trauma Life Support Manual,* physical examination of the patient begins with the ABCDE approach:[3,17]

Airway while maintaining cervical spine

Breathing

Circulation with control of severe hemorrhage

Disability or deficits

Exposure

The common ABC approach includes additional assessments of disability and exposure (figure 4.3).

Glasgow Coma Scale

The Glasgow Coma Scale (GCS) is the gold standard for assessing the level of consciousness in trauma patients (see chapter 8 for more detail). The areas assessed are as follows:[2-4,12,13]

- *Eye opening:* 1 = none to 4 = open spontaneously
- *Verbal stimulus:* 1 = none to 5 = oriented
- *Motor stimulus:* 1 = none to 6 = obeys commands
- *Combined score:* < 8 = unresponsive or comatose

AVPU Scale

The AVPU scale is used to simplify the classification of mental status. The scale uses these 4 possible outcomes:[1,5,8,13]

1. **A**lert: The patient is fully awake (although not necessarily oriented). This patient has spontaneously open eyes, responds to voice (although may be confused) and has bodily motor function. Alert can be subdivided into a scale of 1 to 4, relating to "*Alert and Oriented*" to person, time, place, and event. For example, a fully alert patient might be considered "alert and oriented times 4" (AAO × 4) if the patient could correctly identify his name, time, location, and the event.

2. **V**oice: The patient makes some kind of response when you talk to her, which could be in any of the 3 component measures of eyes, voice, or motor. For example, the patient's eyes open on being asked "Are you OK?" The response could be a grunt, moan, or slight move of a limb when prompted by your voice.

3. **P**ain: The patient makes a response to application of pain stimulus, such as a sternal rub (central pain stimulus) or a peripheral stimulus such as squeezing the fingers. A patient with some LOC (a fully conscious patient would not require a pain stimulus) may respond by using his voice, moving his eyes, or moving part of the body.

4. **U**nresponsive: The patient does not give any eye, voice, or motor response to voice or pain.

To avoid unnecessary tests on patients who are clearly conscious, always start with the best (A) to worst (U) outcomes.

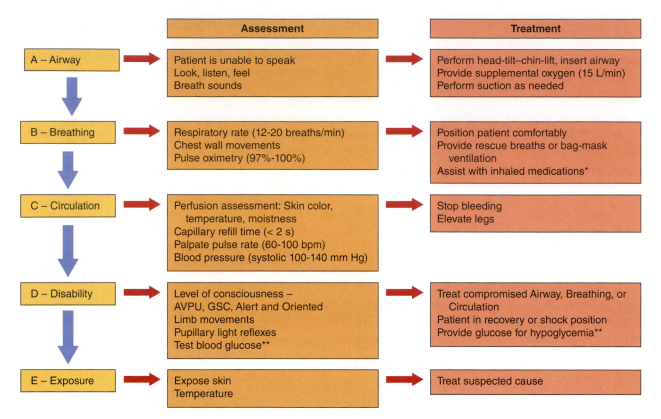

	Assessment		Treatment
A – Airway	Patient is unable to speak Look, listen, feel Breath sounds		Perform head-tilt–chin-lift, insert airway Provide supplemental oxygen (15 L/min) Perform suction as needed
B – Breathing	Respiratory rate (12-20 breaths/min) Chest wall movements Pulse oximetry (97%-100%)		Position patient comfortably Provide rescue breaths or bag-mask ventilation Assist with inhaled medications*
C – Circulation	Perfusion assessment: Skin color, temperature, moistness Capillary refill time (< 2 s) Palpate pulse rate (60-100 bpm) Blood pressure (systolic 100-140 mm Hg)		Stop bleeding Elevate legs
D – Disability	Level of consciousness – AVPU, GSC, Alert and Oriented Limb movements Pupillary light reflexes Test blood glucose**		Treat compromised Airway, Breathing, or Circulation Patient in recovery or shock position Provide glucose for hypoglycemia**
E – Exposure	Expose skin Temperature		Treat suspected cause

FIGURE 4.3 ABCDE approach with important assessments and treatment options. Normal adult ranges are provided, although a patient with values within the given ranges may still be critically ill.

AVPU = Alert, Voice, Pain, Unresponsive; GSC = Glasgow Coma Scale

*Inhaled medications and respiratory conditions are detailed in chapters 5 and 10.

**Blood glucose and hypoglycemic emergencies are detailed in chapter 13.

Disability refers to the patient's level of consciousness that can be affected by profound **hypoxia**, **hypercapnia**, **hypoperfusion**, or drugs such as sedatives or analgesics. *Exposure* in the ABCDE approach refers to removing the patient's uniform or cutting the sleeve, socks, or shoes to allow visualization of the injured area.[3,17] The steps of the initial assessment are described in detail in the following sections and summarized in figure 4.4.

Form a General Impression

The general impression is formed while determining whether the patient has a significant MOI (see the Red Flags earlier in this chapter) or a life-threating condition. In patients with a significant MOI, the general impression may require a rapid trauma assessment (described later in this chapter).[1-4] In patients with no significant MOI who have been determined to have no life-threatening injuries, you form the general impression by observing the overall general appearance; ask yourself, "How does the patient look?" Forming a general impression includes identifying the following:

- Poor **habitus** or general appearance
- Diminished physical appearance
- Difficulty breathing
- Low pulse oximetry (<95% saturation)
- **Cyanosis**

This initial step facilitates the beginning of the physical assessment regarding the patient's general appearance (e.g., anatomical alignment, anxious, or lethargic). If the patient is not familiar to you, introduce yourself to the patient by stating, "Hi, I am [Your name]. I am an athletic trainer, and I am here to help you." After the patient introduction, ask the patient her name and use her name throughout the assessment. The general impression includes taking in as much information as possible, particularly if the patient may lose consciousness. The general impression provides a basis for further assessment and treatment and provides an appropriate sense of urgency. However, it is important to constantly monitor and respond to any changes in the patient's condition. During this phase of the initial assessment, do the following:

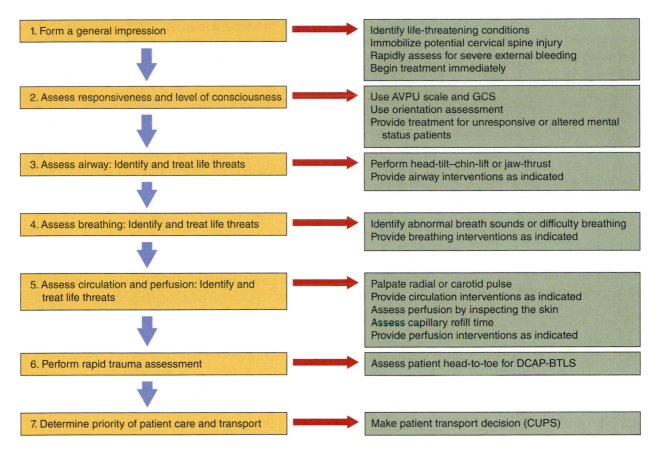

FIGURE 4.4 Overview of initial assessment for all patient situations.

AVPU= **A**wake, **V**erbal, **P**ainful, **U**nresponsive classification of mental status; DCAP-BTLS = **D**eformities, **C**ontusions, **A**brasions, **P**unctures/Penetrations-**B**urns, **T**enderness, **L**acerations, **S**welling; CUPS = **C**ritical, **U**nstable, **P**otentially unstable, **S**table

- Ask (or estimate) age, sex, and sport (or position).
- Establish priorities and chief complaint; ask, "Where does it hurt?"
- Establish responsiveness and mental status using the GCS or AVPU scales.
- Identify and manage immediate life- or limb-threatening conditions.
- Control major bleeding and open wounds.
- Stabilize the cervical spine in patients with a high index of suspicion for cervical spine injury.

Identify and Treat Life-Threatening Conditions

A patient with a life-threatening condition requires immediate recognition and intervention to save her life. Once identified, a life-threatening condition must be treated as soon as possible. While treatment is under way, continue assessing the patient to identify other conditions that require intervention while EMS arrives. It is essential to quickly identify life-threatening conditions, initiate treatment, and make the decision to rapidly transport the patient at any time during the assessment.

Stabilize Potential Cervical Spine Injury

Generally, an ill or injured person should not be moved. The decision to provide **spinal motion restriction** in the prehospital setting depends on the patient presentation and mechanism of injury.[3,18] The spine should be maintained in anatomical alignment and with movement minimized, with or without the use of specific adjuncts such as collars.[18] Any unconscious patient should be

> 🚩 **RED FLAG**
>
> Life-threatening conditions include the following:[1-7]
> - Compromised airway
> - Inadequate breathing or ventilation
> - Impaired circulation or perfusion
> - Severe bleeding

suspected of having a cervical spine injury until otherwise determined. Suspicion of cervical spine injury should be high in any patient with a significant MOI or witnessed trauma to the head or cervical spine, combined with pain or point tenderness on the spine, symptoms of weakness, numbness, or paresthesia bilaterally.[3] A patient with an injury that suggests a neck, back, hip, or pelvic involvement should not be rolled onto her side; instead, she should be left in the position in which she was found in order to avoid potential further injury. If leaving the patient in the position found is causing the airway to be blocked, or if the area is unsafe, move the patient only as needed to open the airway and to reach a safe location.[18] Appropriate spinal motion restriction is discussed further in chapter 9.

Assess and Control Life-Threatening External Bleeding

Trauma patients must be quickly assessed to identify and immediately control major external bleeding that causes a threat to life. You should perform this step before addressing airway or breathing concerns because in some cases, **exsanguinating** blood loss can occur rapidly, quickly resulting in shock or death if not appropriately treated. Signs of severe blood loss include the following:

> 🚩 **RED FLAG**
>
> Indications for spinal motion restriction are as follows:[3,18,19]
>
> - Unconsciousness
> - Pain or tenderness on palpation of the neck or spine
> - Complaint of pain in neck or back
> - Sensory deficit or muscle weakness involving the torso or upper extremities
> - Paralysis or other neurologic complaint such as numbness, tingling, or partial paralysis in the extremities
> - Fall from a greater than standing height
> - Intoxication or lack of alertness
> - Other painful injuries, especially of the head and neck
> - Difficulty or inability to communicate
> - Distracting injury that diverts the patient's attention from other, more severe injuries such as a painful femur fracture that prevents the patient from recognizing pain in the back or neck

- A wound with large volume of bleeding
- Evidence of excessive bleeding such as blood on the patient's uniform or on the turf near the patient
- Steady blood flow from a damaged blood vessel, such as a deep laceration
- Spurting blood from a lacerated artery, such as from an open fracture

An unconscious patient should be rapidly assessed for severe bleeding, and the patient may need to be carefully log-rolled to assess bleeding from wounds on the other side of the body. To perform a rapid assessment for severe external bleeding, do the following:

- Quickly sweep with gloved hands, lightly touching the body from head to toe.
- Pause to check for blood on your gloves.
- Maintaining in-line stabilization with the spine, carefully log-roll the patient and sweep or inspect for severe bleeding on the other side of the body.

Rapid external blood loss must be controlled with appropriate techniques, such as application of firm, direct pressure. When direct pressure is not effective for severe or life-threatening bleeding, the use of a hemostatic dressing combined with direct pressure may be considered.[18] Initially you can control severe bleeding using direct pressure with your gloved hand and then applying a sterile bandage over the wound. Direct pressure usually stops bleeding within a few minutes from the normal process of blood clotting. Minor bleeding should not be addressed at this time. Quickly move on to the next steps of the initial assessment and assess responsiveness, then identify and treat life threats. Hemorrhage control is described in detail in chapter 6.

Assess Responsiveness and Level of Consciousness

The patient's mental status should be determined during the initial assessment by assessing responsiveness and LOC (see chapter 8). Using the GCS or AVPU scale, describing mental status is important so that findings can be relayed in a clear and concise manner to other medical providers. The 3 LOCs are as follows:[5-8,20]

- Unconscious
- Conscious with altered LOC
- Conscious with unaltered LOC

A patient who is responding to questions, forming complete sentences, and appropriately responding to the situation is generally considered to be responsive. Therefore, this patient would be categorized as conscious with unaltered LOC. A patient who is exhibiting altered mental status should be further evaluated using special testing (described in detail in chapter 8).[5-8,20]

Assess Airway

Before moving on to the next steps of the initial assessment, it is essential to recognize and manage any airway obstruction or potential for development of an obstructed airway. An airway obstruction can result in partial or complete blockage of air movement into and out of the lungs, leading to inadequate perfusion of the entire body.[7] To prevent death or permanent disability to the patient, the patient must have a patent airway and adequate perfusion throughout the emergency examination. Patients who are responsive and are talking or crying have an open airway. In patients with difficulty breathing, adequacy of the airway and the status of breathing must be thoroughly evaluated (details in chapter 10). Unresponsive patients require continuous airway maintenance and monitoring until arrival at the emergency department. When it is confirmed that the airway is clear, proceed to the next step of the initial assessment and assess breathing.

Assess Breathing

The ability to speak or hold a brief conversation is a good indicator of the ability of a conscious patient to breathe adequately. However, a patient who can speak only one word at a time or must stop every 2 or 3 words to catch his breath is having significant difficulty breathing. An alert, oriented patient that is talking and not anxious will likely have adequate breathing. A patient with altered mental status, loss of consciousness, or injury to any part of the face, mouth, nose, neck, or chest requires evaluation of the ability to breathe (see chapter 10). Also note that gasping and intermittent breathing, combined with chest pain and absence of external trauma, is associated with a cardiovascular event (agonal breathing), and the HCP should begin CPR and attach an AED to the patient. A patient with injuries to the head, face, neck, or thorax may have difficulty breathing and requires intervention to assist in breathing.[18,21,22] Assessing respiration rate and quality are described in the Monitor the Critically Injured or Ill Patient of this chapter.

For trauma or unresponsive patients, do the following:

- Maintain an open airway, using suction or oral or nasal airway (as described in chapter 10) if necessary.
- Administer **high-concentration oxygen** 10-15 L/min using a face mask with oxygen reservoir.
- Determine the need for **positive-pressure ventilation**.
- Treat critical chest injury.

For a medical or responsive patient with difficulty breathing or poor oxygen saturation, determined with pulse oximetry, do the following:

- Position the patient in a semi-reclined position or other comfortable position that allows improved breathing.
- Provide oxygen via cannula or mask at 6-10 L/min.

Patients who are alert and responsive may be breathing adequately but may be hypoxic. Carefully assess the patient's vital signs (see next section) to ensure adequate breathing and perfusion. Depending on the chief complaint and further assessment findings, supplemental oxygen may be indicated.

Assess Circulation

Circulation is evaluated holistically by assessing the patient's mental status, pulse, and signs of adequate perfusion. Assessing circulation provides information regarding the ability of the cardiovascular system to perfuse blood to major organs, including the brain, lungs, heart, kidneys, and the rest of the body. An unresponsive patient requires quickly checking the carotid pulse and indications of signs of life. A patient who is in cardiac arrest may not have a cardiac rhythm that requires a shock; however, some trauma patients may be in ventricular fibrillation and an AED may indicate shock advised. For example, a shockable rhythm is common in *commotio cordis,* literally "agitation of heart," a condition in which generally young and otherwise healthy individuals are struck on the chest by a baseball or other object and suddenly collapse from trauma-induced ventricular fibrillation.[8] A variety of other conditions can result in impaired circulation, including the following:

- Hemorrhage (chapter 6)
- Shock (chapter 6)
- Cardiac conditions (e.g., myocardial infarction; chapter 11)
- Vascular compromise (e.g., peripheral or extremity trauma; chapter 11)

An absent pulse is an indication to initiate the emergency action plan (as described in chapter 3) and begin CPR (see chapter 11), including applying an AED. In a responsive patient, check the radial pulse to obtain a general pulse rate; however, at this point, do not take the time to get an actual rate. Throughout the initial assessment, continue to monitor the patient while determining interventions (if any) that are required. Assessment of vital signs is described in detail later in the chapter.

- In a stable patient, recheck pulse every 15 minutes.

- In an unstable patient, recheck pulse every 5 minutes.

- A patient who becomes pulseless requires CPR and potentially defibrillation with an AED.

Continue to examine the patient for obvious bleeding; severe, life-threatening bleeding requires management during the initial assessment. Less-severe or minor bleeding should be treated later in the emergency examination. Assessing circulation is an important part of the initial assessment that began with forming a general impression. With practice, the emergency examination can be completed quickly, allowing you to focus on finding and treating other potentially life-threatening conditions. The next step is to assess perfusion to determine whether the patient is experiencing shock so that it can also be treated at this time.

Assess Perfusion

Assessing **perfusion** provides information about the ability of the cardiovascular system to adequately supply the body with blood and oxygen. A normally functioning circulatory system perfuses the skin with oxygenated blood, allowing it to maintain a normal color, temperature, and moisture for the environment. Normal skin should be warm and dry (see Monitor the Critically Injured or Ill Patient). However, exercising athletes usually have warm and moist skin. Inadequate blood flow to the skin results in abnormal findings such as pale, cool skin, which is associated with hypoperfusion of the brain, lungs, heart, or kidneys. In most situations, hypoperfusion is caused by shock, and the degree or duration of hypoperfusion may determine whether a patient will sustain permanent

injuries.[7] Inspecting the skin includes noting the patient's skin color, temperature, moisture, and capillary refill (described later). Other relevant skin conditions combined with current clinical findings could be considered a potential red flag.

Perform a Rapid Trauma Assessment

In patients with MOI consistent with trauma, it is important to rapidly perform an assessment to determine potential life-threatening injuries. In a responsive patient, obtain a symptom history before and during the rapid scan or trauma assessment. During this step of the emergency examination, the severity of the patient's injuries is estimated, and the decision to transport (or not) is reconsidered. To rapidly assess the patient from head to toe, most HCPs use this mnemonic, DCAP-BTLS, to guide the evaluation:[1-7]

Deformities and **D**iscolorations

Crepitus and **C**ontusions

Abrasion and **A**vulsion

Penetrations and **P**unctures

Burns

Tenderness

Lacerations

Swelling and **S**ymmetry

Following the rapid trauma assessment, you must determine the priority of patient care and transport. It should take no more than 90 seconds to perform the assessment and identify other injuries or conditions that must be treated or stabilized before the patient is transported to the AT facility or hospital. During this phase of the examination, a rapid head-to-toe trauma assessment is performed to identify soft-tissue or

---

CLINICAL SKILLS

Performing a Rapid Trauma Assessment

The rapid trauma assessment is performed on patients with significant MOI by examining them from head to toe to determine potential life-threatening injuries. In a patient with no significant MOI who has been determined to have no life-threatening injuries, skip this step and continue to the focused history and physical exam. For example, a patient requiring a rapid trauma assessment would have sustained a fractured arm with no other injuries and no life-threatening conditions. To perform the rapid trauma assessment, quickly identify existing or potentially life-threatening conditions by palpating each of the following areas for DCAP-BTLS:

- Assess the head, face, and neck.
- Assess the chest, abdomen, and pelvis.
- Assess all 4 extremities bilaterally; and include distal pulses and motor and sensory function.
- Assess the back and buttocks in any patient with suspected spine injury; maintain in-line stabilization while rolling the patient on her side in one motion.

musculoskeletal injuries, inspecting and palpating for DCAP-BTLS.

Determine Priority of Patient Care and Transport

In life-threatening situations, the golden hour is the critical time for emergency treatment. Once EMS arrives, the platinum 10 minutes will determine whether to initiate treatment or transport immediately. At this point in the prehospital emergency examination, the priority determination is the point at which all information gathered in the initial assessment is synthesized and the priority and status of the patient are decided.[7] In general, a properly performed initial assessment should provide sufficient information about the status of the patient to make this determination. The standard nomenclature in emergency medicine for priorities in patient transport decisions is CUPS (see table 4.2). In situations not involving triage, using these categories is helpful in determining priority of treatment and emergency transport.

A severe injury or condition that is found during the initial assessment may require immediate treatment or rapid transport. For example, you may identify internal hemorrhage by finding a distended or firm abdomen, deteriorating vital signs, or symptoms of referred pain indicating a lacerated spleen. As soon as these conditions are identified, immediate treatment and rapid transport should be initiated. As with any patient with high-priority condition, protecting the spine or fractured extremities prior to transport is critical. If you have any uncertainty of the need for spinal motion restriction or splinting an extremity, err on the side of caution and provide stabilization. Spend as little time as possible while properly assessing a patient who has sustained significant or severe trauma. For critical or unstable patients, whenever possible attempt to reasonably assess, treat, immobilize, and transport the patient within 10 minutes.[1,7]

Identify the Chief Complaint or Concern

Although the initial assessment and the general impression offer a plethora of information about the patient, the history provides information that will be relevant to the patient's presentation or to identifying complications to treatment. The patient's **chief complaint** or concern is the symptom or condition that is most serious and that is most concerning to the patient. Generally, the chief complaint is the reason the patient has sought help or the reason someone calls for assistance. For example, a coach calls the AT into the locker room where an athlete collapsed and fell onto the floor hitting his head on the bench. The patient may have an underlying cardiac condition that is causing shortness of breath and **syncope**. It is important to talk to anyone who may have witnessed the event and can provide information on the events surrounding the trauma or medical condition. You can obtain information relating to the chief complaint of an unconscious athlete by talking to the following people:

TABLE 4.2   **Standard EMS Nomenclature for Patient Transport Decisions (CUPS)**

Priority	Severity of illness or injury	Transport decision
Critical	Patient receiving CPR, in respiratory arrest, or requiring and receiving life-sustaining ventilatory/circulatory support	High priority; transport immediately. Continue intervention started.
Unstable	Poor general impression Unresponsive with no gag or cough reflexes	High priority; transport as soon as possible. Continue to monitor/assess.
Potentially unstable	Responsive but unable to follow commands Difficulty breathing Pale skin or other signs of poor perfusion (shock) Uncontrolled bleeding Severe pain in any area of the body Severe chest pain, systolic BP <100 mm Hg Unable to move any part of the body	High priority for transport; provide on-site treatment. Transport as soon as practicable.
Stable	Minor illness, minor isolated injury, uncomplicated extremity injuries Any patient not categorized as critical, unstable, or potentially unstable.	Low priority for transport; provide treatment on-site. Continue to reassess for changes in status.

Based on New York Department of Health (2017); Pollack and Beck (2012).

- Teammates
- Coaches
- Parents/guardians or other family members
- Spectators

Ask follow-up questions to thoroughly assess the chief complaint and history of present illness.

Ask SAMPLE Questions

In all patients with trauma or acute medical conditions, ask SAMPLE questions (table 4.3) to ascertain the details of the patient's chief complaint or concern.[1-7,12] These are the questions most commonly used in the prehospital setting on alert, responsive patients. As previously mentioned, these questions may be asked of bystanders, coaches, or parents/guardians, especially in pediatric or adolescent patients. Patients with severe trauma may benefit from a brief or basic version of the questions as appropriate to reduce discomfort or pain. Document all relevant findings from the SAMPLE history on the patient's record or SOAP note.[5,12]

Ask OPQRST Questions

A common mnemonic HCPs use to accurately describe a patient's history of the illness or injury is OPQRST. Each letter stands for an important line of questioning (table 4.4) for the patient assessment of pain or other symptoms as follows:[1,7,23]

- *Onset.* Ask the patient about the onset of the event or what she was doing when the symptoms started (e.g., exercising, resting, stressed) and if that activity prompted the pain. Other aspects of the onset may include a description as a sudden, gradual, or an ongoing chronic problem.

- *Provocation (or palliation).* When determining provocation or palliation, ask the patient if any movement, pressure (i.e., palpation), or other factor makes the problem better or worse, including whether the pain is relieved with rest.

- *Quality.* The patient's description of the quality of the pain should use open-ended questions, such as "Can you describe your pain?" The patient may need examples of pain descriptions such as *sharp, dull, crushing, burning,* or *tearing* or a description of the pain pattern, such as *intermittent, constant,* or *throbbing.*

- *Region and radiation.* Ask the patient to identify exactly where on the body the pain is located and whether it radiates (extends) or travels to other body regions. Many patients need to be instructed to take one finger and point to where it hurts to localize the pain. Radiating pain may be described as shooting pain, such as in sciatic nerve pain traveling down the back of the leg. Referred pain, such as in a myocardial infarction, may radiate through the jaw and arm.

- *Severity.* Severity of pain is usually assessed with a quick pain score on a scale of 0 to 10, where 0 is no pain and 10 is the worst possible pain. The patient may need a relative reference point, such as "compared to the worst pain you have ever experienced." Because pain is a highly subjective and relative experience, it is important to determine the worst injury the patient has had for comparison.

TABLE 4.3   **SAMPLE Questions for Assessing the Patient's Chief Complaint or Concern**

Component	Key questions and follow-up
Signs/**S**ymptoms*	Signs: Observe and document (e.g., vital signs, swelling, deformity). Symptoms: "What hurts? Where does it hurt?"
Allergies	"Do you have any allergies?" Follow up on medication, food, or other environmental factors. Check for medical alert tags.
Medications	"Are you taking any medications? Have you taken medications recently?" Follow-up includes prescriptions, over-the-counter medications, or recreational/illicit drugs; reassure the patient of confidentiality and that the information is needed for treatment purposes.
Past Illnesses	Pertinent or relevant past history: "Have you ever had any illnesses? Operations? Have you ever been admitted to a hospital?" Inquire further about medical problems and past surgical procedures.
Last oral intake	"When did you last eat or drink something? What was it?" A hypoglycemic patient may have skipped breakfast.
Events leading up to present illness/injury	"What happened? How did this happen?" The events leading up to the injury provide information about anatomic structures or mechanisms.

*Added to the traditional AMPLE approach.

TABLE 4.4   **OPQRST Questions for Obtaining History of Present Illness or Injury**

Descriptor	Sample questions
Onset	"What were you doing when the symptoms started?"
Provocation or **P**alliation	"Does anything make the symptoms worse?" "Does anything make the pain feel better?
Quality	"What does the pain or discomfort feel like?" "Can you describe your pain to me? "
Region and **R**adiation	"Where do you feel the pain or discomfort?" "Does the pain or discomfort travel anywhere else?"
Severity	"How bad is the pain?" "How would you rate the severity of your pain?" "Rate it on a scale of 1 to 10; 10 is the worst pain possible."
Time	"How long has the problem been going on?" "How has the pain progressed over time?"

Based on New York Department of Health (2017); Pollack and Beck (2012); Mistovich, Limmer, and Werman (2011).

- *Time*. Length of time the patient has been experiencing symptoms.

Document the findings of the OPQRST history for later reference; it is usually part of the Subjective portion of a SOAP note or medical record.

Determine Trauma or Acute Medical Condition

The patient's chief complaint and the history of illness or injury help determine the rest of the emergency examination as a medical- or trauma-focused assessment. A patient who has sustained a fractured arm who is in severe pain but has no other injuries and no life-threatening conditions will be assessed and treated differently than a patient with a medical complaint such as severe abdominal pain who is conscious, able to adequately relate the chief complaint, and has no life-threatening conditions. After determining the patient's chief complaint and history of present illness or injury, proceed to the focused assessment and perform a full-body exam (for a trauma patient) or a review of systems (for a medical patient) followed by recording **baseline vital signs**. The details of system-specific evaluations are provided in the forthcoming chapters. The following sections in this chapter focus on the general approach to a trauma or acute medical patient.

Focused Assessment

After the initial assessment is complete and life-threatening conditions have been identified and treated, the secondary (focused) assessment should be completed. The purpose of the focused assessment is to perform a systematic physical examination of the patient. In a critical or unstable patient, a rapid full-body exam may

take place in an ambulance. In a stable patient without significant MOI or altered mental status, the focused assessment may take place on the sideline, locker room, athletic training clinic, or other location where the patient can be fully examined. The physical examination may focus on a certain area or system of the body often determined by the chief complaint. Depending on the patient's status (see table 4.2) and determination of a trauma or medical patient, rapid full-body assessment or a focused assessment on a specific injury or body system is warranted. For example, a critical or potentially unstable trauma patient should receive a rapid full-body exam; and a stable or potentially unstable patient should receive a slower, more deliberate focused assessment.

Perform a Full-Body Exam on a Trauma Patient

Assessment of a trauma patient is primarily based on the full-body physical exam (table 4.5) or a focused assessment on a specific body part (addressed in subsequent chapters). If a patient is in stable condition with an isolated complaint, perform a focused assessment on the specific body part before determining priority for transport for further care. For example, for a patient with an isolated ankle injury, perform a focused examination on the specific body part. (Chapter 7 discusses focused assessment of musculoskeletal injures.) An unresponsive patient with unwitnessed collapse or a patient with significant MOI should be quickly assessed from head to toe.[5,12,23] Significant MOI is severe tissue damage resulting from acute direct trauma or delayed indirect injury, defined as follows:

- *Direct:* Severe direct tissue damage to critical organs (e.g., heart, brain, spinal cord) that is responsible for most immediate trauma deaths.

TABLE 4.5 **Full-Body Exam of the Trauma Patient**

Perform a full-body exam on an unresponsive patient with unwitnessed collapse or a patient with significant MOI. Be sure to provide manual spine stabilization as appropriate. In less than 3 minutes, quickly assess the patient from head to toe. Using inspection and palpation, assess the following areas:

Region of the body	Signs of significant MOI
Head and face Eyes and ears	Signs of brain damage such as CSF leakage from the ear or nose (halo test) Signs of brain swelling (altered mental status, **flexion posturing, extension posturing**, fixed or unequal pupils) Signs of skull fracture (Battle's sign or raccoon eyes)
Nose and throat	Airway compromise Facial fracture Severe bleeding on the face, nose, or mouth
Neck	Jugular vein distention Tracheal deviation
Chest and thorax	Open wounds on the chest Paradoxical thorax movement (part of chest moving inward during inhalation) such as flail segments (rib fracture) Absence of or inadequate breath sounds or chest movement
Abdomen	Pain, tenderness, rigidity (tensed abdominal muscles) indicating organ injury identified by quadrant
Pelvis	Pain, tenderness, instability (by assessment through pelvic compression) and deformations or indications of pelvis fracture
Upper and lower extremities	Deformations indicate bone fractures or joint dislocations. Inspect and palpate bilaterally. Assess PMS (distal pulses, motor function, and sensory function) or CMS. Control active bleeding.
Back and spine	Inspect and palpate the posterior body to identify wounds (e.g., gunshot, puncture, bony deformity, discoloration/ecchymosis, or other signs of trauma). Use caution because moving, turning, or rolling the patient is contraindicated if suspected spinal injury exists.

MOI = mechanism of injury; CSF = cerebrospinal fluid; PMS = pulse, motor, sensory and is abbreviated as "PMSx4" if all 4 extremities are intact; CMS = circulation, movement, sensation

Based on Mistovich and Karren (2014); Jordan (2017); Mistovich, Limmer, Werman (2011).

- *Indirect*: Injury effect from external or internal hemorrhage that causes progressive decline in BP and organ perfusion, leading to cellular dysfunction, organ failure, and eventually death (see chapter 6, Shock).[12]

Perform a Review of Systems and Symptoms in the Medical Patient

After immediate life threats are assessed and the patient is stable, a more thorough evaluation is completed. If only limited conversation is possible, use SAMPLE history. In a stable medical patient who is conscious, alert, and can adequately relate her chief complaint, take more time to perform a complete history with a review of systems (symptoms). Based on the chief complaint, use a differential diagnostic approach to identify the signs and symptoms of possible conditions. In medical patients, more information can usually be obtained from the history than from the physical exam. Use the history and physical examination findings (described in subsequent chapters) to rule in or tentatively rule out potential causes of the medical condition and make a treatment decision.[5,12]

The review of systems is a systematic method of assessing the whole body. It consists of a series of questions designed to identify factors contributing to the acute medical condition; see table 4.6. Reviewing questions organized by the main body systems is the opportunity to identify symptoms or concerns that the patient did not mention or did not notice earlier in the assessment. For example, in a patient with a chief complaint of chest pain, you should ask questions about cardiovascular conditions (e.g., shortness of breath, pressure on chest, referred pain,

TABLE 4.6   **Review of Systems and Symptoms**

In a stable medical patient who is conscious, alert, and can adequately relate her chief complaint, complete a review of systems and symptoms. Use questioning for each body system to prompt the patient to reflect on symptoms.

Body systems	Sample question(s) Follow-up questions with description for any positive symptoms
Cardiovascular system	Do you have chest pain? Pressure? Is your heart skipping beats? Do you feel faint? Shortness of breath? Ankle swelling?
Respiratory system	Are you having difficulty breathing? Do you have a cough? Do you have pain when you take a deep breath?
Nervous system	Do you have a headache, loss of consciousness, or dizziness? Have you had difficulty remembering? Thinking? Mood changes? Do you have numbness or tingling? Burning or shooting pain?
Cranial nerve symptoms	Have you had blurry or double vision? Numbness on your face? Weak facial muscles?
Eyes, ears, nose, or throat (EENT)	Have you had any problems with your eyes, such as blurry vision, pain, watery eyes, redness, or itching? Do you wear glasses or contact lenses? Have you had problems with your ears such as hearing problems? Do you have ringing in your ears? Ear pain? Do you have frequent nosebleeds? Frequent sneezing? Any recent sore throat or sores in your mouth? Any problems with your teeth or gums?
Gastrointestinal system	Have you had any weight changes? Heartburn? Painful or difficulty swallowing? Abdominal pain? Nausea or vomiting? Diarrhea or constipation?
Genitourinary system	Have you had frequency, pain, or urgency in urination? Blood in urine?
Endocrine system	Have you been excessively thirsty? Have you experienced increased urination? Increased appetite?
Skin	Do you have any rash? Have you had a spider or other insect bite? Have you had an allergic reaction in the past?
Musculoskeletal system	Do you have joint pain with swelling or tenderness? What makes it feel better? Worse? Does it hurt to move? Do you have a family history of joint disease?

Document the review of systems similar to the following format: "Patient is not currently having problems with headaches, dizziness, visual disturbances, hearing loss, cough or chest pain. She does note shortness of breath after running in the mornings. She denies abdominal pain, nausea, vomiting, diarrhea, blood in the stool, difficulty with urination, weakness or numbness in the legs, but she has had allergy symptoms, which she has difficulty explaining."

Based on Mistovich and Karren (2014); Henry and Stapleton (2012).

or fainting) as well as questions relating to the gastrointestinal system (e.g., nausea, vomiting, or heartburn). The review of systems does not need to be overly detailed, but questioning the patient likely will define the causes of the presenting condition. Questions should reflect a variety of common and important clinical conditions that may have similar symptoms. With practice and experience, you will develop your own particular technique or style to efficiently and thoroughly conduct the review of systems for acute medical conditions.

Monitor the Critically Injured or Ill Patient

After the focused assessment, baseline vital signs should be recorded and reassessed periodically (**serial vitals**), depending on the patient's status. Obtaining vital signs is essential to establish baseline levels, monitor the patient's status, and identify deterioration in the patient's condition. Trends in vital signs are essential in determining the severity and progression of the patient's condition as well as the patient's response to treatment. Monitor vital signs more or less frequently depending on the patient's status as follows:

- *Stable patient*: Reassess vital signs approximately every 15 minutes or at least twice.
- *Unstable patient*: Reassess vital signs every 5 minutes until the patient is transported to the ED.

Baseline vital signs are the first set of measurements while follow-up, repeated sets of vital signs, or serial vitals, are especially important for patients with acute medical conditions. Each of the following vital signs should be performed and documented in the patient record:[7,8]

- Assess perfusion by inspecting skin color, temperature, and condition.
- Assess pulse (heart) rate, rhythm, and quality.
- Assess respiration rate and quality.
- Measure BP using sphygmomanometer and stethoscope.
- Measure blood oxygen saturation using a pulse oximeter.
- Assess pain using a numeric rating scale.

Assess Perfusion by Inspecting Skin Color, Temperature, and Condition

Initially, inspect the skin as an indicator of adequate perfusion and overall condition of the patient. Inspecting the skin is an important part of assessing circulation and provides information about the ability of the cardiovascular system to adequately perfuse tissues with blood. The skin functions as an indication of the overall condition of the patient because of its many functions, including protection from infection, body fluid balance, and body temperature regulation through the surface of skin. Placing the hands on the patient's skin is one of the most important and readily accessible ways of evaluating circulation, perfusion, blood oxygen level, and body temperature. A normally functioning circulatory system perfuses the skin with oxygenated blood, allowing it to maintain a normal color, temperature, and moisture for the environment. Inadequate blood flow to the skin results in abnormal findings such as pale, cool skin, which is associated with hypoperfusion of the brain, lungs, heart, or kidneys. In most situations, hypoperfusion is caused by shock, and the degree or duration of hypoperfusion may determine whether a patient will sustain permanent injuries. Normal skin should be warm, pink, and dry; while skin that is cool, cold, moist, clammy, hot, flushed, or mottled may indicate an acute or emergent condition (see Skin Characteristics and Indications). Any other skin condition combined with relevant clinical findings should be considered a potential red flag.[7]

Inspect Skin Color

Because many blood vessels lie near the surface the skin, inspecting the color of the skin is an easily accessible way of demining the amount of blood circulating through these superficial blood vessels. Blood that has adequate oxygen saturation is red; in lightly pigmented people it

Skin Characteristics and Indications

Characteristic	Indications
Pale or mottled	Early-stage shock
Clammy (cool, wet/diaphoretic)	Uncompensated shock
Cyanotic	Late-stage shock
Red	Anaphylactic shock, poisoning, overdose or other medical condition
Flushed	Exercise, sun exposure, heatstroke
Yellow	**Jaundice**, liver disorder
Pale, white, ashen, or gray	Perfusion, reduced peripheral circulation, or low oxygen saturation
Hot	Fever, heat exposure, localized infection
Warm	Normal
Cool	Inadequate perfusion, shock, or cold exposure
Cold	Hypothermia, frostbite
Wet (diaphoretic) or moist	Shock, sweating, cardiac, or diabetic emergency
Abnormally dry	Severe dehydration, spinal injury

results in a pink color. Various levels of pigmentation do not alter the skin's underlying color. Inspect the fingernail beds, mucous membranes in the mouth, the lips, underside of the arm, and palm (which are usually less pigmented), and the conjunctiva of the eyes. Skin or mucous membranes that appear blue or cyanotic are red flags for uncompensated shock indicating a life-threatening medical emergency.[7,8,24]

Palpate Skin Temperature, Turgor, and Moisture

Assess skin conditions by palpating the patient's skin for temperature, moisture, and **turgor** (deformation). Because skin color, temperature, and moisture are often related, these signs should be considered together. The condition of skin is usually considered as the temperature (i.e., warm, hot, cool) using the back of your hand against the patient's forehead or joint. Include an observation of the amount of moisture on the skin (e.g., dry, moist, or wet). Keep in mind the following:

- Normal skin is generally warm and dry.
- Skin that is slightly moist but not covered excessively with sweat is described as clammy, damp, or moist. In the early stages of shock, the skin will become slightly moist.
- Cool, cold, or clammy (cool and moist) skin indicates hypoperfusion or another life-threatening condition.[8]

You can determine skin's resistance to turgor by grasping a small pinch of skin between the fingers; hold the skin for a few seconds, then release it (figure 4.5). Skin turgor that is **within normal limits (WNL)** snaps rapidly back to its normal position. Skin with poor turgor takes

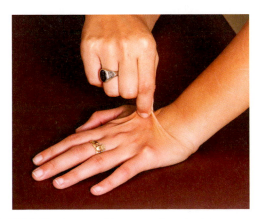

FIGURE 4.5   Assess skin turgor by pinching up a portion of skin (often on the back of the hand) between 2 fingers so that it is raised for a few seconds. Skin with poor turgor takes more than 3 seconds to return to its normal position.

more than 3 seconds to return to its normal position. In a healthy person, when the skin on the back of the hand is grasped between the fingers and released, it returns to its normal appearance either immediately or relatively slowly. Skin turgor is a sign of fluid loss (dehydration), often caused by excessive exercise in the heat, diarrhea, or vomiting. Infants and young children with vomiting or diarrhea can rapidly lose body fluid if insufficient water is ingested, particularly when a fever is present. As a person ages, the skin returns much more slowly to its normal position after having been pinched between the fingers. When assessing turgor in elderly people, you may use skin over the forehead or sternum.[24,25]

When recording or reporting the skin assessment, describe color first, followed by temperature, moisture, and turgor where relevant. For example, write or say, "Skin: pale, cool, clammy, turgor WNL"[7] or "Skin is red, hot, and dry with turgor >3 sec." Assessing skin characteristics during the initial assessment is important, because these findings are associated with hypoperfusion and delaying treatment or ignoring these indications can lead to serious consequences.[24]

Assess Capillary Refill Time

Capillary refill is evaluated in patients to assess the ability of the circulatory system to perfuse the capillaries close to the surface of the nail of the fingers or toes. In an uninjured limb, capillary refill time (CRT) provides an indication of the patient's sufficiency of perfusion. The capillary refill is an indicator of tissue perfusion and, in some cases, severe dehydration. Capillary refill can be affected by the patient's position, age, history as a smoker, history of medical problems such as diabetes, or certain medications. The capillary refill test is important to perform with musculoskeletal injuries to the upper or lower extremity to determine peripheral circulatory compromise, resulting in hypoperfusion of the distal extremity as an indicator of potential hypoxia and necrosis (see chapter 12 for more details).

The capillary refill test, also called the nail blanch test, is performed by placing your thumb on the patient's fingernail with your fingers on the underside of the patient's finger while gently compressing (figure 4.6). The blood will be forced from the capillaries in the nail bed, causing **blanching**. Remove the pressure applied against the tip of the patient's finger. The nail bed will remain blanched for a brief period. As the underlying capillaries refill with blood, the nail bed returns to its normal pink color. Normal capillary refill time is usually less than 2 seconds when there is good blood flow to the nail bed. A positive test will indicate hypoperfusion, shock, peripheral vascular injury, severe dehydration, hypothermia (including frozen tissue; frostbite), and vasoconstriction. Record capillary refill time as CRT = WNL, or CRT = ~5 sec.[7]

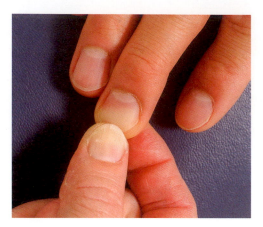

FIGURE 4.6   Capillary refill test. Normal capillary refill time is less than 2 seconds.

Assess Pulse (Heart) Rate, Rhythm, and Quality

The pulse is the heart rate per minute. It is usually measured on the radial artery at the wrist or the carotid artery in the neck. In patients who are in shock or if the radial pulse is difficult or undetectable, use the common carotid artery to assess pulse. You may also obtain the pulse by palpating peripheral pulse points (see chapter 7 for details). Pulse rhythm can be described as regular or irregular. A normal pulse rhythm should have a constant, regular rhythm, and the interval between each contraction should be the same. An irregular rhythm may be indicated by an early or late beat or a missed or "skipped" pulse beat. For an irregular pulse in a patient with signs and symptoms suggesting a cardiovascular problem, the patient likely requires intervention such as advanced cardiac assessment and life support. As with any deviation from expected findings, it is important to determine, if possible, whether the irregular rhythm is new or it represents a normal or chronic condition for the patient.[7] Palpate the radial pulse at the patient's wrist, count the number of beats for 30 seconds, and multiply by 2 to obtain the heart rate in beats per minute (bpm).[7,24,26,27] When recording the heart rate, always report the quality of the pulse. A pulse palpated at the radial or carotid arteries should be strong and easily palpable. Describe a stronger than normal pulse as "bounding" and a pulse that is weak and difficult to feel as "weak" or "thready."[7,24,26,27]

Assess Respiration Rate and Quality

Breathing, or respiration, is the mechanical process of ventilation that includes inhalation and exhalation. Normal breathing is a continuous, uninterrupted, and automatic process that occurs without conscious thought, effort, marked sounds, or pain. Patients with difficulty breathing (**dyspnea**), such as a severe asthma attack or anaphylactic shock, often require significant effort to draw a breath. Additional effort in breathing is indicated by retraction or indentations above the clavicles and intercostal spaces or using accessory muscles of respiration including the sternocleidomastoid, pectoralis major, and abdominal muscles. Nasal flaring and **seesaw breathing** indicate inadequate breathing. Difficulty breathing is also indicated in a patient who can speak only 2 or 3 words without pausing to take a breath (2-to-3-word dyspnea). Patients with significant difficulty breathing often assume a posture allowing easier breathing such as the **tripod position** or sniffing position, in which the patient is sitting and leaning forward on outstretched arms with the head and chin thrust slightly forward.[7] Respiratory rate is the rhythm in which breaths occur, measured in breaths per minute. Quality of respirations can be described as normal, shallow, labored, or noisy.

Assess respirations in a conscious patient after palpating the radial pulse. Assess breathing in an unconscious patient by watching the patient's chest rise and fall while listening for breath sounds with your ear near the patient's mouth and nose and feeling for air through the mouth and nose during exhalation. Chest rise and breath sounds should be equal on both sides of the chest. Identify difficulty breathing, including use of accessory muscles of respiration or tripod position (see chapter 8). To record respiration rate (usually while in position from palpating the radial pulse), count the rise and fall of the patient's chest for 30 seconds and multiply by 2 to obtain the breathing rate per minute. Note breathing rate as respirations per minute (rpm) and quality of respiration.[7,24,26,27]

Measure Blood Pressure

BP measurement is essential during the emergency examination in the prehospital setting. Techniques for measuring BP in the field and other prehospital environments include auscultatory and palpation techniques. Determining blood pressure in the prehospital setting requires a high degree of clinical experience and practice. In this setting, establishing trends in a patient's blood pressure (table 4.7) before transport to a more controlled hospital environment is more important than the absolute value of the blood pressure.[28] Generally, athletes have lower resting blood pressure than sedentary individuals and **hypotension** is nonpathological in these individuals and is considered abnormal only when combined with symptoms of shock or other signs of distress. **Hypertensive crisis** is an emergency with severe elevation in BP (>180/120 mm Hg) associated with evidence of new or worsening target organ damage.[28,29] Hypertensive urgencies are situations associated with severe BP elevation in otherwise stable patients without acute or impending change in target organ damage or dysfunction. The actual BP level may not be as important as the rate

TABLE 4.7   Normal and Abnormal Blood Pressure

Classification	Systolic (mm Hg)	Diastolic (mm Hg)
Child (6-11 yr)	97-120	57-80
Adolescent (12-15 yr)	102-120	61-80
Adult	<120	<80
Hypotension*	<90	<60
Hypertension	>130	>80
Hypertensive crisis	>180	>120

*Only abnormal when combined with symptoms of shock or other signs of distress.

Data from Pollack and Beck (2012); Bickley and Szilagyi (2013); Marx and Rosen (2017); Pickering et al. (2005); Whelton et al. (2017).

of BP rise; patients with chronic hypertension can often tolerate higher BP levels than previously normotensive individuals. Hypertensive emergencies require immediate transport and reduction of BP (not necessarily to normal) to prevent or limit further target organ damage. Examples of target organ damage include hypertensive encephalopathy, acute ischemic stroke, acute myocardial infarction, acute heart failure with pulmonary edema, unstable angina pectoris, dissecting aortic aneurysm, or acute renal failure (see chapter 11). Hypertensive crisis is an indication for referral to the emergency department, immediate reduction in BP in the emergency department, or hospitalization for such patients.[28,29]

The auscultatory technique is the predominant method of clinical measurement and uses a stethoscope and a sphygmomanometer to listen for **Korotkoff sounds**. The standard location for BP assessment is wrapping the cuff around the left arm, with the stethoscope at the antecubital fossa over the brachial artery. While a manometer gauge contains mercury, more commonly an aneroid gauge is used to directly measure the pressure inside the inflatable cuff in the prehospital setting. The mercury manometer is considered the gold standard, but the aneroid or electronic devices are preferred in the field because they are sturdier and do not contain mercury. The well-stocked medical kit should have at least 2 cuff sizes to allow measurements in patients with different arm size (e.g., adolescent female v. adult male). The appropriately sized cuff should be fitted snugly and smoothly, then manually inflated by squeezing the rubber bulb until the artery is completely occluded while using the stethoscope to listen. As the cuff pressure is slowly released, blood begins to flow in the artery and the turbulent flow creates a *whooshing* or pounding (Korotkoff sound).[28] Reading the gauge at this time provides the systolic pressure and, as the pressure in the cuff is further released and no sound can be heard (no Korotkoff sound), reading the gauge at this time provides the diastolic pressure.[7,24,26-29]

In the prehospital setting, many situations make obtaining an accurate BP challenging and may affect the accuracy of the readings. For example, a patient that collapses after running would have a higher blood pressure than a resting adult; however, at rest, athletes generally have a lower blood pressure than untrained individuals. In a high-noise environment such as a football game or noisy AT facility, it may be necessary to estimate BP using a palpation technique; however, only the systolic reading can be obtained. Increasingly, noninvasive blood pressure (NIBP) devices (automatic blood pressure cuffs) are used in the clinical setting and conveniently monitor the patient's BP at automatic intervals. Occasionally, this mechanical device displays incorrect or erroneous reading, especially in hypotensive patients. Therefore, always obtain at least one baseline manual BP and occasionally additional manual readings to compare with the NIBP device and help reduce the impact of the erroneous readings.[7]

Measure Blood Oxygen Saturation

A pulse oximeter is a small, portable, and inexpensive medical device that indirectly monitors peripheral oxygen saturation (SpO_2) of the blood and pulse rate (figure 4.7). This indirect measure is a safe, quick, easy, and convenient determination of peripheral oxygen saturation that is correlated with arterial blood gas or direct measures of oxygen saturation through blood sample analysis. The device uses 2 wavelengths of light that pass through the body part to a photodetector. The pulse oximeter device detects changing absorbance of the wavelengths due to pulsing arterial blood. The device excludes venous blood, skin, bone, muscle, fat, and nail polish (usually).

To measure perfusion or oxygen saturation with a pulse oximeter, place the sensor device on an area of the patient's body with thin skin, usually a fingertip or earlobe. Avoid excessive finger movement, and remove nail polish; with false nails, use the device in a different area, such as the earlobe. Normal blood oxygen (hemoglobin) is 95% to 100% saturated. An abnormal finding of SpO_2 ≤94% indicates hypoxia and should be treated

Measuring Blood Pressure Using the Auscultatory Technique

Step 1: Properly prepare the patient.

1. Adhere to standard precautions as appropriate. Explain the procedure to the patient if possible.
2. Place the patient in a comfortable position (sitting or lying) with forearm supported and the palm upward. Resting heart rate should be measured after the patient has relaxed for 5 minutes.
3. Expose the arm about 5 inches above the elbow by rolling up the sleeve or cutting the garment as needed. Examine the exposed arm for wound, injury, or other reason to not use the arm for BP; otherwise, use the other arm.
4. Place the patient's palm in a supinated position with the elbow extended and at the same level as the heart.

Step 2: Use proper technique for BP measurements.

1. Select the correct size cuff such that the bladder encircles 80% of the arm and note whether a larger- or smaller-than-normal cuff size is used.
   - Small adult: 8-10 inches (22-26 cm) arm circumference
   - Adult: 10-13 inches (27-34 cm) arm circumference
   - Large adult: 14-17 inches (35-44 cm) arm circumference
2. Support the patient's arm (e.g., resting on a desk).
3. Position the middle of the cuff on the patient's upper arm at the level of the right atrium (the midpoint of the sternum).
4. Snugly (not tightly) wrap it around the upper arm with distal edge of the cuff about 1 inch (2.5 cm) above the antecubital space. Ensure the center of the inflatable air bladder (usually marked by an arrow on the cuff) is placed over the brachial artery.

Step 3: Take the proper measurements needed.

1. Using your nondominant hand, palpate the brachial artery in the antecubital fossa to determine where to place the stethoscope. Place the bell of the stethoscope firmly against the artery with the fingers of your nondominant hand. Listen for the pulse.
2. Using your dominant hand, hold the rubber pump and the turn the valve using thumb and first finger.
3. While listening through the stethoscope, close the valve and pump the ball pump until you no longer hear pulse sounds. Continue pumping to increase cuff pressure an additional 20-30 mm Hg above the expected systolic pressure.
4. Slowly deflate the cuff at a rate of 2 mm Hg/sec, watch the gauge, and carefully listen for the first pulse waves (Korotkoff sounds) to be clearly heard; this is the systolic blood pressure. Note the pressure.
5. Continue slowly releasing air until the pulse sound disappears (no Korotkoff sound); this is the diastolic pressure. Note this pressure where the sounds stopped.
6. Open the valve, release the remaining air, and remove the cuff.

Step 4: Properly document accurate BP readings.

1. Document the patient's BP, date, time, and the patient's position when the reading was obtained.

Based on Pollack and Beck (2012); Bickley and Szilagyi (2013); Marx and Rosen (2017); Pickering et al. (2005); Whelton et al. (2017).

Estimating Systolic Blood Pressure Using the Palpation Technique

This technique is most often used in the prehospital setting in which the ambient noise makes it difficult to hear the pulse using the stethoscope. Use these measurements with caution, because only a minimum systolic pressure can be roughly estimated using the palpation technique; diastolic BP cannot be estimated using this method. Whenever possible, use the more accurate auscultatory method for obtaining systolic and diastolic BP.

Follow these procedures:[30]

1. Place the BP cuff around the upper arm.
2. Inflate the cuff rapidly to 70 mm Hg and increase by 10-mm Hg increments while palpating the radial pulse. Note the level of pressure at which the pulse disappears.
3. Slowly release the air from the cuff. Note the pressure when the pulse reappears.
4. When the radial pulse returns, this is the systolic pressure.
5. Use a "p" to note the palpation technique in place of the diastolic pressure.

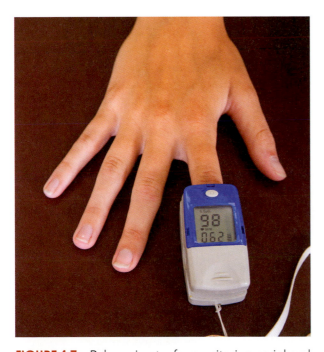

FIGURE 4.7 Pulse oximeter for monitoring peripheral oxygen saturation and pulse rate.

with supplemental oxygen using a nasal cannula or face mask (described in detail in chapter 5).[24,27]

Assess Pain Using a Numeric Rating Scale

Pain is often considered the fifth vital sign, and it is important to determine a baseline level of pain that is subjective for each patient. While pain is a subjectively reported symptom, it is important to be able to assign a number for the patient's level of pain at the beginning of the emergency examination and then repeated throughout the process. Pain level is also essential in determining the effectiveness of the intervention in either reducing the pain or exacerbating it. Using a pain scale is an effective way to measure the patient's pain intensity. Common pain scales are based on self-report subjective data and should be measured and recorded throughout the examination. The most common and widely used pain scale is the numeric pain rating scale (table 4.8). The patient verbally reports pain on a scale from 0 (no pain) to 10 (worst pain imaginable). Document the pain score with other vital signs in the patient care record.

TABLE 4.8   **Numeric Pain Rating Scale**

Rating	Pain intensity	Examples
0	No pain	Normal
1-3	Mild pain	Nagging, annoying, interfering with some ADLs
4-6	Moderate pain	Interfering with most ADLs
7-10	Severe pain	Disabling, worst imaginable, unable to perform any ADLs

ADLs = activities of daily living

Reassessment

Regardless of the priorities assigned to the patient and transport to higher level of care, the final component of the prehospital emergency examination is reassessment. Depending on the condition of the patient, reassessment of vital signs should be performed every 5 minutes for an unstable patient and every 15 minutes for a stable patient. This component of the exam is performed to reassess the following:

- Initial assessment
- Baseline and serial vital signs
- Chief complaint or new complaints
- Response to treatment or interventions

The reassessment aids in determining the effectiveness of interventions started earlier in the process (figure 4.8). Based on findings, treatment should be modified as appropriate, or new treatment should be started. The reassessment is a key time for monitoring the patient for trends indicating improvement or deterioration, and this level of attention continues as the patient is being transported to the hospital. This final step in the process is designed to reassess the patient for changes that may require modification or a new intervention. As transport arrives, be mindful of any new developments or conditions that must be treated. The reassessment is an important step in gathering critical information about condition of the patient in order to provide efficient and effective emergency care and patient hand-off to the next-level care provider.

Patient Hand-Off

Using effective and efficient communication is essential in the intense, fast-paced, emergency transfer of patients. Good communication skills are particularly important for ATs and other providers first on the scene to clearly convey critical patient information to other health care professionals. Documenting and reporting should follow an evidence-based format during these three elements of the handoff process:

- Exchanging information
- Transferring responsibility of care
- Providing continuity of care

SBAR (table 4.9) is a communication tool originally developed for military communication that has been adapted to give HCPs a simple tool for structured communication and reporting. It is critical to document the medical record, medication, and patient history before reporting to the next-level HCP. Rather than speaking in broad terms about the care plan, provide the next-level care provider a clear and succinct clinical bottom line. For example, answer the question "What's the problem,

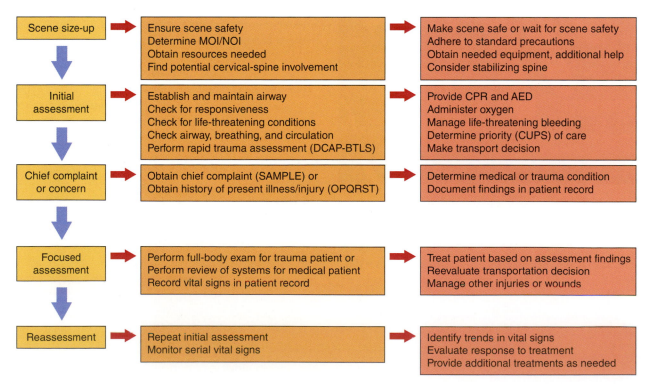

FIGURE 4.8 Patient assessment flow chart.

TABLE 4.9 **Patient Hand-Off SBAR Template**

Use the following template to provide concise, effective communication to other HCPs.

Category of information (Time)	Questions to answer	Data to include	Example
Situation (10 sec)	What is happening?	Your name, title/role, and institution/location Patient's name and current problem	"Hi, I'm Michelle, the head AT here at Springfield High School. This is Jamar. He has a dislocated ankle with a potential bimalleolar fracture."
Background (20 sec)	What is the context and background?	Patient's age, gender MOI/NOI Other pertinent information Recent history Medications, allergies	"Jamar is 17 years old and has chronic ankle instability. He was tackled with his foot planted in the turf. He has no other relevant health history, no drug allergies, and is negative for sickle cell trait. We called his parents who are about 20 minutes away with his health insurance information."
Assessment (20 sec)	What physical assessment data will the physician need to know?	Perform a complete assessment before calling EMS Pertinent physical assessment findings Name the problem	"His vital signs are stable; however, his pain level is 9/10, he has paresthesia distal to the injury, and his capillary refill time is approximately 4 sec in the affected foot."
Recommendation (10 sec)	What actions will correct the problem?	Suggestions to resolve the problem Urgency of transport	"We applied a vacuum splint with his toes exposed to continue to assess distal sensation and circulation. He needs rapid transport to the ED for X-rays and possible surgical reduction and fixation. We can have the parents meet you at the hospital."

ED = emergency department; EMS = emergency medical services; MOI/NOI = mechanism of injury/nature of illness

Based on Eberhardt (2014); Narayan (2013); Pope, Rodzen, and Spross (2008); Powell (2007).

and what is needed?" The SBAR format is helpful because it is a similar to SOAP (**S**ubjective, **O**bjective, **A**ssessment, **P**lan) notes used for medical documentation. Use appropriate assertiveness to concisely communicate SBAR to the EMS team that has just arrived on the scene as follows:[31-35]

• *Situation.* Introduce yourself (name, title or role, and institution or location). Briefly (no longer than 10 seconds) identify the problem or concern and provide a short description of what is happening. Finally, provide the patient's status and major symptoms (e.g., chest pain or syncope).

• *Background.* Provide the patient's name, age, sex, and chief complaint. Provide context of the patient's medical status (no more than 20 seconds) and pertinent medical history (e.g., medical problems, traumatic injuries, or surgical procedures). Indicate most important medical-based information or MOI/NOI to set up the assessment.

• *Assessment.* Survey the situation to determine a course of action (no more than 20 seconds). Provide medical data such as vital signs, test results (e.g., neurological testing), pain intensity score, and other quantitative or qualitative data. Include differential diagnosis and working field diagnosis, avoiding irrelevant or overly detailed information. Specifically mention vital signs outside of normal limits, severity of the patient's status, and additional concerns.

• *Recommendation.* Indicate explicitly (no more than 10 seconds) what actions are required and with what urgency they are needed. Discuss possible solutions for the patient's needs.

Evidence for Injury Scoring Systems

Description of the anatomical severity of injuries in trauma patients is important. In attempts to standardize trauma severity to help trauma centers predict outcomes, a systematic method for scoring injury severity may provide objective information for physicians and trauma centers. Although predicting mortality in trauma patients using a scoring system may be helpful, good clinical judgment is essential. Clinical decisions should never be based solely on a statistically derived injury severity score. However, scoring systems can serve to quantitatively estimate the severity of an injured patient which may be useful in outcome assessments.[36,37]

Following an injury, timely description of the anatomical severity of injuries in trauma patients is important. The Injury Severity Score (ISS) is an anatomical scoring system that provides an overall score for patients with multiple injuries.[38] Baker et al. introduced the ISS in 1974 as a means of summarizing multiple injuries in a single patient.[39] Since that time it has been revised and updated so that it now provides a reasonably accurate ranking of the severity of injury. Each of the 6 body systems' injuries are given an Abbreviated Injury Scale (AIS); the most severe injury in each body system is used for the ISS. Although originally intended for use with vehicular injuries, its scope is increasingly expanded to include other injuries. The AIS is a simple numerical method that trauma physicians use for grading and comparing injuries by severity in this range:

- Minor
- Moderate
- Serious
- Severe
- Critical
- Unsurvivable

To calculate the ISS, only the highest AIS in each body region is used. The three most severely injured body regions have their score squared and added together to produce the ISS (table 4.10). For example, a patient with a cerebral contusion, flail chest, ruptured spleen, and fractured femur would score an ISS of 50. Online ISS calculators can help with the formula.

While the ISS has been regarded as the gold standard since its inception, the system has major limitations. The system is difficult to calculate in the clinical setting; and in a patient with multiple injuries, only one injury per body region is considered, limiting its predictive power. Therefore, in 1997 Osler introduced a modification to the ISS to improve its accuracy and named it the New Severity Injury Score (NISS). The NISS is the sum of the squares of the three highest AIS scores for each patient, regardless of body region.[40] Using meta-analysis, Deng et al. systematically evaluated and compared the accuracy of the ISS and the NISS in predicting mortality.[37] A random effects model resulted in evidence (table 4.11) concluding that the NISS is similar to the ISS in predicting mortality.

However, more research is required to determine the appropriate use of these scoring systems based on specific patient condition and trauma type.

TABLE 4.10   Sample Injury Severity Score (ISS) Calculation

Assess severity of worst injury in each region	Description of injury	Abbreviated Injury Scale	Square top 3
Head and neck	Cerebral contusion	3	9
Face	No injury	0	
Chest	Flail chest	4	16
Abdomen	Ruptured spleen	5	25
Extremity (including pelvis)	Femur fracture	3	
External	No injury	0	
		Injury Severity Score:	50

TABLE 4.11   Evidence From Meta-Analysis on the ISS Compared to the NISS

Evidence	ISS	NISS
Sensitivity	0.64	0.71
Specificity	0.93	0.87
Positive likelihood ratio	5.11	5.22
Negative likelihood ratio	0.27	0.20
Diagnostic odds ratio	27.75	24.74
Area under the summary receiver operator characteristic curve	0.9009	0.9095

Accurately triaging severely injured patients is key to ensuring patients receive the specialized care they need in an appropriate level of trauma center. Many states have unevenly located trauma centers; level I/II trauma centers are found predominantly in urban areas, while rural areas have none. Patients who are severely injured according to the ISS should be appropriately transported to level I/II trauma centers. Triage patterns can be described as follows:[41]

- *Undertriage*. A patient with an ISS > 15 and not transported to a level I/II trauma center
- *Overtriage*. A patient with an ISS < 15 and transported directly from the field to a trauma center

In a study of 60,182 severely injured patients,[41] triage patterns were stratified across these three dimensions: age, MOI, and access to care. Fall-related injuries were frequently undertriaged (52%) compared with injuries from motor vehicle collisions (MVCs) and penetrating trauma (12% and 10%, respectively). This pattern was true for all age groups. Conversely, MVCs and penetrating traumas were associated with high rates of overtriage (>70% for both). The researchers[41] concluded that triage is largely determined by mechanism of injury regardless of injury severity. High rates of undertriage were attributed to fall-related injuries, regardless of age. Patients with MVCs and penetrating trauma were overtriaged and transported to trauma centers regardless of injury severity and at considerable expense to the health care system. Patients with severe injuries (ISS > 15) should be appropriately transported to level I/II trauma centers regardless of age, MOI, or access to care.

Summary

Key to an effective emergency examination is following a routine, systematic approach to ensure each patient is examined in a consistent and appropriate manner without missing critical details. It is essential to practice skills and become competent in conducting each of the steps within a detailed, thorough, and rehearsed emergency action plan (EAP). The decision-making process should be based on performing an efficient scene size-up, a rapid initial assessment, a sound focused assessment, and providing successful patient care. When approaching the patient, pay attention to assess the patient's general appearance and make a determination of "How does the patient look?" These critical details initiate the formation of a plan to identify and treat life threats as quickly as possible. Based on the nature of illness (NOI) or the mechanism of injury (MOI), the HCP on-site must set priorities of patient care and determine whether the patient requires rapid transport to the hospital. The emergency examination requires practice and experience to quickly yet thoroughly perform each step so that a critical injury or condition can be appropriately identified and treated early. As transport arrives, it is essential to monitor the patient and find any new developments or conditions that must be treated. Each of these steps contributes to gathering critical information about condition of the patient in order to provide efficient and effective emergency care and hand-off to the next-level HCP.

 Go to the web study guide to complete the case studies for this chapter.

CHAPTER 5

Emergency Medications and Administration

Eric Fuchs, DA, ATC, AEMT

After reading this chapter, you will be able to do the following:

- Recognize when pharmacologic intervention is needed emergently and determine appropriate medication, dose, and route to administer to a patient.

- Explain the medical direction and oversight regulations by which athletic trainers (ATs) can be authorized to administer a medication.

- Perform proper medication administration via all appropriate routes as patient medical condition dictates for emergency situations.

- Describe and use the medication profiles for the medications identified in the CAATE 2020 standards and identified in various NATA position statements to provide emergent care to patients.

- Properly store and manage emergency medications in an AT facility and while traveling.

This chapter discusses general concepts of all forms of medication administration routes, focusing primarily on administration routes for common medications used in emergency care of a variety of patient conditions. The chapter specifically focuses on the medications identified in the CAATE 2020 standards and the appropriate and common administration routes for these medications in an emergency situation. Neither all medications nor a comprehensive review of pharmacokinetics or dynamics of all medications can be discussed within the pages of this text. However, it is anticipated that the selected medications and routes of administration, in addition to general concepts for medicine administration, will provide the knowledge and skills needed to provide proper medication delivery during a medical emergency. Athletic trainers (ATs) are ultimately responsible for knowing established protocols and dosage for the patient population for which they provide medical services.

Medical Direction and Oversight

ATs work under the direction of a physician as required by the Board of Certification, Inc., or BOC. As discussed in chapter 2, state regulations in the form of licensure, certification, or regulation, which exists in 49 states and the District of Columbia, provide further clarification on scope of practice of an AT.[1] Practice acts vary from state to state and may limit an AT's ability to use a variety of medication administration techniques or specific medications discussed in this chapter. All ATs should review and understand the scope of practice in their state.[3] An AT in one state may be able to use certain methods of administration or specific medications, whereas an AT practicing in another state would violate the state practice act with the use of the same methods or medications; for example, ATs in Kentucky may dispense medication to adult athletes but not to minor athletes (e.g., those in high school).[45]

The AT's roles and responsibility for handling, storing, taking inventory of, and using medications will vary depending on practice setting and state practice act. ATs must take time to understand federal and state laws regarding medication storage, administration, and dispensing. This understanding includes reviewing the AT practice act in relation to other state and federal definitions for administration and dispensing applicable to their state. ATs must develop appropriate policies and procedures to ensure the proper storage and inventory controls for all medications stored and administered to patients in their facility or on the field. One such control that ATs can use is break tabs with codes to secure medications in kits when not in a facility (figure 5.1). A corresponding record sheet indicates the break tab number and date placed on the kit, and when it is used; and who broke the tab and what was used. When it is restocked, a new tab is placed on the kit and the recording process continues. This record is commonly used in emergency medical services (EMS) systems for medications in kits to control inventory and ensure proper documentation when medications are administered.

ATs should develop a comprehensive policy and procedure for all medications in their facility in collaboration with the AT's legal counsel, supervising physician and, when possible, a pharmacist to ensure that established policies and procedures are in compliance with state and federal laws. A common example of improper storage and handling of medication is when an AT collects and holds onto a patient's inhaler medication or epinephrine auto-injector prescribed in the patient's name. An AT may not carry another person's prescription medication for any reason; the medication must be carried and used by the person for whom it was prescribed. Research has shown that collegiate ATs have dispensed medication, improp-

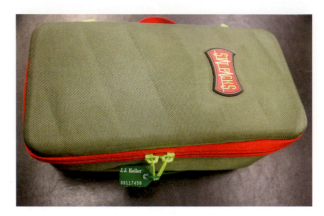

FIGURE 5.1 Break tabs.
Courtesy of Dr. Eric J. Fuchs, ATC, NRAEMT.

erly administered medication, and failed to appropriately document drug administration and dispensation.[2,3]

The CAATE 2020 standards indicate the specific medications ATs are to be able to administer, such as naloxone, glucagon, insulin, epinephrine, baby aspirin, and nitroglycerin.[4] In addition, many NATA position statements[5,6] and the American College of Sports Medicine (2007) Position Stand on Exertional Heat Illness During Training and Competition[7] recommend the administration of intravenous (IV) fluids to manage a variety of emergency medical conditions. Evidence supports the need for ATs to be able to establish intravenous access and provide IV fluid as ordered by a directing physician.

Best practice for handling medication and administering emergency medication for an AT in the clinical setting is to comply with current state practice acts. The AT must also develop a written standing order that is then reviewed by the AT's directing physician or medical director and, when possible, legal counsel (described in chapter 2). The written protocol(s) should then be signed and dated by the directing physician and AT. These protocols should also be reviewed annually by the AT staff and medical director and modified as changes to state law or evidence-based practice are presented.

Mobile Apps

A variety mobile apps are available to help ATs in management of medications. They include the following:

- Epocrates
- Physician Digital Reference (PDR)
- PEPID, LLC

Many health care systems make these tools available to their staff. As an AT you may have access to full versions of Epocrates or PDR apps through your employer.

Best Practices for Safe Administration of Medication

Medication administration is not a stand-alone skill. The medications needed in each emergency situation often vary. The AT must use patient assessment skills and foundational knowledge in anatomy, physiology, pharmacology, chemistry, and pathophysiology to determine whether a patient's current condition warrants administration of a medication or other therapeutic intervention.[4,8] A variety of trauma and general medical conditions common to patients under an AT's care may require the emergent administration of medications. Management of common and other medical conditions such as asthma, anaphylaxis, angina, cardiac arrest, diabetes, exertional sickling, heat exhaustion, heatstroke, and drug overdose is described in future chapters.[4,5,9,10] Trauma conditions where IV fluid access or administration is warranted include treatment of hypovolemic shock, spinal shock, femur and pelvic fractures, and internal hemorrhage. This text provides chapters on the management and treatment of numerous medical and trauma conditions where the immediate administration of medication or IV access is critical for a positive patient outcome.

ATs should have and maintain current training in personal protective equipment (PPE) and Occupational Safety and Health Administration (OSHA) workplace safety with regard to blood-borne pathogens as best practice when administering medications; see chapter 2 for a thorough review.

Six Rights of Patient Medication Administration

1. *Right patient.* In emergent situations at a practice, performance, or other competition, the AT is often providing care to a single patient and thus matching the right medication to the right patient is not a concern. However, ATs who work in physician offices or rehabilitation centers need to follow the protocols of the employer to ensure the right patient is being treated.

2. *Right medication.* As the AT administering medication, confirm that the medication about to be administered is the correct medication. Check the vial, bottle, or auto-injector to ensure both the name of the medication and the concentration are appropriate. For example, epinephrine is available in a concentration of 1:1,000 or 1:10,000. If an AT is administering epinephrine 1:1,000 for anaphylaxis, then it would be administered intramuscularly (IM) and not intravenously (IV). A 1:10,000 concentration would be appropriate for the IV administration route.

3. *Right dose.* Carefully ensure the correct dosage of the medication is administered and double-check dosage calculations. For example, if epinephrine is to be administered for anaphylaxis per standing orders using a non–auto-injector and the patient is a 70-lb (31.75-kg) pediatric patient, then 0.01 mg/kg of the drug should be administered, or 0.32 mg IM. Using mobile apps or standard dose tables for medications can help ensure the right dose.

4. *Right route.* An AT must know the proper route of administration for the medication and ensure that route is used to deliver the medication to the patient. For example, if D25 (dextrose 25%) via IV has been ordered for a patient with diabetes, the AT must ensure the established IV access has an 18ga catheter or greater; otherwise, dextrose will block the IV catheter and will reduce the actual dose the patient receives, if any.

5. *Right time.* In acute care management, medications are often administered as soon as proper assessments have concluded the need for medication. Many medications should be administered only once; however, medications such as nitroglycerin and epinephrine often need repeated doses.

6. *Right documentation.* Documentation of all information regarding the medication administration must be securely maintained. This information includes patient assessment, vital signs, medication name, dose, route of administration, and changes in patient status following administration. The right documentation is necessary for legal protection and to ensure continuity of high-quality patient care during the transfer of the patient to other health care providers (HCPs) or team members.

Once the AT determines, based on the clinical presentation of the patient, that a medication is needed, the 6 rights of patient medication administration should be followed.[8,11] ATs need to take the time to ensure these rights are followed, despite the often-chaotic situations an AT may be faced with while caring for a patient in an emergency situation.

Proper handling of medication is essential for good patient outcomes in emergency situations. The most common type of medication administration error resulting in death of a patient is giving a patient the wrong dosage, which accounts for over 40% of all deaths related to medication administration error.[11,12] ATs must properly store and document the various emergency medications in order to be in compliance with federal and state laws when using prescription medications. An AT must make sure the facility and travel kits comply with local, state, and federal laws to ensure both the AT's legal protection and the patient's safety. Improper storage of medication can lead to decreased medication effectiveness; for example, a vial of in-use insulin may be maintained at room temperature (approx. 15°-25°C or 59°-77°F) for only 28 days, and other vials should be stored in a refrigerator.[8] Temperature extremes in the AT's working environment must be considered when managing medications. ATs must work to ensure that their AT facility is in compliance with all regulations regarding handling, managing, and storing medications by meeting with legal counsel and the medical director to review all applicable state and federal laws.

Medication Administration

Proper medication administration starts with a complete patient assessment, which includes asking the patient about any current prescription or over-the-counter medications or any known allergies. In emergency situations, a patient may be unable to provide this information because of severe pain, altered mental status, or loss of consciousness. Friends or family members, medical alert bracelets (figure 5.2), and tattoos can provide necessary

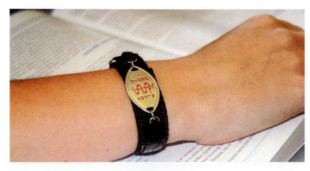

FIGURE 5.2   Medical alert bracelet.

MARK CLARKE/Science Source

information. Mobile apps also allow patients to store medical information on their phones (figure 5.3).

Next, the AT must obtain a complete set of baseline vital signs. (For a thorough discussion, see chapter 4.) This information is needed for indications and contraindications for medication administration. In addition, serial vital signs after medication administration are used to document the medication's effect on the patient.

Administration Routes

The method by which a medication gains access to the body determines the route of administration. The two main routes of medication administration are as follows:[8,11]

1. **Enteral routes:** Medication gains access through the gastrointestinal system.
2. **Parenteral routes:** Medication gains access through all routes that bypass the gastrointestinal tract; medication is usually in the form of liquid, gas, or semisolid form.

Table 5.1 provides common routes of emergency medication administration.

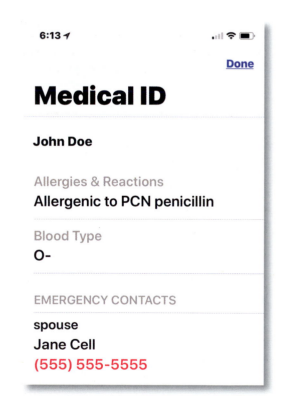

FIGURE 5.3   Medical ID mobile apps, which can be accessed through the Emergency button on a smartphone, allow patients to store medical information (e.g., allergies, blood type) on their phones, which can be accessed by ATs and other health care providers (HCPs) during emergencies.

TABLE 5.1 Emergency Medication Administration Routes

Method	Recommended route	Description	Examples of medications
Enteral	Oral (PO)	• Patient swallows the medication. • Medication onset is slow and depends on drug form, last oral intake by patient, and gastric motility. • It is generally a safe and less expensive form than other forms of delivery. • Skills needed are simple, and most patients tolerate the route well.	Chewable baby aspirin
Parenteral	Sublingual (SL)	• Some sources may consider SL an enteral route. • Medications administered in this manner bypass the liver by being directly absorbed into the bloodstream. • Few medications are available for administration in this form.	Nitroglycerin (tablet and spray) Antihistamine (ready tabs)
Parenteral: percutaneous	Subcutaneous (SubQ)	• Typically use a 3/8-5/8 in. (8-16 mm) and 25ga-27ga fine needle. • Used to deliver a maximum of 1 mL of medication into the subcutaneous tissue below the skin. • Common sites include abdomen, triceps region, and thigh. • Considered slower than IM and IV medication delivery.	Insulin
	Intramuscular (IM)	• Use a 1 to 1-1/2 in. (25-38 mm) 21ga-23ga needle in adults. • Use a 1 to 1-1/2 (25-38 mm) 25ga-27ga needle in pediatric patients. • IM injections result in faster absorption rates than SubQ. • For a medication dose ≤ 2 mL, deltoid or thigh is the preferred site. • For a medication dose of ≥ 5 mL, gluteus maximus is the preferred site.	Epinephrine Naloxone Influenza vaccine
	Intravenous (IV)	• Peripheral IV access is usually established in adult patients with 20ga or 18ga IV catheters. • For pediatric patients it is usually 20ga-22ga. • Larger IV catheters—up to 16ga or 14ga—may be used with some trauma patients. • IV fluids and/or medications are delivered directly into the peripheral circulation via a drip or injection through a saline lock. • IV medication onset of action is immediate.	Normal saline (NS) Naloxone Lactated Ringer's (LR) solution D25—dextrose 25% D50—dextrose 50%
Parenteral: inhalation	Inhalation (INH)	• Medications in the form of gases, mists, and fine powders are administered and absorbed rapidly across the large alveoli surface area. • These medications have a rapid onset. • Often used in patients who have respiratory compromise.	Oxygen Albuterol inhaler 2.5 mg albuterol in 1.5 mL NS via small-volume nebulizer (SVN) Naloxone

Aseptic Technique

Medication administration provides a risk of infection through any injection to a patient and through improper handling of oral or sublingual medication.[8,11] Using and adhering to **aseptic techniques** minimizes the infection risks to a patient. For all **percutaneous techniques** or medication delivery through an IV port, the minimum aseptic technique is the application of an alcohol prep pad to wipe the skin prior to injection. As the clinician, you should move the prep pad from a clean to a dirty area and avoid dragging it back over a clean area; the prep pad must be moved out and away from the selected site for injection.[11,12,13] Solutions such as betadine preps or iodine preps are also options for cleaning the selected site. After preparation of the site, you should not touch the cleaned area. The skin should be allowed to dry fully to complete the disinfecting process. Follow your health care facility standards of practice for any additional requirements.

Additional alcohol prep pads should be available in case the cleaned site becomes recontaminated prior to medication administration (e.g., the patient touches or points to the area before you have delivered the injection). Always clean any medication port on an IV tubing or saline lock prior to administration of medication. Lastly, always avoid contaminating surfaces of aseptic or sterile surfaces of equipment by not touching them or allowing them to come in contact with non-sterile surfaces (e.g., IV catheters, IV tubing connectors, needles).

Oral Medication Administration

Low-dose aspirin is a medication available for oral administration by ATs in an emergency patient.[4] Aspirin is given to patients who are presenting with signs or symptoms of **acute coronary syndrome**. Aspirin for emergency administration is recommended for any patient exhibiting signs or symptoms of cardiac arrest and only contraindicated if signs and symptoms of stroke are present. The American Heart Association currently recommends 160 to 325 mg of chewable baby aspirin for such patients.[11,14-17] Baby aspirin is chewable, which increases the rate of absorption, and it does not require any drink to assist in swallowing.[11,16,18] Baby aspirin comes in generic and brand names in over-the-counter dose of 81-mg tablets; the recommendation is to provide 2 to 4 tablets, which is 162 to 324 mg. Table 5.2 provides information about administering aspirin.

Sublingual Medication Administration

Sublingual medication delivery requires the patient to have the ability to control their own airway and to follow the AT's instructions.[11,15,17] The two most common emergency medications an AT will administer sublingually are nitroglycerin (NTG) and antihistamine.

TABLE 5.2   Aspirin (Acetylsalicylic Acid or ASA) Administration

Indication for emergency use	Acute coronary syndrome (ACS) Acute myocardial infarction (MI) patients
Class	Platelet aggregation inhibitor Nonsteroidal anti-inflammatory Analgesic
Description	Reduces platelet aggregation by inhibiting the release of thromboxane A_2
Mechanism of action	Blocks part of the chemical reaction responsible for activating platelets
Contraindications	Hypersensitivity (i.e., allergic) Not administered to children or adolescents with viral illness that can increase the risk of **Reye's syndrome**
Precautions	Administer with caution in patients with asthma or a history of ulcers, liver disease, alcohol abuse, kidney disease, or coagulopathies
Side effects	GI upset, bleeding, nausea, vomiting, and wheezing
Interactions	Few known when used in single dose for ACS or acute MIs
Dosage	American Heart Association (AHA) recommends 160-325 mg of chewable aspirin[16]
Route	Oral
How supplied	81-mg tablets chewable baby aspirin

Nitroglycerin

NTG is used for the management and treatment of angina and ACS (table 5.3). NTG is administered to dilate coronary arteries by relaxing the smooth muscle, resulting in increased blood flow to the cardiac muscle tissue.[11,14,15] Sublingual administration allows for rapid onset of action. Prior to administering NTG to a patient, the AT must establish baseline vital signs and check systolic blood pressure (BP). Any patient with a 90 mm Hg or less should not receive NTG; doing so will cause an unsafe drop in blood pressure.[11] Any patient who has taken or is taking erectile dysfunction medication within the last 24 to 36 hours (e.g., Cialis, Viagra) should not receive NTG due to a potential catastrophic effect on the patient's BP.[11]

Antihistamine

Antihistamine ready tablets are administered sublingually using the same method described for NTG sublingual tablet administration. Antihistamine ready tablets are often used with patients who suffer from severe allergic reactions such as anaphylaxis. Patients may be instructed to take an antihistamine along with epinephrine auto-injection administration. The patient must be able to protect his own airway (i.e., he must be alert, oriented, and able to drink or swallow fluids) prior to administration of an antihistamine ready tablet.

Metered-Dose Inhaler Administration

Treatment and management of asthma attacks are common for ATs across all clinical practice settings, including athletic fields, factories, and performing arts centers. According to the Centers for Disease Control and Prevention (CDC) National Center for Health Statistics, 6.2 million children under the age of 18 and 18.4 million adults 18 or older have asthma.[18] The CDC statistics show that 2 million visits to emergency departments (EDs) are for patients with asthma as the primary diagnosis. ATs should carry an albuterol metered-dose inhaler (MDI) in their kits to use for patients having an acute asthma attack (see table 5.4).[9,19,20] This habit ensures the right

TABLE 5.3   **Nitroglycerin Sublingual Tablets or Spray**

Indication for emergency use	Supplied in tablets or metered-dose spray Used for treatment or management of chest pain associated with ACS, angina, and suspected acute myocardial infarction (MI) patients
Class	Nitrate Vasodilator
Description	Vasodilator
Mechanism of action	Nitrates are potent vasodilators that increase blood flow to coronary arteries Decrease cardiac workload by dilating the peripheral vasculature, decreasing preload
Contraindications	Hypotension, systolic BP of 90 mm Hg or less Increased ICP (intracranial pressure) or head trauma Use of erectile dysfunction medication (i.e., Cialis, Viagra) within 24-36 h
Precautions	NTG deteriorates rapidly when exposed to light or air Monitor patient's BP and discontinue administration if systolic BP > 90 mm Hg Consider IV access prior to administration
Side effects	NTG is a potent vasodilator and commonly causes a rapid onset of headache Patient may complain of dizziness, weakness, tachycardia, hypotension, or dry mouth; nausea and vomiting may occur after use Spray or tablet may cause burning sensation on administration
Interactions	Effects may be amplified by alcohol use, erectile dysfunction medications, and beta blockers, causing an unsafe drop in blood pressure
Dosage	Administer 0.4 mg sublingually. If chest pain persists and systolic BP remains ≥90 mm Hg, repeat dose every 5 min to maximum 3 doses
Route	Sublingual
How supplied	NTG metered-dose spray delivers 0.4 mg/spray Tablet containing 0.4 mg/tablet

Administering Sublingual Medication

Sublingual Tablets

1. Wear gloves (because moisture on the hand can cause tablets to dissolve and be absorbed into the skin).
2. Check the 6 rights of patient medication administration.
3. Ask the patient to lift her tongue.
4. Place the tablet under the tongue (a), and tell the patient to hold it under the tongue until the tablet dissolves.

Sublingual Spray

1. Wear gloves (because moisture on the hand can cause aerosol contact with skin and subsequent absorption).
2. Check the 6 rights of patient medication administration.
3. Instruct the patient to lift the tongue.
4. Hold the spray just outside the patient's mouth with the spray directed toward the sublingual space (b).
5. Administer the sublingual spray.

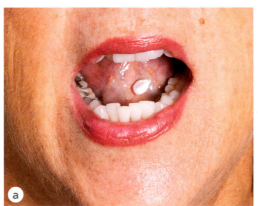 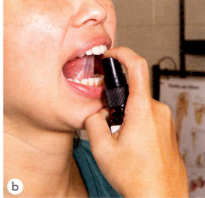

FIGURE 5.4

medication is available and does not rely on patients to have their inhaler with them. ATs must understand that legally they cannot carry another person's prescription medication, so best practice is to have an albuterol MDI in the emergency medications kit and not to collect individual patients' MDIs.

Emergency treatment of asthma attacks commonly uses beta$_2$-agonists such as albuterol. Patients with asthma are often familiar with the use of a MDI, because they are often prescribed a similar device for self-administration.[8,11,18,20] For patients unfamiliar with an MDI (e.g., a youth athlete suffering her first asthma attack), the AT should assist by providing instruction quickly and calmly on how to use the inhaler.

Patients should be monitored following administration of MDI for relief of **respiratory distress**. The patient should have improved pulse oxygen saturation rates and lung sounds, and a decreased use of accessory muscles. An AT can repeat the administration of MDI albuterol every 5 minutes for 3 doses. If a patient's signs and symptoms do not improve by the second administration, EMS should be activated. In addition, the AT should consider using a small-volume nebulizer, also known as a breathing treatment, for the patient; see the later section, Nebulized Medication Administration.

Oxygen Administration

Oxygen is one of the most commonly used prescription medications in the treatment and management of patients having acute medical and trauma-related pathologies (see table 5.5). Oxygen should be available in the AT facility

TABLE 5.4 Albuterol Sulfate Administration

Indication for emergency use	Supplied in MDI or delivered via small volume nebulizers with oxygen for patients having shortness of breath and wheezing associated with asthma, bronchitis, chronic obstructive pulmonary disease (COPD), and other respiratory infections
Class	Beta$_2$-selective sympathomimetic Bronchodilator
Description	Albuterol sulfate (e.g., Proventil, Ventolin) is a sympathetic beta$_2$-agonist that reverses smooth muscle constriction of bronchial tubes in patients with asthma and other COPD
Mechanism of action	Acts on beta$_2$-sympathetic receptors located on the smooth muscle of bronchial passages resulting in relaxation and bronchodilation
Contraindications	Hypersensitivity/known allergy Symptomatic tachycardia
Precautions	Albuterol has minimal beta$_1$-adrenergic effects, but heart rate may increase along with myocardial oxygen demand Use with caution in patients with known cardiovascular disease
Side effects	Anxiety, palpitations, chest discomfort, headache, and diaphoresis
Interactions	Do not concurrently use another beta-agonist with albuterol
Dosage	MDI or 2 90-mcg sprays, preferably with a spacer SVN: Adult dosage 2.5 mg diluted in 2.5 mL over 5-15 min with mask or straw; oxygen flow rate of 12-15 L/min SVN: Pediatric dosage 0.15 mg/kg diluted in 2.5 mL normal saline with mask or straw; oxygen flow rate 12-15 L/min
Route	Inhalation
How supplied	MDI or prepackaged 2.5 mg/0.5 mL nebule

MDI = metered-dose inhaler; SVN = small-volume nebulizer

CLINICAL SKILLS

Using a Metered-Dose Inhaler

1. Shake the MDI.
2. The patient places the mouthpiece in her mouth and seals her lips around it.
3. The patient takes a deep breath and simultaneously depresses the canister and continues inhaling.
4. The patient holds her breath for approximately 5 seconds before exhaling.

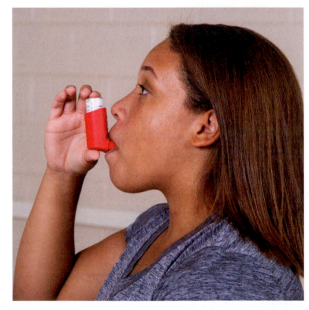

FIGURE 5.5

TABLE 5.5   **Medical Oxygen**

Indication for emergency use	**Dyspnea** **Hypoxia** $SpO_2 < 95\%$ Any patient needing assisted ventilations
Class	Gas
Description	Colorless, odorless, tasteless gas
Mechanism of action	Oxygen is necessary for cellular respiration and energy production to ensure good tissue perfusion. Inhaled oxygen molecules cross the respiratory membrane and attach to hemoglobin for transport to tissues
Contraindications	No absolute contraindications to the use of oxygen exist; however, complications can exist with **hyperoxemia** in patients resuscitated from cardiac arrest, those with acute coronary syndrome (ACS), and neonates
Precautions	Oxygen is a vasoactive drug that can cause cerebral and coronary artery vasoconstriction. Oxygen is not recommend for routine use in ACS patients presenting in an uncomplicated condition with $SpO_2 > 94\%$ and should be titrated to maintain 95% SpO_2 in patients with lower saturation rates[11,14,15,17,21] Do not use near open flame or combustion sources Oxygen tanks contain a compressed gas and can become a projectile hazard if dropped or mishandled; always leave an oxygen tank lying on its side, and use a protective guard over the regulator to prevent damage
Side effects	Few side effects are associated with short-term administration of oxygen; if used for prolonged periods without humidification, it may cause drying out of mucous membranes and lead to nosebleeds
Interactions	None
Dosage	Oxygen administration should be delivered to maintain a patient's SpO_2 at 95%, and flow rate of oxygen should be based on delivery adjunct being used to administer oxygen (see table 5.6)
Route	Inhalation via appropriate adjunct
How supplied	Oxygen comes as a compressed gas in a high-pressure cylinder A range of sizes exist, but D or Jumbo D cylinders commonly are used with portable oxygen kits

and on the sidelines of practices and games as part of the emergency airway or emergency trauma kit or bag.

Oxygen is available in a variety of tank sizes; however, the common sizes used for portable emergency oxygen tanks are sizes D and Jumbo D (see figure 5.6). ATs must become familiar with how to operate an oxygen tank, including knowing how to attach a regulator, how to

RED FLAG

Often special requirements or restrictions exist when traveling on vans, buses, and planes with medical grade oxygen. When flying, ATs should contact the Transportation Security Administration (TSA) for details on how to travel with oxygen tanks in both checked and carry-on luggage.

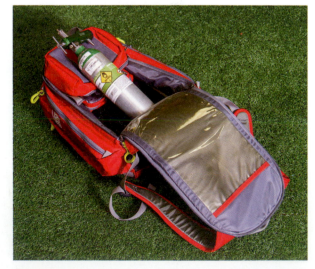

FIGURE 5.6 Portable size D emergency oxygen kit.

check oxygen levels in the tank, and how to operate the regulator of the oxygen cylinder. A variety of regulators, tanks, and gauges exist, so as an AT you must become familiar with the ones used by your health care facility or in the oxygen kit. Always check the oxygen tank to ensure it is full prior to an event. ATs must develop a policy on the minimum tank pressure that is acceptable for use during events; when a tank falls below a certain level, it should be removed from service and a new tank placed in the emergency kit.

The NATA position statement *Preventing Sudden Death in Sports (2012)* recommends the use of oxygen in the treatment and management of patients with asthma and sickle cell trait.[9] As with all medications, oxygen must be administered by acceptable routes and in approved doses. The AT must learn to use supplemental oxygen critically and not just because oxygen is available. Oxygen has specific effects and mechanisms of actions; studies have identified hyperoxemia as a factor that increases morbidity and mortality in patients resuscitated from cardiac arrest.[15-17,21] Oxygen is a vasoactive drug, which causes vasoconstriction, resulting in a decrease in tissue perfusion.[11] Routine practice used to include providing oxygen by non-rebreather (NRB) mask to patients with ACS. The American Heart Association (2010) guidelines cite inadequate evidence to support routine administration of oxygen for patients with uncomplicated ACS with a SpO_2 94% or greater.[16,21] Oxygen is a vasoconstrictor and can potentially decrease perfusion to ischemic tissue in high concentrations, which could increase loss of cardiac muscle tissue in patients.

ATs should not solely rely on SpO_2 values when determining to administer oxygen; while a low value should be assessed as hypoxemia, a high value does not necessarily mean the tissues are receiving oxygen (e.g., a person with carbon monoxide poisoning will register with a high SpO_2 due to the hemoglobin being saturated with carbon monoxide and not oxygen). ATs must use their patient assessment skills in combination with vital signs and instruments to determine whether supplemental oxygen needs to be administered.

Table 5.6 lists common devices used in the emergency care of patients. Each device is capable of delivering varying doses of oxygen based on patients' needs. Several of these devices should be available in the airway bag with the oxygen tank.

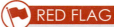

RED FLAG

The following are indicators for oxygen to be administered to patients:

- Respiratory distress or **respiratory failure**
- Cardiac or **respiratory arrest**
- Any patient requiring assisted ventilation
- Adult patients whose respiratory rate is < 8 or > 30
- SpO_2 < 95%
- Patient with an altered mental status or decreased level of consciousness (LOC)
- Shortness of breath or use of accessory muscles
- Patient complaining of chest pain
- Other medical conditions that can cause hypoxia (e.g., seizures, stroke, overdose)
- Signs or symptoms of shock

When administering oxygen to patients who are unable to protect the airway, appropriate use of airway adjuncts is an important consideration. A variety of sizes and types of airway adjuncts should be available in case an airway cannot be maintained with manual techniques. Airway adjuncts include oropharyngeal airways (OPAs), nasopharyngeal airways (NPAs), and supraglottic or blind intubation airways, including but not limited to King LT Airway and iGel Airway. ATs should learn how to properly insert and use these airway adjuncts; chapter 9 provides in-depth discussion about establishing and maintaining an airway. ATs should consult with their medical director and local EMS when determining which devices to carry and use. Consistency of equipment use among providers allows for easier patient transfer and ensures that all those who are involved during an emergency situation are familiar with the equipment.

Nebulized Medication Administration

Patients with asthma or significant lower respiratory infections (e.g., bronchitis) may require the use of a

TABLE 5.6 **Oxygen Delivery Devices**

Device	Oxygen flow rate	Percent oxygen delivered
Nasal cannula	1-6 L/min	24%-44%
Simple oxygen mask	6-10 L/min	Up to 60%
Non-rebreather mask	10 L/min	90%-100%
Bag-valve mask	15+ L/min	Nearly 100%

small-volume nebulizer (SVN) to provide relief of airway constriction and congestion. A SVN consists of tubing that connects oxygen to a small cup that holds the medication and either a mouthpiece or face mask (see figure 5.7). Patients are required to hold the mouthpiece, while the face mask is easily worn. Patients needing a SVN should be administered 2.5 mg of albuterol that is diluted in 2.5 mL of normal saline over 5 to 15 minutes for adult patients. Pediatric dosage is 0.15 mg/kg diluted in 2.5 mL normal saline. Clinicians can order prepackaged dosages for rapid administration. ATs should keep prepackaged albuterol in the airway kit with the SVN equipment.

ATs should carry a SVN set with the oxygen or airway kits, which includes having beta$_2$-agonists such as albuterol (see table 5.4) and levalbuterol, and anticholinergics such as ipratropium bromide (Atrovent; see table 5.7), which can be used alone or in combination with albuterol. These medications are supplied as liquids that are **nebulized** (turned to fine mist) by oxygen flowing through the liquid medication. The mist is inhaled, allowing the medication to come into contact with the lung tissue. ATs should work with their medical directors to develop a written protocol for their place of employment with regard to which medications and type of SVN will be used.

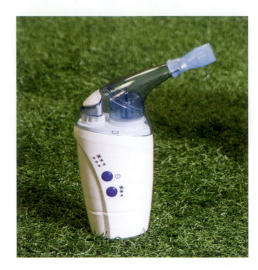

FIGURE 5.7 SVN with mouthpiece attachment.

Emergency Medication Injection

CAATE 2020 Standard 75 states that ATs need to be able to deliver medications by their appropriate route, and in emergency situations several medications need to be administered through injection (see table 5.1). The

TABLE 5.7 **Atrovent or Ipratropium Bromide for SVN**

Indication for emergency use	Moderate to severe asthma exacerbation Chronic obstructive pulmonary disease (COPD) management
Class	Anticholinergics, inhaled
Description	Ipratropium is a bronchodilator that relaxes muscles in the airways and increases airflow to the lungs; ipratropium bromide inhalation is used to prevent bronchospasm (or narrowing airways in the lungs) in people with bronchitis, emphysema, or COPD
Mechanism of action	Antagonizes acetylcholine receptors, producing bronchodilation
Contraindications	Hypersensitivity/known allergy
Precautions	Patients with glaucoma, prostatic hypertrophy, or bladder neck obstruction
Side effects	Blurred vision, eye pain, seeing halos around lights, pain or burning with urination, headache, dizziness, nausea, upset stomach, back pain
Dosage	<6 years old (yo): 0.25 mg SVN q20min prn up to 3 h for adjunct treatment; may mix neb solution with albuterol if used within 1 h of onset 6-12 yo: 0.5 mg SVN q20min prn up to 3 h for adjunct treatment; may mix neb solution with albuterol if used within 1 h of onset 13+ yo: 0.5 mg NEB q20min prn up to 3 h for adjunct treatment; may mix neb solution with albuterol
Route	Inhalation
How supplied	Adult: NEB (0.02%) 0.5 mg per 2.5 mL Pediatric: NEB (0.02%) 0.5 mg per 2.5 mL

NEB = nebule; SVN= small-volume nebulizer

CAATE 2020 standards identify specific emergency medications that ATs should be able to administer, including the following injectable medications: glucagon, insulin, naloxone, epinephrine. The CAATE 2020 standards and some state practice acts do allow for administration of additional medications not specifically identified in the standards, as ordered by the AT's physician or other provider with legal prescribing authority through written, verbal, or pre-established protocols.[4]

ATs must first ensure that they have the equipment and supplies to administer a SubQ, IM, or IV injection. This includes proper PPE (discussed earlier in the chapter) but minimally requires gloves, alcohol prep pad, or other solution to prepare site using aseptic technique, the right medication or fluid, the proper size needle or catheter, syringe size, and sharps container.

Drawing Up Medication

Medications designed to be administered by percutaneous routes usually are supplied in ampules, vials, or prefilled syringes or delivery doses (e.g., epinephrine pen, glucagon pen, insulin pens, flu vaccines). Ampule or vial medications must be drawn into a syringe for patient administration.

- When drawing medication from a vial or ampule, best practice is to use a larger needle than the needle that will be used to administer the medication; this needle is referred to as a fill needle.[11] The fill needle makes drawing the medication easier because it provides a larger diameter needle to pull more volume of fluid through than the smaller diameter syringe.
- When filling the syringe, always make sure the needle stays below the medication level so as to prevent drawing air into the syringe.
- Always draw slightly more than the amount needed. This habit allows for expelling any air in the needle or solution and still having the correct dose.

Subcutaneous Medication Administration

Insulin and epinephrine 1:1,000 (for anaphylaxis) are the two medications administered through a subcutaneous (SubQ) route that are most likely to be administered by an AT. Insulin comes in many forms and types.[8] Insulin protocols for administration in emergency situations with patients who have diabetes should be well defined and reviewed by the medical director. While this chapter does not provide an in-depth discussion on insulin or other medication selections for various diabetic emergencies (as described in chapter 13), you are encouraged to review

other sources.[2,8] Insulin must be properly stored; some forms of insulin need to be kept cool or refrigerated to maintain their effectiveness. Epinephrine 1:1,000 can be administered SubQ for patients in anaphylaxis; however, best practice is to administer IM. The AT must follow the medical director's standing orders or protocols.

The following sites are acceptable for SubQ medication administration (figure 5.8): lateral arm, abdominal region, and lateral thigh. Best practice in emergency situations is the lateral arm, because this site is usually easily accessed and exposed. However, the AT must follow the medical director's orders for site selection.

Intramuscular Medication Administration

Epinephrine 1:1,000, glucagon, and naloxone are medications ATs would administer IM during an emergency situation. Consider having all three of these medications available in the facility and medical kits.

Epinephrine (table 5.8) is used to treat anaphylaxis, which is a serious life-threatening condition that can lead to the death of a patient due to an allergic reaction (details in chapter 6). Common causes of anaphylaxis include allergies to tree nuts, peanuts, shellfish, medications, latex, and bee stings. Many patients who are diagnosed with severe allergies are prescribed and carry epinephrine auto-injectors for self-administration of epinephrine. Any

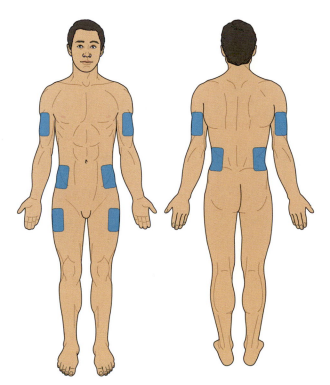

FIGURE 5.8   Sites on the body where SubQ injections can be administered.

Drawing Medication From an Ampule

1. Check for the correct medication and dose.
2. Hold the ampule upright between thumb and fingers.
3. Shake downward or gently tap the top until all medication is below the neck of the ampule.
4. Using a small gauze pad, snap off the top of the ampule *(a)*.
5. Place ampule upside down.
6. Take the syringe (do not prefill with air), and insert the needle into the ampule *(b)*.
7. Draw medication, keeping the needle tip below fluid level in the ampule.
8. Draw slightly more medication than needed.
9. Remove the needle from the ampule, and hold the syringe with the needle pointing up.
10. Tap or flick the syringe to dislodge air bubbles, and allow them to collect at top of syringe.
11. Depress the plunger until the top edge of the black disk is located on the proper dosage level for administration.
12. Dispose of the needle used to draw medication, and attach the needle for medication administration.

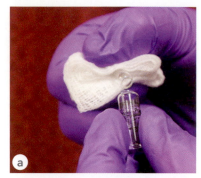
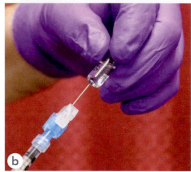

FIGURE 5.9
Courtesy of Dr. Eric J. Fuchs, ATC, NRAEMT.

Drawing Medication From a Vial

1. Check for the correct medication and dose.
2. Clean the top of the medication vial with an alcohol pad.
3. Inject a volume of air equal to the volume of medication you are drawing up from the vial (e.g., if giving 0.5 mg of epinephrine, then you would inject 0.5 mL of air into the epinephrine vial to draw 0.5 mg).
4. Draw medication, keeping the needle tip below the fluid level in the vial *(a)*.
5. Draw slightly more medication than needed.
6. Remove the needle from the vial, and hold the syringe with the needle pointing up.
7. Tap or flick the syringe to dislodge air bubbles, and allow them to collect at the top of syringe *(b)*.
8. Depress the plunger until the top edge of the black disk is located on the proper dosage level for administration.
9. If needed, dispose of the needle used to draw medication, and attach the needle for medication administration.

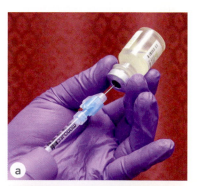
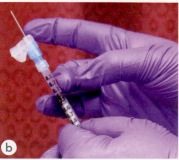

FIGURE 5.10
Courtesy of Dr. Eric J. Fuchs, ATC, NRAEMT.

Administering a Subcutaneous Injection

1. First use proper PPE.

2. Check the 6 rights of patient medication administration.

3. Properly prepare and draw medication for administration into the syringe using draw needle, keeping in mind a SubQ injection dose cannot exceed 1 mL of fluid volume.[11]

4. Select the proper needle for administration—a 25ga-27ga needle with a length of 1/2 to 5/8 inches (13-16 mm)[11]—and attach it to the syringe.

5. Clean the site following established aseptic techniques.

6. Proceed to pinch an approximately 1-inch (2.5-cm) fold of skin between your thumb and forefinger.

7. Position the needle at a 45° angle to the skin, and insert it into the skin you have pinched, injecting the medication.

8. Withdraw the syringe, engaging the needle's safety cap, and dispose of it in the sharps container.

9. Reassess the patient to determine whether the intervention is having the desired effect.

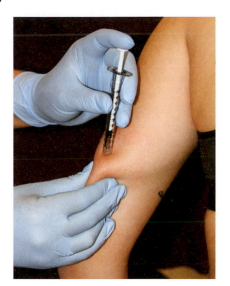

FIGURE 5.11

Courtesy of Dr. Eric J. Fuchs, ATC, NRAEMT.

TABLE 5.8 Epinephrine 1:1,000 Solution

Indication for emergency use	Acute anaphylaxis
Class	Sympathomimetic
Description	Naturally occurring hormone (sometimes called adrenalin) secreted by the adrenal glands in response to sympathetic nervous system stimulation Epinephrine binds with $alpha_1$-, $beta_1$-, and $beta_2$-adrenergic receptors, causing vasoconstriction, increased heart rate, and increased cardiac contractile force and bronchial smooth muscle relaxation
Mechanism of action	Epinephrine 1:1,000 is administered in management of anaphylaxis for vasoconstriction and relaxation of bronchiolar smooth muscle
Contraindications	Use with caution in patients with hypertension or known cardiovascular disease
Precautions	Epinephrine is inactivated by exposure to sunlight; thus, ATs should make sure medication is properly stored and take precaution when the emergency kit will be outside at an event Epinephrine may cause patients to experience chest pain, palpitations, anxiety, nausea, or headache after use; monitor patient's vital signs accordingly
Side effects	Anxiety, palpitations, headache, nausea, and vomiting are common Patients with known cardiac disease may experience chest pain or an acute MI
Interactions	Epinephrine effects can be intensified in patients taking antidepressants
Dosage	Adults: 0.3 to 0.5 mg SubQ or IM q15min as needed Pediatric: 0.01 mg/kg SubQ or IM q15min as needed
Route	SubQ or IM, with IM the preferred route for administration
How supplied	1 mg/1 mL in vials or ampules Prefilled auto-injector devices

patient who receives epinephrine for an anaphylactic reaction must be transported to an emergency department even if symptoms improve, because patients can experience a biphasic anaphylaxis, which is a second reaction from the same exposure.[11,22,23]

Glucagon (table 5.9) is used for patients with **hypoglycemia** who are unable to orally take glucose or drink juices. Glucagon is often prescribed to patients with diabetes for use if they become hypoglycemic. Glucagon's mechanism of action causes the body to release glycogen stores in the liver for utilization. Glucagon is only effective if the patient has not depleted his glycogen stores; ATs must consider this fact with an active patient who may have completed a workout, in which case the AT may need to consider IV dextrose 50% or 25%.[24,25]

The Surgeon General of the United States issued an advisory on naloxone and opioid overdose and recommended all Americans carry lifesaving naloxone (table 5.10).[26] The AT's athletic patient population is at risk for opioid overdose or abuse, because athletes may use such drugs to deal with injuries. Athletic populations have various stressors, such as maintaining a high level of fitness, balancing academic performance with sports, and coping with possible career-ending injuries, along with parental and societal pressures to perform or succeed after injury. These mental and physical stressors may encourage athletes to misuse and abuse pain medication to cope with physical or mental issues. Collegiate and high school athletes with previous mental health problems are more likely to misuse and abuse drugs than the average athlete.[43] Athletes who participate in collision sports have also reported higher opioid use due to increased likelihood of severe injuries.[42]

Once the AT has established a need for administration of a medication for IM injection based on the patient assessment, it is time to administer the medication; see Clinical Skills: Steps for IM Injection Administration.

Epinephrine 1:1,000 also is available in auto-injectors. Medical directors prescribe them for ATs to use on their patients, for emergencies, or as part of emergency action plans (EAPs). Auto-injectors are designed to go through a patient's clothing or outer garments and do not require the patient's skin to be cleaned or clothing removed prior to application. When administering to patients whose activity requires protective equipment, the AT should take steps to ensure no padding or other hard shielding surface would prevent the needle from deploying (e.g., hockey goalie, football thigh pad).

The cost of epinephrine auto-injectors has increased significantly, which can become cost prohibitive for many budgets, especially given that they expire every 2 years or less. Purchasing epinephrine 1:1,000 in ampules or vials, which costs a small fraction of the auto-injector, provides a cost-effective way to ensure the AT's access to epinephrine for emergency situations.

Intravenous Access

Peripheral IV access is indicted in patients when administration of emergency medications or fluids is required

TABLE 5.9 **Glucagon**

Indication for emergency use	Severely hypoglycemic patients who cannot orally take glucose and IV access for glucose administration is not established or available
Class	Hormone with antihypoglycemic action
Description	Pancreatic hormone promotes glycogenolysis and gluconeogenesis while inhibiting glycogenesis
Mechanism of action	Causes release of glycogen stores and their conversion to glucose when released into blood, causing an increase in blood glucose if the patient has significant glycogen stores for conversion to glucose
Contraindications	Hypersensitivity/known drug allergy
Precautions	Not effective in patients whose glycogen stores are depleted. Patients who are involved in physical activity may have depleted glycogen stores
Side effects	Rare, because it is based on a natural hormone; hypotension, dizziness, headache, nausea, and vomiting may occur
Interactions	Few interactions exist when administered in therapeutic doses during emergency situations
Dosage	1 mg
Route	IM
How supplied	In a kit containing powdered medication and solvent that must be combined prior to administration

TABLE 5.10 **Naloxone (Narcan)**

Indication for emergency use	Reversal of respiratory depression or arrest associated with narcotic overdose
Class	Narcotic antagonist
Description	Used to reverse respiratory depression in narcotic overdose patients
Mechanism of action	The medication has a higher affinity for narcotic receptor sites, causing it to displace the narcotic, blocking the effects of the narcotic
Contraindications	Known drug allergy
Precautions	Rapid administration of large doses may cause withdrawal in narcotic-addicted patients Titration of dose: Recommended to use minimum dose needed to establish quality respiratory rate rather than full reversal of narcotic Patient may awake violently or with vomiting; have suction available
Side effects	Hypotension, hypertension, nausea, vomiting, and cardiac arrhythmias
Interactions	May cause withdrawal symptoms if the patient is addicted to narcotics
Dosage	1-2 mg slow IV push titrated to restore respirator rate; if no effect, may be repeated q2-5min; maximum dose 10 mg 1-2 mg IM q2-5min; maximum dose 10 mg Intranasal formulation is available
Route	Slow IV push, IM, or nasal (IN)
How supplied	Prefilled syringe, vial, ampule, or prefilled nasal systems

or anticipated. As HCPs, ATs treat multiple conditions—both medical and trauma—where the establishment of IV access is beneficial to the patient: "When adjusted for illness severity, demographic, dispatch, and transport characteristics, out-of-hospital intravenous access was associated with lower odds of hospital mortality (odds

CLINICAL SKILLS

Steps for IM Injection Administration

1. Select the right medication.
2. Select the proper site based on the dose to be given:
   - Max 1 mL to deltoid
   - Max 2 mL to lateral quad
   - Max 5 mL to gluteal region
3. Properly draw up the medication, and prepare the injection site on the patient.
4. Select the proper gauge and length of needle:
   - 21ga-23ga in adult patients/23ga-25ga in pediatric patients
   - 3/4-1 inch (19-25 mm) for most adults; 3/4 inch (19 mm) for most pediatric patients; 1-1/2 inches (38 mm) for gluteal injection in adults
5. Stabilize the skin over the selected site.
6. Place the needle at a 90° angle to the skin.
7. Insert the needle, then draw back on the syringe slightly, checking for blood.
   - If you see no blood, administer medication.
   - If blood is aspirated into the syringe, do not inject; remove and start over.
8. Place an adhesive bandage over the site.
9. Reassess the patient for effects of medication.

Administering Epinephrine Auto-Injectors

1. Inspect the patient's lateral thigh to ensure that there is no phone or other items in the patient's pocket that would block the needle.

2. Remove the auto-injector from the carrier tube. Check that the medication has not expired. Check the medication viewing window to ensure that the epinephrine is clear.

3. Hold the auto-injector firmly with the orange tip pointing downward. Remove the blue safety cap by pulling straight up. Do not bend or twist.

4. Swing and push the orange tip firmly into the mid-outer thigh until you hear a "click." Hold it on the thigh for several seconds (follow the epinephrine auto-injector's manufacture directions).

5. Call 9-1-1.

Newer models of auto-injectors have built-in needle protection. After injection, the orange cover automatically extends to ensure the needle is never exposed. However, different brands of auto-injectors many not have needle safety engineering. Regardless of the type of auto-injector, the AT should dispose of it in a sharps container or give it to a responding EMS professional for proper disposal.

---

ratio 0.68; 95% confidence interval 0.56-0.81), with the strongest association among seriously ill patients (p. 297)."[27]

Establishing IV access is cited as a treatment method in several AT position statements, including the following:

- *NATA Position Statement on Preventing Sudden Death in Sports*: IV administration is recommended for several conditions (e.g., exertional hyponatremia, exertional sickling cell, exertional heatstroke) that can cause sudden death in sports.[9]

- *ACSM 2007 Position Stand on Exertional Heat Illness During Training and Competition*: IV access and administration are required for treatment of exertional heatstroke—"Preserving intravascular volume with normal saline (NS) infusion improves renal blood flow to protect the kidney from rhabdomyolysis and improves tissue perfusion in all organs for heat exchange, oxygenation, and removal of waste products (p. 561)"[9]; and the position stand continued that for exertional heat exhaustion, treatment recommended IV use and stated, "the most commonly recommended IV fluids for rehydrating athletes are NS or 5% dextrose in NS (p. 563)."[7]

- *NATA Position Statement on Fluid Replacement for the Physically Active* (2017) noted, "If moderate (2%-5%) or severe (>5 %) hypohydration is identified, oral fluids should be administered. Only if oral fluids are not tolerated or fluid losses are ongoing (from vomiting or diarrhea) should

intravenous (IV) fluids be administered by an appropriately trained and licensed medical professional (p. 880)."[28]

Establishing IV access is necessary in a variety of emergency situations, not just those related to fluid replacement or heat illness. Other emergency situations an AT may encounter include medical conditions (e.g., flu, hypoglycemia, seizure disorders), management of hypovolemic shock as a result of trauma, cardiac conditions, or sepsis.[29] An IV access at a rate to keep the vein open (TKO) is often needed but may not push any fluids or medications. The TKO access is primarily performed with patients who have a suspected head trauma; establishing IV access will help decrease transport time so that no delay occurs for EMS personnel to transport the patient to an emergency department. IV fluids are contraindicated for patients with head trauma (except for TKO), because a fluid bolus could cause increase in intracranial pressure. An increase in intracranial pressure would potentially have a negative patient outcome. To keep vein open or TKO IV access is warranted for any patients, including patients with head injuries being transported, as they may need medication or fluids to manage changes in their current vital signs or condition (e.g., seizure patient, trauma patient who is stable but not in shock).

Before administering IV fluids, it is necessary to conduct a thorough patient assessment and obtain baseline vital signs, which includes auscultation of lung sounds. These baseline vitals and auscultations are important when administering IV fluids. First, in patients where large fluid replacement is occurring, the patient can become fluid overloaded. As a result, the patient would develop signs and symptoms, including shortness of breath or the presence of crackles or rales, upon auscultation of the lung. These signs or symptoms need to be noted by the AT, and IV fluids should be discontinued or the rate of infusion slowed.[11] Normal saline (NS), a common IV fluid for use in emergency care, is a **crystalloid** solution. A crystalloid solution contains water and electrolytes and sometimes dextrose. NS is an isotonic crystalloid, which does not cause significant fluid or electrolyte shifts in patients when administered in normal therapeutic amounts. NS is used to temporarily expand a patient's vascular volume, but if administered in large doses it can overload the vascular system with fluid, especially during a short period of time. If lung symptoms occur, then discontinue IV fluids and monitor the patient. Be prepared to assist the patient's breathing with positive pressure ventilations (e.g., bag-valve mask).

For patients with trauma, IV fluids are often used to increase a patient's BP to facilitate the management of shock (described in chapter 6). ATs need to understand that IV fluids must be managed and not overused in cases of hemorrhage shock.[30] The most important treatment for hemorrhagic shock is controlling bleeding. If the AT finds bleeding wounds, she must treat them at the scene (see chapter 6). IV fluids can be used to replace fluid volume in the circulatory system to increase a patient's blood pressure. The physiological basis for shock is poor tissue perfusion, which can result if the body is not circulating oxygen through red blood cells (RBCs), which carry oxygen to the body's tissues and organs. If a patient is bleeding internally or externally, blood volume is lost; this causes a loss of RBCs, which leads to poor tissue perfusion and sends the patient into shock. Because IV

fluid does not contain RBCs, pushing large amounts of IV fluid into a patient who has had large blood volume loss or who is still bleeding may raise blood pressure readings in the patient; however, the patient will still suffer from poor tissue perfusion due to the lack of RBCs in circulation, leading to continued poor tissue perfusion.[11,30] ATs must recognize that IV fluids do not correct the oxygen-carrying deficit caused by the loss of RBCs. The goal in managing a trauma patient with hemorrhagic shock is to establish IV access and to only **bolus** enough fluid to maintain the patient's mean arterial pressure (MAP) at 60 mm Hg.[11,29] MAP is considered a better indicator of perfusion to vital organs than systolic blood pressure (SBP). To calculate MAP, use this equation:

$$MAP = 1/3 \ (SBP - DBP) + DBP$$

where DBP is diastolic blood pressure. For example, a patient with a SBP of 90 mm Hg and a DBP of 60 mm Hg would have a MAP of 70 mm Hg, or

$$MAP \ 70 = 1/3 \ (90 \ mm \ Hg - 60 \ mm \ Hg) + 60 \ mm \ Hg$$

Performing this calculation during an emergency situation may take time, but it is worth the time for a better patient outcome. Most modern electronic vital sign monitors do provide automatic readouts of MAP. ATs should consider making sure the trauma bag or kit has a device that provides MAP.

Supplies for Establishing IV Access

Intravenous access is obtained by using a catheter over a needle device (figure 5.12). The needle is used to puncture the skin and vein; once in the vein, the needle serves as a guide to slide the catheter into the vein. Once the

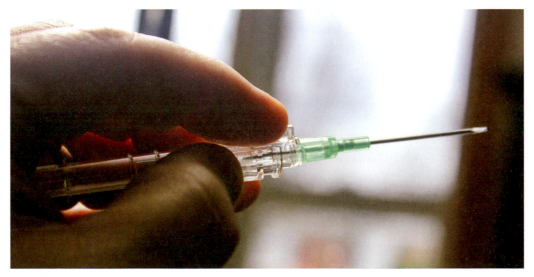

FIGURE 5.12 IV catheter.
Courtesy of Dr. Eric J. Fuchs, ATC, NRAEMT.

catheter is in the vein, the needle is removed and a saline lock or IV tubing is attached to the catheter and secured in place, allowing for medication administration or fluid administration. Based on the previously mentioned studies, most ATs should keep normal saline (NS), lactated Ringer's (LR) solution, and saline locks in the facilities or sideline kits. However, ATs must follow established protocols with the medical director for final determination of which fluids to use.[7,28-32]

Prior to establishing access, best practice is to collect and organize the needed supplies. ATs should create an IV kit that contains all the needed equipment and supplies, which is checked and restocked frequently.[30] This kit will make establishment of IV access more efficient in an emergency. You can purchase commercially prepackaged IV start kits or put them together yourself. Manufactured start packs usually have all the required equipment except for gloves and include the IV catheter, saline lock and flush, and IV fluid and tubing.

These are the supplies needed for starting an IV access kit:

- Gloves
- Tourniquet (constriction band)
- Alcohol prep pad or other cleansing wipe
- Saline lock and saline flush, or IV fluid bag and IV tubing
- Proper IV catheter size
- Small gauze pad for minor bleeding
- Commercial IV dressing
- Adhesive tape strips: Tear tape into 3 or 4 strips (0.5-1 in./12-25 mm × 2-3 in./50-75 mm) to secure IV or saline lock tubing.

IV Catheter Selection

ATs need to properly select the right diameter and length catheter for the patient according to these guidelines:[30]

- The catheter gauge is always an even number.
- The needle gauge is an odd number.
- The numbers are always consecutive for catheter-over-needle devices (e.g., an 18ga catheter uses a 17ga needle).
- Catheters range in size from 14ga (largest) to 24ga (smallest) in diameter.
- The length of a catheter ranges from 3/4 to 1-1/4 inches (19-32 mm).

When using a 20ga diameter or larger catheter, the preferred length is 1-1/4 inches (32 mm). ATs should establish IV access in adult patients commonly using an 18ga and 20ga catheter, with 18ga or larger preferred when medications are going to be administered. When a patient requires a rapid infusion of fluids (e.g., severe dehydration), then a 16ga or 14ga catheter is recommended.[30] For ATs working with pediatric patients or smaller patients with small-diameter veins, the use of larger catheters may be difficult and a 20ga or 22ga catheter should be considered.

IV Fluid, Tubing, and Saline Lock Setup

After gathering the necessary equipment, the AT selects the proper fluid. IV fluid selection is dictated based on medical director protocol and patient assessment and condition. The most common fluid used in emergency situations is normal saline (NS; 0.09% NaCl solution; table 5.11). Other fluids to consider having in the AT emergency medication kit include lactated Ringer's (LR) solution; see table 5.12) or 5% dextrose solution (D5W; see table 5.13).[11,27-30,33] After selecting the fluid, check the IV fluid bag for any damage or leakage and for color, clarity, or visible contaminants.[30]

The AT selects the proper tubing to attach to the IV bag. IV tubing comes in two basic types, macro drip

TABLE 5.11 **Normal Saline (NS) 0.09% NaCl Solution**

Indication for emergency use	Hypovolemia, heat exhaustion, heatstroke, diabetic ketoacidosis
Class	Isotonic crystalloid
Description	Clear fluid containing water (H_2O), 154 mEq/L sodium (Na), and approximately 154 mEq/L chloride (Cl) to match human body concentration
Mechanism of action	Temporary expansion of vascular volume by replacing water and electrolytes in blood
Contraindications	Patients with or in heart failure due to fluid overload
Precautions	Patients provided a large volume of NS should be monitored for fluid overload Patients who have significant electrolyte loss may be better served by administration of lactated Ringer's (LR) solution Hemorrhagic hypovolemic patients should be given bolus to keep MAP at 60 mm Hg to maintain tissue perfusion pressure while avoiding dilution of RBCs within the blood volume

Side effects	Large volumes lead to hemodilution and electrolyte imbalances
Interactions	No known drug interactions **Pyrogenic reaction** can occur due to foreign proteins in fluid; characterized by sudden fever, chills, backache, headache, and nausea/vomiting. If a reaction occurs, discontinue IV and start another IV with new fluid and equipment.
Dosage	Varies with condition; follow your facility's and medical director's protocols A TKO rate is 30 mL/h
Route	Intravenous infusion
How supplied	250-, 500-, and 1,000-mL bags for use with IV drip sets Recommend select bag volume based on patient's condition to prevent fluid overload Macro IV drip sets 10, 15, 20 gtt/mL Micro IV drip sets 60 gtt/mL

TABLE 5.12   Lactated Ringer's (LR) Solution

Indication for emergency use	Hypovolemia with electrolyte imbalances or loss, moderate to severe burns Used to reverse respiratory depression in narcotic overdose patients
Class	Crystalloid solution
Description	Contains 130 mEq/L sodium, 4 mEq/L potassium, 2.7 mEq/L calcium, 109 mEq/L chloride, and 28 mEq/L lactate
Mechanism of action	Used to replace electrolytes and fluid volume
Contraindications	Patients with heart failure, renal failure, or suspected hyperkalemia
Precautions	Monitor for circulatory overload
Side effects	Rare for therapeutic emergency doses
Interactions	Do not use with blood or blood products for infusion
Dosage	Determined by patient condition Follow medical director and written protocols A TKO rate is 30 mL/h
Route	IV infusion
How supplied	LR solution commonly supplied in 1,000-mL bags

TABLE 5.13   5% Dextrose Solution (D5W)

Indication for emergency use	Hypoglycemic patients, prophylactic IV access, or to dilute concentrated medications for IV infusion
Class	Hypotonic carbohydrate-containing solution
Description	Sterile water containing 5% dextrose (5 g/100 mL)
Mechanism of action	D5W is a hypotonic concentration that does not remain in vascular space, reduces danger of fluid overload
Contraindications	Patients who require IV fluid replacement, are hyperglycemic, or with traumatic brain injury (TBI) or stroke
Precautions	D5W is irritating to tissues; closely monitor site for irritation, swelling, or infiltration
Side effects	Rare when used in therapeutic doses
Interactions	Do not use for blood product infusion
Dosage	Normal is at a TKO rate of 30 mL/h
Route	IV infusion
How supplied	250-mL or 500-mL bags

and micro drip. Macro drip sets come in 10 gtt/mL, 15 gtt/mL, 20 gtt/mL; micro drip sets usually come in 60 gtt/mL. When caring for a critically injured patient or patients needing rapid fluid infusion, the macro drip set is appropriate. The AT should keep macro drip sets with IV fluids in the emergency medication kit.[30] Once the IV tubing is selected, it is time to spike the bag.

CLINICAL SKILLS

Spiking the Bag

1. Open the tubing package and ensure the roller clamp is turned off (rolled all the way down to crimp tubing).
2. Remove the seal from the port on the IV fluid bag (a).
3. Remove the cover from the spike on the IV tubing (b), making sure nothing comes into contact with the exposed spike.
4. Apply a slight twisting motion while inserting the exposed spike into the port on the IV fluid bag (c).
5. Proceed to squeeze the clear drip chamber on the IV tubing, filling it one-half to one-third full with IV fluid (d).
6. Release the roller clamp to flush the IV tubing with fluid, and remove all air in the tubing.
7. Place the end of the IV tubing within reach from where you will perform your **venipuncture**, and hang the IV bag.

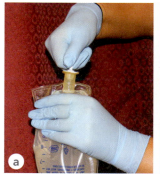 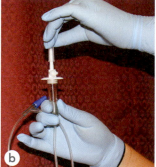 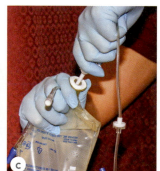 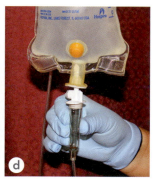

FIGURE 5.13
Courtesy of Dr. Eric J. Fuchs, ATC, NRAEMT.

CLINICAL SKILLS

Saline Lock Setup

Saline locks are commonly used to establish IV access on patients in pre-hospital and inpatient care settings.

1. Select a saline lock, open the package, and open a saline flush.
2. Connect the saline flush to the lock, and flush the lock so that no air is left in the tubing of the lock.
3. Place the lock with the attached flush within reach of where you will perform the venipuncture.

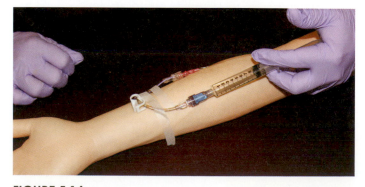

FIGURE 5.14
Courtesy of Dr. Eric J. Fuchs, ATC, NRAEMT.

Vein Selection for IV

ATs must learn how to properly select and identify a suitable vein for IV access; it is a skill that takes practice. Suitable veins for IV access are those on the posterior surface of the hand, forearm, and antecubital fossa region (figure 5.15).[11,29,30] Venipuncture can be performed on the lower extremities in the dorsum of the foot or ankle; however, these sites are not commonly selected due to a higher rate of complications for lower-extremity IVs and should be avoided when another site is available.[11] The AT should consult with the medical director to determine specific protocols or sites for venipuncture selection. The AT and medical director should keep in mind that special circumstances might require lower-extremity access when designing protocols. For example, you may have a patient who, because of a congenital defect, has only a left arm. During a soccer game, she fell and suffered a humeral fracture and dislocated the elbow of her left arm; she is going into decompensatory shock. This situation may require establishing peripheral IV access in the lower extremity. However, for the purposes of this book, the focus is on proper vein selection and establishing access in the hand, forearm, and antecubital fossa region.

The AT begins by applying a venous tourniquet to the patient's arm, which allows the veins to become engorged so that they are easier to locate through palpation and visualization.[30] This band should be placed proximally above the elbow if looking for a vein in the antecubital region (see figure 5.16), or located on the mid-forearm if looking to establish access in the posterior hand or wrist. ATs must learn to palpate for a vein and not completely rely on being able to see it to complete a venipuncture,

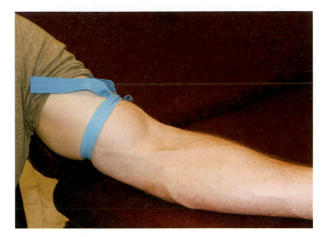

FIGURE 5.16 Tourniquet on the upper arm.

Courtesy of Dr. Eric J. Fuchs, ATC, NRAEMT.

because skin pigment and tattoos can make visualization of veins difficult.[30] The ideal vein is supple, full, and feels spongy or springy upon palpation regardless of visibility.

Venipuncture

The AT uses good aseptic technique to clean the site selected for venipuncture. Open the IV catheter and hold the IV catheter at a 45° angle or less to the skin. A common mistake is to start at too steep an angle to the skin; a 30° angle allows for the best chance of entering a vein and decreases the chance of "blowing the vein" by piercing both sides of the vein.[11,30] ATs should make sure the needle direction is in line with the direction of the vein prior to piercing the skin.

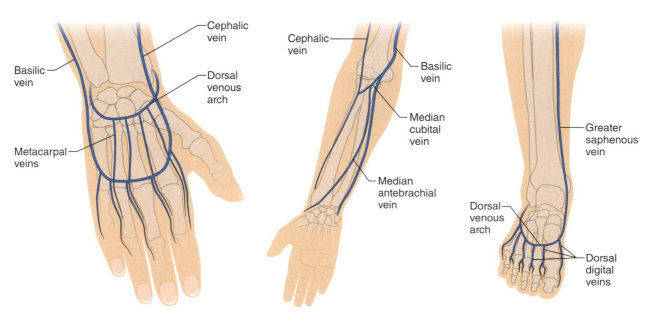

FIGURE 5.15   Veins suitable for peripheral IV access.

Tips for Vein Selection

- Superficial veins, while easily seen, are often more mobile and can move away from the needle tip, which is called "rolling veins." The AT can reduce this tendency of superficial veins from rolling by pulling the skin taut with the non-venipuncture hand to stabilize the vein.[11,30]

- Keep in mind that veins do have valves, which can sometimes be seen or palpated as slight bumps or bulges periodically along the vein. Avoid starting an IV too close to the distal aspect of a valve, because the IV catheter may not easily pass through the valve when you attempt the IV access.

- It is better to work distal to proximal when first starting an IV on a patient; in other words, work from the hand to the antecubital fossa.

- When selecting a vein, consider whether the patient condition warrants large volumes of fluid replacement or needs dextrose 25% or 50% (D25 or D50); if so, then a larger IV catheter and vein will be preferred.[11,30]

As you advance the needle through the skin, you will feel a popping sensation when you enter the vein and see "flash" (figure 5.17), which is blood flowing back through the needle and into a chamber in the catheter. Once you see blood in the flash chamber, you should lower the needle until almost flush with the skin, advance the needle 1 or 2 mm further into the vein, and then advance the catheter into the vein until the catheter hub is resting on the skin.[11,30] Once the catheter is deployed, activate the needle safety engineering on the IV catheter; this may be a button that auto retracts the needle, or once the catheter is advanced, the needle is locked into a sheath.[34,35]

After establishing flash and the catheter hub is resting on the skin, immediately release the tourniquet (which should be tied and able to be released with a single pull of one hand). As you release the tourniquet, you must apply pressure using the fingertips from one hand on the vein proximal to the catheter to occlude blood flow (see

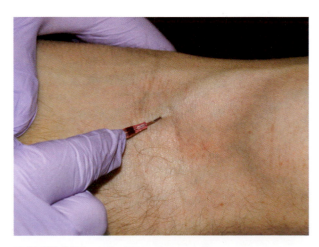

FIGURE 5.17 "Flash" in the needle.

Courtesy of Dr. Eric J. Fuchs, ATC, NRAEMT.

🚩 RED FLAG

Never pull the catheter back over the needle or advance the needle through the catheter. Either of those actions could result in the needle shearing off or tearing the plastic catheter, creating an embolus that can travel through the venous system.[11,30] If your initial attempt is unsuccessful at threading the catheter into the vein, then remove it and restart in a new location. Communicate with your patient and let her know that you will have to look for another vein. Always let your patient know that you will tell her when she will feel a stick. Use a calm, confident, reassuring tone when talking to your patient as this will help reduce her stress and help her to remain calm and reassured through the process.

figure 5.18). Advances in IV catheter design have led to the development of blood control IV catheters, which are recommended for use in sports medicine settings. These catheters will provide flash, but when the needle is disconnected or sheathed, blood will not leak from the hub until a saline lock or IV hub is connected, at which point the blood control barrier will be broken and IV access will occur.[30] This new technology reduces all HCPs' risk of exposure to blood. Make sure to deposit the IV needle into a sharps container.

Next, maintain pressure on the vein (if not using blood control catheters) until you connect the saline lock or IV tubing to the IV catheter hub. Once connected, remove pressure from the vein and proceed to flush the saline lock or check to see that the IV is flowing by looking at the drip chamber and releasing the IV clamp.[11,30] Once you've established flush or flowing, then you secure the

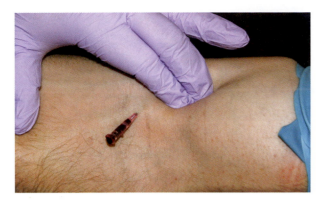

FIGURE 5.18 Occluding blood flow.
Courtesy of Dr. Eric J. Fuchs, ATC, NRAEMT.

catheter hub using a commercial dressing (i.e., Tegaderm, Opsite, etc.) and proceed to secure the tubing or lock with tape strips you previously had prepared. Monitor both the patient and the IV site for signs or symptoms of **infiltration** such as tissue swelling around the area or in ability for the IV to flow or line to flush. If there are issues, check that you removed the tourniquet and make sure all clamps on tubing are open; if you did and there are still issues, then discontinue the IV.[30] If blood backs up into the IV tubing, check to make sure the tourniquet has been released and that the IV bag is hung or placed above the level of the patient's heart.

Changing an IV Bag

In cases where large volumes of fluid are administered to a patient, which may include patients who have become dehydrated or are suffering from exertional heat stress like heat exhaustion or stroke, an AT may need to replace the initial IV bag with a new one. Best practice is to change an IV bag when a few milliliters of fluid are left in the bag rather than allowing the bag to fully empty into the IV tubing.[11,30] This prevents residual air from entering the IV tubing.

Here are the steps to change an IV bag:

1. Select a new bag of IV fluid and check the 6 rights of patient medication administration.
2. Close the roller clamp on the current IV, which prevents air from entering the tubing when you remove the spike from the bag.
3. Pull the tab on the new IV fluid bag.
4. Hold the empty bag upside down.
5. Pull the tubing out of the used IV bag.
6. Spike the new IV bag, and fill the drip chamber 1/2 to 1/3 full.
7. Re-hang the bag, adjust the flow rate, and make sure IV is flowing.

Administering Medication via an Established IV Access Point

Once an IV line has been established, medications can be administered through the IV line or saline lock. The CAATE 2020 standards specifically identify naloxone (see table 5.10) as medication ATs should know how to administer.

Dextrose (D50/D25), which is primarily used emergently for management of patients who have hypoglycemia, is another medication that should be administered via slow IV push (see table 5.14). Dextrose (D25/D50) usually comes in prepackaged emergency needless

TABLE 5.14 **Dextrose 50% (D50) / Dextrose 25% (D25)**

Indication for emergency use	D50—Hypoglycemic adult patient D25—Hypoglycemic pediatric patient
Class	Carbohydrate solution
Description	50 g/100 mL of dextrose in sterile water
Mechanism of action	Increase blood glucose concentrations to reverse acute hypoglycemia
Contraindications	Traumatic brain injury, stroke, and hyperglycemia, IV catheter <18ga
Precautions	Blood glucose level (BGL) should be checked prior to administration Severe tissue necrosis results if IV infiltration occurs
Side effects	Localized irritation of the vein
Interactions	No significant interactions for emergency administration
Dosage	Adult: 5 g slow IV push; repeat every 10-15 min if BGL <70 mL/dL Pediatric: 0.5 g/kg (500 mg/kg) of D25 (25 g/100 mL) If D25 not available, dilute D50 to 1:1 with sterile water or NS
Route	Slow IV push through 18ga IV catheter or greater
How supplied	Prefilled syringe 25 g of dextrose in 50 mL

syringes. Naloxone for IV administration also comes in prefilled emergency syringes. Naloxone IV should be titrated or slowly pushed until the patient's respiratory rate is stabilized.[11,36-39] Naloxone can be administered IV, IM, or intranasally (IN). Best practice for HCPs would be to deliver IM or IV; the Surgeon General of the United States issued a call for everyone to consider carrying naloxone in the form of IN.[26,40] Follow your medical director's established protocols for naloxone administration.

Unsuccessful IV Attempts

ATs will not always be successful with all IV attempts. Some attempts will result in a vein moving or that is difficult to locate; the needle may puncture both sides of

---

CLINICAL SKILLS

Administration of Medication Through an Established IV Line

1. Prepare the medication, and make sure the proper size IV catheter is in place for medication.
2. Clean the IV port with an alcohol prep pad.
3. Attach a syringe to the injection port.
4. Crimp IV tubing above the site of injection.
5. Inject the medication at the proper rate for that medication.
6. Dispose of the syringe in a sharps container.
7. Open IV fluid to flow wide open to flush medication.
8. Adjust the flow rate back to the established rate for the patient's condition.
9. Reassess the patient.

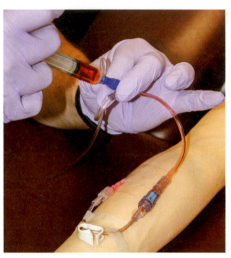

FIGURE 5.19
Courtesy of Dr. Eric J. Fuchs, ATC, NRAEMT.

CLINICAL SKILLS

Administration of Medication Through an Established Saline Lock

1. Prepare the medication by drawing it up, or assemble prefilled emergency medication syringe.
2. Get a minimum of 2 saline flushes.
3. Clean the attachment port on the saline lock with an alcohol swab.
4. Flush the saline lock with 1 saline flush to assure IV access is still patent.
5. Next, attach the medication syringe to the saline lock hub, and administer the medication; disconnect the syringe.
6. Then attach another saline flush, and flush the line.

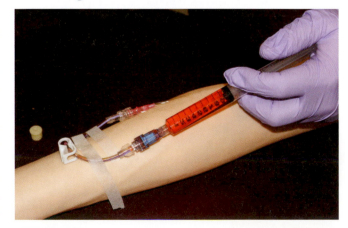

FIGURE 5.20
Courtesy of Dr. Eric J. Fuchs, ATC, NRAEMT.

the vein; or a catheter may meet resistance from a valve. If you make an unsuccessful attempt, then withdraw the IV catheter, dispose of it properly, and apply pressure to the site and a dressing. The AT should proceed to select a new site for attempting IV access on the patient.[11,30] ATs and the medical director should establish guidelines on the maximum number of attempts that an AT should or can make on a patient. However, this number may vary based on patient need and condition. ATs should document all attempts, location, and catheter size in the patient's chart.

Discontinuing an IV

If you need to discontinue an IV, follow these steps:

1. Always begin by closing the roller clamp on the IV tubing or, in the case of saline lock, activating the clamp on the lock.

2. Next, remove the IV catheter dressing and tape on the tubing or saline lock.

3. Place a small or folded 2×2 gauze pad over the insertion site of the skin and catheter hub.

4. Grasp the catheter hub with your other hand, and in one motion smoothly pull the catheter out as you apply pressure over the site with the gauze.

5. Once any bleeding has stopped, place a bandage over the site. Discard the catheter in a sharps container and the tubing and IV bag or saline lock in a biohazard bag.[30,39]

Provide the patient with post-IV care directions, which should include at minimum keeping the site cleaned with soap and water and to watch for any signs of infection, which they should be directed to report immediately to you or their physician.

Summary

ATs in all settings will treat and manage a variety of patients with medical or traumatic injuries, some of whom will benefit from the quick and proper administration of a variety of medications. The CAATE 2020 standards along with several NATA position statements clearly provide guidelines on what emergency medications should be available for use by an AT and the method or techniques by which an AT should be able to administer these medications regardless of enteral or parenteral delivery.[4,28,31,32,41,42] ATs must also recognize that IV access is an important skill that will allow administration of a variety of medications beyond just fluid replacement for management of heat or dehydration patients. ATs must develop written protocols, which should be reviewed and signed by their medical director and reviewed by the facility's or institution's legal counsel.[29,30] These protocols should be reviewed annually for updates or changes based on current evidence-based practice. ATs need to review state practice acts; some skills and medication administration discussed in this chapter and identified in the CAATE 2020 standards may not be within the scope of practice for an AT in some states.[29,30] ATs should advocate for changes to their state practice acts based on current evidence, education, and training of ATs and to ensure that patients are provided the best evidence-based care available when faced with an emergency.

 Go to the web study guide to complete the case studies for this chapter.

PART II

Immediate Management of Acute Injuries and Illnesses

Once the health care team is prepared for emergencies, it can deal with the immediate management of acute injuries and illnesses. Immediate management involves applying the basic concepts of the emergency examination, identifying a chief complaint, monitoring and reassessing the patient as emergency medical services arrive, and handing the patient off to the next level of care. The care provided within the first few minutes of an acute injury or illness can determine the outcome and limit the severity of a potentially limb- or life-threatening condition. Understanding the underlying anatomy and physiology of the body and the etiology of common conditions, and knowing how to respond are important aspects of clinical decision-making during an emergency. The chapters in this section describe how to examine, treat, and manage common acute injuries and illnesses so that the health care practitioner has the knowledge and skills to appropriately manage these potentially life-threatening conditions.

CHAPTER 6

Immediate Management of Bleeding, Shock, and Immunologic Emergencies

After reading this chapter, you will be able to do the following:

- Appropriately identify the indications of excessive external or internal bleeding (hemorrhage).

- Recognize and perform emergency medical care to control bleeding, prevent or treat shock, and prevent contamination of wounds.

- Recognize and manage stages of shock, including emergency medical care for undifferentiated shock.

- Recognize acute anaphylactic reactions, and appropriately treat the patient with anaphylaxis.

For both trauma and medical emergent conditions, prehospital health care providers (HCPs) must be diligent about recognizing the signs of **hemorrhage**, shock, or immunologic dysfunction. For most trauma and medical patients, assessment and management should occur simultaneously while addressing the most life-threatening condition first. The athletic trainer (AT) and other prehospital HCPs should be prepared to appropriately treat a patient with hemorrhage, shock, **anaphylaxis**, or myriad other conditions common in the sports and athletic settings. A rapid assessment of the possible cause of the problem is essential when acute emergent conditions cause hemodynamic instability, and a thorough physical examination should be performed. The prehospital HCP may be required to give an estimate of blood loss, report vital signs, or document when a tourniquet was applied or epinephrine administered. Although the sport and athletic population typically consists of young patients at the peak of their health, a seriously injured or ill patient might present with **tachycardia** and mild hypotension. This patient is potentially in danger of quickly losing compensatory mechanisms and may slip into profound shock unless vigorous therapy is initiated. Reliance on linking the clinical impression with objective data is essential to arriving at a correct diagnosis. The clinical impression is determined by considering the patient's history of present illness, age, underlying health status, and general appearance (described in chapter 4). Objective data needed are not always available in the field, but the prehospital HCP must obtain as much quantitative data as possible, especially vital signs and perfusion. For a patient who presents with a potential life-threatening condition, the HCP must immediately initiate treatment while rapidly identifying the etiology of the condition.

The ability to rapidly assess and identify the cause of the condition is essential so that definitive therapy can be administered to save the patient's life.

Overview of the Circulatory System

The clinical anatomy and physiology of the heart and lungs are presented in chapters 10 and 11. **Perfusion** is the circulation of blood within an organ or tissue with adequate amounts to meet the cells' current needs for oxygen, nutrients, and waste removal. Blood enters an organ or tissue first through the arteries, then the arterioles, and finally the capillary beds.[1] Billions of capillaries are the main site of transport of water, gases, electrolytes, substrates, and waste products between the bloodstream and the extracellular fluid.[2] During emergencies, the autonomic nervous system automatically constricts smooth muscle in arterioles, thereby redirecting blood away from other organs to the heart, brain, lungs, and kidneys. Thus, the cardiovascular system is dynamic, constantly adapting to changing conditions. At times, the system fails to provide sufficient circulation for every body part to perform its function, resulting in **hypoperfusion**, which can lead to death. Knowing which organs need adequate perfusion is the foundation on which your treatment of patients is based.[1,2]

Components of Blood

Blood is a specialized connective tissue that contains these formed elements: red cells, white cells, and platelets (figure 6.1). The average adult has about 5.3 quarts (5 L) of whole blood, with 5.0 to 6.0 L in men and 4.5 to 5.5 L in women. Blood accounts for 6% to 8% of the body weight of a healthy adult.[2] Plasma is the liquid portion of the blood. It comprises mostly water (93%); the remaining 7% is various dissolved solutes (6% organic substances and 1% inorganic substances). Plasma contains key electrolytes and dissolved nutrients, namely, glucose, amino acids, and fatty acids. About 55% of whole blood is made up of plasma, the liquid portion of blood, and it becomes serum after clotting factors are removed.[2]

Determinants of Perfusion

Perfusion occurs when blood circulates through tissues or an organ to provide necessary oxygen and nutrients and remove metabolic waste products. The microcirculation, or capillaries, is the site of exchange of nutrients, water, gas, and small molecules between the plasma and the tissues (figure 6.2). Under normal conditions, the capillaries do not allow exchange of peptides, proteins, and other large molecules between tissues and plasma. Virtually every cell in the body is in close contact with a capillary. Arterioles control blood flow into a region of tissue and, along with precapillary sphincters, control the distribution of blood flow within the capillary network.[2] This microcirculation regulates blood flow to individual organs, the distribution of blood flow within organs, diffusion distances between an organ's blood supply and tissues, as well as the capillary surface area available for exchange of materials between the plasma and tissues. In conjunction with cardiac output, the microcirculation helps maintain arterial blood pressure by altering total peripheral vascular resistance and diastolic filling of the heart.[2]

Reduced perfusion of vital tissues leads to declines in oxygen delivery to cells and is inadequate for aerobic metabolism. As cell function declines, the condition of **shock** can lead to irreversible cell damage and death.[3] The pathophysiologic response to blood loss (hemorrhage) that causes shock is described in detail later in this chapter.

Hemorrhage

Hemorrhage is bleeding that leads to an acute loss of circulating blood volume. Severity of hemorrhage depends on blood volume loss and duration of ongoing bleeding, which may become life-threatening if untreated or uncontrolled. Life-threatening hemorrhage requires a massive transfusion of blood (from a donor) to prevent **sepsis** or **multiple organ failure** (MOF). Controlling hemorrhage, managing shock, and preventing trauma-induced coagulopathy are the foundations of treatment of imminent **exsanguination** in the prehospital and ED settings.[4,5] The goal of prehospital care of bleeding trauma patients is to deliver the patient to a facility for

Red blood cells   Platelets   White blood cell

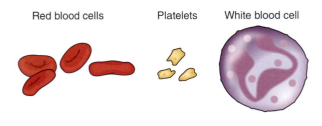

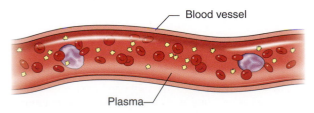

Blood vessel

Plasma

FIGURE 6.1   Components of blood.

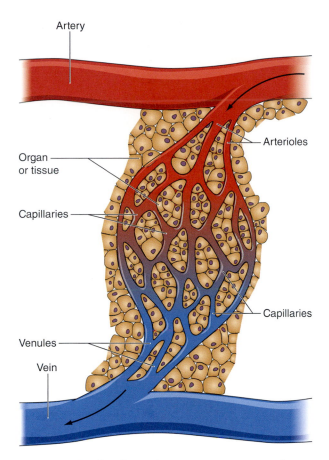

FIGURE 6.2   Capillaries between an artery and vein.

definitive care within the shortest amount of time by rapid transport and minimize out-of-hospital treatment to what is necessary to maintain adequate vital signs.[6] Complications with hemorrhage that the AT may encounter in the prehospital setting include disorders associated with clotting, including **deep vein thrombosis (DVT)** and other **hypercoagulable** conditions.

Epidemiology of Complications With Hemorrhage

Major orthopedic injuries, in particular fractures of large bones (pelvis, femur), that often require surgery carry a high risk for **venous thromboembolism (VTE)**, which includes deep vein thrombosis (DVT) and **pulmonary embolism (PE)**.[7] PE is the most common preventable cause of death among hospital patients in the United Sates, yet VTE is often overlooked as a major public health problem. The potential public health benefit of preventing VTE is large. Data from randomized trials involving general surgical patients suggest that adequate prevention measures in high-risk patients can prevent VTE in 1 of 10 patients and save the life of about 1 of 200 patients.[8] DVT most commonly occurs in the lower

extremities or pelvis and can develop in deep veins of the upper extremities (4%-13% of DVT cases). Lower-extremity DVT is much more likely to cause PE, particularly from the superficial femoral and popliteal veins in the thighs. Posterior tibial and peroneal veins in the calves are most commonly affected by DVT but are less likely to be a source of PE that moves through the proximal thigh veins. Lower-extremity DVT most often results from immobilization, limb trauma, or other causes (see Risk Factors for Deep Vein Thrombosis in Sports Medicine Setting).[7-9]

Upper-extremity DVT is less common in the sports medicine setting but occasionally occurs as a result of a hypercoagulable state or subclavian vein compression at the thoracic outlet, in which blood clots form in the deep veins of the arms, usually in the axillary or subclavian veins (thoracic outlet syndrome) or occur during strenuous arm activity (**effort thrombosis**, or **Paget-Schroetter syndrome**), which accounts for 1% to 4% of upper-extremity DVT cases.[9] In approximately 60% to 80% of effort thrombosis cases, a history of venous obstruction exists with vigorous exercise or activity, with an incidence of 1 to 2 per 100,000 individuals per year.[10] This condition occurs in predominantly upper-extremity sports, such as baseball, softball, and swimming, but it has been reported in wrestling, hockey, martial arts, backpacking, and billiards.[10] A study (more details in Evidence section) identified 32 high-level athletes with effort thrombosis over a 10-year time frame, 14 of whom were baseball players.[11] Overhead workers and manual laborers are considered industrial athletes, subjecting their upper extremities to similar forces, which increases the likelihood of this condition. Clinicians should be aware of this condition and its symptoms, because early intervention can be lifesaving.[10,12]

Pathophysiology of Hemorrhage

Hemodynamic response to an acute blood loss from circulation depends on several confounding factors. These factors must be promptly recognized during the initial assessment and treatment of trauma patients at risk for hemorrhagic shock. Factors that contribute to severity of hemorrhage include the following:[5]

- Patient's age
- Severity of injury, with special attention to type and anatomic location of injury
- Time lapse between injury and initiation of treatment
- Prehospital treatment available
- Medications used for chronic conditions

Hemorrhage results from trauma such as major soft tissue injuries and fractures. Blood is lost into the site

Risk Factors for Deep Vein Thrombosis in the Sports Medicine Setting

More Common

- Immobilization
- Limb trauma
- Recent surgery (past 3 months)
- Obesity
- Oral contraceptives
- Pregnancy and postpartum
- Prior venous thromboembolism

Less Common

- Age > 60 years
- Cigarette smoking*
- Heart failure
- Effort thrombosis, or Paget-Schroetter syndrome
- Hypercoagulability disorders
- Malignancy or cancer
- Estrogen therapy
- Sickle cell anemia

*Including secondhand or passive smoking

Based on Douketis (2017); Kearon and Jauer (2017); Tubbs, Savitt, and Suner (2016).

of injury, particularly in cases of internal bleeding or major fractures (see details in chapter 7). The degree of blood volume loss is related to the magnitude of the tissue injury. Tissue injury results in activation of a systemic inflammatory response and production and release of multiple cytokines. Many of these locally active hormones have profound effects on the vascular endothelium, which increases permeability. Tissue edema is the result of shifts in fluid primarily from the plasma into the extravascular, extracellular space. Such shifts produce an additional depletion in intravascular volume.[3,5]

Cardiovascular Responses to Acute Blood Loss

Three cardiovascular variables—ventricular filling (preload), the resistance to ventricular ejection (afterload), and myocardial contractility—are essential in controlling stroke volume. Cardiac output, the major determinant of tissue perfusion, is the product of stroke volume and heart rate (HR; figure 6.3).[2,5]

Early circulatory responses to blood loss are compensatory; progressive vasoconstriction of cutaneous muscle and visceral circulation preserve blood flow by **shunting** blood toward the kidneys, heart, and brain. The response to acute circulating volume depletion associated

with injury is an increase in heart rate in an attempt to preserve cardiac output. In most cases, tachycardia is the earliest measurable circulatory sign of shock. The release of endogenous catecholamines increases peripheral vascular resistance, which in turn increases diastolic blood pressure and reduces pulse pressure, but it does little to increase organ perfusion.[5,16] Rapid decreases in blood volume can lead to decreases in cardiac output and oxygen delivery because blood flow is preferentially distributed to tissues with greater metabolic requirements. Despite this organ-specific microvascular response, all organs, with the exception of the heart, experience decreases in blood flow during severe hypovolemia.[2,17,18]

Types of Hemorrhage

Hemorrhage, or discharge of blood from the blood vessels, can range from a superficial cut from a piece of equipment, to a spurting artery from an open fracture, or a ruptured spleen from a direct blow to the abdomen during a tackle. External bleeding is visible hemorrhaging that can usually be controlled with direct pressure or a pressure bandage (see Emergency Care for Hemorrhage). Internal bleeding is hemorrhaging that is not visible and is usually not controlled until a surgeon locates the source and sutures the injured structure closed. Any trauma to

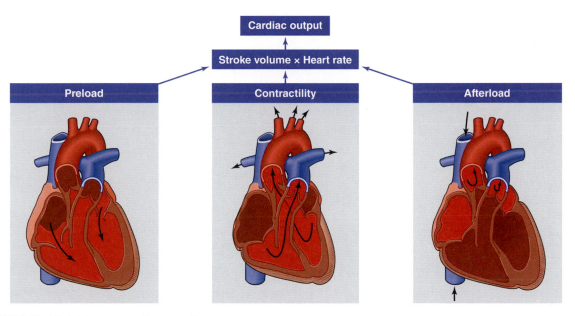

FIGURE 6.3 Variables controlling cardiac output.

the thorax, abdomen, or head that could lead to internal bleeding should be a concern, because the internal hemorrhage is not easily observed or identified. It is essential to depend on signs and symptoms to determine the extent and severity of the hemorrhage. Several signs and symptoms indicate unusual or excessive bleeding, such as the following:[1,3]

- Trauma to the mouth or face, including tooth loss
- Skin wounds with prolonged bleeding
- **Ecchymosis** (collection of blood under skin; bruise)
- **Epistaxis** (unexplained or uncontrolled bleeding from the nose)
- **Hematemesis** (vomiting fresh blood)
- **Hemoptysis** (coughing up blood from the lungs)
- **Menorrhagia** (excessive or prolonged menstrual blood flow)
- **Petechiae** (small intradermal or mucosal hemorrhages)
- **Purpura** (larger areas of mucosal or skin hemorrhage)
- **Telangiectasias** (dilated small vessels visible on skin or mucosa; spider veins)

Classes of Hemorrhage

Estimating blood loss is complicated by several factors, including urinary losses and the development of tissue edema. To help guide volume replacement, the *Advanced Trauma Life Support (ATLS) Manual* divides hemorrhage into four classes (table 6.1), summarized as follows:[5]

RED FLAG

Signs of hemorrhage that should be treated in the prehospital setting and transferred to the emergency department (ED) are the following:[1,22]

- Bleeding is not controlled, requires a tourniquet, or is a result of severe trauma.
- Sutures or other wound closures are needed.
- Cleansing the wound cannot remove debris.
- Mechanism of injury (MOI) may lead to internal bleeding or shock.
- Signs of infection are present (e.g., increased pain, redness, swelling, yellow or brown fluid, enlarged or tender lymph nodes, fever, or red streaks spreading proximally from the wound).
- Wound is from animal or human bite.
- Patient received a tetanus booster more than 10 years ago.

- *Class I*. Class I is a nonshock state, such as occurs when donating a unit of blood. Typically no change occurs in vital signs, and fluid resuscitation is not usually necessary.

- *Class II*. When 15% to 30% of total blood volume is lost, a class II hemorrhage patient is often tachycardic (rapid heartbeat) with a narrowing of the difference

TABLE 6.1 **Classes of Hemorrhage and Estimated Blood Loss Based on Patient's Clinical Presentation**

Clinical sign	Class I	Class II	Class III	Class IV
Blood loss (mL)	< 750	750-1,500	1,500-2,000	> 2,000
Blood loss (% blood volume)	< 15	15-30	30-40	> 40
Pulse rate (bpm)	< 100	↑ 100-120	↑ 120-140	↑ > 140
Blood pressure (mm Hg)	Normal	Normal	↓	↓
Pulse pressure (mm Hg)	Normal or ↓	↓	↓	↓
Respiratory rate (rpm)	14-20	↑ 20-30	↑ 30-40	↑ > 35
Skin appearance	Pink or normal	Pale and cool	Slow capillary refill	Cyanotic or white
CNS/mental status	Slightly anxious	Mildly anxious	Anxious, confused	Confused, lethargic
IV fluid resuscitation	Crystalloid*	Crystalloid	Crystalloid and blood	Crystalloid and blood

*Almost all shock states require large-volume intravenous (IV) fluid resuscitation. Crystalloid solutions (e.g., 0.9% saline or lactated Ringer's solution) are used for intravascular volume replenishment because they are isotonic with blood (described in chapter 5).

Based on Pollack and Beck (2012); de Moya (2013): American College of Surgeons (2012); Gutierrez, Reines, and Wolf-Gutierrez (2004); Bulger et al. (2014); Rossaint et al. (2010); Colwell (2017).

between the systolic and diastolic blood pressures (pulse pressure). The body attempts to compensate with peripheral vasoconstriction such that the skin may start to appear pale and be cool to the touch. The patient may exhibit slight changes in behavior. Volume resuscitation with crystalloids (saline solution or **lactated Ringer's [LR] solution**) is typically required, but blood transfusion is not required.

• *Class III*. When 30% to 40% of circulating blood volume is lost, a class III hemorrhage patient has decreased blood pressure and increased heart rate. Peripheral hypoperfusion (shock) is indicated by slow capillary refill and anxious mental status. Fluid resuscitation with crystalloid and blood transfusion are usually necessary.

• *Class IV*. When more than 40% of circulating blood volume is lost, a class IV hemorrhage reaches the limit of the body's compensation and aggressive resuscitation is required to prevent death.

This system of classification[1,5] represents a continuum of ongoing hemorrhage that should guide initial treatment. This classification system is useful in emphasizing the early signs and pathophysiology of the shock state (described later in this chapter).[1,3,17] Additional conditions that accompany signs of hemorrhage should be immediately treated in the prehospital setting and transported to the nearest trauma center.

Physiologic Response to Hemorrhage

Hemostasis is a series of separate but interrelated steps that occur in response to blood that is outside of the vascular system. This instinctive response stops bleeding and reduces the loss of blood[23] at the site of vascular injury through the formation of an impermeable platelet and fibrin plug.[24] Blood **coagulation** involves the fast formation of a weak platelet plug stabilized by fibrinogen, which is expanded and stabilized into a more robust plug made of cells, platelets, and insoluble fibrin molecules. The process is directed by mediators released by platelets that cause blood coagulation and clotting. Thrombin is necessary for fibrin clot formation, and plasmin for clot dissolution.[2,25] The process of hemostasis (figure 6.4) occurs within 60 seconds of the initial insult to the vascular endothelium.[23] The process of hemostasis involves the following steps:[2,23-26]

1. *Vascular spasm*: This immediate response to blood vessel injury or damage causes vasoconstriction that reduces blood flow through the area and limits blood loss. Damaged endothelium exposes collagen and releases clotting factors that attract platelets to the injury site.

2. *Formation of platelet plug*: Circulating platelets are activated to become sticky and adhere to exposed collagen, forming a loose, temporary platelet plug that limits blood loss. Activated platelets attract other platelets

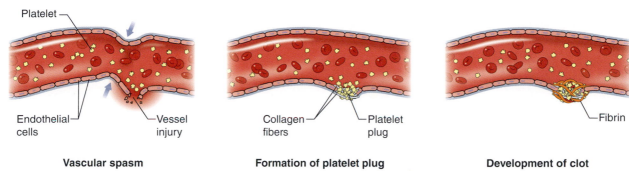

Vascular spasm   Formation of platelet plug   Development of clot

FIGURE 6.4   Process of hemostasis.

to the injury site, producing aggregation and adhesion, thereby continuing the process in a **positive feedback** loop.

3. *Development of clot*: Clotting factors are proteins carried in blood plasma in an inactive state that become activated (coagulation cascade) leading to thrombin, which converts fibrinogen into fibrin. Fibrin forms a mesh that holds the platelet plug in place, forming a more stable, insoluble fibrin clot (**thrombus**). During this process, red and white blood cells may be trapped in the mesh, causing the plug to become harder and resulting in a **thrombosis** (see Deep Vein Thrombosis). If the thrombosis becomes detached from the vessel wall and travels through blood vessel (**embolus**), it may cause a vascular occlusion (**embolism**) that could lead to stroke, heart attack, or pulmonary embolism.

Complications With Hemorrhage

The coagulation system is intricately balanced and designed to stop bleeding at the site of vascular injury through complex interactions between the vascular endothelium, platelets, procoagulant proteins, anticoagulant proteins, and fibrinolytic proteins. Derangements in this system can lead to either bleeding or thrombosis. Bleeding disorders (**coagulopathy**) are the result of a coagulation factor defect, a quantitative or qualitative platelet defect, or enhanced fibrinolytic activity. Abnormal bleeding can result from platelet disorders, coagulation disorders, or blood vessel (vascular) disorders that can be acquired or hereditary. Injury or trauma can impair hemostasis and activation of fibrinolysis. Drug history should be reviewed, because certain medications, such as beta-adrenergic receptor blockers and calcium-channel blockers, can significantly alter a patient's hemodynamic response to hemorrhage.[5] Other drugs (details in chapter 5), such as heparin, warfarin, aspirin, NSAIDs, and some sulfa antibiotics increase the anticoagulant effect.[23]

Generally, any excessive bleeding may lead to complications related to the following:[23]

- Platelet disorders leading to decreased platelet function
- Inadequate production of platelets (e.g., leukemia, some anemias)
- Drug-induced platelet destruction (e.g., by heparin, some sulfa antibiotics)
- Inadequate platelet function (drug-induced dysfunction, e.g., by aspirin or NSAIDs)
- Acquired platelet disorders (e.g., vitamin K deficiency, vitamin C deficiency, vasculitis, liver disease, anticoagulation with warfarin, heparin or direct inhibitors of thrombin or other clotting factors)
- Coagulation disorders
- Deep vein thrombosis (DVT)
- Disseminated intravascular coagulation (DIC)
- Hereditary disorders (e.g., hemophilia, connective tissue disorders such as Marfan syndrome)
- Vascular disorders

In diagnosing coagulation disorders, laboratory testing is not feasible in the prehospital setting. Instead, the focus is to suspect the coagulopathy, refer for evaluation, and appropriately manage acute thrombosis. The diagnostic approach to individual episodes of a suspected hypercoagulant patient is site specific (e.g., cerebral circulation, coronary circulation, or peripheral venous system).[26] This text focuses on these 2 clotting disorders that are likely to be found in the sports medicine or prehospital setting: deep vein thrombosis and disseminated intravascular coagulation (DIC)[26]

Deep Vein Thrombosis   Deep vein thrombosis (DVT) is a condition that may occur in athletic patients, often as a complication of immobilization, surgery, obesity, or oral contraceptive use. A DVT is clotting of blood (figure 6.5) in a deep vein of an extremity (usually calf or thigh) or pelvis.[27] Most deep vein thrombi occur in the small calf veins, are asymptomatic, and may be

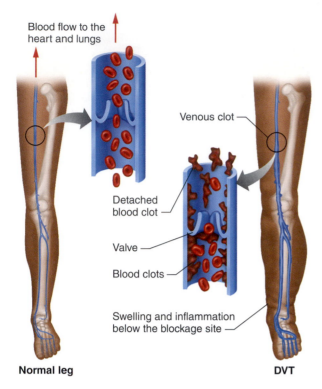

Blood flow to the heart and lungs

Venous clot

Detached blood clot

Valve

Blood clots

Swelling and inflammation below the blockage site

Normal leg   **DVT**

FIGURE 6.5 Swelling and inflammation caused by a DVT.

undetected or misdiagnosed.[13,14] Referral and testing for DVT are crucial, because clinical assessment alone is unreliable and the consequences of misdiagnosis are serious, including fatal pulmonary embolism (PE). Refer to earlier sections, Epidemiology of Complications With Hemorrhage and Risk Factors for Deep Vein Thrombosis in the Sports Medicine Setting.

Clinical features of lower-extremity DVT are non-specific, and many patients are asymptomatic. Therefore, obtaining a thorough history is essential. DVT should be suspected in patients who present with leg swelling, pain, warmth, and erythema. Symptoms are usually unilateral but can be bilateral and are confined to the calf in patients with isolated distal DVT, while patients with proximal DVT may have calf or whole leg symptoms.[14] Although often unrevealing, a physical examination of the legs, abdomen, and pelvis should be performed in patients with suspected DVT to look for the following:[13-15]

- Dilated superficial veins
- Unilateral pitting edema or swelling
- Unilateral warmth, tenderness, or erythema
- Pain and tenderness along the course of the involved major veins
- Low-grade fever

- Local (e.g., inguinal mass) or general signs of malignancy
- Calf swelling (> 1.18 in./3 cm difference in circumference between calves, measured 3.9 in./10 cm below tibial tuberosity)

When present, symptoms and signs (e.g., vague aching pain, tenderness along the distribution of the veins, edema, erythema) are nonspecific, vary in frequency and severity, and are similar in arms and legs. Dilated collateral superficial veins may become visible or palpable. Calf discomfort elicited by ankle dorsiflexion with the knee extended (**Homan's sign**) occasionally occurs with distal leg DVT but is neither sensitive nor specific.[13,15] Tenderness, swelling of the whole leg, pitting edema, and collateral superficial veins may be most specific. A difference in circumference of more than 1.18 inches (3 cm) between calves may be most helpful.[13]

Alternative or differential diagnoses that are more likely than DVT include Baker's cyst, cellulitis, muscle damage, **post-phlebitic syndrome**, inguinal **lymphadenopathy**, or external venous compression. Unfortunately, DVT is often asymptomatic with PE, an immediate complication. Diagnosis is by history and physical examination and is confirmed by objective testing, typically with venous ultrasonography.[13,14,27]

Treatment of lower- and upper-extremity DVT is generally the same. All patients with DVT are prescribed anticoagulants, initially an injectable heparin (see table 6.2) for a brief period, followed by longer-term treatment with an oral drug (e.g., warfarin) within 48 hours. General supportive measures include pain control with analgesics, which may include short (3- to 5-day) courses of a NSAID. Extended treatment with a NSAID and aspirin is often avoided because their antiplatelet effects may increase the risk of bleeding complications. In addition, elevating the legs (supported by a pillow or other soft surface to avoid venous compression) is recommended during periods of inactivity. Patients may be as physically active as they can tolerate; no evidence shows that early activity increases risk of clot dislodgement and PE and may help to reduce the risk of post-phlebitic syndrome.[13,15]

Disseminated Intravascular Coagulation

Normal hemostasis ensures formation of a blood clot at the site of vessel injury, followed by resolution of the clot to allow tissue repair. Multiple feedback mechanisms are built into this system to prevent activation of coagulation in the absence of vessel injury and restrict the clot to the site of injury (see previous section, Physiologic Response to Hemorrhage).[30] However, in **disseminated intravascular coagulation (DIC)**, small blood clots develop throughout the bloodstream, blocking small blood vessels. The increased clotting depletes the platelets

TABLE 6.2 **Pharmacological Agents That Reduce Blood Clots (Anticoagulants and Platelet Aggregation Inhibitors)**

Drug name, route	Brand name	Indications	Adverse reactions*
Heparin, injection	Hep Flush-10	Treatment of DIC, prevention of clotting after surgery	Hypersensitivity/anaphylaxis, uncontrolled bleeding state
Warfarin, oral	Coumadin, Jantoven	Clotting complications (prophylaxis/treatment) or some heart conditions (risk reduction)	Can cause major or fatal bleeding
Acetylsalicylic acid (ASA), tablet	Aspirin, Bayer Aspirin	Prevention and treatment of DVT, arterial thrombosis	Less effective than others, bleeding risk
Other NSAIDs, tablet	Motrin, Voltaren, Naproxen	Conditions requiring blood thinners	Increased risk of fatal heart attack or stroke, and GI bleeding. Avoid while taking other blood thinners

*Patients should be educated to minimize the risk of bleeding and report signs and symptoms of bleeding immediately to their HCP.

Based on Tubbs, Savitt, and Suner (2016); Drugs.com. *Anticoagulants* (2017); Drugs.com. *Nonsteroidal Anti-Inflammatory Agents* (2017).

and clotting factors needed to control bleeding, causing excessive bleeding.[9] Increased platelet aggregation and coagulation factor consumption occur, producing diffuse microvascular thrombosis and hemorrhage.[30,31]

DIC can be an acute, life-threatening emergency with complications that depend on morbidities from the underlying cause.[30] DIC may evolve slowly (over weeks or months) or rapidly (over hours or days), caused primarily by bleeding. Severe, rapidly evolving DIC causes **thrombocytopenia** and depletion of plasma coagulation factors and fibrinogen, which cause bleeding. Bleeding into organs, along with microvascular thromboses, may cause dysfunction and failure in multiple organs. The most common cause of DIC in the prehospital setting is shock due to any condition that causes ischemic tissue injury and release of tissue factor.[31] Other common causes of DIC in the sports medicine setting include the following:[30]

- Sepsis from a variety of organisms (bacterial, fungal, viral, and parasitic)
- Trauma, especially to the central nervous system
- Heatstroke
- Crush injuries (in addition to **rhabdomyolysis**)
- Amphetamine overdose
- Fat embolism
- Vascular abnormalities (e.g., aortic aneurysm)
- Rattlesnake or other snake bite
- Malignancy (e.g., leukemia, tumors)

Diagnosis of severe, rapidly evolving DIC in the prehospital setting is not feasible, because this condition is diagnosed by testing platelet count and prothrombin clotting time. Findings consistent with acute DIC include the following, although none of these findings are highly specific for DIC:[30]

- Recent history of trauma, sepsis, or malignancy
- Bleeding, especially oozing from sites of trauma
- Abnormalities of coagulation testing (in the hospital setting)

Treatment of acute DIC requires rapid transfer to the hospital setting for correction of the cause and replacement of platelets, coagulation factors, and fibrinogen to control severe bleeding. Heparin is used as therapy (or prophylaxis) in patients with slowly evolving DIC who have (or are at risk of) venous thromboembolism.[31]

Systemic Responses to Acute Hemorrhage (Transition to Shock)

The first response to blood loss is an attempt to form a clot at the local site of hemorrhage. As hemorrhage progresses, catecholamines, antidiuretic hormone, and atrial natriuretic receptors respond to the perceived loss of volume by vasoconstriction of arterioles and muscular arteries and by increasing the heart rate. The aim of these compensatory mechanisms is to increase cardiac output and maintain perfusion pressure. Urine output decreases and thirst is stimulated to maintain circulating blood volume.[17] Internal abdominal bleeding should be suspected in a patient with referred pain or slowly deteriorating vital signs. The first sign of hypovolemic shock (hypoperfusion) is a change in mental status, such as anxiety, restlessness, or combativeness. In nontrauma patients, weakness, faintness, or dizziness on standing are other early signs. Changes in skin color or pallor are often found in both trauma and medical patients.[1] Anxiety may be related to the release of catecholamines and to mild decreases in cerebral blood flow. A person who is bleeding briskly also may develop **tachypnea** and hypotension. As hypovolemia worsens and tissue hypoxia ensues, increases in ventilation compensate for the metabolic acidosis produced by increased carbon dioxide production. Compensatory mechanisms are eventually overwhelmed by volume losses; and blood flow to the viscera decreases and systolic blood pressure declines. The loss of coronary perfusion pressure adversely affects myocardial contractility; cerebral blood flow decreases, resulting in the loss of consciousness, coma, and eventually death.[17]

Assessment of the Patient With Hemorrhage

A rapid assessment of the possible source of bleeding is essential when acute hemorrhage is the suspected cause for hemodynamic instability, and a thorough physical examination should be performed. Emergency personnel may give an estimate of blood loss at the scene, but one should always be wary of such estimates because they are notoriously inaccurate. In general, young patients who present with tachycardia and mild hypotension (see table 4.7 for BP classification) are in danger of losing their compensatory mechanisms and may well slip into profound shock unless vigorous therapy is initiated. Reliance on systolic blood pressure alone may delay recognition of the shock state (see text that follows). Most practitioners can palpate a carotid pulse in an adult. This is equivalent to a systolic pressure of 60 mm Hg. A femoral pulse is produced by a systolic pressure of 60 to 70 mm Hg. A palpable radial pulse usually requires slightly higher pressures.[17]

Ideally, shock is recognized before hypotension develops. The clinical presentation of traumatic shock depends on the rate, volume, and duration of bleeding, the patient's baseline physiology, and the presence of other acute pathologic processes (e.g., tension pneumothorax, myocardial ischemia). Large-scale bleeding occurs at these 5 possible locations:

- External hemorrhage
- Thoracic cavity
- Peritoneal cavity
- Retroperitoneal space (often from a pelvic fracture)
- Muscle or subcutaneous tissue (usually from a long-bone fracture)

Bleeding that can be controlled (such as external bleeding that responds to a pressure bandage) and bleeding that cannot be controlled (such as a femur fracture) are serious emergencies. Consequently, the primary assessment of the patient includes identifying life-threatening bleeding. If found, the hemorrhaging must be controlled; if the hemorrhaging cannot be controlled in the field, rapidly transport the patient to the ED.[1]

Indications of Excessive Bleeding

Vital signs and general appearance can indicate hypovolemia (tachycardia, hypotension, pallor, and **diaphoresis**) or infection (fever, tachycardia, hypotension with sepsis). The skin and mucous membranes (nose, mouth) are examined for petechiae, purpura, and telangiectasias. Signs of bleeding in deeper tissues may include tenderness during movement and local swelling, muscle hematomas and, for intracranial bleeding, confusion, stiff neck, focal neurologic abnormalities, or a combination of these findings.[32]

Indications of Internal Bleeding

Internal hemorrhage is one of the most serious consequences of trauma. Usually, hemorrhage results from obvious injuries that require rapid medical attention. However, internal bleeding may occur after a less severe MOI or may be delayed by hours or days.[20] Most cases of internal bleeding result from trauma to the thorax, abdomen, retroperitoneum, and from major external wounds. For example, the thigh can hold up to approximately 1 to 2 L of blood following femur fracture.[21] Because it is difficult to identify internal bleeding, a high index of suspicion should be maintained while actively identifying signs and symptoms of blood loss (details follow). A patient with an unidentified source of bleeding should undergo immediate further assessment of the chest, abdominal cavity, and pelvic ring, which represent the major sources

 RED FLAG

The following findings are of particular concern for excessive bleeding:[1,32]

- Significant mechanism of injury (MOI), especially when the MOI suggests that severe forces affected the abdomen, chest, or both
- Significant or rapid blood loss
- Poor general appearance of the patient
- Signs of shock, hypoperfusion, hypovolemia, or hemorrhagic shock
- Abdominal tenderness or rigidity
- Local swelling, muscle hematomas
- Confusion, stiff neck, focal neurologic abnormalities
- Signs of infection or sepsis

of acute blood loss in trauma.[20] Prompt transport to the ED is necessary for controlling internal bleeding,[33] which often requires surgical bleeding control.[20]

Internal bleeding may occur after any significant physical injury. Two main types of trauma can occur, and either may cause internal bleeding.

- *Blunt trauma* involves a body part colliding with another object, usually at high speed. Blood vessels inside the body are torn or crushed by a shear force or a blunt object. Examples include a blast from an improvised explosive device (IED), fall from a high place, physical assault, or car accident.

- *Penetrating trauma* occurs when a foreign object penetrates the body, tearing a hole in one or more blood vessels. Examples include bomb shrapnel, gunshot wounds, stabbings, or falling onto a sharp object.[21]

In the prehospital setting, the HCP should clinically assess the extent of traumatic hemorrhage using a combination of MOI, patient physiology, anatomical injury pattern, and the patient's response to initial treatment. The MOI represents an important screening tool to identify patients at risk for significant traumatic hemorrhage.[20] Almost any organ or blood vessel can be damaged by trauma and cause internal bleeding. The most serious sources of internal bleeding due to trauma are the following:[21]

- Head trauma with internal bleeding (intracranial hemorrhage; discussed in chapter 8)

- Thoracic bleeding around the lungs (hemothorax) or heart (hemopericardium and cardiac tamponade; discussed in chapter 10)

- Tears in the large blood vessels near the center of the body (aorta, superior and inferior vena cava, and their major branches; discussed in chapter 11)

- Damage to organs such as liver or spleen lacerations or perforation of other organs caused by abdominal trauma (discussed in chapter 12)

Any of these signs of internal bleeding after a trauma should be treated as a medical emergency. The patient requires urgent evaluation and treatment in the ED. Delayed signs and symptoms of internal bleeding in both trauma and medical patients include the following:[1,20,21]

- *Abdominal pain or swelling:* Often caused by internal bleeding from trauma to the liver or spleen; these symptoms increase as bleeding continues.

- *Kehr's sign:* Referred pain at the left shoulder from trauma to the spleen; discussed further in chapter 12.

- *McBurney's point:* Pain in the right lower quadrant one-third of the distance from the anterior superior iliac spine to the umbilicus, indicating possible appendix rupture; discussed in chapter 12.

- *Hematemesis:* Vomited blood that may be bright red or dark red; or, if the blood has been partially digested, it may appear like coffee grounds.

- *Hemoptysis:* Bright red blood that is coughed up by the patient.

- *Melena:* Black, foul-smelling, tarry stool that contains digested blood.

- *Hematochezia:* Bloody stools containing bright red blood may indicate bleeding near the external opening of the colon; often caused by hemorrhoids in the lower colon.

- *Pain, tenderness, bruising, guarding, or swelling:* Signs that a closed fracture is bleeding.

- *Bruises or ecchymosis:* In the chest or with a rigid, distended abdomen indicating bleeding into the thoracic or abdominal cavities, respectively.

The prehospital management of the bleeding patient at the scene has a major impact on the overall care of the patient. The focus of prehospital care of the trauma patient should be on a rapid primary assessment and management of life-threatening injuries.[34] It is important to complete a thorough evaluation to avoid treating a fracture or other more obvious injury and missing internal bleeding that may be life-threatening. The severely injured patient arriving to the ED with continuous bleeding that progresses to hemorrhagic shock generally has a poor

🚩 RED FLAG

Internal bleeding that occurs after a less severe trauma may have symptom progression as the bleeding continues. Delayed symptoms of internal bleeding depend on the type of trauma and body part(s) involved, as in these examples:[1,20,21]

- Lightheadedness, dizziness, or fainting from any source of internal bleeding once enough blood is lost

- Large area of ecchymosis from bleeding into soft tissues under the skin

- Swelling, tightness, and pain from internal bleeding in the thigh from a fractured femur

- Headache, seizures, and loss of consciousness from internal bleeding in the brain

chance of survival without early control of bleeding, proper resuscitation, and blood transfusion. This is particularly true for patients with uncontrolled bleeding due to multiple penetrating injuries, or patients who have multiple injuries and unstable pelvic fractures with ongoing bleeding from fracture sites and retroperitoneal vessels.[20] Significant loss of intravascular volume may lead sequentially to hemodynamic instability, decreased tissue perfusion, cellular hypoxia, shock, MOF, and death.[17]

Emergency Care for Hemorrhage

The aim of prehospital care of bleeding trauma patients is to deliver the patient to a facility for definitive care within the shortest amount of time by rapid transport and minimize therapy to what is necessary to maintain adequate vital signs. The order and means of treatment of bleeding patients may differ between patients in

the prehospital phase. Rapid decisions must be made using algorithms based on best evidence (figure 6.6). Treatment of bleeding patients should begin in the prehospital setting, although noncompressible bleeding may be difficult to treat or not at all be treatable in the field.[6]

Direct Pressure

External bleeding from the extremity, and particularly bleeding from the junctional segment of the extremity vasculature (e.g., axillary artery, common femoral artery), is life-threatening and should be controlled as soon as possible.[19] Most bleeding can usually be controlled using direct pressure or a pressure dressing (figure 6.7). However, prolonged application of direct pressure, particularly bleeding from junctional vessels, is not practical during transport in the prehospital or tactical environment. Therefore, other approaches are necessary, including top-

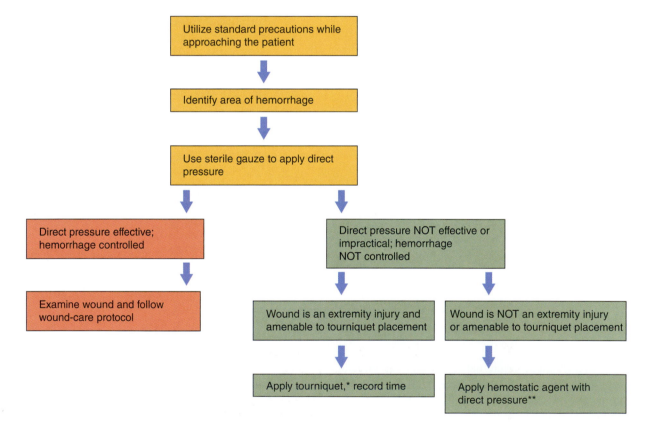

FIGURE 6.6 Algorithm for prehospital control of external hemorrhage.

*Use a tourniquet for extremity hemorrhage if sustained direct pressure is ineffective or impractical. Use a commercial windlass pneumatic device demonstrated to occlude arterial blood flow. Avoid narrow, elastic, or bungee-type devices. Improvised tourniquets should only be used when a commercial device is not available. Do not release the tourniquet until the patient reaches definitive care.

**Use a topical hemostatic agent that has been determined effective and safe in literature. Use hemostatic agents in gauze format that supports wound packing.

Based on Bulger (2014); Cannon and Rasmussen (2017).

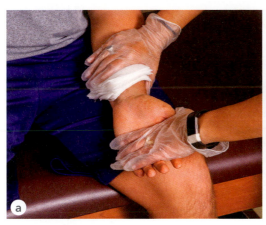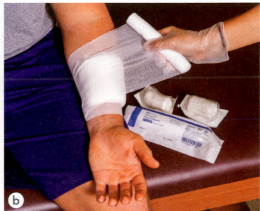

FIGURE 6.7   Most external bleeding can be controlled with *(a)* direct pressure or *(b)* a pressure dressing.

ical hemostatic agents and tourniquets (details follow).[19,35] If an object is protruding from the wound, apply a bulky dressing to stabilize the object in place, and apply pressure as well as possible. Never remove an impaled object from a wound unless it is through the cheek and interferes with bleeding control, or in the chest and interferes with chest compression. Hold uninterrupted pressure until the bleeding is controlled.[1]

Hemostatic Agents

Advanced hemostatic products can be used as adjuncts to the direct compressive techniques in severe external bleeding through local application on or in the wound. When controlling bleeding from noncompressible injuries in anatomical areas such the groin, axilla, or neck, these products may be helpful. However, in the prehospital environment, depending on the available expertise, uncontrolled bleeding from large lacerations can be stopped more effectively with rapid suturing or stapling of the wounds prior to the application of a pressure bandage.[6] Hemostatic agents (e.g., Celox, HemCon, Quik-Clot) are primarily used in the military to promote hemostasis. The agent consists of granules poured into a wound or contained in a dressing. The agent absorbs the water component of blood, thereby concentrating the clotting factors, activating platelets, and enhancing the coagulation cascade.[21] Hemostatic agents are non-prescription topical products that form an artificial scab when in contact with blood. The powder does not react with or bind to the skin and can be removed by soaking it with hydrogen peroxide. For this reason, it can be used for temporary hemostasis until definitive wound care can be performed.[43]

Wound Closure

Although the ED routinely treats acute trauma, HCPs with appropriate training should be prepared to manage acute lacerations. Doing so requires knowledge of

> ### 🚩 RED FLAG
>
> Emergent wounds requiring urgent referral to the ED include the following:[37-39]
>
> - Deep wounds of the hand or foot
> - Full-thickness lacerations of the eyelid, lip, or ear
> - Lacerations involving nerves, arteries, bones, or joints
> - Penetrating wounds of unknown depth
> - Severe crush injuries
> - Severely contaminated wounds requiring drainage
> - Wounds leading to a strong concern about cosmetic outcome
>
> Physician consultation should be considered for these wounds; however, referral decisions are ultimately based on the HCP's level of expertise, experience, and comfort with managing the wound.

wound evaluation, preparation, and appropriate repair techniques; when to refer for surgical treatment; and how to provide follow-up care.[38] Depending on the state practice act or the direction of the physician, the AT may be trained in wound closure or may be asked to assist in the preparation of materials and the patient to expedite the closure process.[36] Evaluating the wound involves finding and treating serious associated injuries, obtaining hemostasis, and looking for damage to underlying structures.[37] The goals of wound closure are to do the following:[38,39]

- Achieve hemostasis.
- Avoid infection.

Steps for Controlling External Bleeding

To control external bleeding, manual direct pressure should be applied first. You can use a pressure dressing to maintain the pressure by firmly wrapping a sterile, self-adhering roller bandage around the entire wound. Bleeding often stops when the pressure of the dressing exceeds arterial pressure and assists in controlling bleeding and facilitating blood clotting. If direct pressure or pressure dressing fails to immediately stop the hemorrhaging, consider applying a hemostatic agent or apply a tourniquet above the level of the bleeding. Follow these steps:

1. Use standard precautions.
2. Maintain the airway with spinal motion restriction (see chapter 9) if the MOI suggests the possibility of spinal injury.
3. Apply direct pressure over the wound with a dry, sterile dressing; if appropriate, the patient can hold the dressing in place.
4. If bleeding continues, do not remove the dressing; instead, apply additional dressing with manual pressure through the dressing.
5. To apply a pressure bandage, cover the entire dressing, above and below the wound. Stretch the bandage tight enough to control bleeding, but not so tight as to decrease blood flow to the extremity.
6. Palpate a distal pulse on the injured extremity before and after applying the pressure dressing.
7. If the wound is still bleeding, apply additional dressing without removing the first dressing. Secure it with a second, tighter, roller bandage.
8. If direct pressure and a pressure dressing are not immediately effective, apply a tourniquet above the level of the bleeding or use a hemostatic agent (described next).
9. If a tourniquet is not possible because the bleeding is too far proximally or a hemostatic agent is unavailable, apply direct pressure and hold it; the patient is transferred to the ED.
10. Apply high-flow oxygen (10-15 L/min) as necessary, once hemorrhaging is controlled.
11. Do not remove the dressing until a physician has evaluated the patient.
12. Prior to the application of a pressure bandage, uncontrolled bleeding from large lacerations may be controlled with rapid suturing or stapling of the wounds (see Wound Closure section).

Based on Pollack and Beck (2012); American College of Surgeons (2012); Bulger (2014); Harper, Young, and McNaught (2014); Cannon and Rasmussen (2017).

- Restore function to the involved tissues.
- Achieve optimal cosmetic results with minimal scarring.

Immediately upon presentation, the wound should be evaluated and the bleeding controlled using direct pressure, hemostatic agents, or a tourniquet (see Tourniquets, later in the chapter).[37] A patient history should be obtained, including mechanism and time of injury and personal health information (e.g., human immunodeficiency virus and diabetes status; tetanus immunization history; allergies to latex, local anesthesia, tape, or antibiotics). A careful exploration of the laceration is necessary to determine severity and whether it involves muscle, tendons, nerves, blood vessels, or bone. Baseline neurovascular and functional status of the involved body part should be evaluated before repair.[38] Wound evaluation requires good lighting; a headlamp is often useful.[37]

Wound care involves cleansing and local anesthesia (sequence can vary), exploration, debridement, and closure. Throughout the wound care process, tissue should be handled as gently as possible.[37,39] Injectable local anesthetics are generally used before or after cleaning and irrigation. Topical anesthetics are beneficial in certain cases, especially for wounds of the face and scalp and when topical skin adhesives are used to close wounds.

Local anesthesia with lidocaine 1% (Xylocaine; 10 mg/mL) or bupivacaine 0.25% (Marcaine; 2.5 mg/mL) is appropriate for small wounds.[37-39]

The wound and the surrounding skin must be cleaned prior to wound closure. Subepidermal tissue in the wound is relatively delicate and should not be exposed to harsh substances (e.g., full-strength povidone-iodine, chlorhexidine, hydrogen peroxide) or vigorous scrubbing. Isotonic (normal) saline or tap water is frequently used to irrigate uncomplicated wounds. Normal saline or a 1:10 mixture of povidone-iodine solution and isotonic saline (e.g., Betadine solution) provides useful antiseptic activity for contaminated wounds. Irrigation should be performed by using a 19ga syringe or catheter on a 60-cc syringe or a pressurized bag of normal saline solution (e.g., 1-L bag under a 400-mm Hg BP cuff). The volume of irrigation solution depends on the location and cause of the wound. Using a splash shield decreases splatter and minimizes the clinician's exposure to potentially infectious fluids.[40]

The HCP should explore the full extent of the wound to find foreign material and possible nerve, joint, or tendon injury. **Debridement** of the wound should be performed using a scalpel, scissors, or both to remove dead tissue, devitalized tissue (e.g., tissue with a narrow base and no viable blood supply), and sometimes firmly adherent wound contaminants (e.g., turf, dirt, pebbles).[37,39] Most wounds can be closed immediately, and it is usually appropriate to do so for uninfected and relatively uncontaminated wounds less than 6 to 8 hours

old (<12-24 hours for face and scalp wounds).[37] Wound repair is accomplished in the prehospital setting using skin adhesives, adhesive strips, metal staples, and sutures.

Skin Adhesives and Adhesive Strips   Topical skin adhesives (figure 6.8*a*) usually contain octyl cyanoacrylate, butyl cyanoacrylate, or both (e.g., Dermabond). These products harden within a minute; are strong, nontoxic, and waterproof; form a microbial barrier; and have some antibacterial properties. Tissue adhesives can be applied more quickly, require no anesthesia, and slough off within 5 to 10 days.[38] Adhesives are best for simple, regular lacerations; however, the adhesive should not be

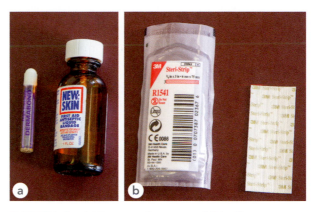

FIGURE 6.8   *(a)* Tissue adhesive and *(b)* adhesive strips can be used to close minor wounds.

CLINICAL SKILLS

Laceration Repair With Adhesive Tape

1. After the initial cleansing of the skin, clean the skin surface with acetone or alcohol to remove any surface oils. Allow the skin to dry. Apply benzoin solution (e.g., Tuf-Skin) to the skin on both sides of the wound with a cotton applicator.

2. Cut the skin closure tapes to the proper length.

3. Gently tear the end tab off the back of the card to prevent the strips from deforming.

4. Remove a strip from the card.

5. Firmly secure the tape to one side of the wound.

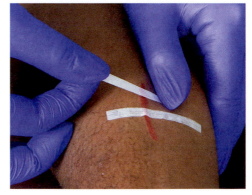

FIGURE 6.9

6. Use the nondominant hand to oppose the wound edges as the tape is brought over and secured to the skin on the opposite wound edge.

7. Place additional tapes at 2- to 3-mm intervals until the wound edges are apposed.

8. Place pieces of tape across the tape edges to prevent premature removal and skin blistering from the tape ends.

allowed into the wound or used for wounds under tension. Adhesives are not appropriate for wounds requiring debridement, deep dermal suturing, or exploration under local anesthesia. With long lacerations, skin edges can be held together by a second person or with adhesive strips (e.g., Steri-Strips) while the adhesive is applied. Generally, only one layer is applied as recommended by the manufacturer. The adhesive sloughs spontaneously in about a week. Excess or inadvertently applied adhesive can be removed with any petrolatum-based ointment or acetone in areas away from the eyes or open wounds.[37,39]

Using adhesive strips (figure 6.8b) is a convenient and quick method for wound closure, and they have a low infection rate. Steri-Strips and other adhesive strips are useful for wounds not subject to tension or hairy areas. HCPs can also use adhesive strips to reinforce wounds after suture or staple removal; skin must be dry before application. Many ATs use tincture of benzoin (e.g., Tuf-Skin) applied with a cotton swab (not sprayed near the wound) to improve adhesion. The patient may remove adhesive strips, although they eventually will fall off on their own.[37]

Staples   Minor wound closure using staples is acceptable for linear lacerations through the dermis that have straight, sharp edges and are located on the scalp, trunk, arms, and legs.[42] Metal staples are durable, have minimal tissue reactivity, and can be placed relatively quickly. Because of their width, they are not recommended in body parts where a cosmetic closure is needed. Staples have been shown to be faster, less expensive, and possibly less painful for repair of scalp lacerations.[41] Newly developed subcuticular absorbable staples may be comparable to traditional subcuticular sutures.[39,42]

Because staples can be placed more rapidly than sutures can, they are especially useful in urgent or emergent situations.[39,42] Where skin staples are used to seal a skin wound it will be necessary to remove the staples after an appropriate healing period, usually between 5 and 10 days, depending on the location of the wound and other factors. The skin staple remover is a small manual device used with hand pressure to push down on the staple and to deform it into an M shape to facilitate its removal.[41]

Sutures   **Sutures** provide wound edge approximation and are the best choice for the following:[36,37]

- Irregular, heavy bleeding, or complex lacerations
- Areas of loose skin
- Areas under tension
- Wounds requiring deep dermal closure

CLINICAL SKILLS

Applying and Removing Staples

Applying Staples

After wound assessment and preparation with appropriate local anesthesia, perform staple closure as follows:

1. Approximate the adjacent skin margins with eversion of the skin edges using forceps with teeth (e.g., Adson forceps) or the thumb and forefinger. Eversion is necessary to avoid the tendency of the stapler to invert the edges of the wound, which can cause a less aesthetically pleasing scar. An assistant may aid in eversion of the wound edges, possibly permitting more accurate staple positioning.
2. Place the stapler firmly on the skin surface but without indenting the skin.
3. Align the center mark on the stapler with the center of the wound margin.
4. Gently squeeze the stapler handle to eject the staple into the skin.
5. If the stapler does not automatically release, then release the staple from the stapler by pulling the stapler back. When properly placed, the crossbar of the staple is elevated a few millimeters above the skin surface.
6. Place staples about 1/2 to 1 cm apart.
7. Place enough staples to allow for proper apposition of the wound edges.

Removing Staples

1. Place both jaws of the skin staple remover symmetrically under the staple.
2. Depress the handle, which unbends the staple and permits removal.

Sutures are left in place depending on how much healing time is needed to allow the natural properties of the skin to hold the wound together:[36]

- Facial: 3 to 5 days
- Extremities and trunk: 5 to 7 days
- Scalp, back, feet, hands, and over the joints: 10 to 14 days

Suturing technique depends on the type of wound, the area to be sutured, and the preference and experience of the person suturing. Four suturing techniques are illustrated in figure 6.10. For excellent descriptions and illustrations of suturing techniques, see *Medical Conditions in the Athlete*.[36]

Tourniquets

Tourniquets are recommended in the prehospital setting for the control of significant extremity hemorrhage if direct pressure is ineffective or impractical. Expert panelists advise that using a tourniquet to treat severe extremity hemorrhage has a clear survival benefit, demonstrated by a large and consistent effect size across several studies.[19] A tourniquet is especially useful if a patient has substantial bleeding from an extremity injury below the axilla or groin. Commercially produced windlass (figure 6.11), pneumatic, or ratcheting devices have been demonstrated to occlude arterial flow and are recommended. The use of narrow, elastic, or bungee-type devices should be avoided; they are associated with adverse outcomes such as soft tissue or nerve damage, or uncontrolled or excessively high extremity vascular pressure.[19,20]

When applying a tourniquet, observe these precautions:

- Do not apply a tourniquet directly over any joint. Keep it as close to the injury as possible.
- Make sure the tourniquet is tightened securely.
- Never use wire, rope, a belt, or any other narrow material; it could cut into the skin.
- Use wide padding under the tourniquet if possible. It will protect the tissues and help with arterial compression.
- Never cover a tourniquet with a bandage; leave it open and in full view.
- Write the day and time the tourniquet was applied on the tourniquet or on the patient's skin.

Once a tourniquet has been properly applied in the prehospital setting, never release it until the patient has reached definitive care. Given the relatively short transport times for most civilian EMS agencies, the safest option is to leave a tourniquet in place until the patient can be assessed in the hospital. Exceptions to this approach may exist for prolonged transport times or austere environments. In these circumstances, prehospital providers should consult direct (online) physician medical direction.[19] Be aware that bleeding may rapidly return upon tourniquet release and that you should be prepared to reapply it immediately if necessary.

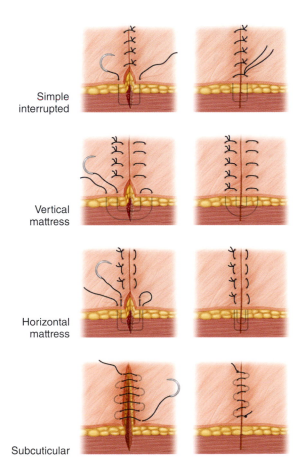

Simple interrupted

Vertical mattress

Horizontal mattress

Subcuticular

FIGURE 6.10   Types of sutures.

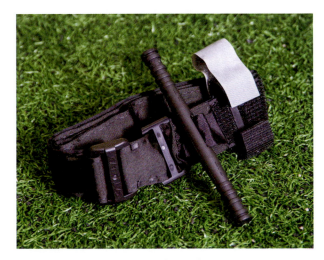

FIGURE 6.11   Commercial windlass tourniquet.

Applying a Tourniquet

Commercial Tourniquet

1. Hold direct pressure over the bleeding site.
2. Place a tourniquet around the extremity just proximal to the bleeding site.
3. Click the buckle into place, and pull the strap tight (a).
4. Turn the tightening dial clockwise until pulses are no longer palpable distal to the tourniquet or until bleeding has been controlled (b).

Blood Pressure Cuff

As an alternative method, a BP cuff can function as an effective tourniquet.

1. Position the cuff proximal to the bleeding point, and inflate it just enough to stop the bleeding.
2. Leave the cuff inflated, and monitor the gauge continuously to make sure that the pressure is not gradually dropping.
3. To prevent loss of pressure, the tube can be clamped with a hemostat leading from the cuff to the inflating bulb.

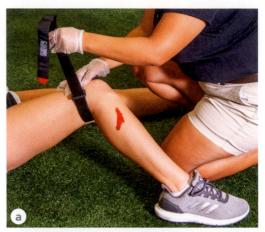

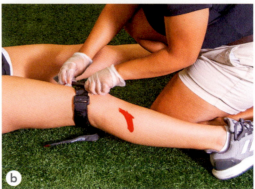

FIGURE 6.12

Shock

Shock is a clinical syndrome resulting from inadequate tissue perfusion. The effects of shock are initially reversible, but they can become a life-threatening, irreversible condition of circulatory failure, MOF, and death. In the prehospital setting, the most common etiology of shock is trauma resulting from loss of circulating blood volume from hemorrhage. Other contributing factors of shock include the following:[3,5,17,44,45]

- Decreased circulating blood volume
- Decreased cardiac output
- Inadequate oxygenation
- Vasodilation
- Low organ perfusion pressure
- Shunting of blood to bypass capillary exchange beds
- Impaired delivery of oxygen and nutrients to the tissues

- Pulmonary dysfunction (e.g., pulmonary contusion, hemothorax)
- Mechanical obstruction (e.g., cardiac tamponade, tension pneumothorax)
- Neurologic dysfunction (e.g., spinal cord injury)
- Cardiac dysfunction (e.g., myocardial damage)
- Pharmacologic or toxicologic agents

Epidemiology of Shock

Shock is a common and frequently treatable cause of death in injured patients and is second only to traumatic brain injury (TBI; see chapter 8) as the leading cause of death from trauma.[44] In the trauma setting, loss of circulating blood volume from hemorrhage is the most common cause of shock. Inadequate oxygenation, mechanical obstruction (e.g., cardiac tamponade, tension pneumothorax), neurologic dysfunction (e.g., high–spinal cord injury), and cardiac dysfunction represent other potential causes or contributing factors.[21] Most deaths from trauma with shock occur within 24 hours from hypovolemic shock.[46] Trauma patients present in various stages of physiologic dysfunction and dysregulation; 5% to 15% of trauma admissions are considered to be in shock on arrival to the ED.[47] In the sports medicine setting, according to the most recent report from National Center for Catastrophic Sport Injury Research (NCCSIR) the majority of sport-related catastrophic cases are at the high school level (81%).[95] Overall 28% of cases of catastrophic sport-related injuries were fatal, 19% were nonfatal, and 55% were serious with recovery. Direct trauma injury caused 61% of sport-related catastrophic cases; 15% of direct events were fatal, 31% were nonfatal, and 54% serious with recovery. Most (84%) direct trauma injuries were in football. Of all sport-related trauma, the most common were to the cervical spine (51%) and head/brain (31%).[95] Although catastrophic injuries are not common in the sports medicine setting, the AT should be prepared to recognize and treat concomitant conditions such as shock.

Pathophysiology of Shock

Physiologically, shock is a transition between life and death.[45] Hypoperfusion leads to an imbalance between the delivery of and requirements for oxygen and substrate which leads to cellular dysfunction (figure 6.13). The cellular injury created by the inadequate delivery of oxygen and substrates releases proteins and other inflammatory mediators that further compromise perfusion through functional and structural changes within the microvasculature. This response leads to a vicious cycle in which impaired perfusion is responsible for cellular dysfunction, which leads to death.[16]

In the prehospital setting, vital signs, including BP and heart rate, are the initial parameters necessary to assess for possible shock in trauma patients. The early recognition of shock using vital signs alone may be difficult, even in the presence of significant blood loss, due to compensatory mechanisms in otherwise healthy patients. According to the guidelines from Advanced Trauma Life Support (ATLS[5]), only hemorrhage classes III and IV include a decrease in BP, requiring blood loss of greater than 30% of the total blood volume. Patients with this severity of illness also begin to display evidence of MOF, including altered mental status and decreased urine output. Thus, the goal of trauma assessment should be the early recognition of circulatory dysfunction, prior to the development of hypotension and end-organ dysfunction.[17,48,49]

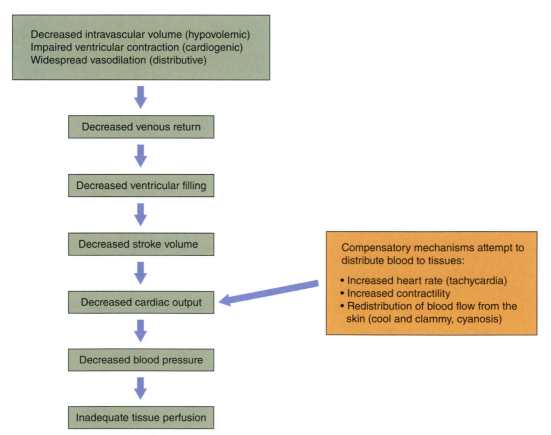

FIGURE 6.13   Pathophysiology of shock.

Based on de Moya (2013); American College of Surgeons (2012); Gutierrez, Reines, and Wolf-Gutierrez (2004); Rosen (2001); Marx and Rosen (2017).

Stages of Shock

Shock is a physiologic continuum that begins with a precipitating event, such as trauma or a severe infection (e.g., abscess) that progresses through several stages. The early stages of shock (pre-shock, shock) in which compensatory mechanisms maintain homeostasis, are responsive to treatment and are more likely to be reversible, compared with end-stage shock, associated with irreversible end-organ damage and death. End-organ dysfunction results from progressive shock that leads to irreversible organ damage, MOF, and death. The four stages of shock listed here are continuous with a progression from one stage to the next; the fifth stage is death.[45]

1. Pre-shock or compensated shock
2. Uncompensated shock
3. Reperfusion
4. Multiple organ failure
5. Death

Pre-Shock or Compensated Shock

Pre-shock involves compensatory responses to diminished tissue perfusion. These compensatory physiologic responses to acute hemorrhage attempt to maintain adequate oxygen delivery to tissues. In early hypovolemic pre-shock, compensatory tachycardia and peripheral vasoconstriction may allow an otherwise healthy adult to be asymptomatic and preserve a normal BP. In addition, when oxygen delivery is decreased, tissues compensate by extracting a greater percentage of delivered oxygen. Low arterial pressure stimulates the sympathetic nervous system, resulting in increased heart rate, vasoconstriction, and increased ventricular contractility.[45,50]

During this stage, hypoperfusion causes cell hypoxia and lactate accumulation, resulting in lactic acidosis. Cellular function is maintained as long as energy is produced in the cell. Skeletal and smooth muscles are highly resistant to hypoxia, while liver cells can survive 2.5 hours of ischemia without irreversible damage. However, brain cells sustain permanent damage after only a few minutes of hypoxia.[17,49] With timely and appropriate management, deterioration can be prevented, and signs of impending deterioration can be reversed (e.g., normalization of serum lactate levels).[45]

Uncompensated Shock

As the process of shock progresses, the compensatory mechanisms become overwhelmed, the combined aerobic and anaerobic supplies of ATP are not sufficient to maintain cellular function, and irreversible tissue damage occurs. Failure of membrane-associated ion transport pumps, especially pumps associated with the regulation of calcium and sodium, results in the loss of membrane integrity and in cellular swelling. Among other mechanisms that lead to irreversible cellular injury during hypoxia are depletion of cellular energy, cellular acidosis, oxygen free radical generation, and loss of adenine nucleotides from the cell.[17] As the shock state progresses, vital organ (e.g., brain and heart) perfusion can only be maintained at the expense of nonvital organs. If the process is not reversed, progressive lactate production leads to worsening systemic metabolic acidosis, which along with hypoxemia ultimately causes the loss of peripheral vasoconstriction and cardiovascular collapse.[17,49,50]

Reperfusion

Reperfusion of ischemic cells can cause further injury. As substrate is reintroduced, neutrophil activity may increase, thereby increasing production of damaging superoxide and hydroxyl radicals. After blood flow is restored, inflammatory mediators may be circulated to other organs. Vascular responses to hemorrhagic and traumatic shock can result in functionally important reductions in visceral blood flow. Damaged intestinal cells may trigger the production of inflammatory mediators, such as cytokines. This response initiates of a chain of events leading to a process of systemic inflammation that ultimately produces multiple organ failure.[2,49,50]

Multiple Organ Failure

During MOF, also known as multiple organ dysfunction syndrome (MODS), total organ failure (TOF), or multisystem organ failure (MSOF), altered organ function in an acutely ill patient requires medical intervention to achieve homeostasis. The combination of direct and reperfusion tissue injury may cause MODS and progressive dysfunction of 2 or more organs leading to life-threatening illness or injury. MODS can follow any type of shock, but it is most common when infection is involved; organ failure is one of the defining features of septic shock (see Distributive Shock). Death is common in this phase of shock.[3,17,18,49,50]

Types of Shock

Life-threatening decreases in blood pressure result in shock or tissue perfusion that is not capable of sustaining aerobic metabolism. Many patients with circulatory failure have a combination of more than one form of shock (multifactorial shock). These four types of shock are recognized:[3,17,18,45]

1. *Hypovolemic shock:* Low circulating volume as a result of hemorrhagic or nonhemorrhagic fluid losses.
2. *Distributive shock:* Vasodilation that may have septic or nonseptic causes, including anaphylaxis and neurogenic etiologies.
3. *Cardiogenic shock:* Decrease in cardiac output that may have cardiomyopathic, arrhythmogenic, or mechanical causes.
4. *Obstructive shock:* Pulmonary or mechanical cause of reduced preload or other etiologies.

Hypovolemic Shock Hypovolemic shock is caused by a critical decrease in intravascular volume from hemorrhagic or nonhemorrhagic causes (table 6.3). This type of shock occurs when diminished venous return (preload) occurs resulting in decreased ventricular filling and reduced stroke volume. Unless increased heart rate compensates for it, cardiac output decreases.[3,51] Hemorrhagic shock is a condition produced by rapid and significant loss of intravascular volume, which may lead sequentially to hemodynamic instability, decreased oxygen delivery, decreased tissue perfusion, cellular hypoxia, organ damage, and death. Hemorrhagic shock resulting from severe external or internal bleeding can be rapidly fatal.[16,17] Nonhemorrhagic shock is caused by reduced intravascular volume from fluid loss other than blood. The loss of plasma (the fluid part of the blood) occurs when fluid in blood leaves the vascular compartment and subsequently is lost from the body through cutaneous routes. Displaced plasma fluid can be lost from exposed areas, such as burns or excessive sweating leading to heatstroke, gastrointestinal, or renal losses. Sufficiently large external losses of body fluid from any cause can result in hypovolemic shock.[18]

Distributive Shock Distributive shock occurs when circulating blood volume is normal, but a relative inadequacy of intravascular volume exists, caused by arterial or venous vasodilation. In some cases, cardiac output distribution of oxygen is high, but increased blood flow through arteriovenous shunts bypasses capillary beds; this bypass plus uncoupled cellular oxygen transport causes cellular hypoperfusion. In other situations, blood pools in venous capacitance beds and cardiac output is decreased. Distributive shock may be caused by bacterial infection with endotoxin release (septic shock); severe injury to the spinal cord, usually above T4 (neurogenic shock); or anaphylaxis (anaphylactic shock; described in detail later in this chapter) (table 6.4).[51,52]

TABLE 6.3 **Etiology of Hypovolemic Shock**

Etiology	Pathology	Examples
Hemorrhagic	External bleeding	Trauma, lacerations, contusions, fractures
	Internal bleeding	Intrathoracic, intraperitoneal, retroperitoneal
Nonhemorrhagic	Gastrointestinal losses	Diarrhea, vomiting, external drainage
	Skin losses	Heatstroke, burns, dermatologic conditions
	Renal losses	Excessive drug-induced or osmotic diuresis, salt-wasting nephropathies, hypoaldosteronism
	Third space losses into extravascular space or body cavities	Postoperative and trauma, intestinal obstruction, crush injury, pancreatitis, cirrhosis

Based on de Moya (2017); Maier (2015); Gutierrez, Reines, and Wolf-Gutierrez (2004); Rice (1991); Marx and Rosen (2017); Nicks and Gaillard (2016).

TABLE 6.4 **Etiology of Distributive Shock**

Etiology	Examples
Septic	Inflammatory shock • Systemic inflammatory response syndrome (SIRS)
	Infections • Gram-positive or gram-negative bacterial • Fungal, viral, or parasitic
Nonseptic	Neurogenic • Traumatic brain injury (TBI) • Spinal cord injury
	Anaphylactic shock • IgE mediated (e.g., foods, medications, insect bites or stings) • IgE independent (e.g., iron dextran) • Nonimmunologic (e.g., exercise or heat induced, idiopathic)
	Other • Liver failure, transfusion reactions • Toxic shock syndrome • Ingestion of certain drugs or poisons, such as nitrates, opioids, and adrenergic blockers

Based on de Moya (2017); Maier (2015); Gutierrez, Reines, and Wolf-Gutierrez (2004); Rice (1991); Marx and Rosen (2017); Nicks and Gaillard (2016); Singer et al. (2016).

Sepsis, or septic shock, is the most common form of distributive shock and is the primary cause of death from infection, especially when the infection is not recognized and treated promptly. Septic shock is the progression from its precursor conditions—**systemic inflammatory response syndrome** (SIRS), sepsis, and severe sepsis. SIRS is a clinical syndrome characterized by a robust inflammatory response, usually induced by a major body insult that can be infectious.[45,50] SIRS requires urgent medical intervention. Septic shock can be produced by infection with any microbe, although in at least half of cases of septic shock, no organism is identified.[45] Sepsis is a syndrome shaped by pathogen factors and host factors (e.g., sex, race and other genetic determinants, age, comorbidities, environment) that result from a systematic infection that is aberrant or dysregulated, leading to organ dysfunction. Unrecognized infection (see chapter 2) may be the cause of septic organ dysfunction. Specific infections may result in local organ dysfunction without generating a dysregulated systemic host response.[52]

Neurogenic shock results from severe, traumatic injury to the brain or spinal cord, usually above T4. Hypotension and, in some cases, overt shock are common in patients with severe TBI and spinal cord injury.[3] Interruption of autonomic pathways, causing decreased vascular resistance and altered vagal tone, may be responsible for distributive shock in patients with spinal cord injury. However, hypovolemia from blood loss and myocardial depression may also contribute to shock in this population.[50] In neurogenic shock, massive unopposed vasodilation causes arterioles to dilate and reduce peripheral vascular resistance.[3] As venules and veins dilate, blood pools in the venous side of the circulation, causing a decrease in venous return to the right side of the heart. Decreased venous return reduces ventricular filling pressure, stroke volume, cardiac output, and BP, reducing tissue perfusion.[18]

Cardiogenic Shock   Cardiogenic shock (table 6.5) is a relative or absolute reduction in cardiac output due to a primary cardiac disorder. Cardiogenic shock is due to intracardiac causes of cardiac pump failure that result in reduced cardiac output.[51] Cardiomyopathic shock is caused by myocardial infarction (see chapter 11) often accompanied by severe extensive ischemia. Patients with hypertrophic cardiomyopathy (see chapter 11) or severe diastolic heart failure rarely present with cardiogenic shock, but these underlying conditions may contribute to hypotension and shock from other causes (e.g., sepsis, hypovolemia).[3,50] Myocardial infarction is the most common cause of cardiogenic shock. **Dysrhythmias** are another common cause because they can lead to a decreased cardiac output. **Bradyarrhythmias** result in low cardiac output, and **tachyarrhythmias** can result in decreased preload and stroke volume. Mechanical causes of cardiogenic shock include severe valve insufficiency or defects, or aortic insufficiency.[3,45]

Obstructive Shock   Obstructive shock (table 6.6) is primarily related to **extracardiac** causes of cardiac pump failure that is often associated with poor right ventricle output. The causes of obstructive shock can be divided into pulmonary vascular and mechanical causes that interfere with filling or emptying of the heart or great vessels.[3,51] Pericardial tamponade and tension pneumothorax are common causes.[51]

Assessment of the Patient With Undifferentiated Shock

Shock is a life-threatening condition of circulatory failure. When a patient presents with undifferentiated shock,

TABLE 6.5   Etiology of Cardiogenic Shock

Etiology	Examples
Cardiomyopathic	Myocardial infarction Severe heart failure from dilated cardiomyopathy Myocarditis Pericardial tamponade Myocardial contusion
Arrhythmogenic	Tachyarrhythmia Atrial tachycardias (fibrillation, flutter, reentrant tachycardia) Ventricular tachycardia and fibrillation Bradyarrhythmia Complete heart block, second-degree heart block
Mechanical	Severe valvular insufficiency Critical valvular stenosis Acute or severe ventricular septal wall defect Ruptured ventricular wall aneurysm

Based on de Moya (2013); Gutierrez, Reines, and Wolf-Gutierrez (2004); Rice (1991); Marx and Rosen (2017).

TABLE 6.6 **Etiology of Obstructive Shock**

Etiology	Examples
Pulmonary or venous vasculature	Hemodynamically significant pulmonary embolus Severe pulmonary hypertension Severe or acute obstruction of the pulmonic or tricuspid valve Venous air embolus
Mechanical	Tension pneumothorax or hemothorax Pericardial tamponade Constrictive pericarditis Restrictive cardiomyopathy
Endocrine	Adrenal insufficiency, thyrotoxicosis, myxedema coma Other
Metabolic	Acidosis, hypothermia
Polytrauma	More than one shock category Acute shock etiology with preexisting cardiac disease Late underresuscitated shock Poisonings, drug overdose

Based on de Moya (2013); Gutierrez, Reines, and Wolf-Gutierrez (2004); Rice (1991); Marx and Rosen (2017); Gaieski and Mikkelsen (2017).

the clinician must immediately initiate therapy while rapidly identifying the etiology so that definitive therapy can be administered to reverse shock and prevent MOF and death. Undifferentiated shock refers to the situation where shock is recognized but the cause is unclear.[50] Regardless of the underlying cause, shock manifests clinically as hemodynamic disturbances and organ dysfunction.[3] Because a patient may have shock with no obvious cause, rapid recognition of shock requires the integration of information from immediate history and physical examination. Shock should be suspected when the patient appears to exhibit a stress response; the patient appears ill; is **asthenic**, pale, often sweating, and usually tachypneic or grunting; and often has a rapid, weak, or thready pulse.[45] Initial assessment of a patient in shock requires careful physical examination, inspecting for signs of tension pneumothorax, cardiac tamponade (discussed in chapters 10 and 11, respectively), and other causes of the shock state.

Upon initial examination, prehospital health care providers can provide the history, vital signs, and physical examination documentation that is valuable for management in ED. On physical examination, diagnosis is mostly clinical, based on evidence of insufficient tissue perfusion (**obtundation, oliguria**, peripheral cyanosis) and signs of compensatory mechanisms (tachycardia, tachypnea, diaphoresis). None of these findings alone is diagnostic, and each must be evaluated by its trend (i.e., worsening or improving) and in the overall clinical context, including physical signs.[3,45,53] Most clinical features are neither sensitive nor specific for the diagnosis of shock. However, many of the clinical manifestations provide clues to the underlying etiology and are primarily used to narrow

the differential diagnosis so that empiric therapies can be administered in a timely manner.[53]

Physical examination of the patient provides essential information regarding the ability of the cardiovascular

 RED FLAG

Red flags for recognition of shock are the following:[3,45,53]

- Cool, clammy skin, diaphoresis, pallor, cyanosis, restlessness
- Ill appearance, altered mental status (lethargy or confusion), or obtundation
- Tachycardia (heart rate >100 bpm)
- Tachypnea (respiratory rate > 20 breaths/min)
- Hypotension (systolic < 90 mm Hg, a 30-mm Hg deterioration from baseline BP, or low BP > 30 min of continuous duration)
- Weak peripheral pulses, narrowing of the pulse pressure (<25 mm Hg)
- Prolonged capillary refill (>2 seconds)

In the ED, laboratory findings that support the diagnosis include the following:

- Oliguria (urine output < 0.5 mL/kg/h)
- Lactate > 3 mmol/L
- Base deficit < −4 mEq/L
- $PaCO_2$ < 32 mm Hg

system to perfuse major organs, including the brain, lungs, heart, and kidneys, and the rest of the body. As with any assessment, begin with the initial assessment as described in chapter 4. Circulation should be initially checked; an absent pulse is an indication to begin CPR (see chapter 11) and initiate the emergency action plan (EAP; see chapter 3), including applying an automated external defibrillator (AED). In a responsive patient, check the radial pulse to obtain a general pulse rate; however, at this point, do not take the time to get an actual rate. The next step is to assess perfusion (capillary refill test or pulse oximeter; refer to chapter 4) to determine whether the patient is experiencing shock so that it can also be treated at this time. Throughout the emergency examination, continue to monitor the patient while determining interventions (if any) that are required.

Shock may exist even with normal vital signs, but the patient may have more subtle signs or symptoms of shock depending on the cause and severity of the shock. In addition to the Red Flags, symptoms of shock include the following:

- Altered mental status (i.e., agitation, confusion, irritability, or inattention)
- Cyanotic earlobes, nose, or nail beds
- Skin that appears grayish or dusky and moist (distributive shock)
- Skin that appears warm or flushed, and a bounding pulse with fever preceded by chills (septic shock)
- Urticaria or wheezing (anaphylactic shock; described in the next section)
- Numerous other symptoms (e.g., chest pain, dyspnea, abdominal pain) that may be caused by an underlying disease or secondary organ failure[3]

Young, otherwise healthy patients can maintain a BP within the normal range despite substantial blood loss; subtle mental status alterations, such as agitation, confusion, irritability, or inattention, may be their only signs of early shock. Altered mental status from inadequate cerebral perfusion can be difficult to distinguish from drug or alcohol intoxication or associated head injury. Altered mental status on presentation or a subsequent decline in mental status, particularly in patients without obvious evidence of head injury, should raise suspicion for cerebral hypoperfusion. On the other hand, hypotension is not always an indication of the early stages of shock; although as shock progresses to uncompensated shock, marked hypotension eventually occurs. Athletes without underlying comorbidities can often maintain normal blood pressure despite substantial blood loss by compensatory vasoconstriction and increased heart rate.[3]

In the prehospital setting, the HCP must recognize shock by linking the clinical impression with objective data. The clinical impression of shock is determined by considering the patient's history of present illness, age, underlying health status, and general appearance. Objective data needed to identify shock are not always available in the field, but the HCP must obtain as much quantitative data as possible, including vital signs and perfusion.[44] With a patient that presents with potential diagnosis of shock, the HCP must immediately initiate treatment while rapidly identifying the etiology of the condition. Rapid assessment and identification of the etiology of shock are essential so that definitive therapy can be administered to reverse shock and prevent MOF and death.[3,17,49]

Emergency Care for Undifferentiated Shock

Prehospital HCPs must be diligent about recognizing the signs of hypoperfusion, ideally before traumatic shock and hypotension develop. For most trauma patients, assessment and management should occur simultaneously, addressing the most life-threatening condition first. The HCP should appropriately treat the patient in shock according to her level of skill by performing the following immediate interventions listed in order of priority:[3,5,17,53]

- Recognizing the state of shock
- Establishing a patent and protected airway (chapter 10) while protecting the cervical spine
- Maintaining adequate oxygen delivery and maximizing oxygenation
- Limiting ongoing blood loss by controlling external hemorrhage
- Restoring intravascular volume by gaining intravenous (IV) access and initiating fluid resuscitation by ATs and other HCPs trained in this skill (see chapter 5)
- Covering the patient to maintain normal body temperature
- Rapidly transporting the patient to an appropriate level trauma center[3]

Initial Care of the Patient in Undifferentiated Shock

Initial management of the patient in shock is focused on restoring intravascular volume, maintaining adequate oxygen delivery, and limiting ongoing blood loss. In undifferentiated shock, the patient should be treated as if he has hypovolemic shock, unless clear evidence shows that the shock state has a different cause (figure

6.14). When the clinical impression and the quantitative data suggest widespread organ hypoperfusion, emergent resuscitation is necessary to restore normal tissue oxygenation and substrate delivery to prevent deterioration into systemic inflammation, organ dysfunction, and death.[44]

In prehospital trauma patient care, it is crucial to recognize and treat hemorrhage early and limit the consequences of hemorrhagic shock. Initial treatment for undifferentiated shock involves controlling external hemorrhage, checking airway, and providing ventilation if necessary. Intravascular volume loss should be replaced with IV fluid resuscitation (see chapter 5) by HCPs trained in this skill.[3,5,54] For HCPs trained in IV fluid administration, normal saline (NS) or lactated Ringer's (LR) solution should be infused.[3,5,17] For patients with severe hemorrhage (internal or external), IV NS should be established immediately to prevent delay in patient care by administration of blood products by arriving EMS, receiving ED, or trauma center. Supplemental oxygen should be provided by face mask and, if shock is severe or if ventilation is inadequate, airway intubation with mechanical ventilation with a bag-valve mask should be initiated. The patient should be covered with a blanket or jacket to maintain normal body temperature, and nothing should be given by mouth. The patient's head should be turned to one side to avoid aspiration if **emesis** occurs. For a patient with evidence of shock, who is responsive, and who is breathing normally, it is considered reasonable to place or maintain the patient in a supine position. If no evidence of trauma or injury (e.g., simple fainting, shock from nontraumatic bleeding, sepsis, dehydration) exists, raising the feet about 30° to 60° from the supine position is an option that may be considered while awaiting arrival of EMS. Do not raise the feet of a person in shock if the movement or the position causes pain.[55]

Reassess and Monitor Perfusion Status

In all patients with shock, continuously monitor heart rate, BP, and oxygen saturation.[5,45] As transport arrives, look for any new developments or conditions that must be treated. The reassessment is an important step in gathering critical information about the condition of the patient; it contributes to providing efficient and effective emergency care and hand-off to the next-level care provider. For the ongoing assessment, continue to reassess mental status, reestablish patient priorities, reassess vital

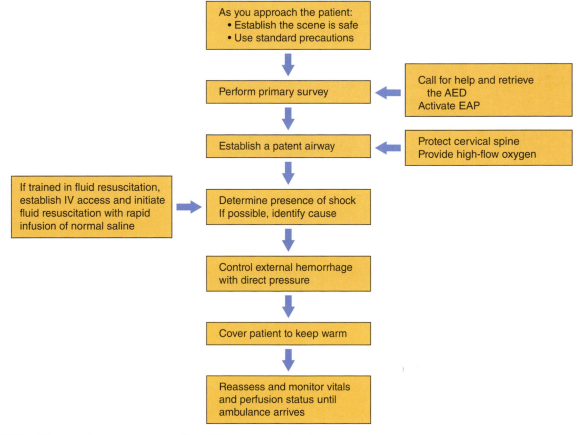

FIGURE 6.14   Initial management of undifferentiated shock.

Based on de Moya (2013); American College of Surgeons (2012); Gutierrez, Reines, and Wolf-Gutierrez (2004); Gaieski and Mikkelsen (2017).

signs, repeat the focused assessment, and continually recheck adequacy of interventions. Determine whether the treatment is improving the patient's condition or if the patient seems to be deteriorating. In all patients with shock, HR, BP, and oxyhemoglobin saturation must be continuously monitored until higher-level HCPs arrive.[45]

Anaphylactic Reactions and Immunologic Emergencies

Immunologic disorders can become a clinical emergency that all HCPs should be able to recognize and manage. Most immunologic emergency conditions are clinical diagnoses based on a constellation of presenting features and triggers.[56] The most serious and potentially fatal immunologic emergency is anaphylaxis that occurs in the out-of-hospital or physician's office settings. Anaphylaxis is an acute, potentially life-threatening multisystem syndrome caused by the sudden release of mast cell and basophil-derived mediators into the systemic circulation.[57] This condition most often results from immunologic reactions to foods, medications, and insect stings, but any agent is capable of producing a sudden, systemic degranulation of mast cells or **basophils**, which releases **histamine** from their granules into the surrounding tissue. Histamine and other inflammatory mediators cause several systemic effects, such as vasodilation, mucous secretion, nerve stimulation, and smooth muscle contraction resulting in **rhinorrhea**, itchiness, dyspnea, and anaphylaxis.[57-60] The term **anaphylactoid** has been used in the past to indicate adverse reactions that are not mediated and typically are not life-threatening.[61] Anaphylactic shock represents the most dramatic and severe form of immediate **hypersensitivity reactions**.[62,63] Anaphylactic shock is a result of anaphylaxis, which is an acute, severe, life-threatening multisystem allergic reaction resulting from the sudden systemic release of biochemical mediators and chemotactic substances.[62,64] This section focuses on recognizing and treating acute or emergency conditions of the immune system. While the focus is on anaphylactic shock and respiratory insufficiency, other immunologic disorders may require acute care in the prehospital setting, including the following:

- **Atopic** disorders, such as latex or food allergies
- Allergic drug reactions
- Exercise-induced anaphylaxis and food-dependent, exercise-induced anaphylaxis
- Insect bites and stings
- **Urticaria** (both cholinergic, cold urticaria, and **dermographism**)
- Angioedema
- Flush syndrome
- Syncope

Pathophysiology of Anaphylactic and Hypersensitivity Reactions

Allergic, atopic, and hypersensitivity disorders are inappropriate, exaggerated immune system responses to generally harmless antigens, manifesting on a continuum from minor to severe disorders.[63,65] Exaggerated immune reactions include those that are misdirected against intrinsic body components, leading to **autoimmune disorders**. Inappropriate immune responses involve **immunoglobulin E antibody (IgE)**, a protein antibody produced by the immune system's plasma cells primarily to fight parasites. However, IgE also has an essential role in **type I** (immediate) **hypersensitivity reactions** most commonly encountered in the prehospital setting such as allergic asthma, most types of sinusitis, allergic rhinitis, food allergies, and specific types of chronic urticaria and atopic dermatitis (see table 6.7). Interaction of an antigen with IgE triggers basophils and mast cells to degranulate and release histamine, leukotrienes, and other mediators that cause diffuse smooth muscle contraction resulting in bronchoconstriction and vasodilation with plasma leakage (e.g., resulting in urticaria or angioedema).[66] Mast cells, basophils, and their mediators are the central effectors in **allergy** and anaphylaxis. Exposure of a genetically predisposed person to an **allergen** leads to the synthesis and release of allergen-specific IgE by plasma cells into the circulation.[62,64]

In immunologic emergencies, there is an immunologically triggered inflammatory response that attacks the body's own tissues. A variety of foreign substances (e.g., dust, pollen, viruses, bacteria) provoke protective immune responses. In certain situations, the protective effects of an immune response lead to harmful consequences, which can range from temporary discomfort to substantial injury. For example, in the process of ingesting and destroying bacteria, phagocytic cells (neutrophils and macrophages) often cause injury to surrounding tissue. A hypersensitivity reaction is an immune response that leads to tissue injury. Many diseases are categorized as immune disorders or immunologically mediated conditions, in which an immune response to a foreign or self-antigen causes injury. Immune- or hypersensitivity-mediated disorders are common and include urticaria, asthma, hay fever, hepatitis, and arthritis.[67]

Classification of Anaphylactic or Hypersensitivity Reactions

Anaphylactic or hypersensitivity reactions are classified according to immune mechanism as type I, II and III hypersensitivity reactions (table 6.7). All involve antibodies specific for exogenous (foreign) or endogenous

TABLE 6.7   **Classification of Anaphylactic or Hypersensitivity Reactions**

Type	Mechanism	Examples
Type 1 anaphylactic: immediate hypersensitivity	IgE antibody–mediated mast cell activation and degranulation	Rhinitis, food allergies, aspirin, asthma, urticarial, anaphylaxis, drug allergy, bee and other insect stings
Type II cytotoxic: cytotoxic antibodies	Cytotoxic (IgG, IgM) antibodies formed against cell surface antigens; complement usually involved	Autoimmune hemolytic anemias, Graves' disease
Type III immune complex: complement or immune-mediated diseases	Antibodies (IgG, IgM, IgA) formed against exogenous or endogenous antigens; complement and leukocytes (neutrophils, macrophages) often involved	Autoimmune diseases (SLE, rheumatoid arthritis), many types of glomerulonephritis
Type IV delayed hypersensitivity: cell mediated	Mononuclear cells (T lymphocytes, macrophages) with interleukin and lymphokine production	Granulomatous disease (tuberculosis), delayed skin reactions (poison ivy) No relationship to anaphylaxis

SLE = systemic lupus erythematosus

Based on Rowe and Gaeta (2016); Tran and Muelleman (2017); Warren and Strayer (2017).

(self) antigens (except a subset of type I reactions). Antibody isotype influences the mechanism of tissue injury.[67,62] Antigen-specific IgE antibodies are a key risk factor for the development of allergy and anaphylaxis. Quantification of specific IgE levels is used as part of the diagnostic evaluation of those thought to have allergic disorders and to identify potential triggers of anaphylaxis in patients with a history of anaphylaxis.[62,68] Type I reactions (immediate hypersensitivity) are IgE mediated. Exposure to sensitizing allergens causes histamine and other mediators from mast cells and basophils to be released through IgE-dependent mast cell degranulation mechanisms. Examples of the IgE-dependent mechanism include rhinitis caused by ragweed pollen and anaphylaxis caused by foods.[62,64] Because the type I mechanism accounts for most allergic and anaphylactic reactions, the chapter focuses on this hypersensitivity mechanism.

Risk Factors for Anaphylaxis

Anaphylaxis represents one of the most urgent of medical emergencies, in which rapid diagnosis and prompt and appropriate treatment can mean the difference between life and death.[68] The International Consensus on Anaphylaxis defines anaphylaxis as a severe systemic hypersensitivity reaction that is rapid in onset; characterized by life-threatening airway, breathing, or circulatory problems; and usually associated with skin and mucosal changes.[56,68,69] Because in some people allergic or hypersensitivity reactions can be triggered by minute amounts of antigen such as certain foods or single insect stings, anaphylaxis can be considered the most aberrant example of an imbalance between the cost and benefit of an immune response.[68] Foods, medications, insect stings, and allergen immunotherapy injections are the most common provoking factors for anaphylaxis, but any agent capable of producing a sudden degranulation of mast cells or basophils can induce anaphylaxis.[62] The more rapid an anaphylaxis reaction is after an exposure, the more likely it is to be severe and potentially fatal.[64]

Risk factors for increased severity and mortality of an anaphylaxis reaction include the following:[62,64]

- Recent episode of anaphylaxis
- Extremes of age (very young or very old)
- Presence of atopy or cardiopulmonary conditions
- Taking medications that may influence timely recognition of symptoms or impede treatment of anaphylaxis
- Rapid onset of symptoms after exposure

The rate of occurrence of anaphylaxis is increasing, especially in young people.[59,62,69] Unfortunately, anaphylaxis is not a reportable disorder, and both its morbidity and mortality are probably underestimated.[57,62] The lifetime individual risk of anaphylaxis is estimated to be 1% to 3%;[60,62] however, allergic reactions are a common cause for ED visits.[62] The true rate of occurrence of anaphylaxis from all triggers in the general population is unknown because of underrecognition by patients and caregivers and underdiagnosis by health care professionals.[62,69] In addition, underreporting, use of a variety of case definitions, use of different measures of occurrence such as incidence or prevalence, and undercoding are problematic in many epidemiologic studies. Despite this problem and although anaphylaxis is not rare, death from anaphylaxis is considered uncommon. However, case fatality rate is difficult to ascertain with accuracy.[69] Understanding potential triggers, mechanisms, and patient-specific risk factors for severity and fatality is the key to performing appropriate risk assessment in those who have previously experienced an acute anaphylactic episode.[59,69]

Patient factors including age-related factors, concomitant diseases, and concurrent medications potentially contribute to severe or fatal anaphylaxis. Cofactors potentially amplify anaphylaxis. Multiple factors and cofactors likely contribute to some anaphylactic episodes. Atopic diseases are a risk factor for anaphylaxis triggered by food, exercise, and latex (details follow), but not for anaphylaxis triggered by insect stings and medications.[64,69]

Etiology of Anaphylaxis

Anaphylaxis typically occurs through an IgE-dependent immunologic mechanism, most commonly triggered by foods, stinging insect venoms, or medications. Medications can also trigger anaphylaxis through an IgE-independent immunologic mechanism and through direct mast cell activation. In patients with idiopathic

Patient Factors That Contribute to Anaphylaxis

Age-Related Factors*

- Infants
- Adolescents and young adults
- Labor and delivery
- Elderly

Concomitant Diseases

- Asthma and other respiratory diseases
- Cardiovascular diseases
- Mastocytosis/clonal mast cell disorders
- Allergic rhinitis and eczema**
- Psychiatric illnesses

Concurrent Medication, Alcohol, and Recreational Drug Use

- Beta-adrenergic blockers and ACE inhibitors***
- Alcohol
- Sedatives
- Hypnotics
- Antidepressants
- Recreational drugs

Cofactors That Amplify Anaphylaxis

- Exercise
- Acute infection
- Emotional stress
- Disruption of routine
- Premenstrual status

* Age-related factors, concomitant diseases, and concurrent medications potentially contribute to severe or fatal anaphylaxis. Cofactors potentially amplify anaphylaxis. Multiple factors and cofactors likely contribute to some anaphylactic episodes.

** Atopic diseases are a risk factor for anaphylaxis triggered by food, exercise, and latex, but not for anaphylaxis triggered by insect stings.

*** ACE = angiotensin-converting enzyme

Based on Simons (2011).

anaphylaxis, the possibility of a novel allergen trigger or of underlying mast cell disorder should be considered.[69] The relative importance of specific anaphylaxis triggers in different age groups appears to be universal. Foods are the most common trigger in children, adolescents, and young adults. Insect stings and medications are relatively common triggers in middle-aged and elderly adults; in these age groups, idiopathic anaphylaxis, a diagnosis of exclusion, is also relatively common.[56,69] Common causes for anaphylaxis, anaphylactoid, and allergic reactions are the following:[56,62,69,70]

- Foods and additives: Shellfish, soybeans, nuts (peanuts and tree nuts), seeds, wheat, milk, eggs, salicylates, sulfites

- Venoms: Hymenoptera stings, insect parts

- Drugs: Beta-lactam antibiotics, acetylsalicylic acid (aspirin or ASA), vancomycin, nonsteroidal anti-inflammatory drugs (NSAIDs), insulin, virtually any drug

- Proteins: Tetanus antitoxin, blood products or transfusions

- Others: Latex, molds, radiographic contrast material, vaccines

Clinical Features of Anaphylaxis

Anaphylaxis is a serious allergic reaction with a rapid onset; it may cause death and requires emergent diagnosis and treatment. Consensus clinical criteria have been developed to provide consistency for diagnosis.[71] The diagnosis of anaphylaxis remains clinical (details follow in Assessment of the Patient in Anaphylactic Shock). A good history and physical examination provide the HCP the best tools in diagnosis of anaphylaxis.[64,69]

Skin signs are present in 80% to 90% of all patients; when they are absent, anaphylaxis is harder to recognize.[69] Cutaneous symptoms are described as generalized warmth and tingling of the face, mouth, upper chest, palms, soles, or the site of antigenic exposure. **Pruritus** is a nearly universal feature and may be accompanied by generalized flushing and urticaria. Patients presenting

Anaphylaxis Mechanisms and Triggers

Immunologic Mechanisms (IgE Dependent)
- Food: Peanuts, tree nuts, shellfish, fish, milk, eggs, soybeans, peaches, sesame
- Venoms: Stinging insects
- Medications: Beta-lactam antibiotics, NSAIDS, biologic agents
- Natural rubber latex
- Occupational allergens
- Seminal fluid
- Aeroallergens
- Radiocontrast media

Immunologic Mechanisms (IgE Independent)
- Radiocontrast media
- NSAIDs
- Dextrans
- Biologic agents

Nonimmunologic Mechanisms (Direct Mast Cell Activation)
- Physical factors
- Alcohol
- Medications

Idiopathic Anaphylaxis (No Apparent Trigger)
- Previously unrecognized allergen
- Mastocytosis/clonal mast cell disorder

Based on Simons (2011).

with angioedema may complain of swelling and a sensation of burning under the skin but no itchy rash.[57,64] Generalized urticaria and angioedema are the most common manifestations of anaphylaxis and occur as the initial signs and symptoms or accompany severe anaphylaxis. Cutaneous manifestations might be delayed or absent in rapidly progressive anaphylaxis.[57] A patient presenting with skin symptoms (itchy urticaria, flushing, and swollen lips, tongue, or throat) and either respiratory difficulty (dyspnea, wheezing, and stridor) or reduced blood pressure, after an acute exposure is considered highly likely to have the diagnosis of anaphylaxis.[56,64,69] Other symptoms can occur, such as nausea and vomiting,[56] a generalized flushing sensation, headache, lightheadedness, uterine cramps, and feeling of impending doom.[58] The classic presentation of anaphylaxis helps clinicians identify likely anaphylaxis and emphasize the rapid onset of its multiple symptoms and signs.[56]

Anaphylactic reactions vary in duration and severity, affecting organs that are rich in mast cells—the cutaneous, upper and lower respiratory, cardiovascular, neurologic, and gastrointestinal systems.[64] The pattern (onset, number, and course) of symptoms and signs differ from one patient to another, and even in the same patient from one anaphylactic episode to another. At the beginning of an episode, it can be difficult to predict the rate of progression or the ultimate severity. Fatality can occur within minutes.[69] Clinical presentations of anaphylaxis depend on the following:[64,69]

- Degree of hypersensitivity
- Quantity, route, and rate of antigen exposure
- Pattern of mediator release
- Target organ sensitivity and responsiveness

Signs and symptoms of anaphylaxis begin suddenly, and they usually occur minutes after an exposure, although some reactions take longer (usually within 30 minutes to 2 hours after exposure to the allergen for food allergy) and even faster with parenteral medication or insect stings. In general, the faster the onset of symptoms, the more severe is the reaction; 50% of anaphylactic fatalities occur within the first hour.[56,58,62,64,72] In a large case series of fatal anaphylaxis, the median time from symptoms to arrest has been reported as 30, 15, and 5 minutes for food, insect venom, and parenteral medication, respectively.[56,74] Respiratory compromise and cardiovascular collapse are responsible for most fatalities.[58,64] The more rapid the onset of the signs and symptoms of anaphylaxis following exposure to an offending stimulus, the more likely the reaction will be life-threatening.[58]

Differential Diagnosis

Anaphylaxis is difficult to diagnose and manage. Severe reactions are unexpected and may progress so quickly

 RED FLAG

In a patient with anaphylaxis, symptoms begin immediately, usually within 15 minutes of exposure and involve the skin, upper or lower airways, cardiovascular system, or GI tract.[56,57,64,66,69,71-73] In quickly progressing anaphylaxis, early symptoms may be missed and symptoms do not necessarily progress from mild (e.g., urticaria) to severe (e.g., airway obstruction, refractory shock). Anaphylaxis that is left untreated will lead to anaphylactic shock, a state of systemic hypoperfusion that may progress to multiple organ failure and death. Cardiovascular collapse can occur without respiratory or other symptoms. In severe cases, the patient may become unresponsive and die. Hypersensitivity reactions can be categorized as follows:[73]

- *Mild:* Skin and subcutaneous tissues only including flushing, pruritus, urticaria, erythema, edema or angioedema, sneezing, rhinorrhea, conjunctivitis, bronchospasm.

- *Moderate:* Features suggesting respiratory, cardiovascular, or gastrointestinal involvement including dyspnea, stridor, wheezing, nausea, vomiting, dizziness, (presyncope), diaphoresis, chest or throat tightness, or abdominal pain.

- *Severe:* Indications of hypoxia, hypotension, or neurologic compromise including hypotension, tachycardia, urticaria, angioedema, wheezing, stridor, cyanosis, and **syncope** (fainting).

- *Life-threatening:* Laryngeal edema may be indicated by a sense of choking, complaint of a "lump in the throat," a sense of fullness in the throat, dyspnea, a sensation of chest tightness, shortness of breath, anxiety, and lightheadedness.

- *Late-phase:* Reactions that occur 4 to 8 hours after the exposure or later.

that no treatment can be administered before respiratory or cardiac arrest.[74] The diagnosis of anaphylaxis is clinical.[69] Consider anaphylaxis when involvement of any 2 or more body systems is observed, with or without hypotension or airway compromise. The diagnosis is easily made if a clear history of exposure exists, such as a bee sting, shortly followed by the multisystem signs and symptoms described previously. Unfortunately, diagnosis is not always easy or clear, because symptom onset may be delayed, symptoms may mimic other presentations (e.g., syncope, gastroenteritis, anxiety), or anaphylaxis may be a component of other diseases (e.g., asthma).[62]

In anaphylaxis, some of the most common diagnostic dilemmas involve acute asthma, syncope, and anxiety or panic attacks. A severe asthma episode can cause diagnostic confusion because wheezing, coughing, and shortness of breath can occur in both asthma and anaphylaxis; however, itching, urticaria, angioedema, abdominal pain, and hypotension are unlikely in acute asthma. An anxiety or panic attack can cause diagnostic confusion because a sense of impending doom, breathlessness, flushing, tachycardia, and gastrointestinal symptoms can occur in both anxiety or panic attacks and in anaphylaxis; however, urticaria, angioedema, wheezing, and hypotension are unlikely during an anxiety or panic attack. Syncope can cause diagnostic confusion because hypotension can occur in both syncope and anaphylaxis; however, syncope is relieved by **recumbence** and is usually associated with pallor and sweating, and absence of urticaria, flushing, respiratory symptoms, and gastrointestinal symptoms.[69] The differential diagnosis of anaphylactic reactions is extensive, including myocardial ischemia, arrhythmias, severe acute asthma, seizure, vocal cord dysfunction, foreign body airway obstruction, and non–IgE-mediated drug reactions.[62] The most likely anaphylactic reactions to encounter in the sports medicine setting include food sensitivities and allergies, latex allergy, bites and stings, urticaria, angioedema, allergic drug reactions, syncope, and exercise-induced anaphylaxis.

Food Sensitivities and Allergies   Food is the most common cause of anaphylaxis in the outpatient setting, and food allergens account for 30% of fatal cases of anaphylaxis.[62,75] Between 2001 and 2010, a 9.8% increase per year in the incidence rate of food-related anaphylaxis occurred. Food-related anaphylaxis was most common in children aged 0 to 9 years. The most commonly implicated foods responsible for food-induced anaphylaxis include peanuts, tree nuts, fish, shellfish, cow's milk, soy, and egg.[62,75,76] In addition, sesame seeds have been identified as a significant cause of food-induced anaphylaxis.[75] As is the case of anaphylaxis following other agents,

Signs and Symptoms of Anaphylaxis or Anaphylactic Shock

Skin and Mucosal Tissue (Most Common)
- Generalized hives or urticaria
- Pruritus
- Angioedema
- Flushing/diaphoresis

Respiratory Compromise
- Dyspnea
- Wheezing/bronchospasm/reduced PEF
- Stridor
- Cough
- Voice change
- Cyanosis/hypoxemia

Reduced BP or Associated End-Organ Dysfunction Involvement
- Hypotension
- Hypotonia/collapse/presyncope/sudden weakness
- Syncope

Gastrointestinal Symptoms (Least Common)
- Crampy abdominal pain
- Nausea
- Vomiting
- Diarrhea

BP = blood pressure; PEF = peak expiratory flow

Based on Simons (2014); Tran and Muelleman (2017); Simons (2011); Campbell et al. (2012).

asthma is a risk factor for more severe food-induced anaphylaxis.[75,77] It is essential to identify the trigger or causative agent and provide effective recommendations on important aspects of care that need to be improved.[77] Common themes associated with fatal food anaphylaxis include the following:[74,75]

- Reactions commonly involve peanuts and tree nuts.
- Cutaneous and respiratory symptoms are frequently observed.
- Victims are typically teenagers and young adults.
- Patients have a previous history of food allergy and asthma.
- Failure to promptly administer epinephrine to relieve symptoms

Food allergy is a major cause of anaphylaxis in children, and the rates of both food allergy and anaphylaxis are increasing in developed countries.[77] Food allergy may coexist with asthma, atopic dermatitis, **eosinophilic esophagitis**, and exercise-induced anaphylaxis. In patients with asthma, the coexistence of food allergy may be a risk factor for severe asthma exacerbations. Elimination of food allergens in sensitized individuals can improve symptoms of some comorbid conditions. Atopic dermatitis and food allergy are highly associated,[76] and recognizing food-induced anaphylaxis is essential in appropriately treating the episode.

Hypersensitivity reactions to ingested foods are generally caused by IgE-coated mast cells lining the GI tract reacting to ingested food proteins and, rarely, to additives.[62,76] Symptoms of food allergy include the following:

- Swelling and itching of the lips, mouth, and pharynx
- Nausea
- Abdominal cramps
- Vomiting
- Diarrhea
- Angioedema
- Urticaria
- Anaphylaxis

Treatment for mild food reactions is supportive; antihistamines are administered to lessen symptoms. More severe reactions or anaphylaxis are managed as described next.[62] The first treatment for immediate allergic reactions to food is often provided by ATs, school nurses, paramedics, or other prehospital providers. Because all food-related reactions cause difficulty breathing, often HCPs experience difficulty deciding whether to use the protocol for anaphylaxis or for asthma. This difficulty may lead to delayed or inappropriate treatment that may contribute to a fatality. Prehospital acute care protocols and EAPs should account for the difficulty in diagnosing food hypersensitivity and anaphylactic reaction. Often a similarity exists between panic attacks and breathing difficulty because of food allergy. For example, a patient with symptoms attributed to a panic attack may be confused with symptoms of anaphylaxis and epinephrine is not administered, leading to fatal respiratory arrest.[74] A detailed dietary history within the 24 hours of allergic symptoms may provide the best clues to food allergy, with particular attention to other allergic history and prior reactions. However, diagnosis is often difficult, and multiple episodes might need to occur before an offending agent is identified.[62,76]

Latex Allergy   Latex in gloves, condoms, and surgical materials may induce anaphylaxis. The diagnosis of latex or natural rubber latex allergy relies on specific IgE measurement, which has poor sensitivity, and materials for skin testing have not been standardized.[59] A latex-safe environment is an environment in which no latex gloves are used in the room or treatment area and the latex accessories that contact the patient (e.g., catheters, adhesives, tourniquets, and anesthesia equipment or devices) are limited. In health care settings, general use of latex gloves with negligible allergen content, powder-free latex gloves, and nonlatex gloves and medical supplies should be considered in an effort to minimize patient exposure to latex. Such an approach can minimize latex sensitization of health care workers and patients and reduce the risk of reactions to latex in previously sensitized individuals. Patients with a diagnosis of latex allergy by history or skin testing can wear a medical identification bracelet, carry a medical identification card, or both. If patients have a history of anaphylaxis to latex, they should carry auto-injectable epinephrine.[75] However, with the recent introduction of latex-free facilities and the use of nonlatex gloves, the incidence of anaphylaxis related to this allergy has dramatically decreased.[59]

Exercise-Induced Anaphylaxis and Food-Dependent Exercise-Induced Anaphylaxis

Exercise is the immediate trigger for the development of symptoms in **exercise-induced anaphylaxis (EIA)**. Attacks occur sporadically and unpredictably, even though most patients with this disorder exercise regularly. Vigorous exercises, such as jogging, racquet sports, dancing, and aerobics, are most often implicated, although lower levels of exertion, such as brisk walking or yard work, are capable of triggering attacks in some patients.[75] Typical symptoms of EIA include the following:[61,62,75]

- Extreme fatigue
- Warmth
- Flushing

- Pruritus
- Urticaria

Occasionally, symptoms progress to the following:[61,62,75]

- Angioedema
- Wheezing
- Upper airway obstruction
- Collapse

Some patients experience disabling headache that persists for several days after an episode. Cessation of exercise usually results in improvement or resolution of symptoms, although patients often do not instinctively stop exercising when they first experience symptoms. Instead, many try to run for help or sprint home, which precipitates a dramatic worsening of symptoms.[75] Once the patient either stops exercise or receives treatment (description follows), symptoms may dissipate rapidly or last for several hours. It is not known how often this disorder results in fatal anaphylaxis, although at least one death has been reported. Such events are likely underdiagnosed and misdiagnosed, as with other causes of fatal anaphylaxis.[75]

Exercise-induced anaphylaxis is defined by 4 criteria:[61,76,78-80]

- Episodes of syncope or obstruction of upper airways with "flush" or recurring generalized urticaria (at least twice)
- Urticaria papules greater than 0.39 inches (10 mm)
- Collapse is not due to cardiac, pulmonary, or cerebral dysfunction
- Anaphylaxis is not secondary to an elevation in body temperature (hot bath, shower, fever)

Food-dependent exercise-induced anaphylaxis (FDEIA), or augmentation factor-triggered food allergy, is a unique clinical syndrome in which anaphylaxis occurs within a few hours of specific food ingestion or any meal, and exercise (details in Evidence section).[75,79] This condition is triggered by foods in about one-third of patients and has a natural history marked by frequent recurrence of the episodes.[61,76] Typically this syndrome presents in adolescence or in individuals in their 20s, but it can occur at any age.[77] The time between consumption of the food and onset of symptoms is frequently longer than in other kinds of food-induced anaphylaxis; reactions have been reported hours after eating the food. Usually, symptoms begin within 30 minutes of the start of exercise but can occur at any time during the workout and with any intensity of exercise. This syndrome can be life-threatening, but most common symptoms are urticaria, flushing, fatigue, pruritus, and angioedema.[77,80,81]

FDEIA includes the criteria for EIA, in addition to an association between ingestion of food and physical exercise, and the following:[59,75,81]

- The reaction occurs 15 to 30 minutes after initiation of physical effort.
- The maximal delay between food ingestion and onset of symptoms is 3.5 hours or less.
- The delay between initiation of exercise and onset of the first signs varies from 5 to 15 minutes.

Management of FDEIA must be individualized depending on the severity of symptoms, the presence of co-triggers, and the patient's desire to continue exercise. For exercisers with wheat or gluten sensitivity, eliminating wheat ingestion 4 to 6 hours before exercise is recommended to avoid anaphylaxis.[59,75,81] Patients with exercise-induced anaphylaxis must be advised to stop exercising immediately at the first sign of symptoms, because continued exertion causes the attacks to worsen. Patients must be vigilant for early signs (e.g., flushing, pruritus) and stop exercise immediately if these signs develop. Patients must understand the importance of immediately stopping exercise at the first sign of symptoms. All patients should carry epinephrine auto-injectors and exercise with a partner who can both recognize symptoms and administer epinephrine if necessary. Prophylactic medications are not effective for preventing attacks in most patients, although a small subset does appear to benefit from daily administration of antihistamines.[75] The prognosis of patients with EIA or FDEIA is generally favorable, and most patients experience fewer and less-severe attacks over time. It is unclear whether this improvement is the result of trigger avoidance or a change in the underlying condition.[75,78,81] For patients with identifiable co-triggers, avoidance of these factors may allow them to resume exercise safely. Most patients do well, reporting fewer attacks over time. With proper counseling and careful self-monitoring, most patients are able to continue exercise.[75] Improvement may be attributable to recognition of early symptoms, modifications in exercise habits, and improved avoidance of triggering food and augmenting factors.[80]

Insect Bites and Stings   Venomous bites and stings from a variety of insects are a significant problem in the United States; the American Association of Poison Control Centers[82] reported that the most common bites were from scorpion stings, but bee, wasp, or hornet stings were more likely to be fatal; yellow jackets cause the most allergic sting reactions in the United States.[82] In the United States, bee stings cause 3 to 4 times more deaths than do venomous snakebites.[83] Bites and stings from the following hymenoptera and arachnids can cause anaphylaxis:

- *Apids*: Honeybees, bumblebees
- *Vespids*: Yellow jackets, hornets, wasps
- *Formacids*: Stinging or fire ants
- *Arachnids*: Spiders, scorpions

Insect bites and stings can cause systemic allergic reactions, including tissue necrosis, anaphylaxis, and death (table 6.8).[75,84] The venom of the brown recluse spider contains multiple enzymes that cause extensive tissue necrosis. Significant necrotic wounds are rare but possible through neutrophil activation, platelet aggregation, and thrombosis.[84] The black widow spider includes varieties that are predominantly brown with an orange-red

hourglass-shaped marking and injures the patient with highly potent venom.

Allergic reactions to insect bites (table 6.8) are IgE mediated, causing local and systemic (generalized) reactions that may include any one or more of the signs and symptoms of anaphylaxis (see Signs and Symptoms of Anaphylaxis or Anaphylactic Shock, earlier in the chapter).[75] In general, the shorter the interval between the sting and the onset of symptoms, the more severe is the reaction. Fatalities that occur within the first hour after the sting usually result from airway obstruction or hypotension.[84] Large local sting reactions can cause delayed and prolonged local inflammation, increasing

TABLE 6.8 Insects and the Reaction to Bites and Stings

Insect	Reaction	Description
Yellow jacket		Initial: Mild symptoms Progresses quickly to anaphylactic shock Similar reaction from other stinging insects
Brown recluse spider		Initial: Mild to severe pain, localized erythema, pruritus, and swelling May progress to hemorrhagic blister surrounded by vasoconstriction-induced blanched skin Progresses over days to hemorrhagic area that may become necrotic with extensive tissue necrosis
Black widow spider		Initial: Small <5-mm erythematous macule develops that evolves into larger lesion with a blanched center and surrounding erythema Progresses to pain, cramping, hypertension and tachycardia, and systemic symptoms include headache, nausea, vomiting, diaphoresis, photophobia, and dyspnea

Yellow jacket: Ted Kinsman/Science Source; yellow jacket reaction: Dr. P. Marazzi/Science Source; brown recluse spider: Smith Collection/Gado/Getty Images; brown recluse spider bite: Francesco Tomasinelli/Science Source; black widow spider: Ian Waldie/Getty Images; black widow spider bite: Dr. P. Marazzi/Science Source

Based on Lieberman et al. (2010); Barish and Arnold (2016); Schneir and Clark (2016).

over 24 to 48 hours and resolving in 3 to 10 days.[75,84] Clinical features of anaphylaxis from an insect sting are identical to those due to other causes of anaphylaxis.[75] Most reactions develop within the first 15 minutes, and nearly all occur within 6 hours. Initial mild symptoms may progress quickly to anaphylactic shock. Symptoms include the following:[75,83,84]

- *Local*: Immediate burning, transient pain, itching, erythema, swelling
- *Mild systemic*: Nausea, vomiting, and diarrhea; lightheadedness and syncope
- *Moderate systemic*: Muscle spasms, edema without urticaria, seizures (rare)
- *Serious systemic anaphylaxis:* Angioedema, bronchospasm, refractory hypotension, respiratory distress, and cardiac arrest

Urticaria and bronchospasm need not be present.

General treatment for insect bites and stings is to remove the stinger immediately if it is present in the wound; scrape the stinger out or remove it with tweezers. Wash the sting site thoroughly with soap and water to minimize infection. For local reactions, intermittent application of ice packs at the site diminishes swelling and delays the absorption of venom while limiting edema. Oral antihistamines and analgesics may limit discomfort and pruritus. Nonsteroidal anti-inflammatory drugs (NSAIDs) can be effective in relieving pain. Transport to the hospital is recommended for victims with over 100 stings, for those with substantial comorbidities, and for those at extremes of age.[83,84] Spider bites should be observed and referred if serious symptoms arise. For severe spider **envenomations**, hospital admission is required for analgesia, supportive care, and treatment with antivenom (if available).[84]

The initial signs and symptoms of a systemic anaphylactic reaction may be mild initially, but the patient's condition can deteriorate rapidly in a matter of minutes. For treating anaphylaxis from bites or stings, administer an epinephrine auto-injector. Massage the injection site to hasten absorption,[84] and immediately transfer the patient to the ED for definitive treatment. Similarly, patients with systemic symptoms following a spider bite warrant hospitalization.

Urticaria Urticaria is a cutaneous reaction marked by acute onset of pruritic, erythemic **wheals** of varying size (figure 6.15); it is also called **hives**. Generalized urticaria is usually allergic in nature (i.e., mast cell mediated), and in half of the cases urticaria is accompanied by angioedema and may have serious findings that meet the criteria for anaphylaxis.[61,62,64,79,85] Urticaria results from the release of histamine, bradykinin, kallikrein, and other vasoactive substances from mast cells and basophils in the superficial dermis, resulting in intradermal edema caused by capillary and venous vasodilation and occasionally leukocyte infiltration. Acute urticaria most often results from type I hypersensitivity reactions but may have non–IgE-mediated mechanisms. Additional etiologies of urticaria result from a trigger (e.g., drug, food ingestion, insect bite or sting, infection) that is the cause of the reaction.[62,79,85]

Additional etiologies of urticaria include the following:[61,64,79]

- *Dermographism:* Occurs in 1% to 4% of the population, is defined by the appearance of a linear wheal at the site of a brisk stroke with a firm object or by any configuration appropriate to the eliciting event.
- *Pressure urticaria:* Presents in response to a sustained stimulus such as a shoulder strap or belt, running (feet), or manual labor (hands).
- *Cholinergic urticaria:* Distinctive with pruritic wheals that are of small size (1-2 mm) surrounded

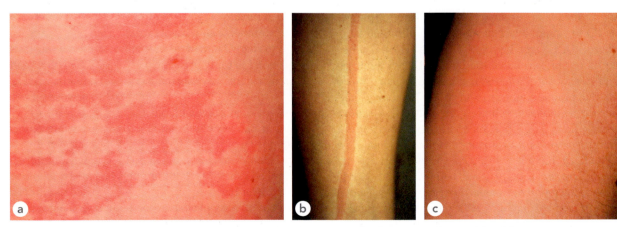

FIGURE 6.15 Etiologies of urticaria: *(a)* generalized urticaria; *(b)* dermographism; *(c)* cold urticaria.
Courtesy of Dr. Charles Phillips.

by a large area of erythema; attacks are precipitated by fever, a hot bath or shower, or exercise and are presumptively attributed to a rise in core body temperature.

- *Exercise-induced anaphylaxis:* Discussed in previous section.
- *Cold urticaria:* Local areas exposed to low ambient temperature, cold objects, and ice or other cryotherapy, and can progress to vascular collapse with immersion in cold water (swimming).
- *Solar urticaria:* Response to specific portions of the light spectrum that promptly (generally within 1-3 minutes) have urticaria with exposure of skin to sunlight.
- *Physical urticaria:* Physical allergy always defined by stimulus-specific elicitation.

Physical examination of urticaria should include vital signs and inspection for any signs of respiratory distress, jaundice, or agitation. Examination of the head should note any swelling of the face, lips, or tongue; scleral **icterus**; facial rash; tender and enlarged thyroid; lymphadenopathy; or dry eyes and dry mouth. Skin examination should note the presence and distribution of urticarial lesions as well as any cutaneous ulceration, hyperpigmentation, small papules, or jaundice.[61,62,85]

Treatment of urticarial reactions is generally supportive and symptomatic, with attempts to identify and remove the trigger agent. First-line therapy is antihistamines, with or without corticosteroids, although epinephrine should be considered in severe cases or if the diagnosis of anaphylaxis has not been excluded.[62,79] Nonspecific symptomatic treatment such as taking cool baths, avoiding hot water and scratching, or wearing loose clothing may be helpful.[85]

Angioedema   Angioedema is edema of the deep dermis and subcutaneous tissues that can be life-threatening with swelling of the tongue, lips, and face with potential for airway obstruction (figure 6.16). Angioedema is a similar reaction as urticaria, but with deeper involvement characterized by edema formation in the dermis, generally involving the face and neck as well as distal extremities. Most cases of angioedema are allergic and usually associated with urticaria.[61,62,64,86] In over 90% of cases, acute angioedema is an acute IgE-mediated mast cell allergic reaction caused by exposure to specific allergens.[62,64,86] IgE-mediated angioedema is usually accompanied by acute urticaria and is often caused by the same allergens (e.g., drug, venom, dietary, and other allergens).

Management of angioedema is supportive with special attention to the airway, which can become occluded rapidly and unpredictably.[62,64] If angioedema involves the airway, a supraglottic airway (see chapter 11) may be required, and epinephrine is given as for anaphylaxis. Treatment of angioedema also includes removing or avoiding the allergen and using drugs that relieve symptoms. Patients with severe mast cell–mediated reactions should be advised to always carry a prefilled, self-injecting syringe of epinephrine and oral antihistamines and, if a severe reaction occurs, to use these treatments as quickly as possible and then go to the ED.[61,86]

Allergic Drug Reactions   Adverse reactions to drugs are a common clinical problem, but true hypersensitivity reactions probably account for less than 10% of these occurrences, with the majority of anaphylaxis from IgE-mediated drug reactions.[62,64] Many drugs and treatments can cause allergic reactions and anaphylaxis.[62]

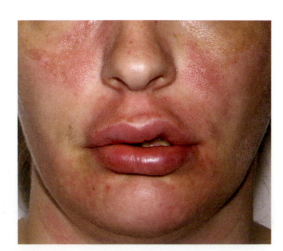

FIGURE 6.16   Angioedema of the lips.

Dr. P. Marazzi / Science Source

Penicillin is the drug most commonly implicated in eliciting true allergic reactions and accounts for approximately 90% of all reported allergic drug reactions and about 75% of fatal anaphylactic drug reactions. After antibiotics, aspirin and other NSAIDs (including COX-2–specific inhibitors) are the second most common cause of drug-induced anaphylaxis.[75]

It is important to appreciate that fatal anaphylactic reactions can occur without a prior allergic history; less than 25% of patients who die of penicillin-induced anaphylaxis exhibited allergic reactions during previous treatment with the drug.[62] Anaphylactic reactions to NSAIDs may involve respiratory reactions and exacerbations of urticaria.[64,75] The clinical manifestations of drug allergy vary widely, and diagnosis is determined by a careful history. Treatment is supportive, with oral or parenteral antihistamines and corticosteroids. Drug cessation is important, but reactions can continue. Referral to an allergy specialist is indicated for severe reactions.[62,64]

Assessment of the Patient in Anaphylactic Shock

This form of distributive shock is characterized by massive vasodilation and increased capillary permeability. It is a severe systemic form of anaphylaxis or immediate hypersensitivity and presents a very dramatic clinical picture that is potentially life-threatening. Anaphylactic shock follows a severe allergic reaction when the patient ingests or is injected with an antigen to which he has been previously sensitized.[69] These criteria for diagnosis of anaphylaxis or anaphylactic shock (figure 6.17) significantly improve the identification of anaphylaxis and demonstrated excellent sensitivity (96.7%) and good specificity (82.4%) for the diagnosis of anaphylaxis in a retrospective ED study.[56,72]

In all patients with shock, continuously monitor heart rate, blood pressure, and oxygen saturation.[5,45] As transport arrives, it is important to find any new developments or conditions that must be treated. The reassessment is an important step in gathering critical information about the condition of the patient to provide efficient and effective emergency care and hand-off to the next-level care provider. For the ongoing assessment, continue to reassess mental status, reestablish patient priorities, reassess vital signs, repeat the focused assessment, and continually recheck adequacy of interventions. Determine whether the treatment is improving the patient's condition or if the patient seems to be deteriorating. In all patients with

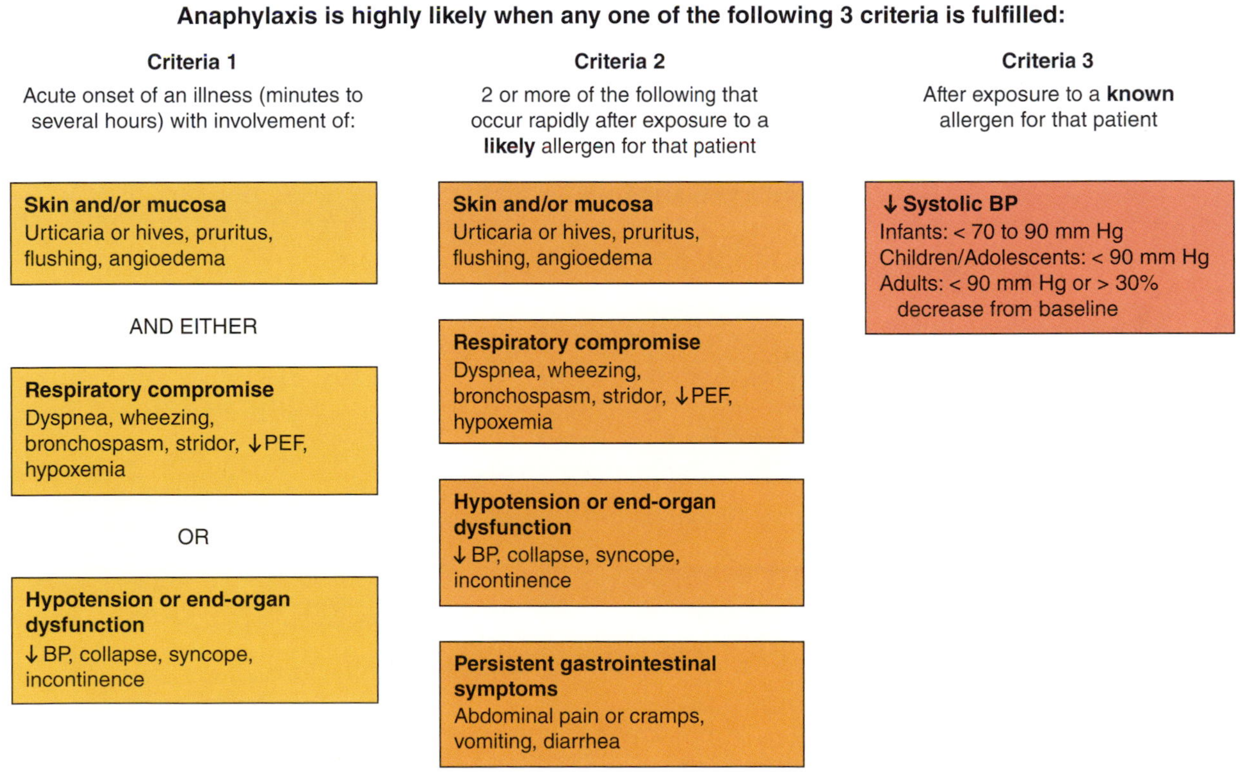

Anaphylaxis is highly likely when any one of the following 3 criteria is fulfilled:

Criteria 1

Acute onset of an illness (minutes to several hours) with involvement of:

Skin and/or mucosa
Urticaria or hives, pruritus, flushing, angioedema

AND EITHER

Respiratory compromise
Dyspnea, wheezing, bronchospasm, stridor, ↓PEF, hypoxemia

OR

Hypotension or end-organ dysfunction
↓ BP, collapse, syncope, incontinence

Criteria 2

2 or more of the following that occur rapidly after exposure to a **likely** allergen for that patient

Skin and/or mucosa
Urticaria or hives, pruritus, flushing, angioedema

Respiratory compromise
Dyspnea, wheezing, bronchospasm, stridor, ↓PEF, hypoxemia

Hypotension or end-organ dysfunction
↓ BP, collapse, syncope, incontinence

Persistent gastrointestinal symptoms
Abdominal pain or cramps, vomiting, diarrhea

Criteria 3

After exposure to a **known** allergen for that patient

↓ Systolic BP
Infants: < 70 to 90 mm Hg
Children/Adolescents: < 90 mm Hg
Adults: < 90 mm Hg or > 30% decrease from baseline

FIGURE 6.17 Clinical criteria for anaphylaxis.

BP = blood pressure; PEF = peak expiratory flow

Based on Simons et al. (2014); Rowe and Gaeta (2016); Tran and Muelleman (2017); Simons et al. (2011); Sampson et al. (2006); Lieberman et al. (2010); Manivannan et al. (2009); Campbell et al; (2014).

shock, HR, BP, and blood oxygen saturation must be continuously monitored until higher-level HCPs arrive.[45]

Emergency Care for Anaphylactic Reactions

Emergency management of anaphylaxis requires immediate assessment using an airway, breathing, circulation, disability and exposure (ABCDE) approach (see chapter 4). Problems should be treated as they are found and with a call for emergency services. Deaths result from upper airway, lower respiratory, or cardiovascular compromise, so emergency management must focus on these manifestations. First-line treatment is intramuscular epinephrine (as described in chapter 5) before instituting other interventions, because it is potentially lifesaving treatment. CPR should be immediately instituted if cardiorespiratory arrest occurs.[56] Base the diagnosis of anaphylaxis on the history and physical examination, but recognize that a broad spectrum of anaphylaxis presentations occur that require clinical judgment. Do not rely on signs of shock for the diagnosis of anaphylaxis.[70,88] Figure 6.18 presents an emergency care algorithm.

A systematic approach to treating anaphylaxis is critically important. The principles of treatment apply to all patients with anaphylaxis from all triggers, who present at any time during an acute episode. Basic initial treatment (what all HCPs should be able to provide, even in a low resource environment), is listed here:

- Create a written emergency protocol in the form of an EAP (see chapter 3), post it, and rehearse it regularly.[56]

- In severe anaphylaxis, securing the airway is the first priority. Carefully examine the mouth, pharynx, and neck for signs and symptoms of angioedema including uvula edema, audible stridor, respiratory distress, and hypoxia. If angioedema is producing respiratory distress, intubate early (see chapter 9), because delay may result in complete airway obstruction secondary to progression of angioedema.[62]

- After rapid assessment of the patient, treatment begins with implementation of the protocol. Remove exposure to the trigger, if possible; rapidly assess the patient's circulation, airway, breathing, mental status, and skin; and estimate the body weight (mass).

- Promptly and simultaneously, call EMS, inject epinephrine intramuscularly in the mid-anterolateral thigh, and place the patient on the back (or in a position of comfort if respiratory distress or vomiting occurs), with the lower extremities elevated.

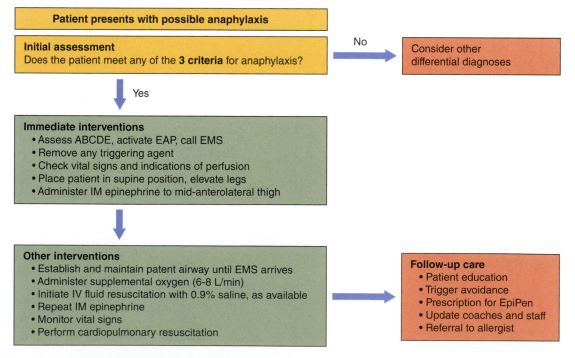

FIGURE 6.18 Treatment algorithm for anaphylaxis emergency measures (taken simultaneously).

ABCDE = airway, breathing, circulation, disability, exposure; EAP = emergency action plan; EMS = emergency medical services; IM = intramuscular; IV = intravenous

Based on Simons et al. (2014); Rowe and Gaeta (2016); Tran and Muelleman (2017); Simons et al. (2015); Campbell (2017).

- When indicated at any point in time, as soon as the need is recognized, administer supplemental oxygen, insert an intravenous catheter, give intravenous fluid resuscitation (as available), and initiate CPR with continuous chest compressions.
- At frequent and regular intervals, monitor the patient's blood pressure, heart rate, respiratory status, and oxygenation; and, if possible, obtain an electrocardiogram (ECG).[56,69]

In many sport and athletic settings, lack of availability of supplemental oxygen and pulse oximetry for detecting hypoxemia and guiding oxygen therapy remains a concern. Basic management of anaphylaxis is relatively inexpensive to implement and should be possible even in a low-resource environment. Limited-resource areas can be found in inner cities, some rural areas, many public venues, and situations such as anaphylaxis on airplanes. Steps in the algorithm should be performed promptly and simultaneously as soon as anaphylaxis is diagnosed. If precious minutes are lost early in the treatment of an acute anaphylactic episode, subsequent management can become more difficult.[69] In limited-resource situations, lack of availability of basic essentials such as epinephrine, supplemental oxygen, and IV fluid resuscitation is more critical than lack of second-line medications such as antihistamines and glucocorticoids. Lack of availability of advanced life support management can be a major barrier to survival. In any limited-resource situation, resuscitation efforts prolonged over hours using a handheld bag-valve mask (manual resuscitator) are often successful in anaphylaxis.[64,69]

Pharmacological Intervention: Epinephrine as First-Line Treatment

Also known as adrenaline, epinephrine is the cornerstone of treatment and drug of choice for anaphylaxis; it may help relieve all symptoms and signs and should be administered immediately at the first suspicion of an anaphylactic reaction (see figure 6.15).[45,66] The World Health Organization[90] classifies epinephrine as an essential medication for the treatment of anaphylaxis. All guidelines consistently emphasize prompt injection of epinephrine as the first-line medication of choice in anaphylaxis.[69]

Epinephrine is lifesaving because of its alpha$_1$-adrenergic vasoconstrictor effects in most body organ systems (skeletal muscle is an important exception) and its ability to prevent and relieve airway obstruction caused by mucosal edema, and to prevent and relieve hypotension and shock.[62,64,69] Other relevant properties in anaphylaxis include its beta$_1$-adrenergic agonist properties leading to increased force and rate of cardiac contractions and its beta$_2$-adrenergic agonist properties leading to decreased mediator release, bronchodilation,

and relief of urticaria.[62,64,69] Epinephrine decreases mediator release from mast cells (and basophils), improves hives and bronchospasm, decreases mucosa edema and swelling, and reverses systemic hypotension. Epinephrine therefore works directly to improve the clinical features most commonly observed in a fatal anaphylactic reaction.[62,64]

Epinephrine must be administered to all patients experiencing anaphylaxis, and it should also be administered to those with clinical features that are likely to evolve into anaphylaxis. Treatment with epinephrine in a patient experiencing anaphylaxis has no absolute contraindications; the benefits outweigh the risks.[56,61] Most patients with anaphylaxis need only a single epinephrine dose;[62,69] however, depending on the severity of the episode and the response to the initial injection, if no improvement is observed, one additional dose may be repeated after 5 to 15 minutes.[45,69] Most patients respond to 1 or 2 doses of epinephrine injected intramuscularly promptly; however, more than 2 doses are occasionally required.[45,61,69] Supplemental oxygen should be administered by face mask or by oropharyngeal airway at a flow rate of 6 to 8 L/min to all patients with respiratory distress and those receiving repeated doses of epinephrine. Oxygen should also be considered for any patient with anaphylaxis who has concomitant asthma, other chronic respiratory disease, or cardiovascular disease. Continuous monitoring of oxygenation by pulse oximetry is desirable, if possible.[69]

Maximal absorption of epinephrine occurs when the drug is administered intramuscularly (IM) in the lateral thigh.[56,61,66] The intramuscular route allows shorter time to peak plasma epinephrine concentration (8 minutes) versus subcutaneous administration (34 minutes).[45,64] The safety profile of intramuscular adrenaline is excellent, although patients may experience transient pallor, palpitations, and headache.[56,61] To avoid mishaps in dosing, many schools, clinics, and facilities stock adult and pediatric auto-injectors (e.g., EpiPen).[45,56,66,84,91] Auto-injectors are indicated in the emergency treatment of type I allergic reactions, including anaphylaxis, to allergens, idiopathic and exercise-induced anaphylaxis, and in patients with a history or increased risk of anaphylactic reactions.[91]

Epinephrine is the first-line treatment in all cases of anaphylaxis,[61,64,69] and it is underused in anaphylaxis treatment. Failure to inject it promptly is potentially associated with fatality, encephalopathy because of hypoxia or ischemia, and biphasic anaphylaxis in which symptoms recur within 1 to 72 hours (usually within 8-10 hours) after the initial symptoms have resolved, despite no further exposure to the trigger.[45,69] When a susceptible patient is reexposed to an antigen to which a previous reaction has occurred, self-administered epinephrine is recommended at the first onset of clinical manifestations of anaphylaxis. Delayed administration of epinephrine is associated with increased risks of adverse outcomes.[61,64] The use of antihistamines is the most common reason reported for not using epinephrine and may place a patient at significantly increased risk for progression toward a life-threatening reaction.[61] Antihistamines should be used only as a secondary treatment. Giving antihistamines instead of epinephrine may increase the risk of a life-threatening allergic reaction.[63] All other drugs have a delayed onset of action, and epinephrine dosing remains first-line therapy over adjunctive treatments.[61]

Education and Communication on Anaphylaxis and Immunologic Emergencies

Medical facilities should have an established and regularly practiced plan of action to deal with anaphylaxis and the appropriate equipment to treat it. Athletic trainers and other staff should maintain clinical proficiency in anaphylaxis management.[75] Anaphylaxis management plans should cover avoidance advice, contact details for advice, and an anaphylaxis EAP with likely presenting symptoms and how to respond to each of them. Anaphylaxis EAPs should be used from diagnosis to aid recognition and treatment of any further reactions and should be regularly updated.[56] Additional recommendations for education and communication include the following:[92]

- Coaches should be educated about the major signs and symptoms of anaphylaxis after the athlete is exposed to a likely or known allergen.

- Parents or guardians of all athletes should be encouraged to complete a form that discloses all known medical conditions. This form should also include a treatment plan for these individuals, consisting of the medications used as well as who will be responsible for ensuring these medications are present during practices and competitions.

- Member organizations should educate parents and guardians on the dangers of not disclosing such conditions.

Anaphylaxis education should be personalized according to the needs of the individual patient, taking into consideration their age, concomitant diseases, concurrent medications, relevant anaphylaxis trigger(s), and likelihood of encountering such trigger(s) in the facility.[69] For prevention of exercise-induced anaphylaxis, strict avoidance of the relevant co-trigger such as food(s), ethanol, and NSAID(s) should be recommended. Exercise under ambient conditions of high humidity, extreme heat or cold, or high pollen counts should be avoided, if relevant. Additional precautions should include never exercising alone, discontinuing exertion immediately when the first symptom of anaphylaxis occurs, and carrying a mobile phone and epinephrine auto-injector.[69]

As with all forms of anaphylaxis, patient education is an ongoing process that should take place at regular follow-up visits and after any recurrent symptoms. The anaphylaxis EAP should be provided, listing the most common symptoms and signs of anaphylaxis and providing instructions for prompt epinephrine injection. Athletes usually have a strong desire to continue to exercise, and every attempt should be made to construct a management plan that allows them to do so. However, modifications in the patient's choice of activities may be required, and several precautions involving exercise are advised.[80]

For many patients, the standard prescription and formal instruction on how to prevent and treat anaphylaxis by a physician are insufficient to achieve compliance with respective practical measures, including carrying an epinephrine auto-injector and appropriately using it.[74] This problem is compounded by the inability of many clinicians to correctly use an auto-injector. Training should be offered to all professionals dealing with patients at risk of anaphylaxis. Educational training programs are especially effective when using a written EAP, having a multidimensional and multidisciplinary approach, and involving repeated regular practice of the EAP.[56,75] A retrospective study revealed how avoidance, self-treatment, and medical management failed to prevent anaphylactic death. This insight should lead to better management of severe allergies by encouraging more effective advice on allergen avoidance, more appropriate prescribing of a self-treatment kit, and improved training in its use. Improving protocols for prehospital practitioners will increase awareness of the correct dose of epinephrine used in treatment of anaphylactic reactions.[74] A multidisciplinary approach and the provision of educational printed and online materials for food allergy have both been shown to improve knowledge, correct use of auto-injectors, and reduce adverse reactions.[56,75]

An anaphylaxis EAP should follow a sample plan[56,63] that should be individualized. For example, patients with previous rapid-onset life-threatening anaphylaxis may be instructed to use their self-injectable epinephrine earlier in the development of any subsequent allergic reaction.[56,63] Refer patients with severe or frequent allergic reactions to an allergist for in-depth preventive management and attempts at allergen identification. Offer patients information about this syndrome (e.g., from websites), advice on advocacy groups, and education regarding food contamination for food allergies, and encourage wearing of personal identification alerts about this condition (e.g., MedicAlert bracelets).[62]

Long-term management of patients at risk of anaphylaxis is essential to prevent a reoccurrence of the episode. An individualized anaphylaxis-specific acute care protocol or plan should be written clearly in simple, nonmedical language (figure 6.19); the protocol and an

Clinical Recommendations for Athletes With Exercise-Induced or Food-Dependent Exercise-Induced Anaphylaxis

As with prevention of anaphylaxis of any etiology, athletes should be informed about the risks of certain medications, such as beta blockers and triggers. Develop an anaphylaxis action plan to provide education to the athlete, coach, or other staff as appropriate. The athlete should exercise with other informed people, at least initially until it is clear to the patient and the clinician that the situations that induce symptoms can be successfully avoided. Exercising with a companion, in a gym, or under the supervision of a coach or AT who has been taught to recognize early signs and administer epinephrine is appropriate. Long-term management of patients at risk of anaphylaxis is essential to preventing a recurrence of the episode.

An individualized management plan should be written clearly in simple, nonmedical language; it should include the following:[56,80]

- Have an epinephrine auto-injector and mobile phone available in all exercise settings.
- Identify who will carry the auto-injector and where it will be (patient, coach, companion). This person must be trained in how and when to administer and be able to recognize early signs and symptoms.
- Runners can be reluctant to carry auto-injectors and mobile phones, which they may find bulky. Auto-injectors should not be left in lockers or cars away from the patient.
- Provide the patient and others with an anaphylaxis action plan.
- If any symptoms occur, stop exertion immediately; never push through. Identify situations in which the patient might be reluctant or unable to stop. Adolescents involved in team sports may be reluctant to stop for fear of disappointing others or interrupting a game. Discuss this possibility and make a plan with the coach.
- For patients with high-activity jobs such as military personnel or pilots, work conditions may need to be adjusted.
- The triggering food may need to be avoided altogether or avoided for 4-6 hours before exercise, at least initially. Time may be reduced going forward, although most patients must avoid the food for a minimum of 2 hours.
- Patients in school or teams whose mealtimes and activity are structured should plan to have foods recognized as safe available for snacking. Planning lists of safe foods with parents or caregivers is particularly helpful for children and adolescents. Avoid possible augmenting factors, and pay close attention to circumstances surrounding symptoms to detect other factors that might be important.
- Provide the patient with a list of possible augmenting factors. Review it periodically, especially if new symptoms occur. When new symptoms occur, instruct the patient to contact the athletic training clinic and review circumstances surrounding her symptoms while the details are fresh in her memory.
- Review the patient's medication list regularly to make sure medications have not been added.

emergency kit should include the following specific to the patient with life-threatening allergies:[56]

- Personal identification data: Name and address; contact details of the parents, guardian, or next of kin; allergist; family doctor; and the local ambulance service
- A photograph clearly identifying the source of the allergen(s) to be avoided and any non-allergen triggers or cofactors, such as exercise

- Instructions on prompt recognition of symptoms of anaphylaxis
- Epinephrine auto-injector and instructions on when and how to use an adrenaline auto-injector, where appropriate; when in doubt, the adrenaline auto-injector should be administered
- Contact information for psychological support as required

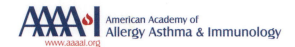

American Academy of
Allergy Asthma & Immunology
www.aaaai.org

Anaphylaxis Emergency Action Plan

Patient Name: _____ Age: _____

Allergies: _____

Asthma ☐ Yes *(high risk for severe reaction)*   ☐ No

Additional health problems besides anaphylaxis: _____

_____

Concurrent medications: _____

_____

Symptoms of Anaphylaxis

MOUTH	itching, swelling of lips and/or tongue
THROAT*	itching, tightness/closure, hoarseness
SKIN	itching, hives, redness, swelling
GUT	vomiting, diarrhea, cramps
LUNG*	shortness of breath, cough, wheeze
HEART*	weak pulse, dizziness, passing out

Only a few symptoms may be present. Severity of symptoms can change quickly.
*Some symptoms can be life-threatening. ACT FAST!

Emergency Action Steps - DO NOT HESITATE TO GIVE EPINEPHRINE!

1. Inject epinephrine in thigh using (check one):   ☐ Adrenaclick (0.15 mg)   ☐ Adrenaclick (0.3 mg)

☐ Auvi-Q (0.15 mg)   ☐ Auvi-Q (0.3 mg)

☐ EpiPen Jr (0.15 mg)   ☐ EpiPen (0.3 mg)

Epinephrine Injection, USP Auto-injector- authorized generic
☐ (0.15 mg)   ☐ (0.3 mg)

☐ Other (0.15 mg)   ☐ Other (0.3 mg)

Specify others: _____

IMPORTANT: ASTHMA INHALERS AND/OR ANTIHISTAMINES CAN'T BE DEPENDED ON IN ANAPHYLAXIS.

2. Call 911 or rescue squad (before calling contact)

3. Emergency contact #1: home_____ work_____ cell_____

Emergency contact #2: home_____ work_____ cell_____

Emergency contact #3: home_____ work_____ cell_____

Comments: _____

_____

_____

Doctor's Signature/Date/Phone Number

_____

Parent's Signature (for individuals under age 18 yrs)/Date

This information is for general purposes and is not intended to replace the advice of a qualified health professional. For more information, visit www.aaaai.org. © 2017 American Academy of Allergy, Asthma & Immunology   4/2017

FIGURE 6.19   Sample anaphylaxis EAP.

Reprinted with permission from the American Academy of Allergy, Asthma & Immunology (AAAAI). Visit AAAAI.org for additional information and updates.

The emergency kit should be checked regularly and the auto-injector replaced if expired. Extra copies of the plan should be distributed to the patient, any coaches, school staff, and parents or guardians.

Evidence

FDEIA is uncommon, but cases are reported around the world. The disorder most commonly affects young adults, but patients of all ages are reported.[80] The most common trigger foods are wheat in the West and shellfish in Asia. The exact mechanism of FDEIA is unknown, although several hypotheses exist. Cofactors such as NSAID use, alcohol consumption, and others have been associated with reported cases.[93]

A few large-scale epidemiological studies of FDEIA have been done. An epidemiological study of Japanese school children was conducted to clarify the frequency and characteristic of FDEIA.[94] This strict definition was used to classify children with FDEIA:

- Symptoms provoked by physical exercise after eating a specific food, but not by that food or exercise alone;
- Symptoms involving more than two organs; and
- Cutaneous symptoms that must include severe symptoms only, such as generalized urticaria or angioedema of the face.

In patients who have a history of severe immediate food allergy, anaphylaxis may be triggered by exercise after consumption of the food to which they had acquired unresponsiveness; this phenomenon is especially observed in patients who have been treated with **oral immunotherapy (OIT)** for food allergy, which is considered different from FDEIA. A survey of 317 public school nurses reported that 8 of 170,146 (1/20,000) children met the criteria for diagnosis with FDEIA, which was significantly lower than the prevalence in junior high school students (0.0047% v. 0.018%, $P = 0.0009$). The causative foods were wheat ($n = 4$), and soy, fruit, crustaceans, and squid ($n = 1$ each). Four children had EIA, and the causative foods were wheat and milk ($n = 2$ each). Multiple episodes occurred in 5 children with FDEIA and in 3 children with EIA. The condition of FDEIA was far less common in elementary school than in junior high school, and wheat was the major causative food. Proper assessment and education in medical settings at the first episode is important to decrease the recurrence of FDEIA. Patients with a history of severe immediate food allergy should be educated about the potential risk of FDEIA. If they develop FDEIA, they should avoid the causative food before exercise. The medical staff must be provided with adequate information about how to manage these patients and improve their care.[94]

Summary

The prehospital HCP must be able to recognize the signs of emergent conditions including hemorrhage, shock, or anaphylaxis. Rapid assessment and management of these life-threatening conditions requires skills including classifying hemorrhage and estimating blood loss, monitoring and recording vital signs, applying a tourniquet or hemostatic agent, and administering epinephrine. Recognizing signs of excessive external or internal hemorrhage requires maintaining a high index of suspicion based on MOI while actively identifying signs and symptoms of blood loss. Although diagnosis of severe, rapidly evolving complications of hemorrhage in the prehospital setting is unlikely, the prehospital HCP must be able to promptly recognize DVT and DIC. These acute, life-threatening emergency complications have serious potential morbidity and mortality. Similarly, sufficiently large losses of body fluid from severe external or internal bleeding can result in hypovolemic shock that can be rapidly fatal. The prehospital HCP must quickly perform the initial assessment and rapid trauma assessment, obtain the history or MOI, record vital signs, and provide documentation that will be valuable for managing the patient's condition in the ED. Treatment of acute anaphylaxis may be challenging in limited-resource settings; essentials such as epinephrine, supplemental oxygen, and IV fluid resuscitation are critical in the management of this life-threatening condition. Epinephrine is the cornerstone of treatment and drug of choice for anaphylaxis or anaphylactic shock and should be administered immediately at the first suspicion of an anaphylactic reaction. This lifesaving medication should be available in all sport and athletic settings.

 Go to the web study guide to complete the case studies for this chapter.

CHAPTER 7

Immediate Management of Musculoskeletal Injuries

Dewayne DuBose, PhD, ATC, LAT, NCPT
Dominique Francis DuBose, PhD
Laura Zdziarski-Horodyski, PhD, LAT, ATC

OBJECTIVES

After reading this chapter, you will be able to do the following:

- Evaluate signs and symptoms of acute injuries, traumatic fractures, and dislocations.

- Analyze life- or limb-threatening injuries and complications.

- Apply initial and secondary injury assessment to determine the urgency for which a patient needs to be transported in the case of acute traumatic fractures and dislocations.

- Know about wound care in the case of an open fracture or fracture–dislocation.

- Apply appropriate care to acute, traumatic fractures and dislocations.

We acknowledge the contributions of Michelle Cleary and Lindsey Eberman to this chapter.

This chapter discusses general concepts as well as specific musculoskeletal emergencies. Not all possible injuries can be discussed within the pages of this text. However, the selected injuries in addition to the general concepts provide the knowledge and skills needed to care for a variety of musculoskeletal injuries.

Overview of the Structures

When evaluating musculoskeletal trauma, the athletic trainer (AT) or other health care provider (HCP) must carefully consider major functional components of the body area individually and together for the best patient outcomes. The major functional components of the limbs are the bones, nerves, blood vessels, and soft tissues. Properly evaluating each of these components is essential in achieving the best outcome in patients with severe extremity injuries.

- *Bones.* The bones create a structural support system for other tissues such as muscle and ligaments, while also protecting major organ systems such as the cardiovascular and respiratory organs contained within the thorax. Bones come together to make joints, or **articulations**, which allow movement and provide attachment sites for ligaments, tendons, and muscles. When muscles contract, bones serve as levers that allow the joint angles to change and provide movement for the body.[1]

- *Ligaments.* Often associated with synovial joints, ligaments are composed of dense regular connective tissue that connects bone to bone while crossing a joint space. Ligaments can be thickenings within the synovial capsule itself (intrinsic ligaments, such as the anterior cruciate ligament) or physically separate from the capsule (extrinsic ligaments, such as the medial collateral ligament).

• *Muscles.* Skeletal muscle includes epithelial, connective, muscle, and nervous tissue and is highly vascularized. Muscles serve to produce body movement, maintain posture, store protein, and provide support for the body The connective tissue surrounding muscle is continuous with the dense, fibrous tendon that connects the muscle to bone.[1]

• *Tendons.* Tendons are tough bands of dense, regular connective tissue that are continuous with the connective tissue coverings of muscle and firmly attach muscle to bone. These dense, fibrous bands are composed mostly of parallel arrays of collagen fibers closely packed together that can withstand tension.[1]

Clinical Anatomy of the Upper Extremity

The bony anatomy of the upper extremity includes the scapula, clavicle, humerus, radius, ulna, and small bones of the wrist and hand. The muscles of the forearm are contained within defined anterior and posterior compartments. The delicate arteries and nerves surrounding the bones and joints of the upper extremity can pose challenges in managing acute or emergent injuries.[1] A working knowledge of the clinical anatomy of the upper extremity is essential in properly recognizing and treating patients with trauma to this area of the body.

Nerves of the Upper Extremity

The ventral rami of the lower cervical and upper thoracic nerve roots (C5-T1) form the brachial plexus that supplies sensory and motor innervation to the upper extremity (figure 7.1). The five major nerves that arise from the cords of the brachial plexus and supply the upper extremity are as follows:

• Axillary
• Musculocutaneous
• Radial
• Median
• Ulnar

The axillary nerve supplies only sensory input to the arm, while the musculocutaneous nerve lies on the lateral side of the arm and innervates shoulder and elbow flexor muscles (coracobrachialis, brachialis, and biceps brachii) as well as sensory input to the lateral forearm. The radial nerve lies deep and winds around the humerus as it innervates the muscles on the posterior arm (triceps, anconeus) and the extensor muscles of the wrist and hand. The median nerve passes through the cubital fossa into the

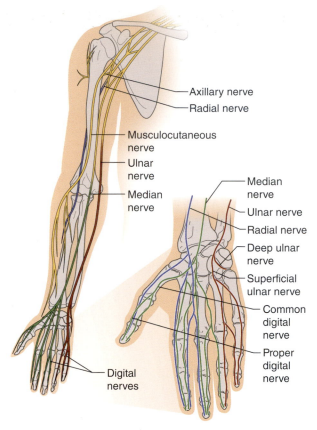

FIGURE 7.1   Nerves of the upper extremity.

forearm, branches off the anterior interosseous nerve, and then enters the hand through the carpal tunnel, providing motor input to the radial side of the hand. The ulnar nerve is the largest unprotected (not covered by muscle or bone) nerve in the body as it lies in the groove posterior to the medial epicondyle and innervates the flexor muscles of the wrist and hand.[1]

Blood Vessels and Pulse Points of the Upper Extremity

The upper extremity is supplied with blood from the subclavian artery as it passes beneath the clavicle and becomes the axillary artery (figure 7.2). As the axillary artery passes the head of the humerus, the circumflex artery branches off to encircle the neck of the humerus while the vessel continues as the brachial artery into the arm. The circumflex arteries of the shoulder and the arteries of the elbow provide robust collateral circulation around these joints. As the brachial artery continues close to the anteromedial humerus, it passes through the cubital fossa with the median nerve. The brachial artery divides into the radial and ulnar arteries in the forearm, which pass distally to the wrist lying close to the radius and ulna, respectively.[1]

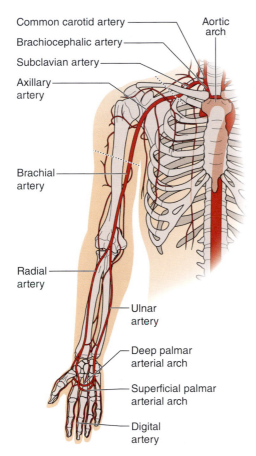

Common carotid artery
Aortic arch
Brachiocephalic artery
Subclavian artery
Axillary artery
Brachial artery
Radial artery
Ulnar artery
Deep palmar arterial arch
Superficial palmar arterial arch
Digital artery

FIGURE 7.2   Arteries of the upper extremity.

The **pulse points** of the upper extremity are found on the brachial and the radial arteries. In infants the brachial artery is most frequently palpated.

- To palpate the brachial artery (figure 7.3*a*), your hand supports the patient's forearm with the patient's upper arm abducted, the elbow slightly

flexed, and the forearm externally rotated. The brachial artery is palpated by pressing the artery against the humerus by curling the fingers on the medial side of the upper arm into the space between the biceps brachii and triceps.

- To palpate the radial artery (figure 7.3*b*), support the patient's forearm with one of your hands; the other hand supports the wrist. To palpate the radial pulse, curl your fingers around the distal radius from the dorsal toward the volar aspect, with the tips of the first, second, and third fingers aligned longitudinally over the course of the artery.[2]

Clinical Anatomy of the Lower Extremity

The bony anatomy of the lower extremity includes the femur, patella, tibia, fibula, and the smaller bones of the ankle and foot. Muscles, tendons, blood vessels and nerves are contained within defined compartments of the lower extremity, which include the anterior, posterior, and medial compartments of the thigh and the anterior, lateral, posterior, and deep posterior compartments of the lower leg.

Nerves of the Lower Extremity

These nerves arise from the lumbar plexus (figure 7.4):

- The femoral nerve (L2-L4) lies within the femoral triangle lateral to the common femoral artery. The femoral nerve innervates the hip and knee extensors (quadriceps) and provides sensory input from the anterior thigh, femur, knee joint, and medial leg.

- The sciatic nerve (L4-S3), the largest and longest nerve in the body, is found in the posterior compartment of the thigh; it continues posterior to

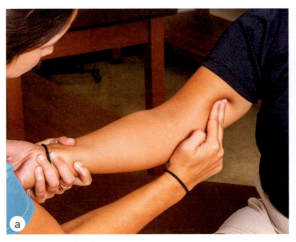
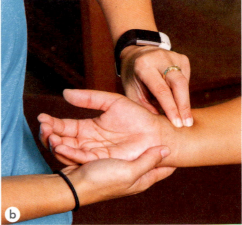

FIGURE 7.3   Pulse points of the upper extremity: *(a)* brachial artery and *(b)* radial artery.

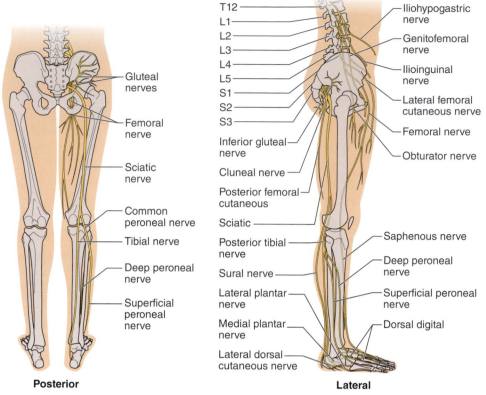

FIGURE 7.4   Nerves of the lower extremity.

the knee, then divides into the tibial and common peroneal nerves. The sciatic nerve supplies the hip flexors, hamstrings, and lower-leg muscles and almost all sensory input from the lower extremity.

- The common peroneal nerve lies on the lateral knee, close to the fibular head, and then divides into the superficial and deep peroneal nerves.

- The deep peroneal nerve, along with the anterior tibial artery, lies in the anterior compartment of the lower leg and innervates the anterior tibial and foot extensor muscles.

- The superficial peroneal nerve lies in the lateral compartment of the lower leg, innervating the peroneal muscle group, while the tibial nerve lies in the deep posterior compartment, along with the peroneal and posterior tibial arteries and innervates the ankle plantar flexors (triceps surae) and the foot flexor muscles.[1]

Blood Vessels and Pulse Points of the Lower Extremity

The arterial supply to the lower extremity is provided by the external iliac artery as it passes through the femoral canal and becomes the common femoral artery, which branches into the deep and superficial femoral arteries (figure 7.5).

- The deep femoral artery lies close to the femur and has branches (medial and lateral femoral circumflex arteries) that surround the hip joint, creating **collateral circulation** around the neck of the femur.

- The superficial femoral artery is found within the anterior compartment of the thigh between the adductor and quadriceps muscles. At the distal third of the femur, the superficial femoral artery lies in close proximity to the femur, then passes through the adductor canal and to the posterior knee to become the popliteal artery.

- Posterior to the tibial tuberosity, the popliteal artery divides into the anterior tibial, posterior tibial, and peroneal arteries.

- In the leg, close to the tibia lie the anterior tibial artery and the deep peroneal nerve, and within the deep posterior compartment lie the posterior tibial artery and the tibial nerve. As the peroneal artery passes distally through the leg, it lies close to the medial side of the fibula.[1]

The pulse points found on the lower limb are the femoral, popliteal, posterior tibialis, and dorsalis pedis.

- The femoral artery (figure 7.6a) is located just distal to the inguinal ligament one-third of the

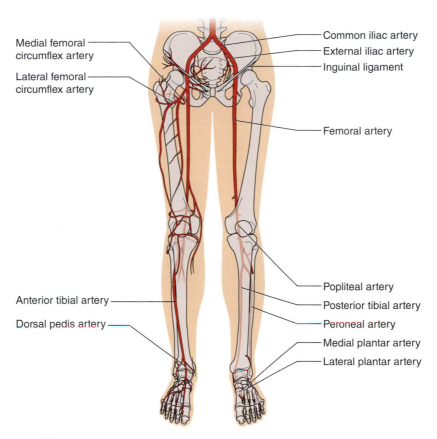

FIGURE 7.5 Arteries of the lower extremity.

distance from the pubis to the anterior superior iliac spine (ASIS). It is best to palpate standing on the ipsilateral side of the patient and the fingertips of your hand pressed firmly into the groin.

- The popliteal artery (figure 7.6*b*) passes vertically through the deep portion of the popliteal space just lateral to the midline. It may be difficult or impossible to palpate in patients who are obese or very muscular. This pulse is palpated with the patient in the supine position and your hands encircling and supporting the knee from each side. Instruct the patient to let the leg go limp in order to relax the surrounding musculature. Detect the pulse by pressing deeply into the popliteal space with the supporting fingertips.

- The posterior tibial artery (figure 7.6*c*) is found just posterior to the medial malleolus. This pulse point is most readily palpated by curling the fingers of the examining hand anteriorly around the ankle, indenting the soft tissues in the space between the medial malleolus and the Achilles tendon, superior to the calcaneus. The thumb grasps the opposite side of the ankle to provide stability. The posterior tibialis pulse is palpated

by placing three fingers on the distal tibia on the medial side of the ankle.

- The dorsalis pedis artery (figure 7.6*d*) is found on the dorsum of the foot, immediately lateral to the extensor hallucis longus tendon, and along the proximal first metatarsal-cuneiform joint. This artery may be in an aberrant in location or congenitally absent in approximately 10% of people.[1]

Classification of Injuries

In the broadest categorization of fracture types, *open* and *closed* are used to describe the osseous, soft tissue, and skin interaction. **Open fractures** are usually the result of high-energy mechanisms, causing a disruption in the osseous tissue and the surrounding soft tissue. Muscles, tendons, ligaments, vasculature, and nerves are all susceptible to injury. The so-called openness of the injury can vary from a poke hole the size of a pen to significant portions of soft tissue loss. In the event of an open fracture, it should be managed with universal precautions, and the fracture site should be covered before splinting (details in the Immobilization section).[3] The injury site should be immediately and serially irrigated

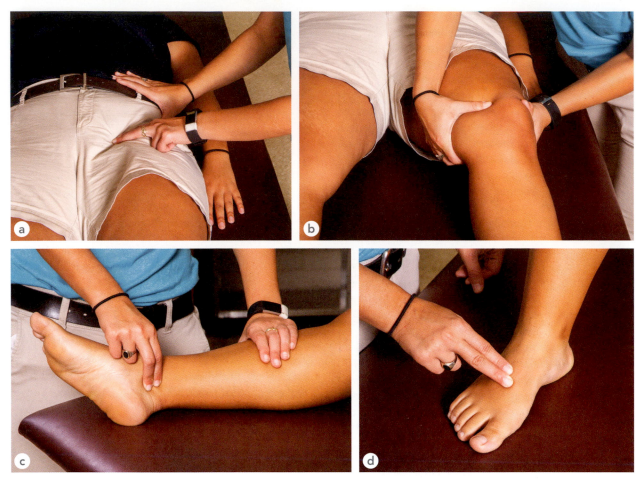

FIGURE 7.6   Pulse points of the lower extremity: *(a)* femoral artery, *(b)* popliteal artery, *(c)* posterior tibial artery, and *(d)* dorsalis pedis artery.

and debrided.[4] The patient should be given antibiotics and definitive wound care until he reaches the hospital for further treatment.[4] While **closed fractures** may seem less severe, significant soft tissue damage can still result. The important distinction is that the risk for infection is significantly reduced with a closed fracture. Patient outcomes following an open fracture are highly dependent on degree of soft-tissue damage, wound size, and amount of **comminution**.[5]

General Classification of Fractures

Fractures are a common daily health issue, and improperly managing them can lead to long-term disability. Most fractures are the result of significant trauma to healthy bone. Fractures are a result of a direct traumatic blow to the bone. Fractures can also form in an area away from traumatic force; they are called indirect fractures.[3] The bony cortex may be disrupted by a variety of forces, including a direct blow, indirect blow, axial loading, angular (bending) forces, torque (twisting stress), or a

combination of them.[6] Fractures may occur as a result of a violent muscle contraction or abnormal stress placed on the bone.[3]

Fractures are classified based on approximation of the segments, the deformation and magnitude of tissue injury, and location. The complexity of a fracture may require more advanced intervention and management for complete healing to occur.[3,7] The most common fractures are detailed in table 7.1. Epiphyseal fractures are fractures that occur along the growth plates in children and adolescents. They are classified by Salter-Harris into five types (see table 7.2).[8]

Subluxations and Dislocations

When two bones separate and form an articulation, **subluxations** and **dislocations** result. A dislocation is the result of one bone in an articulation being forced out of its proper alignment completely. The bone must be reduced to the proper alignment manually or surgically. When a bone is dislocated, usually a deformity appears

TABLE 7.1 Classification of Common Fractures

Classification	Illustration	Description
Transverse		Fracture splits perpendicular to the shaft of the bone.
Linear (longitudinal)		Fracture splits down the length of the bone.
Oblique		Fractures have a spiral shape, but they occur when one end of the bone is twisting while the other end of the bone is in a fixed position. Oblique fractures can be displaced or nondisplaced.
Spiral		Fractures have an S-shaped separation and occur when the ends of the bones are twisted in opposite directions.
Greenstick		Fracture is an incomplete break of a bone that has not fully ossified. The fracture resembles a break in a green twig of a tree.
Comminuted		Fracture consists of > 3 fragments at the fracture site and can be caused by a hard blow of fall in an awkward position.
Avulsion		Fractures occur when a ligament or tendon pulls off a piece of bone from its attachment site.
Impacted (compression)		Fracture results from a fall from a height that causes the bone to be compressed.
Blow		Fracture occurs at the orbital wall of the eye.

> continued

Table 7.1 > *continued*

Classification	Illustration	Description
Serrated		In this fracture, the bony fragments have a sawtooth fracture line.
Stress		Fracture is caused by repetitive microtraumas that exceed the stress-bearing capacity of the bone, leading to a vibratory summation point in the bone.

TABLE 7.2 Salter-Harris Classification of Epiphyseal Fractures

Classification	Illustration	Description
Type I		Complete separation of the physis occurs in relation to the metaphysis with no fracture to the bone.
Type II		Separation of the growth plate occurs along with a small portion of the metaphysis.
Type III		Epiphysis fractures.

Classification	Illustration	Description
Type IV		Portions of both the epiphysis and metaphysis fracture.
Type V		Crushing force causes a growth deformity without displacing the physis.

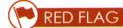
RED FLAG

See chapter 10 for a discussion of posterior sternoclavicular injuries.

that is not present on the uninjured side. A subluxation is similar to dislocation; however, the bone that is out of proper alignment reduces on its own.[3]

Shoulder Dislocation

Two types of glenohumeral shoulder dislocations can occur:

- *Anterior/inferior shoulder dislocation:* The shoulder is forced out of the glenoid capsule in an anterior direction past the labrum and then downward to rest under the coracoid process.[3] The labrum, which is a connective tissue ring around the glenoid cavity, can tear, causing Bankart lesions.[15,16] These lesions allow for the humeral head to dislocate more easily, and patients are prone to dislocate the shoulder after the first traumatic dislocation takes place.[17]

- *Posterior dislocation:* The shoulder is forced out of the glenoid capsule in a posterior direction, which often results in fractures of the lesser tuber-

cle as the subscapular tendon avulses.[3] Posterior dislocation can also result in reverse Hill-Sachs lesion, a defect that can occur on the anteromedial portion of the humeral head.[3,11]

Incidence and Epidemiology

Sir Astley Cooper first described shoulder dislocations in 1838.[18] These dislocations occur at the glenohumeral joint where the head of the humerus meets the glenoid fossa of the scapula. It is reported that 1.7% of the general population experiences shoulder dislocations, and of that percentage, 95% of the dislocations occur anteriorly. Posterior dislocations make up the other 5% of shoulder dislocations.[19] A person is 15 to 21.7 times more likely to have the shoulder dislocate anteriorly as opposed to the shoulder dislocating posteriorly.[20] Mechanism of injuries (MOIs) for shoulder dislocation vary. First, any athlete playing a contact or overhead sports may dislocate the shoulder.[15] Second, anterior dislocations may occur when the shoulder moves through excessive external rotation with hyperextension of the arm while it is over the athlete's head. Third, posterior dislocations may occur as a result of a seizure causing a muscle imbalance in the shoulder region.[21] Finally, high-energy trauma such as a motor vehicle accident can cause the shoulder to dislocate posteriorly when forced into a combination of adduction, flexion, and internal rotation.[22]

Secondary Survey for Musculoskeletal Trauma

HCPs can use this guide of the clinical evaluation process for an injured patient as a reference for obtaining the proper information to diagnose a musculoskeletal injury.

History
- Chief complaint
  - Consider other possible injury sites
- Mechanism of injury (MOI)
  - Playing surface
  - Equipment using
- Previous injury to the area

Observation
- Deformity
  - While gross deformity may have been identified in the primary survey, a smaller or less obvious deformity may be identified.
- Skin color
  - Hematoma
  - Pallor
- Patient's disposition
  - Excessive amount of agony
  - Signs of shock
- Ambulatory ability
  - Weight bearing or not (lower extremity)

Palpation
- Tenderness to palpation (TTP)
- **Crepitus**
- Deformity or loose bodies
- Swelling
  - Joint effusion
  - Localized swelling
- Pulse and sensation
  - Above and below the suspected injury

Special Tests
- Range of motion (ROM)—if possible
  - Above and below the suspected injury
- Manual muscle test (MMT)—if possible
- Joint-specific tests—as able
  - If an obvious fracture exists, no extra movement is recommended.

Risk Factors

Several risk factors are associated with shoulder dislocations. Males are 2.64 times more likely than females to dislocate the shoulder. Almost half of the dislocations occur between the ages of 15 and 29 years.[23] Overall, nearly 50% of all dislocations occur during sports or recreation. In fact, competing in contact sports is a prime factor for shoulder dislocations.

The shoulder has few bony constraints and relies on soft tissue structures for support.[24] The shoulder lacks the type of deep socket that is located at the hip joint. The joint is a shallow ball-and-socket joint that sacrifices stability for increased mobility,[1] and only 30% of the head of the humerus makes contact with the glenoid fossa.[16] Shoulder stability is maintained by the rotator cuff muscles (supraspinatus, infraspinatus, teres minor, and subscapularis), deltoid muscle, and ligamentous structures.[1] Weakness in any of these structures can lead to a shoulder dislocation.

Ligaments and connective tissue damage are risk factors in a shoulder dislocation, because the ligaments develop more laxity and the shoulder becomes hypermobile over time.[15] These anatomical structures create the risk factors seen in a shoulder injury. Previous injuries to the shoulder such as Bankart lesions and Hill-Sachs lesions can increase the chance of anterior and posterior dislocations, respectively.[11]

Signs and Symptoms

The initial sign for a shoulder dislocation will be the humeral head not being in the correct anatomic position (figure 7.7). Patients may also report a popping sensation or sound at the time of the injury. An obvious deformity will show, and the deltoid will appear to be flattened.[11] Once a shoulder dislocation has occurred, the patient may display some of the following symptoms:

- Pain and a decreased ROM or no ROM
- More prominent acromion and coracoid processes
- Decrease in neurovascular deficits if nerves and arteries have been damaged

When a shoulder becomes dislocated, the axillary artery that supplies blood to the arm may become damaged.[25] Damage to the axillary artery can lead to a decrease or even a stoppage in blood flow to the tissue in the arm. The

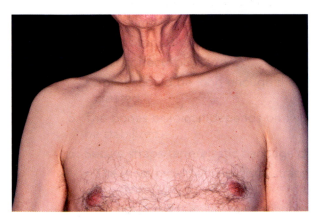

FIGURE 7.7   Shoulder dislocation.
Dr. P. Marazzi/Science Source

brachial plexus or axillary nerve may become damaged during this injury,[15,16,25] which can lead to a decrease or loss of function in the injured arm.

Field Assessment Techniques

When assessing a possible shoulder dislocation, medical personnel need to determine the location of the pain. The pain will typically be along the acromioclavicular joint with pain remaining in the upper shoulder region. The MOI will help determine the type of dislocation of the shoulder. Arm posture should be assessed, because the position of the arm indicates the type of dislocation that has occurred. The arm position and the corresponding dislocations are as follows:[11]

- Abducted and externally rotated indicates anterior dislocation.
- Limited abduction indicates inferior dislocation.
- Internally rotated arm with adduction indicates a posterior dislocation.

Immediate Management Techniques

Prior to reduction, the patient will need to be helped off the field with medical staff supporting the injured arm as they walk to the sidelines or athletic training clinic. The patient may need analgesic medicine to relieve the pain before the reduction.[15,25] The patient may also need reassurance before the shoulder reduction can take place.[25]

Anterior shoulder dislocations should be reduced as soon as possible to reduce the pain and suffering of an athlete.[11] ATs can reduce a dislocated shoulder in the following ways:

- *Hippocratic method.* When using this method, the AT applies traction while axial countertraction is applied (figure 7.8a).[17]
- *Stimson's hanging arm technique.* The patient lays in the prone position while holding a weight in the injured arm hanging downward (figure 7.8b). Eventually the muscle spasms fatigue and the shoulder reduces on its own.[17]
- *Milch technique.* In the event that an AT is working alone, the Milch technique can be used to reduce the shoulder dislocation. When performing this technique, the patient is in the supine or prone position, and the shoulder is abducted behind the patient's head. Longitudinal traction with external rotation is applied (figure 7.8c), and the shoulder is reduced.[26]
- *Spaso technique.* This technique is another option in the event that the AT is working alone. The patient is supine, and the AT lifts the injured arm

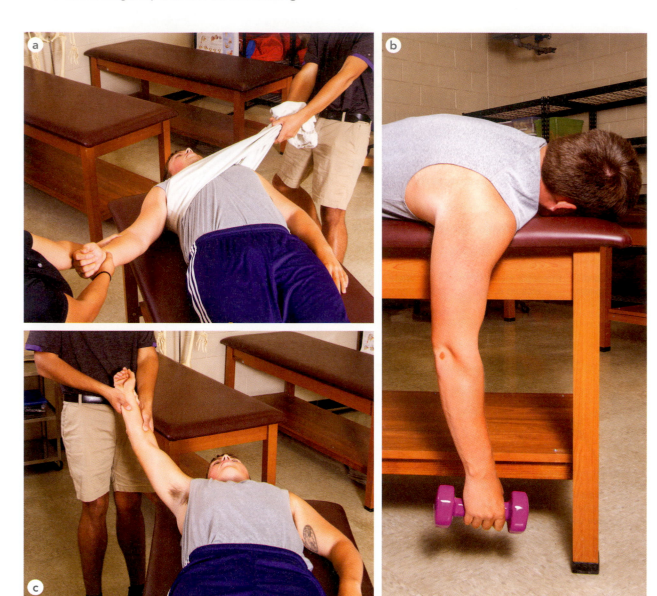

FIGURE 7.8   Shoulder reductions: *(a)* Hippocratic method, *(b)* Stimson's hanging arm technique, and *(c)* Milch technique.

vertically by the wrist or distal forearm. Gentle traction is applied while slightly externally rotating the shoulder.[26]

AT staff can reduce a shoulder dislocation based on CAATE Standard 70; however, the reduction must be in accordance with collaborating physicians (CAATE Standard 90).

AT staff should not reduce a posterior shoulder dislocation, because the patient will have to be placed under anesthesia. Traction is applied at the elbow, then the arm is abducted with posterior pressure applied to the head of the humerus. The arm is internally and externally rotated while traction is applied.[3]

After the shoulder has been reduced, a neurovascular evaluation should be performed along with active ROM. However, abduction and external rotation should be avoided.[11] The axillary nerve or brachial plexus will need to be assessed by testing dermatomes from the shoulder to the fingertips.[25] Damage to the vascular structures can be managed by checking the color of the skin and temperature of the skin at the fingertips of the injured arm. The arm should then be placed in a sling with the fingers and hands exposed for neurovascular monitoring. The arm should remain in the sling until further evaluation.[11]

In the event that the shoulder cannot be reduced, it should not be forced back into the glenoid fossa. This action may damage the fossa and other structures such as the neurovascular network.[11] The shoulder should be placed in a sling, and the patient should be transported to the hospital for further assistance. Other criteria for transporting to the hospital include the patient has a weak pulse or has no pulse at all in the injured arm. Weak or no pulse can indicate a transection of the axillary artery.[11,25,27] If medical personnel suspect neurological damage to the axillary nerve or brachial plexus, the patient should be transported to the hospital.[25,28,29] When it comes to posterior shoulder dislocations, patients must be taken to the hospital for X-ray imaging to rule out a possible fracture before the shoulder can be reduced.[30] A decision tree for shoulder dislocations is presented in figure 7.9.

Elbow Dislocation

The bony anatomy of the elbow is made up of the humerus, the ulna, and the radius. The olecranon process of the ulna articulates at the trochlea of the humerus to form the humeroulnar joint.[1] The radius articulates with the humerus at the capitulum of the humerus, forming the humeroradial joint.[11] The ulnar ligament bundles support the elbow on the medial side and radial ligament bundles support the elbow on the lateral side (figure 7.10). The ulnar nerve passes down the medial side of the elbow and forearm while the radial nerve and median nerve pass through the elbow laterally and cuboidal space, respectively.[1,11]

Incidence and Epidemiology

The incidence of elbow dislocations is reported to be 6 to 8 per 100,000 individuals,[31] and 10% to 25% of elbow injuries.[32] The elbow is the second most dislocated joint in the upper extremity behind the shoulder.[33] When it comes to dislocations, 80% of the dislocations are posterior and 20% are anterior, medial, and lateral dislocations.[34] The dislocation of the elbow is a result of the shallow olecranon fossa and prominent olecranon tip.[35] The most common MOI is **FOOSH** when the elbow is extended and the arm is abducted, causing an axial load down the arm.[11,36] Additional MOIs are motor vehicle accidents, sports injuries, and other high-energy mechanisms for young people.[33]

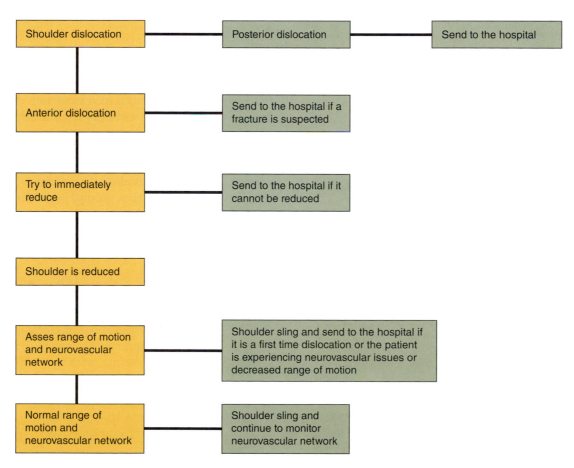

FIGURE 7.9 Decision tree for shoulder dislocations.

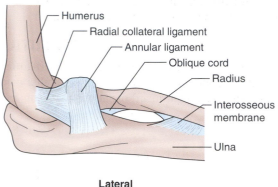
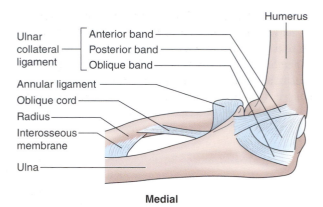

Lateral

Medial

FIGURE 7.10   Anatomy of the elbow.

Risk Factors

The stabilizing anatomy of the elbow involves humeroulnar articulation, the anterior bundle of the ulnar collateral ligament, and the radial collateral ligament complex.[37] Damage to any of these structures predisposes a person to elbow dislocations. Elbow dislocations occur more often in males than females. Younger age groups between 10 and 19 years old are also at more of a risk to have elbow dislocations when compared to other age groups.[38] The next highest age group is 20 to 29 years old. In the athletic realm, wrestling has the highest incidence of elbow dislocation, followed by gymnastics and football.[39]

Signs and Symptoms

The initial signs and symptoms of an elbow dislocation are an obvious deformity (figure 7.11), loss of function

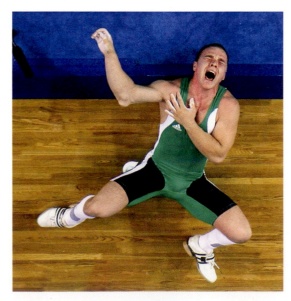

FIGURE 7.11   Elbow dislocation.
AP Photo/Andres Leighton/FILE

at the elbow, and pain. Often, the patient may be hysterical. The patient may be experiencing compromised vascularity around the elbow and the distal portion of the elbow. Neurological deficit may be experienced as a result of damage to the ulnar, medial, or radial nerve.[11] Lastly, some swelling may occur in the elbow after the dislocation as a result of profuse hemorrhage. Because of the swelling that may occur from the elbow dislocation, there is a risk of developing **compartment syndrome**.[40] The elbow dislocation is often associated with a fracture of the radial head.

Field Assessment Techniques

FOOSH with the elbow in hyperextension or twisting the elbow while flexing forces the ulna and radius anteriorly, laterally, or posteriorly. The most common elbow dislocation is the posterior dislocation. The forward-displaced humerus and olecranon process extend posteriorly, creating an obvious deformity. Medical personnel can distinguish the type or dislocation by the alignment of the lateral and medial epicondyle with the humerus.[3]

Once on the field, observe the position of the arm. The elbow and its supporting structures absorb the forces, increasing the suspicions of an acute injury. The type of force can help describe the nature of injury to the elbow. An axial force from landing on an outstretched hand can help diagnose an elbow dislocation. Inspection of the elbow area can help determine the presence of a gross deformity from an elbow dislocation, or the deformity may be palpated. No ROM test should occur at the injured elbow. A neurovascular screening should be performed to ensure that these structures are not compromised.[11] Any ecchymosis should be noted at this time also.

The posterior triangle of the elbow is the alignment of the medial epicondyle, lateral epicondyle, and olecranon process. These structures should make an isosceles triangle when the elbow is flexed to 90°. If a posterior dislocation exists, the olecranon process becomes more prominent. In this case, stop the evaluation immediately, and immobilize the patient's elbow; the patient must be referred to a physician.[11]

Immediate Management Techniques

Qualified HCPs should reduce the elbow dislocation on the field or in the emergency department (ED).[11] Reductions require the patient's muscles to be relaxed, so intramuscular or intravenous analgesia may need to be administered to the patient in the ED. Elbow reduction can be performed by applying force posteriorly to the olecranon to bring it distally and anteriorly around the humeral trochlea (figure 7.12). The patient will feel a clunking sensation when the elbow is reduced. After the reduction, the elbow should be taken through the ROM to ensure the elbow does not dislocate again during extension.[33] X-rays should be taken to rule out the possibility of a fracture.[11,33] The elbow should be placed in a hinge brace, and checking sensations and distal pulses in the fingers can help with neurovascular assessments.[11] In the event that the pulse or sensation cannot be detected, the patient should be taken to the ED (if not already in the ED for the reduction).

Finger Dislocation

The hand is made up of 5 metacarpals numbering I (thumb) to V (little finger), and these bones make up the palm of the hand. The proximal end of a metacarpal articulates with a carpal in the wrist, while the distal end of the metacarpal articulates with the proximal phalanx, forming a metacarpophalangeal (MCP) joint. Fingers II through V are made up of 3 phalanges (proximal, intermediate, and distal, respectively), but the thumb only has 2 phalanges (proximal and distal). The proximal and intermediate phalanx form a proximal interphalangeal

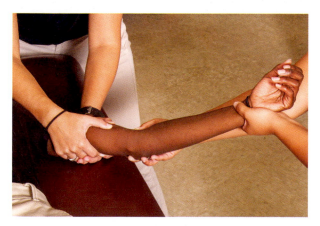

FIGURE 7.12   Elbow reduction.

(PIP) joint, and the intermediate and distal phalanx form the distal interphalangeal (DIP) joint.[1]

Incidence and Epidemiology

When it comes to dislocations in the finger, the PIP is the most common articulation to be dislocated, and the MCP is commonly dislocated at the thumb.[41] The MOI for a dislocation is hyperextension or an axial load impacting intermediate phalanx condyles against the proximal phalanx condyles.[42]

Risk Factors

Finger dislocations are a common injury for people who participate in sports and recreation activities; basketball leads the way, followed by football.[43-45] Participants in volleyball are likely to experience a finger dislocation. Age is a risk factor for finger dislocations; people between 10 and 19 years old are most likely to experience this injury.[43,44] As the age groups progress, the likelihood of this injury occurring decreases as a result of a decrease in the amount of sports participation.[43] The incidence rate is higher in males (17.8/100,000) than females (11.1/100,000).[43]

Field Assessment Techniques

When assessing a finger dislocation, pain and an obvious deformity will be at the injured joint. For PIP dislocations, the deformity can indicate a dorsal, volar, or lateral dislocation. With a dorsal dislocation, the intermediate phalanx dislocates dorsally over the proximal phalanx; it is the most common type of dislocation. When the intermediate phalanx dislocates anteriorly, it is called a volar dislocation.[41] The least common dislocation is the lateral dislocation, which occurs when the intermediate phalanx dislocates to the side of the proximal phalanx.[42] DIP dislocations can be categorized similar to the PIP dislocations. An MCP dislocation frequently occurs at the thumb; it is primarily a dorsal dislocation.[41]

Immediate Management Techniques

Once a finger dislocation has been diagnosed, the finger can be reduced to its proper alignment based on CAATE Standard 70 and the standing orders provided by the overseeing physician (CAATE Standard 90). For dorsal dislocations, longitudinal traction is applied along with pressure on the dorsal aspect of the base of the intermediate or distal phalange. The PIP or DIP should reduce to the proper position. The same technique can be used for dorsal dislocations of the MCP. For volar dislocations, reduction can be more difficult because of the extensor tendon. Longitudinal traction with pressure on the palmar aspect of the base of the intermediate or distal phalange should reduce the dislocation. However, the volar dislocation may require surgery for a proper reduction.[42] For lateral dislocations, similar techniques may be used to reduce the dislocation.

After the dislocation has been reduced, the patient should be further evaluated. Check for neurovascular status such as sensation and capillary refill. Soft tissue structures should be checked for injuries. In a dorsal dislocation, the volar plate should be assessed and the central slip should be checked after reducing a volar dislocation. No matter the type of dislocation, imaging should be performed in order to check for a possible fracture.[41]

Hip Dislocation

The head of the femur articulates within the acetabulum, which is supported by the labrum, a thick capsule, capsular ligaments, and strong musculature. The hip is a ball-and-socket joint that is inherently stable and not likely to dislocate. Just to distract the femoral head from the acetabulum, more than 400 Newtons of force is needed.[46] Therefore, hip dislocations are uncommon injuries in the sports medicine setting and substantial forces are needed for these injuries to occur.[47]

Incidence and Epidemiology

Hip dislocations almost exclusively occur following a traumatic injury.[47] Motor vehicle and motorcycle accidents are typically the cause of injury, and males aged 16 to 40 are the most commonly injured.[48,49] This injury has also been reported during collisions in skiing, football, and other contact sports.[50] Dislocations in the posterior direction occur most frequently; anterior dislocations represent only 8% to 15% of the total number of dislocations.[51]

Risk Factors

Factors that increase the risk of hip dislocation include advanced age, poor muscular conditioning, participation in high-impact sports, total hip replacement, previous hip dislocation, and arthritis of the hip.[52]

Signs and Symptoms

A complete trauma evaluation is necessary to rule out concomitant injuries. If there are no femoral shaft or neck fractures, then the position of the leg determines the diagnosis as follows:

- In posterior dislocations, the leg is in a flexed, adducted, and internally rotated position.

- In anterior dislocations, the leg is in a flexed, abducted, and externally rotated position.

Concomitant injuries occur with nearly every (95%) hip dislocation. Fractures to the acetabulum were reported in 70% of patients with traumatic hip dislocations.[53] Capsular, ligamentous, labral, and muscular damage also typically occur in a hip dislocation.[54] Other reported injuries included fractures to the femur (head, neck or shaft), pelvis, and patella, as well injuries to the sciatic nerve, patellar tendon, abdomen, upper extremity, thorax, and head.[49,53,55]

Field Assessment Techniques

Advanced trauma life support (ATLS) should be initiated immediately because of the high-energy nature of hip dislocations.[54,56] During ATLS, the physical examination typically identifies the direction of the dislocation—anterior or posterior—through observation. During the exam, palpations may reveal the femoral head in the buttocks for a posterior dislocation. For an anterior dislocation, you may palpate the femoral head in the femoral triangle.[56] A neurovascular examination is crucial because damage to the sciatic nerve or femoral neurovascular structures (artery, vein, or nerve) may occur during dislocations and should be noted. Patients may also present with ipsilateral femoral, patellar, or tibial fractures.[54]

Primarily, all dislocations are classified as either anterior or posterior. Next, commonly used classification systems are implemented. The most commonly used classification systems are the Thompson-Epstein, Epstein, and Steven-Milford. Classification systems have prognostic value; dislocations with femoral or acetabular fractures have a worse prognosis than the others.[54,57]

Diagnostic Accuracy

A single anteroposterior plain radiograph is the only radiograph needed to confirm a diagnosis of a hip dislocation.[56,57] For a posterior dislocation, the radiograph will demonstrate a femoral head that is small, shifted superiorly, and no longer in line with the acetabulum (figure 7.13a).[56] For an anterior dislocation the radiograph will reveal an abducted femur with the femoral head situated inferior to the acetabulum (figure 7.13b).[56] However, if the anteroposterior radiograph is inconclusive, then additional lateral radiographs are necessary.

Immediate Management Techniques

Treatment for hip dislocations is reduction by trained medical professionals. Therefore, following a full trauma evaluation, patients are stabilized and immediately sent to the ED for further treatment.

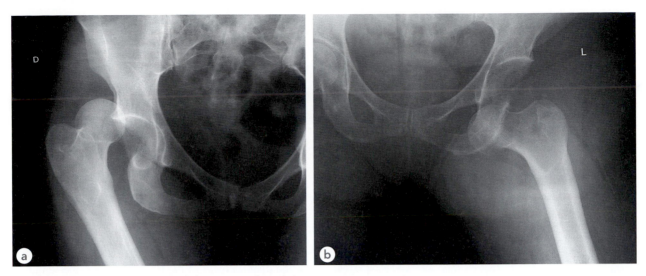

FIGURE 7.13   *(a)* Posterior and *(b)* anterior hip dislocation.

Miodrag Vranjes/Medical Images

Knee Dislocation

The knee is an articulation between the femur and the tibia, and the joint is supported by 4 ligaments (anterior and posterior cruciate ligaments and medial and lateral collateral ligaments; figure 7.14). The main muscle groups that also provide support for the knee are the quadriceps and hamstrings.[1]

Incidence and Epidemiology

A knee dislocation is the disruption of the integrity of the tibiofemoral joint (figure 7.15). When it comes to dislocations of the knee, these injuries are uncommon; however, the neurological and vascular damage as a result these dislocations can be limb threatening.[4] The occurrence of a knee dislocation is less than 0.02% to

2%,[4,58] but it is difficult to measure because of spontaneous reduction.[4] Of the dislocations of the knee, 5% to 17% are open dislocations.[59] The MOI is hyperextension or exaggeration of the pivot shift mechanism in the knee.[4]

Risk Factors

Risk factors for a knee dislocation include motor vehicle accidents, which are considered to be high-energy mechanisms. Low-energy mechanisms include falling during extreme sports.[4] Participating in nonextreme sports such as football creates a risk of knee dislocation.[60] Because of higher rates of participation in these types of sports, males are more likely to dislocate their knee than females.[58] This injury predominantly occurs in males between the age of 19 and 29 years.[61] Ultra–low-energy mechanisms occur

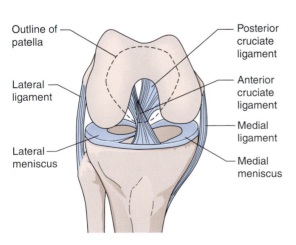

FIGURE 7.14   Ligaments of the knee.

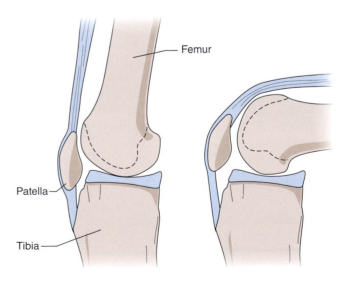

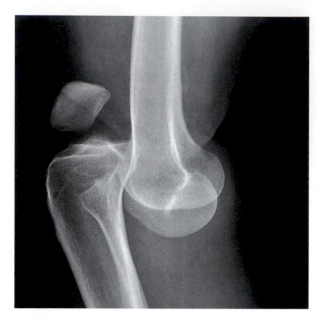

FIGURE 7.15   Knee dislocation.

Steven Needell/Science Source

in obese individuals as a result of physiological stress placed on the knee joint.[60]

Signs and Symptoms

Signs and symptoms of a dislocated knee include a deformity or malalignment at the tibiofemoral joint. A "dimple sign" may be visible over the medial femoral condyle, which represents buttonholing of the medial condyle through the anteromedial joint capsule. This dimpling occurs after a posterolateral rotatory injury mechanism.[4]

Patients may have vascular and neurological damage, which occurs in 23% to 32% of dislocations.[60] The damage to the popliteal artery and peroneal nerve may lead to limb amputation.[60,62] Signs of active hemorrhaging include an expanding hematoma and distal ischemia. The injured limb may start to lose color, and the patient may have diminished or absent capillary refill.[4] A periarticular fracture may occur during the dislocation of the knee,[4] and the patient may exhibit damage to soft tissues such as ligaments and menisci.[63]

Field Assessment Techniques

The first method of determining the type of knee dislocation is the Kennedy classification method, which was developed in 1963. This method is based on the direction of the displacement of the tibia relative to the femur.[4,60] However, this method is difficult to use in the event of a spontaneous reduction of the dislocated knee.[60] The next classification of a knee dislocation is based on the Schenck System[64] that has been modified by Wascher et al., which is the most widely accepted method.[4] This classification system is based on the ligaments that have been injured, presence of fracture, and neurovascular injury.

The anterior dislocation (figure 7.16) is the most common type of knee dislocation that leads to stretching of the nerves and arteries, and posterior dislocation is the second most common.[4,60] The posterior dislocation leads to a shearing force on the nerves and arteries.[60] Medial knee dislocation results from a valgus load, while lateral dislocation results from a varus load. Both tend to result in a tibial plateau fracture.[58] Vascular damage can be monitored with Doppler ultrasound to measure the ankle-brachial index (ABI) at the dorsal pedis and

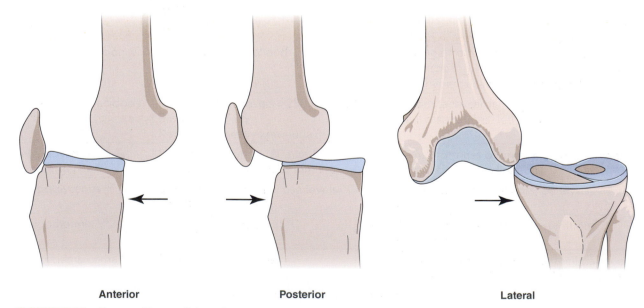

Anterior   Posterior   Lateral

FIGURE 7.16   Types of knee dislocation.

posterior tibial location. ABI is a measurement of systolic pressure in the affected leg proximal to the ankle divided by systolic pressure in the ipsilateral arm. A value greater than 0.9 is normal arterial flow; a value less than 0.9 requires further examination into possible vascular damage. Using the ABI has a sensitivity of 100% when it comes to clinical relevance.[4]

Immediate Management Techniques

In the event of a knee dislocation, proper precaution must be taken to manage a knee dislocation, and a physician must evaluate knee dislocations immediately.[11] If a motor vehicle accident is the cause for the knee dislocation, you must follow the ATLS. Life-threatening injuries must be managed before non–life-threatening injures such as a knee dislocation are managed.[4] After the patient is placed under conscious sedation in the prehospital setting, the dislocation should be reduced as soon as possible.[4,58] A dislocation is reduced by applying gentle traction and countertraction combined with deformity correction (figure 7.17).[4] If the closed reduction is not possible, the patient should be taken to the operating room for an open reduction procedure.[58]

After the reduction has occurred, the patient should be placed into a knee immobilizer and transported to the hospital for further evaluation and imaging.[4,58] Neurovascular presence should be documented before the patient is transported to the hospital. Damage to the popliteal artery must be repaired within 8 hours to avoid limb amputation. Medical personnel must assess fascial compartment pressure to rule out compartment syndrome.[4] Lastly, soft tissue, ligament, and meniscus integrity should be managed, because they are the least emergent injuries associated with a knee dislocation.[63]

Ankle Dislocation

The fibular articulation with the tibia is considered a **syndesmotic joint**. The tibia and fibula are connected via the interosseous membrane or ligament along their diaphyses. The distal space between the tibia and fibula is referred to as the syndesmosis, and it allows for about 2.5 to 4.0 mm of translation during normal gait.[65]

The tibia and fibula articulate with the talus to form the true ankle joint, **ankle mortise**, which is a hinge joint. The distal tubercle of both the tibia and fibula are called the medial and lateral malleolus, respectively. The **tibial plafond** articulates with the talus at the **talar dome**. Figure 7.18 depicts the various articulation and ligamentous structures that form the ankle mortise.

Disassociation of the talus, medial/lateral or anterior/posterior, from the tibia describes an ankle dislocation. Due to the high force required to produce this injury, concomitant injuries are frequently observed. Facture to the talar dome and medial and lateral malleoli, and disruption of ligamentous structures are a few of the more common associated injuries. Neurovascular injury can also arise with ankle dislocations. Ankle dislocations without fracture or other injuries are very rare.

Incidence and Epidemiology

Based on data from the NCAA surveillance system, between 2004 and 2009, only 18 (0.08/10,000 athlete

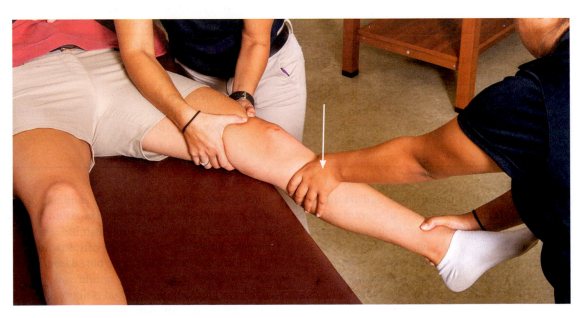

FIGURE 7.17 Knee reduction.

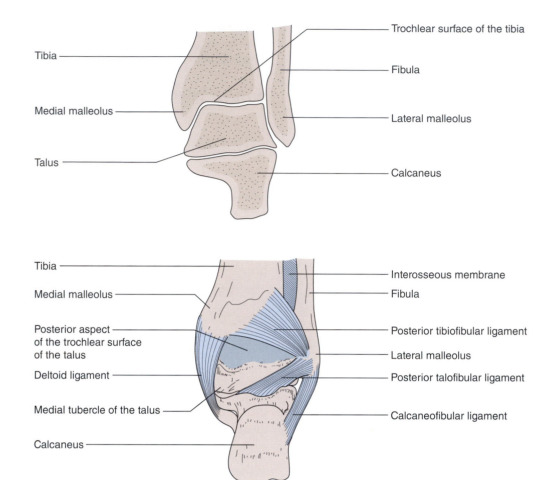

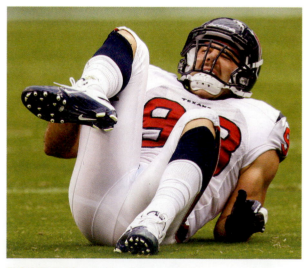

FIGURE 7.18   Ankle anatomy.

exposures) ankle dislocations occurred during participation in American football.[66] A systematic review indicated that 31% of all pure ankle dislocations were the result of participating in sports; other high-impact traumas and motor vehicle accidents had the second and third highest incidence, accounting for 26% and 23%, respectively. Pure ankle dislocations have equal incidences of open versus closed injury (50% split).[67]

Risk Factors

Risk factors are similar to other severe fractures. Participation in athletic activities that produce high force and contact place the athlete at an increased risk. Contact with another participant is not the only MOI; forceful landing on or into a surface (i.e., the boards in hockey, the wall in baseball) can produce the directional force responsible for ankle dislocations.

Signs and Symptoms

Obvious and gross deformity is typically associated with ankle dislocations (figure 7.19). The forefoot may be

FIGURE 7.19   Ankle dislocation.
Bob Levey/Getty Images

severely inverted and plantar flexed or other variations of malalignment. The patient may describe hearing or feeling a "pop" in their ankle. With closed dislocations, skin discoloration or tightening may occur due to the proximity of the osseous structure and the skin. Swelling within or around the ankle joint may be visible.

Field Assessment Techniques

Careful palpation of the osseous structures helps HCPs determine whether the injury is a pure ankle dislocation (no associated fracture), a true ankle dislocation (talus not articulated with the tibia and fibula), or a subtalar dislocation (dislocation of the talus and calcaneus; table 7.3). This distinction is important for deciding which joint is involved and whether or not to reduce. Attempts to reduce the subtalar joint are less successful and can cause further damage to the articular surfaces of the talus and calcaneus. In addition, if a fracture is suspected, reduction should not be attempted unless neurovascular structures are compromised. Reduction of the ankle should take place in the AT clinic or the ED.

Immediate Management Techniques

The joint should be reduced as quickly as possible in order to minimize neurovascular compromise or additional soft-tissue damage. According to the 2020 CAATE Standards, HCPs can reduce dislocations; however, HCPs can reduce joints only in accordance with the standing orders given by the physician. Ideally, radiographs should be obtained prior to reducing the ankle; however, if obtaining images results in extended delays for reduction, reduction should take priority. If the ankle cannot be reduced on the first few attempts, the lower leg should be splinted in the position found and prepared for transport. Prior to attempting reduction or splinting, a neurovascular exam of the lower leg and foot should be conducted. Furthermore, after every attempt to reduce or after reduction has been achieved, a follow-up neurovascular exam should be conducted. The purpose of the sequential exams is to assess for neurologic and vascular changes. All neurologic and vascular exam results should be documented. In many situations reduction may be more easily achieved if the patient has received some form of anesthetic, which is typically delivered by the EMS or hospital physician. Decisions to reduce depend on the neurovascular status and presence of fracture.

When splinting either a reduced or unreduced ankle dislocation, the HCP should assess the pulse, movement, and sensation before and after splinting. A splint should be applied so that the foot and lower leg are supported. If a vacuum splint is available, the splint should be molded so that the ankle cannot move but does not compromise neurovascular structures. The splint should be snug to provide adequate motion restriction, but not so tight that the patient has increased pain. Other splints such as a

TABLE 7.3   Classification of Ankle Dislocation

Classification	Description
Posterior	Talus is located posterior to tibia; associated with fracture to the lateral malleolus and tibiofibular ligament disruption; it is the most common ankle dislocation.
Anterior	Talus is anterior to tibia.
Lateral	Talus is lateral to tibia; associated with bimalleolar fracture or distal fibular fracture.
Medial	Less common than lateral dislocations; associated with bimalleolar fracture or distal fibular fracture.
Superior or diastasis injury	Talus is superiorly located within the mortise (separation of the syndesmosis).

CLINICAL SKILLS

Reduction Technique

1. The patient is supine on the exam table.
2. Flex the patient's knee to alleviate tension of the Achilles tendon.
3. Place one hand on the dorsum of the foot and the other hand on the heel. Perform countertraction at the knee.
4. Apply inline traction (based on the direction of dislocation); the goal is to create a force that is opposite of the deforming force (the dislocation).[68]

structural aluminum malleable (SAM) splint and compression bandages, padded splints, or flexible splints can be used. Regardless of splint choice the same principle applies; provide rigid support to the bones above and below the ankle joint.

Because of the high risk of associated fracture with ankle dislocation, patients should be transported to a medical facility for further evaluation. No attempt should be made to reduce any dislocation if a fracture is suspected. Risk of neurologic injury is high with medial and lateral dislocations because of their proximity of the peroneal nerve. Therefore, activation of emergency medical services (EMS) should occur immediately if the sports medicine team suspects neurologic or vascular compromise. The patient should refrain from weight bearing on the affected limb even if reduction was achieved. Soft-tissue ligamentous structures were most likely damaged, leaving the ankle vulnerable to dislocating again or causing further injury.

Humeral Fractures

The humerus is the largest and longest bone in the upper arm. It articulates with the scapula at the proximal end to form the glenoid humeral joint. At the proximal end are the greater and lesser tubercles, which are attachment sites for the rotator cuff muscles. Between the tubercles is the bicipital groove, which guides the biceps tendon to its attachment at the rim of the glenoid cavity. Midway down the shaft is the deltoid tuberosity on the lateral side. At the distal end, the humerus articulates with the radius and ulna to form the elbow. Medial and lateral epicondyles are the attachment site for wrist flexors and wrist extensors, respectively (figure 7.20).[3]

Incidence and Epidemiology

Proximal humeral fractures are common fractures and make up 5% of appendicular fractures.[69,70] Of these fractures, 15% are significantly displaced fractures.[69] These humeral fractures are seen in the elderly population and are usually caused by a low-energy impact when an elderly person falls. However, in the young population, these humeral fractures are caused by high-energy traumas.[71] These high-energy traumas are usually related to a contact sport such as football. The young population is also at risk of humeral fractures caused by FOOSH or by motor vehicle accidents.[72] In rare cases, pitchers have been known to have spontaneous humeral fractures in

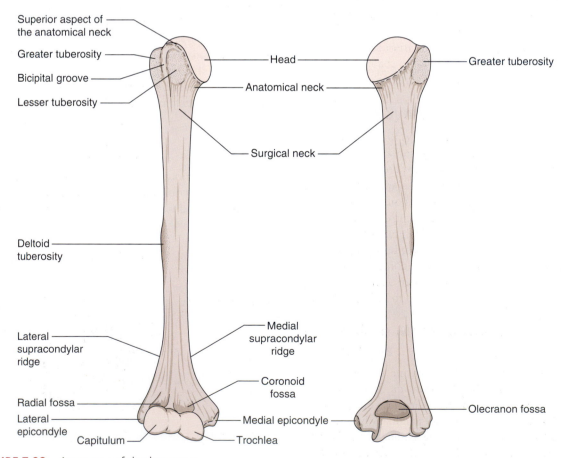

FIGURE 7.20   Anatomy of the humerus.

the middle of their arm swings while pitching a baseball. These spontaneous breaks may be caused by the torques and forces placed on the humerus while pitching.[73]

Risk Factors

Several risk factors can influence the possibility of a humeral fracture. People with low bone mass are susceptible to humeral fractures. The level of activity such as sports participation can affect risk for a fracture. Other risk factors include previous histories of fractures and a low body mass index. When it comes to age, women who are older are more likely to have a humeral fracture because of the change in bone density after menopause. In addition, women are more likely to have a humeral fracture than men are. Diet can influence the chance of a fracture; poor intake of calcium can weaken bones. Poor vision is a risk factor for a humeral fracture because it increases the likelihood to trip and fall.[74] People of Caucasian descent are more likely to have humeral fractures than people of African descent.[75] In children, those going through puberty are more likely to have fractures because of the constant high rate of bone turnover.[76]

Signs and Symptoms

The signs and symptoms of a humeral fracture may vary from person to person. One possible sign is an obvious deformity or displacement of the humerus (figure 7.21).[11] The symptoms may include **ischemia** as a result of damage to the vessels around the fracture site.[77] Due to the swelling and compression a patient may experience, the axillary artery may become a false aneurysm and

rupture, a potentially fatal event. A fractured humerus may cause a brachial plexus neuropathy issue resulting in pain or numbness of the limb.[71]

Field Assessment Techniques

This text discusses three types of humeral fractures that can cause neurovascular damage to the patient[3]:

1. Humeral shaft fracture (figure 7.22) is the result of a direct blow or fall on the arm. This fracture can be comminuted or transverse with a possible deformity. Because of the location of this type of fracture, a risk exists for the radial nerve to be severed by jagged bone, which causes radial nerve paralysis. This event causes wrist drop and the inability to supinate the forearm.

2. The proximal humeral fracture may result from a direct blow, shoulder dislocation, or fall on an outstretched hand. The proximal fracture can occur at the anatomical neck, surgical neck, or tuberosities (figure 7.23). Because of the location of the proximal fracture, it is often mistaken for a shoulder dislocation.

3. The epiphyseal fracture of the distal end of the humerus occurs in patients 10 years old or younger. It is caused by a direct blow or indirect force traveling along the length of the humerus and damages the epiphyseal plate. It leads to a shortening of the arm, disability, swelling, and point tenderness of the arm. An immature cartilaginous joint known as a false joint may be present when this injury occurs.[3] The epiphyseal

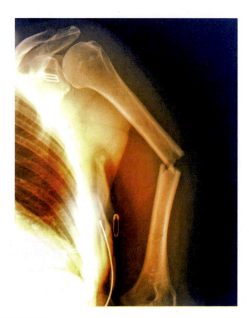

FIGURE 7.21   Humeral fracture deformity.

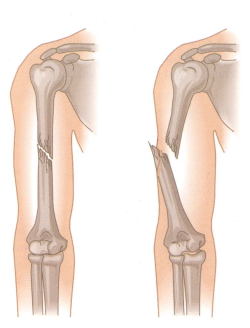

FIGURE 7.22   Humeral shaft fracture.

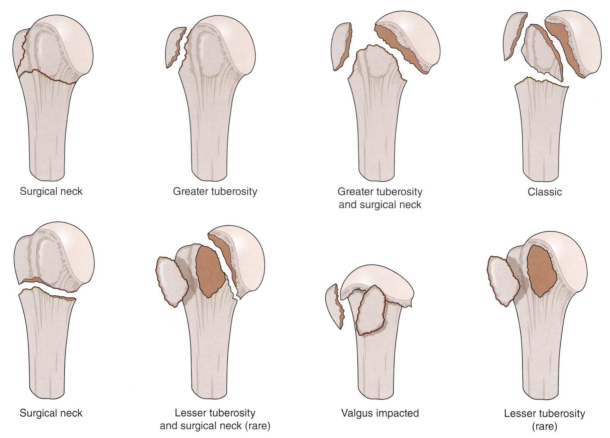

Surgical neck   Greater tuberosity   Greater tuberosity   Classic
                                                  and surgical neck

Surgical neck   Lesser tuberosity   Valgus impacted   Lesser tuberosity
                       and surgical neck (rare)   (rare)

FIGURE 7.23 Proximal humeral fracture.

fractures can be broken down into 5 Salter-Harris classifications (see table 7.2).

During the field assessment of a possible humeral fracture, the HCP will need to determine the location of pain. HCPs should perform an evaluation similar to the evaluation of a shoulder dislocation. The possibility of a gross deformity can be an indication of a humeral fracture. The palpations should extend the length of the humerus for any signs of a fracture. The surgical neck is the main area to palpate for a possible fracture.[11] Any ecchymosis should be noted at this time also.

Immediate Management Techniques

The fractured humerus should be splinted in the position that it is found. If it is displaced, the humerus should not be returned to a neutral position. A vacuum splint or a moldable aluminum splint should be used to immobilize that fractured humerus. The wrist and fingers should be exposed after splinting to monitor radial pulse, circulation to the fingers, and neurological sensation.[11] The patient should be referred to a physician for imaging to confirm the humerus fracture has occurred. The fractured humerus can be treated with a surgical fixation or nonoperatively.[72]

However, indications for immediate surgery are an open fracture and fractures with vascular injuries or reparable neurological injuries.[78]

Colles' Fracture

The wrist is composed of several structures. The radius and ulna come together to make the distal radioulnar joint. The distal radioulnar joint allows for pronation and supination with the help of the proximal radioulnar joint. The radiocarpal joint is an articulation formed by the radius, scaphoid, and lunate carpal bones in the wrist. This joint allows for radial and ulnar deviation, and flexion and extension of the wrist.[11]

Incidence and Epidemiology

Distal radial fractures make up 14% of all extremity injuries and 17% of all fractures treated in the ED.[79] The MOI of a Colles' fracture is typically FOOSH or hyperextension of the wrist.[3] This type of injury displaces the radius dorsally (figure 7.24). A reverse Colles' fracture (Smith fracture) is less common; it is caused by falling on a flexed wrist, which displaces the distal radial metaphysis anteriorly.[3]

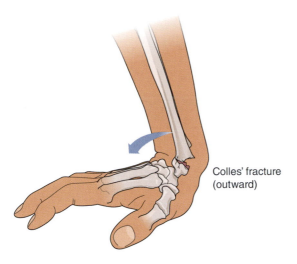
Colles' fracture
(outward)

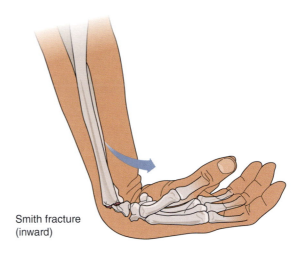
Smith fracture
(inward)

FIGURE 7.24 Colles' fracture and Smith fracture.

Risk Factors

Children and adolescents (6-10 years old) put themselves at risk for a Colles' fracture because of their typical level of activity such as riding a bike, playing football, and playing on playground equipment.[81] In this age group, boys are more likely to have a Colles' fracture than girls in the same age group. In the elderly population, chances of a fracture increase in the 50- to 70-year-old age group. Women in this age group are more likely to have a fracture as a result of menopause, which may lead to osteoporosis or osteopenia.

Signs and Symptoms

Pain at the distal radial site is an indication of a possible sprain. Other signs and symptoms of a Colles' fracture include displacement of the radius that leads to visible deformity called a dinner fork deformity. The displacement can be dorsal for a Colles' fracture or palmar for a reverse Colles' fracture. However, at times a deformity may not be present at the fracture site and may be evaluated as a bad sprain. Blood and other fluids in the area can cause profuse swelling in the wrist, hands, and fingers.[3] These fluids can compress nervous tissue such as the median, ulnar, and radial nerves.[3,82] This fracture can also lead to avulsion of tendons from the bone while the ligamentous tissue is typically unharmed.[3]

Field Management Techniques

When managing a Colles' fracture, it is important to evaluate the pulse of the radial and ulnar artery prior to splinting the injury. The fingers should be checked for any neurological deficits in the event that the Colles' fracture damaged any of the three major nerves in the wrist. The injury should be splinted in the position that it is found. A vacuum splint or any other type of splint can be used to stabilize above and below the fracture site. The splinted limb may be placed in a sling if necessary. An ice pack may also be placed on the injury site. The patient should then be transported to the ED for X-rays and further treatment.[3,11]

Pelvis Fracture

Hip fractures involve the pelvic girdle, which is also known as the pelvic ring. The pelvic ring is made up of the coccyx and sacrum posteriorly. The lateral and anterior borders of the pelvic ring are made up of hip bones (ilium, ischium, and pubis). In adolescents, these three bones are separated; they fuse together in adulthood. Strong ligament structures add to the bony stability of the pelvic girdle (figure 7.25). The weight of the upper body transfers from the upper body to the lower body through the pelvic girdle.[1]

Incidence and Epidemiology

Fractures to the hip are an immediate emergency situation for a patient. The incidence of pelvic ring fractures in children is 1 case per 100,000, and hip fractures make up 1% to 2% of all fractures in children. In adults, pelvic ring fractures make up roughly 10 cases per 100,000.[91]

Risk Factors

Adults in high-energy collisions such as a motor vehicle accident or being hit by a car are at risk for pelvic ring fractures.[83] Other MOIs are falls and sports; however, sports makes up less than 10% of pelvic ring fractures,[84] and these sports include skiing,[85] motorcycle riding,[85] and rodeo.[86] Sports injuries are rare because of the amount of padding and muscles protecting the hips.[11]

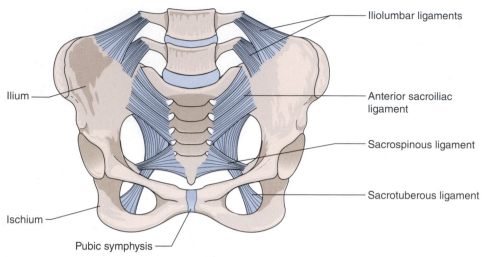

FIGURE 7.25 Pelvic ring.

Signs and Symptoms

Pain in the hip region is one of the main signs or symptoms of a pelvic ring fracture. Other signs and symptoms of a pelvic ring fracture include the presence of blood and swelling in the flank, scrotum, or perineal areas. Labial hematoma is also indicative of a pelvic ring fracture in women. Lacerations to the midsection areas may indicate a possible open fracture. The patient may have a leg length discrepancy as a result of the pelvic ring fracture. The patient may exhibit a rotational deformity of the lower extremity as a result of the asymmetry of the hips without a lower-extremity fracture.[87]

In adults, hemorrhaging of blood vessels is concomitant with pelvic ring fractures.[83] It is the result of the fractured bone edges damaging arteries such as the internal iliac artery.[88] Hemorrhaging in children is less common, because their blood vessels have a smaller diameter than adults.[83] Other soft tissue is at risk of being damaged with pelvic ring fractures. The fractured bone edges may perforate the gastrointestinal organs, bladder, or urethra.[89] Pelvic ring fractures in children can have long-term effects on their bones. They may experience long-term disability from residual deformities and pain.[90] Possible occurrence of growth disturbances can lead to leg length discrepancies and compensatory scoliosis resulting from the fracture.[83,90] Lastly, death may result from the hemorrhaging blood vessels around the pelvic ring fracture. The mortality rate is 8% in adults[89] and 3% to 5% in children.[91]

Field Assessment Techniques

In the adult population, the pelvic ring fracture occurs with anteroposterior (AP) compression from the force of the seatbelt during a car accident (figure 7.26). This MOI leads to serious blood loss. In children, the MOI tends to be a lateral force, which can be the result of being hit by a car. This force causes a single bone fracture, because the flexibility and higher elasticity of bones in children leads to less vascular damage.[83,91]

Assessment of a pelvic ring fracture should be conducted according to the ATLS. The patient's pelvis should be examined for vertical rotational instability; the patient will experience pain during the palpation of the pelvic ring. For an unconscious patient, check mobility by gently applying anteroposterior and lateral-medial compression to the anterosuperior pelvic crest. For axial stability, gently push and pull on the lower extremity. All these assessment techniques should be performed once; repetitive testing can dislodge any blood clots around the fracture, which could increase the bleeding within the pubis. The patient's abdomen should be examined for muscle guarding. When tapping on the suprapelvic

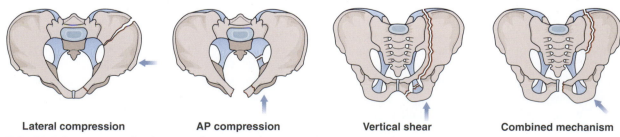

FIGURE 7.26 Types of pelvic ring fractures; the arrow illustrates the force of direction.

region, a dull sound can be an indication of a hematoma in the pelvis.[87]

Immediate Management Techniques

Suspected pelvic ring fractures should be transported to the hospital because of the mortality rate associated with the injury. Prehospital devices such as circumferential compression devices and SAM pelvic binders should be used to stabilize the possible pelvic fracture (figure 7.27). These devices help stabilize the pelvis and allow for the formation of a clot, which controls the hemorrhaging that is associated with pelvic ring fractures. Once these devices are applied, then the patient should be transported to the hospital for further evaluation.[92]

Femur Fracture

Fractures to the femur are uncommon in the healthy athletic population. The femur is one of the strongest bones in the body, and a considerable amount of force is necessary to fracture it. Age and rates of femur fracture have a positive relationship; with increasing age are increased rates of femur fractures. In addition, a negative relationship exists between force necessary to

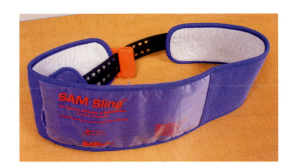

FIGURE 7.27   Pelvic binding.
Courtesy of Dr. Eric J. Fuchs, ATC, NRAEMT.

elicit injury and increasing age; as age increases, force decreases. These associations are related to osseous structural changes throughout the human life cycle. All traumatic femur fractures are emergent situations and require immediate attention. Due to the low incidence of femur fractures in young, apparently healthy patients, pathologic fractures should be considered when the patient receives treatment.[93]

Proximal Femur Fractures

Proximal femur fractures are often called hip fractures. Figure 7.28 depicts the various proximal femur fractures

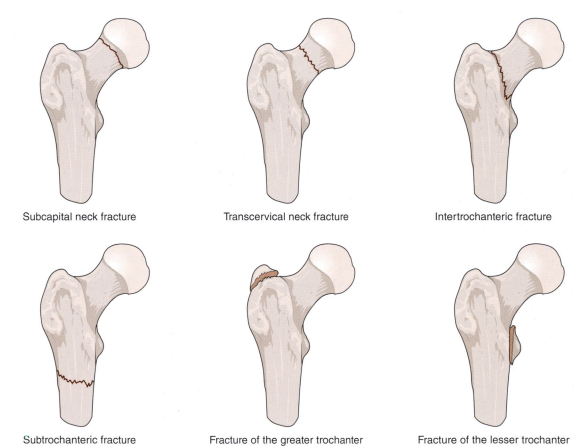

Subcapital neck fracture   Transcervical neck fracture   Intertrochanteric fracture

Subtrochanteric fracture   Fracture of the greater trochanter   Fracture of the lesser trochanter

FIGURE 7.28   Proximal femur fractures.

based on fracture location. The medial circumflex and lateral femoral circumflex are the primary vascular supply to proximal femur. Fractures to the proximal femur, specifically the femoral head, disrupt the vascular supply of the proximal femur. Therefore, these fractures are emergent due to the risk of **avascular necrosis**. Subtrochanteric femur fractures are at high risk of hemorrhage.

Low-energy mechanisms such as falls are the most common MOI in older patients. Younger patients are typically the victims of motor vehicle accidents or falls from a considerable height. Highly active patients (athletes, military recruits) may experience fractures resulting from repetitive loading, typically resulting in stress fractures to the femoral neck. As previously discussed, femur fractures are more commonly observed in the older population; more specifically for proximal femur fractures. Proximal femur fractures are more prevalent in women (63.3 per 100,000) than in men (27.7 per 100,000). As women increase in age, the incidence doubles, beginning after age 30. Of all proximal femur fractures, subtrochanteric fractures are more commonly observed in patients aged 20 to 40 years.[94] Pathologic fractures account for 17% to 35% of all subtrochanteric fractures.

Femoral Shaft Fractures

Shaft (diaphyseal) fractures are injuries occurring to a long bone, along the length of the bone between the two epiphyses. Diaphyseal fractures are categorized based on proximal, middle, or distal thirds. A 2015 study reported that only 4 femoral fractures had occurred in the past 20 years in professional athletes.[95] The NCAA surveillance data do not mention femur fracture, indicating that the incidence of traumatic femur fractures in the athletic setting and population is very uncommon.[96] Males between

the ages of 15 and 24 years have the highest incidence of high-energy MOI femoral shaft fractures. At age 25, males have an incidence of 10 per 100,000 per year.[94]

Stress fractures of the femur (rather than acute traumatic femur fractures) are more commonly observed in athletes, particularly female runners. Athletics-related femoral stress fractures are reported to occur at an overall incidence of 20.6%.[97] Stress fractures may not be emergent medical conditions; however, left untreated, these injuries can become acute traumatic injuries.

While femoral fractures may be uncommon, isolated case reports of these injuries do exist and should therefore be discussed. In addition, due to the MOI typically associated with femur fractures, the likelihood of concomitant injury is high. Compartment syndrome is not as common in femur fractures.

Distal Femur Fractures

Axial loading with a valgus, varus, or rotational force can fracture the distal femur (figure 7.29). The popliteal artery and vein, common peroneal nerve, and tibial nerve are neurovascular structures that are in very close proximity to distal femur fractures. While only about 2% of distal femur fractures are associated with neurovascular injury, a neurovascular exam should be completed.[94]

Distal femur fractures include injuries to the physis, condyles, and joint surface. Physeal fractures occur in younger patients and present great clinical concerns. While distal femur physeal fractures account for only 1% of all physeal fractures, this physis is responsible for approximately one-third of longitudinal growth in the leg.[98] Seven percent of all femur fractures are attributed to distal femur fractures.[94] Distal femur fractures in younger patients are more frequently observed in male patients. As age progresses, the frequency of distal femur fractures

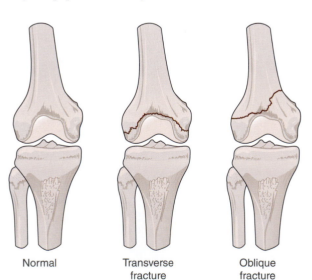
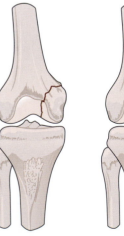
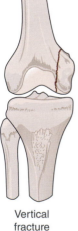
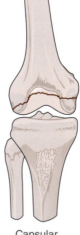
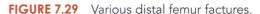

| Normal | Transverse fracture | Oblique fracture | Semivertical fracture | Vertical fracture | Capsular fracture |

FIGURE 7.29 Various distal femur factures.

in males significantly decreases, while the prevalence in females increases.[99]

Risk Factors for Femur Fractures

With the limited evidence as to prevalence of all femur fractures, it is difficult to identify specific risk factors. In general, participation in sports that require the body to withstand considerable amounts of force increases the chance of sustaining a femur fracture. In addition, some reports indicate that males sustain acute traumatic femur fractures at elevated rates compared to their female counterparts. This difference could be equated to males more commonly participating in higher-impact sports such as American football and lacrosse. A 2017 retrospective analysis by Pennock et al.[98] indicated that 50% of their distal intra-articular femur fractures were the result of receiving a tackle in American football. Pharmacologic risk factors also exist. Patients taking certain medications may be at an increased risk of fractures (in any bone). Glucocorticoids have the highest a relative risk of fracture, at 1.67 compared to the other drugs. Fracture risk while taking a selective serotonin reuptake inhibitor (SSRI) is 1.45. Anticonvulsants such as topiramate, often used to treat migraines, have a relative risk of 1.19.[100]

Tibia-Fibula Fractures

The tibial plateau articulates with the femoral epicondyles and serves as an attachment site for multiple soft tissue structures of the knee. Proximal articulation of the tibia and fibula occurs at the inferior surface of the lateral tibial condyle. This articulation is often called the proximal tibiofibular joint (PTFJ) and is a sliding or diarthrodial joint. The PTFJ is surrounded by a fibrous capsule with two additional ligaments to provide stability; anterosuperior and posterosuperior tibiofibular ligaments. An interosseous membrane (thick, fibrous tissue) attaches the tibia and fibula along their diaphyses. This intricate articulation can provide increased stability to this complex, but it can also complicate repair and recovery from tibia-fibular fractures.

Proximal Tibia Fractures

Proximal tibia fractures are also known as tibial plateau fractures. Classifying fractures to the proximal tibia is based on fracture location, fibula involvement, and degree of comminution. Two commonly used classification systems are the Schatzker classification and the Orthopaedic Trauma Association Classification of Tibial Plateau Fractures.

Proximal tibia fractures are relatively uncommon in athletics; however, one study reported 7.5% of their population sustained plateau fractures from sport participa-

tion.[101] In the general population, tibial plateau fractures account for 1% of all fractures.[94] Fractures to the lateral plateau are more prevalent compared to medial plateau fractures. MOIs are as follows:

- Valgus force—lateral plateau
- Varus force—medial plateau
- Axial force—bicondylar plateau
- Combined (high force)—bicondylar plateau, with soft tissue injuries

Tibia-Fibula Shaft Fractures

Diaphyseal fractures can occur anywhere along the length of a long bone between the two epiphyses. Unlike femur fractures, tibia-fibula shaft fractures are the most prevalent long-bone fractures in the general population and athletic population.[5,11] Regardless of openness, soft tissue damage can be significant depending on the direction of fracture displacement. Closed posterior fracture displacement can disrupt the posterior soft-tissue (e.g., soleus, gastrocnemius); anterior fracture displacement can injure the anterior tibialis. Anterior fracture displacement has increased propensity to result in open fractures.[94,98]

Incidence and Epidemiology

Incidence of injury for the entire population is 26 per 100,000 per year, but young males experience an increased incidence of 109 per 100,000 per year. The highest incidence rates are seen in elderly women (90-99 years of age).[94] Fractures to the fibular shaft typically occur in the middle third.[3] Conversely, tibial shaft fractures occur in the distal third.[102] As discussed previously, compartment syndrome may be a complication in lower-extremity fractures. Of all the cases of acute compartment syndrome, 40% are the result of tibial shaft fractures.[103,104]

Risk Factors

No specific risk factors are associated with proximal tibial fractures. Some studies have indicated that the incidence of plateau fractures is higher in the elderly; it is 8% of all fractures. Therefore, it could be argued that increased age is a risk factor. The group at highest risk for tibial shaft fractures is males between the ages of 15 and 19.[94]

As it relates to sport, most studies examining proximal tibia fractures are in winter sports. Recent changes to skiing equipment have coincided with increased prevalence of proximal tibia fractures. Based on Stenroos et al., alpine snowboarding would create an increased risk of proximal tibia fracture.[105] As a whole, tibial plateau fractures are the result of high-force mechanisms; therefore, any sport activity that increases the potential force applied to the tibia would be an increased risk.

Ankle Fractures

Ankle fractures are fractures to the distal portions of the tibia and fibula and the talus. Ankle fractures can be isolated to one of these osseous structures, or all three bones can be injured. The most common classification system of ankle fractures is the Weber classification; however, a more detailed classification system is the Lauge-Hansen classification for rotational ankle fractures. The Lauge-Hansen system accounts for foot position and force direction during injury.

Pilon fractures are a variant of ankle fractures that accounts for about 7% to 10% of all ankle fractures. The articular surface of the tibial plafond is disrupted and can result in injury to the talar dome. Pilon fractures are categorized as follows:[94]

- Type I: Nondisplaced fracture
- Type II: Displaced fracture with minimal comminution or impaction
- Type III: Displaced fracture that significantly disrupts the metaphysis and articular surface

Incidence and Epidemiology

A study of the United States trauma database, which includes data from all participating level I trauma hospitals across the country, stated that 280,933 foot and ankle fractures and ankle dislocations were reported between 2007 and 2011. About 56% of the total fractures reported were ankle fractures. Only 5.47% of these fractures occurred at recreational locations; 53.4% occurred on the street.[106] A European study indicated that ankle fractures represent 10% of all acute sport-related fractures. The incidence of sport-related ankle fractures in the European population is about 0.19 per 1,000 people.[107] The incidences of ankle fractures in the United States and Europe are quite similar.

The most common ankle fractures based on epidemiologic studies are isolated malleolar fractures (66.6% of all ankle fractures) and bimalleolar fractures, accounting for 25%.[94,106] Open ankle fractures comprise about 2% of all ankle fractures.[94] Ankle fractures in American football have an incidence of 0.22 per 10,000 athlete exposures.[66]

In children, ankle fractures are the most common physeal fractures at 15% to 20%. The most common MOI in children is playing basketball, football, or soccer, and playing on a scooter.[108]

Similar to proximal femur fractures, when looking at the population as a whole, older women account for the majority of ankle fractures. As the AT profession continues to expand, ATs are working with a variety of populations, not just the young active population.

Risk Factors

High-energy mechanisms are a risk factor for ankle fractures and open[106] ankle fractures in the younger athletic population. High-energy mechanisms can occur in many sports, but most commonly American football, soccer, volleyball, and basketball. In European sport, soccer players sustained the most ankle fractures compared to all other sports; while American football in the U.S. population has the highest reported number of ankle fractures.[107] Level of sport participation (professional, amateur, primary school) may also be associated with increased risk of ankle fractures. People participating in sports for leisure or amateur leagues are at increased risk of sustaining ankle fractures.[107] In addition, young males were more likely to sustain a sport-related ankle fracture at the amateur level.

Signs and Symptoms

Depending on severity, patient signs and symptoms vary. Severe ankle fractures may present with deformity, swelling, and severe pain. Other fractures may not present as apparently. Inability to walk immediately and after transport to hospital or a physician's office indicates potential fracture. Tenderness to palpation on the medial and lateral malleolus or proximal fibular head may also indicate a fracture is present. The articulations and interosseous membrane of the tibia and fibula connect to form a ring-like structure. Therefore, fracture to the distal tibia should create high suspicion of a proximal fibular fracture. This type of fracture is known as the Maisonneuve fracture (figure 7.30); it can also be observed in the forearm. The Ottawa ankle rules are used to help decide if further

Risk Factors for Ankle Fractures

- High-energy MOI potential
  - Football
  - Soccer
  - Basketball
  - Volleyball
- Younger males
- Level of sport participation
- High body mass index (BMI)

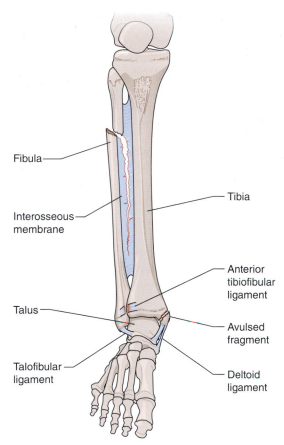

FIGURE 7.30 Maisonneuve fracture of the lower extremity.

imaging is necessary (see Clinical Decision Rules for Lower-Extremity Fractures for more information).

Management of Lower-Leg Fractures

In general, signs and symptoms are similar to any fracture, including tenderness to palpation (TTP), swelling, **ecchymosis**, inability to bear weight, potential gross deformity, and open versus closed injury. Proximal tibia fractures can be accompanied by **hemarthrosis** or **lipohemarthrosis**. In approximately one-third of knees with an intra-articular fracture (tibial plateau), lipohemarthrosis can be seen on imaging.

A neurovascular exam should always be completed. Compromise to neurovascular structures can indicate severe trauma, signifying increased suspicion for compartment syndrome. The peroneal nerve, tibial nerve, popliteal artery, and anterior tibial artery may be injured in lower-extremity fractures. The peroneal nerve is the most frequently injured nerve in the lower extremity due to its proximity and location to the lateral tibial plateau and fibular head. Proximal tibial-fibular fractures may produce signs and symptoms of peroneal nerve or tibial artery injury. Patients with an injury to the peroneal nerve my present with **drop foot** and the inability to evert the foot. The tibial nerve may be injured in severe trauma or more commonly in the athletic population, as a result of compartment syndrome.[109] The anterior tibial artery passes through a gap in the interosseous membrane, and therefore is at an increased risk of injury in tibial-fibular shaft fractures. As previously mentioned, compartment syndrome may be present. While compartment syndrome can occur in open fractures, more commonly it is associated with closed fractures. **Volkmann's contracture** may be a late indication that compartment syndrome should be assessed. While most reports of Volkmann's contracture are in the upper extremity and the younger population, cases of lower-extremity presentation do exist.

Ninety percent of tibial plateau injuries are associated with surrounding soft tissue injuries; and the younger the patient, the increased propensity for ligamentous damage.[94] Decreased ROM or inability to flex and extend the knee may be observed in patients presenting with a proximal tibia-fibula fracture. During the advanced imaging evaluation using radiographs or computed tomography (CT), ligamentous injury may be indicated by the **Segond sign**.

In summary, signs and symptoms associated with lower-extremity fractures are fairly similar. A few signs and symptoms are unique to the various injuries and may be beneficial in ruling out other conditions in same body region. While the signs and symptoms listed in Common Signs and Symptoms for Lower-Extremity Fractures attempt to include the most common signs and symptoms, it is possible that additional signs or symptoms based on the severity or patient condition are not listed.

Field Assessment Techniques for Lower-Extremity Fractures

Lower-extremity fractures are typically diagnosed in the field based on signs and symptoms. In situations where gross deformity is not present, radiographic or CT evaluation is necessary for definitive diagnosis. All suspected fractures should receive advanced imaging to properly classify and diagnose or assess for concomitant injury. Management of all lower-extremity fractures and dislocations will follow very similar procedures; therefore, the procedures described are applicable in all situations with minor variations. Specifics for injury management are described where special considerations should be observed. Keep in mind that all injuries can vary from their typical presentation; and patient, environment, or personnel circumstances may alter your management strategies. As with all clinical and emergent situations, management and care decisions must be critically evaluated

Common Signs and Symptoms for Lower-Extremity Fractures

Proximal Femur Fracture

TTP

Severe pain

Swelling

Ecchymosis

Inability to bear weight

Decreased ROM

External rotation with some abduction

Shortened limb

Groin pain

Pain with axial compression

Femoral Shaft Fracture

TTP

Severe pain

Swelling

Ecchymosis

Inability to bear weight

Gross deformity

Distal Femur Fracture

TTP

Severe pain

Swelling

Ecchymosis

Inability to bear weight

Gross deformity

Decreased ROM

Lipohemarthrosis

Profuse swelling in popliteal fossa

Proximal Tibia-Fibula Fracture

TTP

Severe pain

Swelling

Ecchymosis

Inability to bear weight

Gross deformity

Decreased ROM

Drop foot

Ligamentous laxity/Segond sign

Lipohemarthrosis

Tibial-Fibular Shaft Fracture

TTP

Severe pain

Swelling

Ecchymosis

Inability to bear weight

Gross deformity

Compartment syndrome

Ankle Fracture

TTP

Severe pain

Swelling

Ecchymosis

Inability to bear weight

Gross deformity

so that the best and proper procedures are used for that injury and setting.

Types and Sequencing

ATs and other HCPs caring for patients in emergent situations will have to make quick decisions. Following a systematic approach to determine whether the situation is emergent or not can facilitate better and quicker identification of emergent conditions in musculoskeletal injury.

The goal of the primary survey is to establish whether a medical emergency is present. Airway, breathing, circulation, disability, and exposure (ABCDE) should all be evaluated (see chapter 4). With respect to lower-extremity fractures or dislocations, these 5 assessments should all be completed to ensure the patient is stable so that a

RED FLAGS

When completing the primary survey, check for these red flags to lower-extremity fractures:

- Pallor in extremity
- Temperature differences between extremities
- Loss of movement or sensation
- Gross deformity
- Open fracture or open wound
- Profuse bleeding

secondary assessment can be completed. Some emergencies may not be as apparent, not all severe fractures will produce gross deformity, and they are not always obvious open fractures. Poke holes can be disguised by dermal abrasions, dirt, or other environmental substances. Equipment can prevent immediate identification of open fractures. Therefore circulation, not only to the heart but also to the involved extremities, is crucial.

When caring for open fractures, hemorrhage control should be addressed with utmost concern. Stabilizing the patient and activating EMS are the priorities. Once the hemorrhage has been adequately addressed, further evaluation (secondary survey) can continue. If possible, the injured extremity should be evaluated without clothing or equipment. Shoes, socks, long compression pants, shin guards, knee pads, and other clothing and equipment should be removed or cut off so that the skin may be examined and direct palpation achieved. When evaluating a hip fracture or upper femur injury, modesty should be respected. This chapter provides a brief outline of the secondary survey for musculoskeletal trauma; for more detailed information on application of the secondary survey, see chapter 4.

Clinical Decision Rules for Lower-Extremity Fractures

Knee fractures and further decisions for imaging can be ruled in or ruled out using the Ottawa knee decision rule. Unlike the ankle rules, the knee decision rule does not have as strong evidence for ruling in or out a knee fracture. Bachmann et al.[110] stated that using the Ottawa knee decision rule had decent evidence to support its use in ruling out the need for knee imaging. The Pittsburgh decision rule is another clinical decision algorithm used

Decision Rules for Lower-Extremity Fractures

Ottawa Knee Decision Rule Criteria

Positive test = presence of any one of the following characteristics

- >55 years of age
- TTP on head of fibula
- Isolated TTP on patella
- Knee flexion < 90°
- Inability to bear weight immediately or in the emergency department (ED; at time of evaluation) to perform 4 steps

Pittsburgh Decision Rule

Positive test = history (for current injury) of blunt trauma or fall AND any one of the other criteria

- History of blunt trauma or fall as MOI
- Inability to bear weight immediately after injury or in the ED (at time of evaluation) to perform 4 steps
- <12 years of age or >50 years of age

Knee Decision Rule of Bauer

Positive test = presence of any one of the 3 listed characteristics

- Inability to bear weight immediately after injury or in the ED (at time of evaluation) to perform 4 steps
- Presence of knee effusion
- Presence of ecchymosis

to determine whether X-rays are needed. Similar to the Ottawa knee rule, the Pittsburgh rule provides minor support to rule in the need for imaging and has moderate evidence to support its use in ruling out X-rays.[111,112] The knee decision rule of Bauer is a third set of criteria developed to help clinicians determine whether knee imaging is advised. Similar to the other two criteria described, the rule of Bauer has a small positive likelihood ratio (+LR) and a moderate negative likelihood ratio (–LR), indicating that it may be more useful in ruling out the need for knee imaging.[113,114]

The Ottawa ankle rule is used to determine need for further imaging in ankle fractures (figure 7.31). This clinical decision rule is helpful when an ankle fracture may not be as apparent. The Ottawa ankle rules have a sensitivity of 97% to 98%, but they have a specificity that has greater disagreement between studies 7 and 32. Furthermore, the Ottawa ankle rules have a +LR of 2 and a –LR of .03 to .06, indicating that this rule is somewhat helpful to rule in and quite helpful to rule out the need for ankle X-rays.[115,116] These rules have been validated in both pediatric (>5 years) and adult populations.[117]

A tuning fork is often used to determine whether a fracture is present in many body regions. In the lower extremity, the tuning fork is frequently used to assess for a malleolar fracture. A systematic review of the literature indicates that not enough clinical evidence exists to support the use of a tuning fork to rule in a fracture, but a decent amount of evidence exists to support its use in ruling out a fracture.[118] For most lower-extremity fractures (excluding open fractures or dislocations), some form of imaging is necessary to accurately diagnose the injury. Tibial plateau fractures can be diagnosed quite accurately using X-rays and CT scans. However, MRIs are more accurate to assess potential soft tissue injuries (97%-99% specificity).[119]

Immediate Management Techniques for Lower-Extremity Fractures

Any open fracture should be transported by EMS to the nearest facility for definitive treatment. The risk of infection in open fractures is extremely high. The quicker the antibiotic treatment is administered, the more significantly the infection risk decreases. The primary and secondary survey should have alerted the AT and sports medicine team to the severity of the injury. Open fractures or a significant deformity will dictate immediate management of the injury.

A key principle in immediate management of fractures (all fractures) is protection, rest, ice, compression, and elevation (PRICE). First, protect the suspected fracture with a splint, brace, or other form of immobilization device. Support or immobilization should be applied to the bones or joints above and below the injury. The patient should be moved (if safe and possible) to a location where she can rest while transportation is arranged. If the fracture is not open, you may immediately apply ice in conjunction with compression and elevation. Open fractures need to have proper wound coverings or dressings and compression to cease blood loss. Compression and elevation are two options for stopping blood loss. Exercise caution when elevating an open fracture, because unsupported movement of the injury could cause further injury. This decision should be based on severity of blood

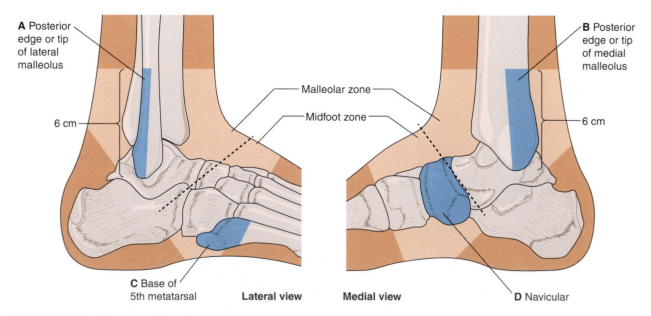

FIGURE 7.31   Ottawa ankle rules.

loss versus risk of further injury. (See chapter 6 for information about hemorrhage control.)

Displaced lower-extremity fractures should be evaluated for neurovascular compromise. If the neurologic exam is abnormal, EMS or advanced life support (ALS) should be activated immediately. The longer neurologic or vascular structures are compromised, the higher the risk for loss of function or limb.

Immobilization

All fractures should be splinted prior to transport, regardless if the patient is being transported via EMS, ALS, or by family. Splinting not only provides protection for the fracture, it also can ease the pain and discomfort of the patient. A variety of splints are available to ATs and the sports medicine team. Vacuum splints are commonly used but can be expensive. In settings where budgets may be a limiting factor, access to vacuum splints or other high-end splints may be difficult, but keeping rigid materials and compression bandages on hand can aid in making splints. The key to splinting is providing stability above and below the injury so that excess movement is limited.

Traction Splint

Traction splints are most commonly used with femur fractures or acetabular (pelvic) fractures. While they

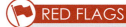

RED FLAGS

The following are red flags for avoiding vacuum splints:

- Open fracture
- Significant bleeding
- Neurologic compromise
- Decreased or absent pulse
- Changes in patient's status

are available, the efficacy of these splints is not widely agreed upon. Some reports indicate that a traction splint may not provide any additional benefit compared to standard splinting techniques.[120] Traction splints are more commonly used in the military setting because of the extended duration of transport to medical facilities.

Adequate traction and continued traction can also be difficult to achieve in the lower extremity with just a traction splint. Similar to prolonged joint dislocations, displaced femur fractures induce significant muscle spasm. Therefore, substantial force may be required to achieve the traction necessary. This application can be especially difficult in larger patients.

CLINICAL SKILLS

Step-by-Step Splinting

1. Remove protective equipment and other garments.
2. Identify location of injury.
   - If open fracture: control hemorrhage.
   - Cover wound.
3. Assess and document pulse, movement, and sensation (PMS).
   - Assess pulse by testing capillary refill.
   - Assess movement by asking the patient to move the toes or fingers.
   - Assess sensation by touching the distal extremities below the fracture.
4. Select correct splint size.
   - Splint should be long enough that the fracture is well covered and a fulcrum is not created.
5. The bones or joints (depends on injury location) above and below the injury should be stabilized.
6. Secure straps/tape/elastic bandage distal to proximal.
   - The most proximal and distal straps or anchors should be snug to prevent slipping of splint.
   - Do not prevent ability to continually monitor PMS.
7. Reassess and document PMS.

Criteria for Decision to Transport for Further Medical Examination

Decisions to transport for lower-extremity fractures are similar for upper-extremity fractures and joint dislocations. Any fracture to a major long bone should be transported for definitive medical treatment. The risk of significant bleeding is high in femur fractures. Depending on the severity and displacement of femur and acetabular fractures, percutaneous traction pins may be necessary. This type of traction can only be applied in the hospital (in most situations). Any suspicion of vascular or neurologic injury, lower and upper extremity, is reason to transport immediately. As previously described, any open fracture, dislocation, or other injury should be transported for further medical treatment. If a patient is showing signs of shock or hemorrhage (internal or external), he should be transported via EMS. Changes in patient status are better addressed and cared for in the hands of trained medical personnel rather than parents. Therefore, if you are concerned that the patient's condition may change during transport, use EMS.

Immediate Management of Musculoskeletal Injuries: General Steps

Musculoskeletal emergencies should undergo initial evaluation as any other patient would be assessed. Conduct the primary survey (ABCDE). For injuries involving open fractures or other open wounds, hemorrhage control and reducing the risk of shock is crucial. Chapters 4 and 6 specifically discuss the types of hemorrhage and shock a patient could experience from an open musculoskeletal injury. Remember that stabilizing the patient (stopping the bleeding or managing shock) is the priority. Once the patient is stabilized and hemorrhage has been controlled, you can stabilize the fracture and prepare the patient for transport. Open fractures should *always* be sent to a definitive care facility; risk of infection significantly increases if the open fracture is not treated within 6 hours of injury.[121]

Compartment Syndrome

While predominantly observed in lower-extremity fractures, compartment syndrome can occur in any region of the body where fascia may prevent fluid from exiting, therefore increasing the internal pressure. When intra-compartmental pressures approach diastolic blood pressure (BP), vascular perfusion is significantly impaired[122] and neurological tissue is at risk for damage. It is crucial to monitor serial neurovascular exams for changes in patient symptoms in order to identify compartment syndrome early. Figure 7.32 illustrates the anatomy within each compartment of the lower leg.

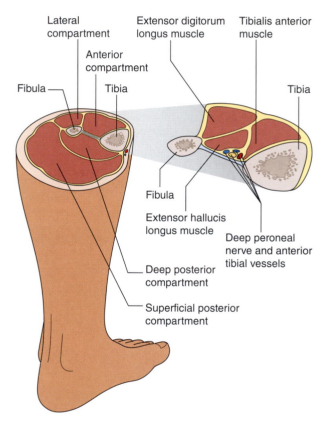

FIGURE 7.32   Compartments of the lower leg.

General Steps for Managing Musculoskeletal Injuries

- Asses and establish ABCs.
- Evaluate D and E.
- Check the need for hemorrhage control; warranted in the event of an open fracture or bleeding wound.
- Extricate if necessary.
- Monitor and stabilize (shock management).
- Stabilize the fracture.
- Prepare the patient for transport.

Compartment syndrome has these 3 categories:[3]

1. *Acute compartment syndrome*: A secondary injury to direct trauma to the area, such as being kicked in the anterior portion of the leg, it is considered to be a medical emergency because of compression to the neurovascular network.

2. *Acute exertional compartment syndrome*: It occurs without the direct trauma and is a result of minimal to moderate exercise.

3. *Chronic compartment syndrome:* Related to activity, it occurs during running and jumping activities.

Signs and Symptoms

The patient presents with a deep and aching pain along with tightness and swelling of the involved compartment. In addition, passive stretching of the muscles causes pain. Another sign is reduced circulation and sensation in the distal portion of the affected limb. Measuring intracompartmental pressure helps the HCP to determine the severity of the injury.[3]

Immediate Management

When an athlete experiences acute compartment syndrome, apply ice and elevate the limb, but never apply compression. The affected limb already has too much pressure, so using a compression wrap makes the injury worse. In the case of both acute and exertional compartment syndromes, a physician performs an emergency **fasciotomy** after the intracompartmental pressure confirms that it is compartment syndrome. The fasciotomy will relieve the pressure in the affected compartment.[3] Chronic compartment syndrome is managed conservatively at first by changing activity, icing, and stretching the affected compartment. A fasciotomy is a last resort for treating chronic compartment syndrome if the conservative approach fails.[3]

Ring Avulsion

Everyday activity can place the digits at great risk for injury. Whether in sports or when working with heavy machinery, fingers can be crushed, broken, or dislocated. These forces can shear, stretch, scrape, or even avulse a finger.[3] Even wearing protective equipment cannot protect fingers from injuries from these type of forces.

Incidence and Epidemiology

Ring avulsion injuries can range from soft tissue injuries to complete amputations.[123] Ring avulsion injuries are uncommon despite the fact that small forces are needed for a complete amputation to occur.[124] The MOI for a ring avulsion tends be a crushing, pulling, or rotational force. These forces tend to lead to nerve and vascular damage to the structure.[125] Acute hand traumas such as these account for over 1 million visits to the ED.[126]

Risk Factors

People aged 25 to 35 are more likely to experience a ring avulsion of the finger. People who work with machinery such as power saws, meat grinders, and rolling presses are at risk for an avulsion injury. Another risk factor is people who do not wear protective equipment such as gloves while working with this type of machinery.[126] People with more experience in these related fields tend to take more risks with these machines because they have worked with the machines longer, which leads to increasing the chances of a ring avulsion.[127]

Field Assessment and Immediate Management

Signs and symptoms of a ring avulsion range from a simple wound to profuse bleeding from an amputation.[3] The types of ring avulsions are as follows:[128]

- *Class I*: Adequate profusion with some circumferential skin loss and possible damage to the flexor and extensor apparatus. Treating this injury requires wound assessment and wound care.

- *Class II*: Inadequate circulation needing vessel repair. The patient must be sent to the hospital for treatment of this injury because it requires microvascular surgery.

- *Class III*: Complete degloving of the skin or complete amputation. When treating this injury, the avulsed tissue should be wrapped in gauze soaked in saline and placed into a watertight bag. The bag should be placed in ice water or on a bag of ice.

The 6 Ps of Compartment Syndrome	
Pain in compartment	Pulseless
Pain with passive stretch	Pallor
Paresthesia	Paralysis

That bag should be sent to the ED with the patient for further evaluation and possible reattachment.[3]

Summary

Traumatic musculoskeletal injuries have severe and potentially life-altering consequences. The injuries range from dislocating joints to fracturing bones. The injuries can result in neurovascular injuries, amputation, or even death. HCPs must be able to recognize these types of injuries and provide adequate care to patients based on evidence-based medicine. With proper treatment, the potential for exacerbating the injury can be decreased and the patient can have a better chance of recovery and returning to daily activities.

 Go to the web study guide to complete the case studies for this chapter.

CHAPTER 8

Traumatic Injuries to the Head and Face

Priscilla Maghrabi, PhD, ATC

Kristan Erdmann, EdD, ATC, EMT

OBJECTIVES

After reading this chapter, you will be able to do the following:

- Differentiate between various types of head injuries.
- Classify headaches into primary and secondary based on signs and symptoms.
- Recommend acute care procedures for patients who are having a stroke.
- Prioritize acute care procedures for patients who are having a seizure.
- Prioritize neurological medical conditions that warrant immediate treatment.
- Formulate acute care procedures for patients who are experiencing facial trauma.

Traumatic injuries to the head and face often warrant immediate medical attention. Injuries and conditions to the head and face are common in certain sporting events, such as concussions in football, while other conditions are rare, such as febrile seizures. Traumatic injuries to the head and face account for some of the most severe injuries in sport. A significant impact to the head requires immediate attention and evaluation; recognition and assessment are vital to properly treating these conditions. This chapter presents some of the more common conditions associated with traumatic injuries to the head and face along with recommendations for acute and emergent medical care.

Overview of the Head and Face

Head and face injuries are often the result of direct trauma. The severity of the condition can be masked by the protective mechanism of the skull or worsened by the delicate nature of the soft tissue. Health care providers (HCPs) who have an understanding of the anatomy and physiology of the head and face, along with the mechanism of injury (MOI), are able to provide patients with optimal care.

Anatomy and Physiology

Many pathological conditions exist regarding the head; some are more life-threatening than others. Due to the wide range of injuries to the head as well as the face, an understanding of structural and functional complexities is necessary for adequate evaluation. Foundational concepts of anatomy and physiology allow a clinician to develop and strengthen such skills.

The anatomy of the head consists of the skull and brain. The skull functions as a protective barrier to the brain and face. The skull is divided into the cranial and facial skeleton. Ethmoid, frontal, occipital, parietal, sphenoid, and temporal bones comprise the cranium. The facial skeleton includes the lacrimal, mandible, maxilla, and nasal bones (figure 8.1).

Within the skull is the brain, the body's control center. The brain is divided into 3 major areas as illustrated in figure 8.2 and described here:

- *The cerebrum* comprises about 75% of the total brain volume and controls voluntary muscle activ-

ities, sensation, and higher-level brain functions such as emotion, hearing, learning, memory, personality, and vision.

- *The cerebellum* lies under the cerebrum and is responsible for coordinated body movement.

- *The brain stem* lies posterior to the cerebellum and controls basic life functions, including sleeping, eating, and cardiorespiratory functioning. Specifically, the pons is responsible for respiration and swallowing while the medulla oblongata controls blood pressure, breathing, and heart rate. The brain stem also provides the majority of movement and sensation to the face and neck; 10 of the 12 pairs of cranial nerves are housed in the brain stem.

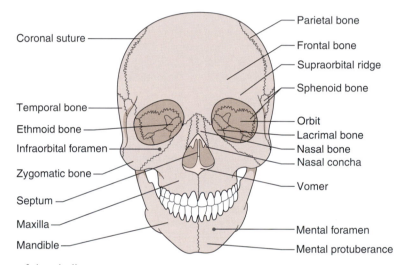

FIGURE 8.1   Anatomy of the skull.

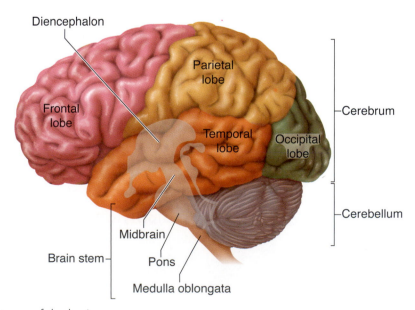

FIGURE 8.2   Anatomy of the brain.

The meninges, 3 layers of tissue surrounding the brain and spinal cord, provide further protection.

1. The outer layer, separated from the cranium by the epidural space, is known as the *dura mater*. Latin for "hard mother," the dura is named for its toughness.

2. The second layer is the *arachnoid mater*, separated from the dura by the subdural space. Latin for "spider mother," the arachnoid is named due to its weblike appearance.

3. The third layer, separated from the arachnoid by the subarachnoid space, is the *pia mater*. Latin

for "tender mother," the pia is named for its delicateness.

Eye anatomy and dental anatomy are presented in figures 8.3 and 8.4, respectively. Additional information regarding specific eye and dental injuries is presented later in the chapter. Laryngeal anatomy is presented in figure 8.5. Functions of laryngeal anatomy are threefold, as follows:[1]

1. Provide an airway.
2. Provide a mechanism for speech.
3. Provide a sphincter for swallowing.

Laryngeal injuries are presented later in the chapter.

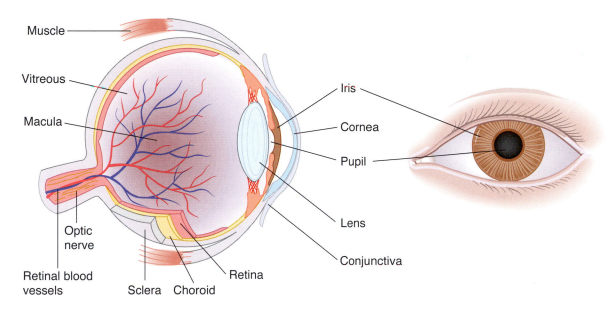

FIGURE 8.3   Anatomy of the eye.

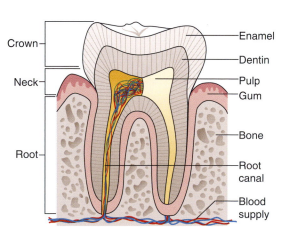

FIGURE 8.4   Anatomy of tooth structures.

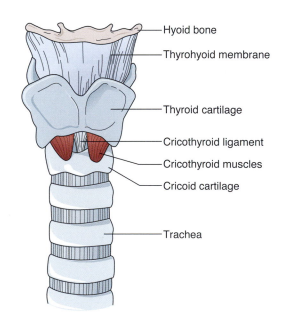

FIGURE 8.5   Anatomy of the larynx.

Overview of Head Injuries

Due to their potential severity (ranging from minor to life-threatening), a proper evaluation of head injuries is paramount. Head injury classification can be based on anatomic location, mechanism of injury (MOI; coup, contrecoup, linear, or rotational), distribution (focal or diffuse), and clinical presentation.[2] The injuries occur when an athlete collides with either an object or another athlete, exposing the brain to a combination of biomechanical impact forces. When injury to the brain occurs at the site of impact, it is known as a **coup injury**. When injury occurs opposite the side of impact, it is known as a **contrecoup injury**. Prevention of head injury centers on development of protective equipment to minimize the magnitude of impact forces.[2,3]

Affecting millions of people worldwide, traumatic brain injuries (TBIs) are considered a major cause of death and disability.[4] TBIs are typically categorized along a severity spectrum as mild, moderate, or severe. Classification is based on several factors, including neurological symptoms, amnesia, imaging scan results, and duration or severity of unconsciousness (if present). Historically, classification has also been based on the Glasgow Coma Scale (GCS) score,[5] which provides standardization of level of consciousness (LOC) in patients with head injury.[6] The GCS is divided into 3 components—eye opening, verbal response, and motor response (table 8.1). Each component is summed to produce a total score. A GCS score of 13 to 15 indicates mild TBI; 9 to 12 is moderate TBI; and 3 to 8 is severe TBI.[7]

From 2001 to 2010, 5 of every 1,000 people experienced a TBI per year; in 2010, 2.5 million people were either treated in emergency departments (EDs), admitted to hospitals, or died as a result of a TBI.[8] In the general population, the most common cause of TBIs in adolescents and elderly is falls. In young adults, however, the most common causes are motor vehicle accidents and assaults.[9] In the military setting, the majority of TBIs are associated with accidents (74%), while battle-related trauma accounts for only 11%.[10]

Scalp Lacerations

Lacerations to the scalp are common and can be minor or major. Because of the great vascularity of the scalp and face, small lacerations can lead to significant blood loss in a short amount of time. Healing times are shorter when compared to other areas of the body, and infections are less common, also because of the extensive vascularity.

Field Assessment Techniques

As with all head traumas, initial clinical assessment should rapidly identify life-threatening conditions, followed by a thorough secondary survey. Any patients with visible or palpable bony defects should be transported and referred for additional diagnostic testing. Most scalp lacerations should be identified during the secondary survey.

Immediate Management Techniques

Initial treatment of scalp lacerations should begin with removal of foreign debris via pressure irrigation (5-8 PSI) with tap water or 0.9% normal saline (NS) followed by application of direct pressure for approximately 10 to 15 minutes, which leads to adequate control in most cases.[11] Place sterile gauze over the laceration, taking care to replace any torn flaps over the area. Apply pressure

TABLE 8.1   **Glasgow Coma Scale**

Behavior	Response	Score
Eye-opening response	Spontaneously	4
	To speech	3
	To pain	2
	No response	1
Verbal response	Oriented to time, place, and person	5
	Confused	4
	Inappropriate words	3
	Incomprehensible sounds	2
	No response	1
Motor response	Obeys commands	6
	Moves to localized pain	5
	Flexion withdrawal from pain	4
	Abnormal flexion (decorticate)	3
	Abnormal extension (decerebrate)	2
	No response	1

for several minutes until bleeding subsides. Antiseptic solutions of hydrogen peroxide or povidone-iodine (Betadine) may be toxic to wound tissue and impede wound healing;[12] however, diluted solutions of povidone-iodine may be acceptable. Scalp lacerations are often jagged or irregularly shaped and may require approximation with wound closure strips, sutures, or staples. In these instances, wound closure may occur up to 24 hours after injury, again due to the extensive vascularity of the face and scalp. For more information regarding wound closure, see chapter 6.

Skull Fracture

Any significant impact or blow to the head could cause a skull fracture. The 4 categories of skull fractures are as follows:

1. *Depressed fractures* occur most often in penetrating traumas[6] and may cause indentations and bony fragments to enter the brain cavity.

2. *Linear fractures* are the most common, occurring as a result of minor blunt trauma over a relatively wide bony area.

3. *Basilar fractures* occur at the floor or base of the skull.

4. *Diastatic fractures* occur at the suture lines and usually affect young children.

Treatment considerations include fracture type and severity, and may range from pain medication to neurosurgery. Skull fractures require surgery when other brain injuries exist. For example, basilar fractures may result in excessive leakage of cerebrospinal fluid. Depressed skull fractures may require surgery if the depression is severe. As with other fracture sites, most skull fractures heal over time, usually within a period of 6 weeks.

Incidence and Epidemiology

Skull fractures represent the third highest fracture site among children and adolescents (21%-24%), and the lowest fracture site among adults (12%-23%) and the elderly (3%-4%).[13] The likelihood of sustaining a skull fracture tends to diminish with age. Linear skull fracture incidence rates are highest in the young as well as the elderly. Motor vehicle accidents and falls account for the majority of skull fractures.[14]

Signs and Symptoms

Symptomology of a skull fracture include

- bleeding,
- ecchymosis,
- pain,
- swelling, and
- redness or warmth.

Less severe symptomology may include headache, nausea, blurred vision, diminished pupillary reaction to light, excessive drowsiness, and fainting. Basilar skull fractures (located in the posterior skull) are associated with a higher rate of intracerebral bleeding.[6] Bilateral periorbital bruising (raccoon eyes), bruising in the mastoid area (Battle's sign), blood pooling behind the eardrum, and leakage of cerebrospinal fluid are indicative of a basilar skull fracture.

Field Assessment Techniques

As with all head traumas, initial clinical assessment should rapidly identify life-threatening conditions, followed by a thorough secondary survey. Any patients with visible or palpable bony defects should be transported and referred for additional diagnostic testing.

Immediate Management Techniques

If a skull fracture is suspected, do not apply a great amount of pressure, because bone fragments may invade the brain or intracranial pressure may increase. Bleeding can be controlled with indirect pressure to the wound edges and by placing sterile cloth or gauze over the injury site. Skull fractures require immediate transportation of the patient, and they are best evaluated with further diagnostic imaging, such as computed tomography (CT) scans.

Concussion

Concussions are a subset of mild TBI.[2,5,15] Some of the more common activities associated with concussions are sports related and include cycling, rugby, hockey, American football, women's soccer, baseball, and softball.[17] Given the individualized nature of concussion presentation and treatment, it is important for HCPs to develop a systematic and comprehensive sideline evaluation technique.

Incidence and Epidemiology

Almost two-thirds of emergency room visits related to concussion occur in children and young adults younger than 19 years old.[17] In youth, sports-related concussions (SRCs) are the most common subset of mild TBI, accounting for approximately one-third of all concussions.[18] Limitations in concussion surveillance in sport include the patient not seeking care, the hidden symptoms of concussions, medical coding, and the variability of terms such as concussion, athlete exposure, and asymptomatic.[19]

Risk Factors

As with other injuries, the best predictor of sustaining subsequent concussions is previous history of concussion.[20] Recurrence is likely to occur within the first 10 days of initial injury. In addition to previous concussion history, younger patients may be more susceptible to sustaining a concussion because of their stage of development and longer recovery rates.[16] High-risk sport participation is a considering factor, as is gender. Evidence suggests that female soccer players sustain a high number of concussions, due in part to the large number of participants, but also due to physiological predisposition, symptom reporting frequency, and style of play.[22]

Signs and Symptoms

Concussion symptoms are usually transient and can be identified through witnesses or self-reported by the patient. Physical, cognitive, and behavioral symptoms may be present. In the vast majority of cases, symptoms typically resolve within 7 to 10 days. Athletic patients may recover in a shorter period of time, partly because of better physical conditioning when compared to patients with a concussion mechanism not related to sport.[4] Loss of consciousness may or may not be associated with concussions.[23] Common signs and symptoms of concussion include the following:

- Headache
- Fatigue
- Blurred vision
- Irritability
- Inappropriate emotions or behaviors
- Nausea
- Vomiting
- Poor concentration and memory
- Drowsiness

A diagnosis of **post-concussive syndrome** is made when a patient's concussive symptoms persist for greater than 3 months. It is estimated that 10% to 15% of patients with concussion will develop post-concussive syndrome.[4] Challenges exist when attempting to diagnose post-concussive syndrome, however, because symptoms are also common in healthy people as well as those with preexisting conditions such as anxiety and depression.[5]

Second impact syndrome occurs when a patient sustains repetitive head injuries with short recovery periods between episodes. Returning to play too soon and receiving a second impact while still exhibiting signs and symptoms of the first head injury is the primary concern. A patient with a recent history of concussion who receives a second impact may initially exhibit signs and symptoms of a second concussion; however, within minutes the patient collapses and exhibits signs of cranial nerve and brain stem damage. Mortality and morbidity rates associated with second impact syndrome are high (50% and 100%, respectively).[24] Furthermore, all documented cases occurred in people under 20 years of age.[25] Although the overall incidence of second impact syndrome is unknown,[26] researchers agree that the rareness of the condition does not lessen its devastation, in that death can occur within minutes[25,27]—even more rapidly than with an epidural hematoma. This fact is significant, because there may not be time to transport the patient from the playing field to an ED. Malignant cerebral **edema** is classically associated with second impact syndrome, which is most common in younger athletes as opposed to adults.[2,5,20]

Field Assessment Techniques

A concussion is one of the most difficult sports-related injuries to evaluate, diagnose, and manage.[28] Concussion assessment typically involves a series of quick screenings. Baseline testing provides a measure of pre-established cognitive and neuromuscular function, which is a reference for post-injury comparison. Baseline testing should be conducted in a manner that allows for repeatability for each sport or environment. Use of video review to determine MOI is becoming more widespread for sideline evaluation and assessment at all levels of sport.

At the time of injury, the patient should be evaluated for cervical spine involvement and more serious brain injury such as intracranial hemorrhage or skull fracture. An unconscious patient should be treated as though a cervical spine injury exists and transported accordingly. If the patient is conscious, cranial nerve function (table 8.2) and mental status checks using the GCS should be performed. The GCS is useful in ruling out moderate to severe TBI.[29] Initial questions should assess alertness, orientation, and memory. Using a symptom checklist in combination with clinical indicators and knowledge of concussive history is helpful during the evaluation process. Because of the challenges of evaluating for a concussion on the sideline, caution is preferable; treat symptoms as concussion related until otherwise known, and remove the patient from play to conduct a more comprehensive evaluation.[29]

Types and Sequencing

Depending on the response to the screenings, further evaluation is essential to provide optimal and time-sensitive care to the injured patient. No definitive diagnostic test exists; no consensus indicates what specific tests should

TABLE 8.2 **Cranial Nerve Function**

Cranial nerve	Function	Testing procedure
I. Olfactory	S; Smell	Close eyes and identify smell
II. Optic	S; Vision	Read object both near and far away Test peripheral vision; test each eye separately and together Use Snellen chart (office setting)
*III. Oculomotor	M; Eye movement and pupillary reaction; vision	PEARLA (pupils equal and responsive to light; accommodating): Use a penlight to compare pupil size bilaterally and bring light toward nose to assess accommodation
*IV. Trochlear	M; Lateral and inferior eye movement	Using eyes only, follow movement of penlight in bowtie pattern
V. Trigeminal	B; Mastication and facial sensation	S: Light touch over jaw, cheeks, forehead M: Speech, jaw clench, jaw movement
*VI. Abducens	M; Lateral eye movement	Using eyes only, follow movement of penlight in "H" pattern
VII. Facial	B; Taste; facial expression	S: Not normally tested on sideline M: Facial symmetry of expressions
VIII. Vestibulocochlear	S; Hearing and balance	Hearing: Rub fingers together near each ear; snap; perform Weber's test (tuning fork) Balance—Romberg's test: Finger to nose with eyes closed
**IX. Glossopharyngeal	B; Swallowing; gag reflex; tongue sensation	S: Not normally tested on sideline M: Voice tone and quality; say "ahhh"; swallow
**X. Vagus	B; Speech; swallowing	S: Not normally tested on sideline M: Voice tone and quality; say "ahhh"; swallow
XI. Accessory	M; Innervation of trapezius and sternocleidomastoid	Test bilateral comparison of shoulder shrug against resistance (trapezius); neck rotation against resistance (SCM)
XII. Hypoglossal	M; Tongue movement	Waggle tongue; tongue in each cheek

B = both sensory and motor; M = motor; S = sensory

*CN III, IV, and VI can be tested simultaneously.

**CN IX and X can be tested simultaneously.

comprise an assessment. Typical management includes a multidimensional approach through a screening tool or multiple screening tools, with traditional or computerized neurocognitive testing, postural stability, self-report symptom instruments, and physical and neurological examination components. One such recommended framework is the Sport Concussion Assessment Tool (SCAT-5).[30] In 2016, the 5th International Consensus Conference on Concussion in Sport published the recommendation to use the SCAT-5 assessment tool for assistance in identifying and managing concussion.[31,32] The SCAT-5 is used in patients 13 years of age and older;

a Child SCAT-5 version is available for patients aged 5 to 12. The SCAT-5 is also available for free as a smartphone application. For additional information on each section of the SCAT-5, see appendix B.

The SCAT-5 has 6 steps, the first of which is performed either on-field (sideline) or off-field.

Step 1:
- On-field:
  - Red flags
  - Observable signs
  - Maddocks questions
  - GCS

- Cervical spine assessment
- Off-field:
  - Patient background

Step 2: Symptom Evaluation

Step 3: Cognitive Screening

- Orientation
- Memory
- Concentration

Step 4: Neurological Screening

- Passive cervical range of motion (ROM)
- Cranial nerve III, IV, and VI
- Finger to nose coordination
- Gait
- Balance

Step 5: Delayed Recall

Step 6: Scoring and Clinical Decision

Additional popular tools for concussion assessment include the Standardized Assessment of Concussion (SAC) and the Concussion Assessment & Response: Sport Version (CARE). The SAC includes tests for orientation, immediate and delayed recall, concentration, and exertional maneuvers. Unscored components of the SAC include a graded symptom checklist, brief neurologic examination, and presence of retrograde amnesia. When results of the SAC are compared with baseline measurements prior to injury, better information may be elicited.[33] The CARE is a smartphone application available for a small fee and to assist HCPs in concussion evaluation. The CARE app includes primary emergency survey information, cranial nerve function, cardiopulmonary resuscitation prompts, balance testing, the SAC, a graded symptom checklist, return-to-play guide, post-concussion home and school instructions, and frequently asked questions.

Currently in development are assessment tools such as the King-Devick test and head impact sensors. The King-Devick test consists of printed cards designed to assess saccadic eye movement. This test may be promising as a sideline assessment tool, but additional research is warranted.[30] Head impact sensors placed in helmets, mouth guards, headbands, or adhered directly to the skin provide minimal helpful information to sideline personnel about concussion.[30,34]

Diagnostic Accuracy

Some patients will present with elevated scores on baseline testing, indicating a lack of asymptomatic status.[19] The elevated scores could be due to a lack of motivation[35] or physical fitness;[35,36] or a history of anxiety, depression, learning disorders,[37] or concussion.[38] The accuracy of comparing post-concussion testing results to baseline data is patient specific. All details of the assessment process must be taken into consideration to adequately use and interpret diagnostic testing, including assessment techniques and the patient's medical history.

To maximize diagnostic accuracy and account for various patient presentations and preexisting symptoms, a combination of multiple tests should be conducted at baseline and during post-concussive care. While individual components have good sensitivity values (table 8.3), the diagnostic accuracy increases when multiple components are included. As a recently revised assessment tool, the SCAT-5 does not have any diagnostic accuracy values as of the date of publication.

Immediate Management Techniques

If no HCP (e.g., athletic trainer [AT] or a physician) is available, the patient should be removed from participation and immediately referred to a HCP for additional evaluation. If a concussion is suspected, the patient should not be left alone; additional monitoring is essential over the next few hours to determine whether the patient's condition is deteriorating. Furthermore, the patient should not be permitted to return to activity on the day of the injury.

Procedures and Protocols

Since the First International Conference on Concussion in Sport, held in Vienna in 2001, treatment strategies have varied greatly. The most repeated factor in TBI recovery

TABLE 8.3 **Diagnostic Accuracy of Concussion Field Tests**

Test	Specificity	Sensitivity	Reference
SSS >7; or SSS ≤7 with a SAC ≤22	96%	77%	Bin Zahid, Hubbard, Dammavalam, et al.[140]
BESS	—	60%	Buckley, Munkasy, Clouse[141]
Modified BESS	—	71%	Buckley, Munkasy, Clouse[141]
Combination*	98%	80%	Resch, Brown, Macciocchi, et al.[142]

BESS = balance error scoring system; SSS = symptom severity scale; SAC = standardized assessment of concussion

*Combination of assessments including Immediate Post-Concussion Assessment and Cognitive Test (ImPACT), Sensory Organization Test (SOT), and Revised Head Injury Scale (HIS-r)

is rest. Physical rest is designed to protect the brain from repeat injury; cognitive rest (including no schoolwork, no television or computer screens, even social limitations) protects the brain from neural activity and stimulation. Recent studies, however, have begun to examine the use of physical activity earlier in concussive treatment,[39,40] because the necessity of waiting until the patient is completely asymptomatic has led to periods of weeks or months without activity.[41] The recommended process from the Fifth International Conference on Concussion in Sport, held in Berlin in October 2016[42] suggested that, although earlier physical activity (<7 days) post-concussion may be beneficial,[40] additional studies are needed to address the challenges of early physical activity and the ethical considerations.[40,42] Until further evidence can produce additional guidelines, HCPs should use common sense regarding limiting physical activity and use caution when resting an active patient for long periods.[42]

The additional material provided with the SCAT-5 includes a stepwise return to play progression.[31] Each step cannot start until 24 hours have passed from the previous step. If any symptoms appear or worsen, a regression to the previous step is warranted.

> Step 1: Symptom-limited activity—activities of daily living
>
> Step 2: Light aerobic conditioning
>
> Step 3: Sport-specific activity—earliest attempt at resistance training
>
> Step 4: Noncontact sport training
>
> Step 5: Full-contact practice
>
> Step 6: Return to competition

As a means of continuing to emphasize the health and safety of young athletes, the Centers for Disease Control and Prevention (CDC) developed the HEADS UP Concussion in Youth Sports Initiative.[9] HEADS UP offers concussion information to youth sport parents, athletes, coaches, and officials by providing resources on prevention, recognition, and response to a concussion.

Criteria for Deciding to Transport for Further Medical Examination

Most concussions do not present with outright neurologic signs such as loss of consciousness, posturing, or clear disorientation. The decision to send a patient to the ED should be based on the likelihood of a significant injury other than a concussion, such as an intracranial hemorrhage, skull fracture, or cervical spine injury. If, after careful clinical evaluation, more significant injury is not suspected, the associated cost and potential harm (additional cognitive stimuli and radiation exposure) of sending a concussed patient to the ED should be considered.

Clinical presentation, indicating immediate transfer by ambulance to the nearest ED, includes the following:

- Prolonged loss of consciousness >1 minute
- Suspected c-spine injury
- High-impact or high-risk MOI for intracranial bleed
- Suspected skull fracture
- Post-traumatic seizure
- Significant acute worsening of condition:
  - Persistent nausea and vomiting
  - Focal neurologic deficits
  - Deteriorating neurologic status including slurred speech, inability or difficulty with walking, worsening mental status, or progressive **somnolence**

Chronic Traumatic Encephalopathy

Chronic traumatic encephalopathy (CTE) is a degenerative brain disease seen in athletes, military veterans, and other people with a significant history of repetitive head trauma. An official diagnosis of CTE is made during autopsy. Physiologically, brain degeneration is caused by a protein known as tau, which forms clumps in the brain tissue that spread over time.

Incidence and Epidemiology

The development of CTE is thought to occur from repeated mild TBIs or subconcussive impacts, specifically in patients who participate in contact sports (e.g., football, ice hockey, soccer, rugby, wrestling)[4] and in military veterans.[43] However, current limitations include the lack of epidemiological evidence on this association as well as the lack of knowledge on risk increase in patients who sustain multiple head impacts during a competitive season.[4] Patients who are ultimately diagnosed with CTE typically began participating in their sport as children and adolescents and played for at least 5 years.[4] It is thought that 33% of athletic individuals who develop CTE are symptomatic at retirement, and the condition advances over time.[44]

Signs and Symptoms

As of the date of publication, researchers have categorized CTE into these 4 stages of severity:[45]

- *Stage I symptomology* includes headaches and attention and concentration issues.
- *Stage II symptomology* includes depression, short-term memory loss, and explosivity.

- *Stage III symptomology* includes cognitive impairment and executive function shortfalls in planning, organization, multitasking, and judgment.
- *Stage IV symptomology* includes full-blown dementia (memory and cognitive impairment significant enough to impede daily living).[45]

Next steps in research include the development of methods to diagnose CTE during life.

Intracranial Pressure

When a head injury occurs, the presence of swollen brain tissue, blood, or cerebrospinal fluid may cause an increase in pressure exerted on the skull because the skull is unable to expand. Intracranial pressure (ICP) is a measurement of this pressure. Measured in millimeters of mercury (mm Hg), typical resting ICP is 7 to 15 mm Hg.[46] An increase in ICP is usually indicative of underlying brain injury.

In addition to a blow to the head, possible causes of ICP include the following:

- Infection
- Tumor
- Stroke
- Aneurysm
- Epilepsy
- Hypoxemia
- Meningitis

Signs and Symptoms

Signs and symptoms similar to a concussion may indicate an increase in ICP, including headache, nausea or vomiting, confusion, double vision, unequal pupil size, and seizures. Later signs of ICP include motor changes, high blood pressure, and a slow, irregular pulse. Classically, headaches associated with ICP are typically worse in the morning, perhaps due in part to the recumbent sleeping position.[47]

Immediate Management Techniques

Suspected brain hemorrhaging should lead to immediate transport of the patient to an ED for additional evaluation, because the hemorrhaging could lead to an increase in ICP. Magnetic resonance imaging (MRI) or a CT scan can determine the cause of ICP, and ICP itself can be measured during a lumbar puncture (spinal tap). Placement of a shunt, antihypertensives, or diuretics may be used to decrease ICP in the ED.

Intracerebral Contusion

The cause of intracerebral contusion is associated with a direct blow or acceleration–deceleration injury.[2] Contusions can vary in size. A contusion differs from a laceration in that with a contusion, the pia mater remains intact. A contusion differs from a hematoma in that with a contusion, blood is intermixed with brain tissue.[48] Contusions can occur in combination with skull fractures or hematomas.

Signs and Symptoms

Contusions can be present in any area of the brain but are more common in the frontal and temporal regions.[49] Depending on the severity of the contusion, signs and symptoms of intracerebral contusions may differ.

Typical indications of contusions include the following:

- Sleepiness
- Dizziness
- Confusion
- Nausea or vomiting
- Coordination difficulties
- Seizures
- Tinnitus
- Loss of consciousness

Immediate Management Techniques

Immediate medical referral and emergency management due to possible intracranial hemorrhage include the following signs: drowsiness (somnolence), posttraumatic amnesia, altered level of consciousness or alertness, abnormal behavior, disorientation longer than 5 minutes, changes in mental status, and seizures.[50] Research also suggests that patients 16 years and younger undergo close evaluation, because they may be at a higher risk of intracranial pathology based on symptoms such as loss of consciousness, focal deficits, and the presence of a skull fracture.[50,51]

Epidural Hematoma

Epidural hematomas are focal injuries often caused by a linear and direct impact force (e.g., hit with baseball or bat) in patients who aren't wearing a helmet.[2,4] Epidural hematomas are usually associated with skull fractures and lacerations.[2] The vessels closest to the impact site are the sources of the hemorrhage that forms the hematoma; blood accumulates between the inner layer of the skull and the dural membrane. Classically, a patient who has sustained an epidural hematoma may exhibit a **lucid**

interval, or an initial loss of consciousness upon impact followed by a regaining of consciousness and temporary improvement, after which the condition deteriorates.[2] The bleeding into the epidural space can be shunted out through veins, delaying accumulation of the hematoma and rise in intracranial pressure and ultimately slowing down the development of symptoms.[52]

Incidence and Epidemiology

Intracranial epidural hematoma is a serious complication of head injury and primarily occurs as a result of acute trauma (58%).[53] The vast majority of epidural hematomas are associated with arterial bleeding. Approximately one-third of patients experience venous bleeds. Venous epidural hematomas form mainly with depressed skull fractures. The lucid period of transient neurological recovery occurs in 10% to 33% of patients with epidural hematomas and can last from minutes or hours to a few days.[52]

Risk Factors

In a sports setting, the absence of protective headgear can increase the risk of epidural hematomas. Other risk factors include the use of anticoagulant medications, alcohol use leading to an increased risk of fall and other accidents, and the absence of a seat belt when riding in a vehicle. In addition, because the dural adherence to the skull increases with advanced age, younger patients could be at an increased risk for epidural hematoma.[54]

Signs and Symptoms

Symptoms of epidural hematoma include headache, nausea or vomiting, seizures, and focal neurologic deficits (e.g., aphasia, weakness, numbness, visual field disturbances). Keep in mind that an epidural hematoma can cause death within minutes.

Immediate Management Techniques

Initial efforts should include stabilization of airway, breathing, and circulation (ABC). A thorough trauma evaluation should be performed, including inspection of skull fractures and an appreciation of the MOI. The patient should be immobilized and transferred to the nearest level I trauma center for further neurological and surgical evaluation. Subsequent management may be tailored to the patient based on the degree of neurological impairment at presentation.

Subdural Hematoma

Subdural hematomas are the leading cause of sports-related fatalities and are frequently reported in football.[2] Bleeding collects under the inner layer of the dura mater but external to the brain and arachnoid membrane. Subdural hematomas can become life-threatening very quickly.

Incidence and Epidemiology

A subdural hematoma results most often from a severe head injury. Acceleration–deceleration forces cause injuries as the patient's momentum is stopped suddenly by a solid object and the brain makes contact with the inside of the skull.[2] Subdural hematomas can present either acutely or chronically based on the time since symptoms first appeared. Acute subdural hematomas occur within 72 hours after injury, while chronic subdural hematomas may take as long 3 weeks to show signs.

Risk Factors

Risk factors associated with acute subdural hematoma include head trauma, postsurgical complications, anticoagulation drug therapy, and nontraumatic cerebral aneurysm. As with epidural hematomas, decreased risk is associated with appropriate use of protective headgear in athletic environments.

Signs and Symptoms

Immediate medical referral and emergency management are recommended for any of the signs presented in the Red Flag box. Subsequent impacts to the head during the development of a chronic subdural hematoma may put patients at a higher risk of experiencing a life-threaten-

 RED FLAG

The following are possible indicators of intracranial injury, in which case immediate medical referral is warranted:[20,50]

- Worsening headache
- Increased drowsiness or sleep
- Changes in mental status or confusion
- Repetitive nausea and vomiting
- Posttraumatic seizure
- Perseveration
- Focal neurologic deficits
- Visual changes
- Signs of basilar skull fracture
- Abnormal behavior
- Progressive loss of consciousness
- Numbness or tingling in extremities
- Unequal pupil size
- Seizures
- Inability to speak or slurred speech
- GCS score <15

ing situation; as such, continued monitoring and serial assessment is important.

Field Assessment Techniques

In the pre-competition season, athletes participating in at-risk sports (e.g., football, soccer, rugby) should undergo baseline neurocognitive testing, either as a component of a pre-participation physical exam or an adjunct to such an exam. The importance of an established emergency care plan (ECP) cannot be overemphasized; the ECP provides for a standard of care and ensures rapid and efficient treatment measures are in place.

The Canadian CT Head Rule is a clinical prediction rule that uses CT scans to identify head injuries that could require neurosurgical intervention.[55] Inclusion criteria include patients with a GCS score of 13 to 15; injury within 24 hours; and blunt head trauma resulting in loss of consciousness, definite amnesia, or disorientation. Exclusion criteria include patients under 16 years of age, nontraumatic cases, patients using anticoagulants or with a bleeding disorder, obvious skull fracture, GCS score of less than 13, and pregnancy.

Immediate Management Techniques

Emergency management of any sports-related injury should first address a primary survey assessment of the patient's mental status, followed by ensuring proper ABC. Knowledge of the patient's neurocognitive baseline may be critical for both short-term and long-term

management, and it is helpful when conducting a sideline assessment. Although uncommon, possible differential diagnoses should include intracranial hemorrhage, because the signs and symptoms of a concussion and an intracranial injury are differentiated.[50,56] Incorporating potential clinical signs of intracranial injury into the assessment of a patient with a suspected concussion is important.[50] Injuries to the head can escalate into medical emergencies quickly, therefore an efficient process of providing immediate care based on signs and symptoms is required (figure 8.6).

Headaches

Headaches affect most people at some point in their life span; however, some people are disabled by the headache frequency and severity.[57] Headaches, in and of themselves, are not medical emergencies, but they may be a symptom of a medical emergency, particularly after a TBI where the primary complaint is a headache. The headache could also be a warning sign to a more serious medical condition. Therefore, a thorough evaluation is essential to provide the patient with optimal care.

Headache disorders can be divided into 2 main categories, primary and secondary. Primary headaches, which include migraines, are those that are the pathology; the headache is the primary complaint, and no other medical condition could have caused the pain.[57] Secondary headaches are those felt as the result or symptom of a separate pathology or injury, such as TBI, whiplash, or environmental changes.

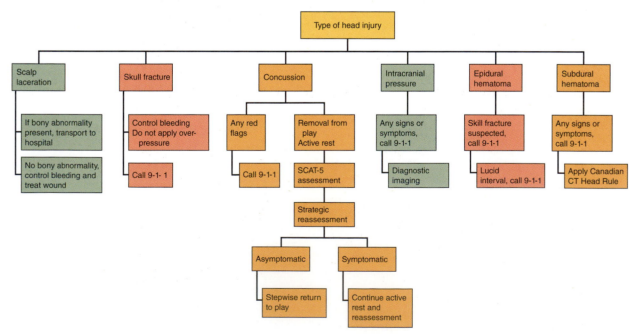

FIGURE 8.6 Head injury algorithm.

Incidence and Epidemiology

The diagnosis of a primary headache disorder is made when the patient has no medical history or a current condition that could have caused the headache; and the patient has an unremarkable neurological exam.[58] Tension headaches, trigeminal autonomic cephalalgias, and migraines are primary headaches (figure 8.7). Primary headaches are extremely common; the vast majority of people experience tension headaches at least once during their lifetime.[59] Migraine headaches affect approximately 13% of adults.[60] Generally, more women experience primary headaches than men,[60-62] especially tension and migraine headaches.[63] While primary headaches are not the result of sport or exercise, they may impact the baseline symptoms reported during preseason testing, therefore it is important to evaluate the frequency and symptom severity of the athlete's headaches prior to the start of the season.

Secondary headache disorders, however, are documented as the result of a separate but possibly related health condition. Secondary headaches traditionally develop, worsen, and dissipate as the primary condition develops, worsens, and dissipates; however, the headache may also develop with a delayed onset to the primary condition.[57]

Tension Headache

Tension headaches typically present as bilateral, mild to moderate pain.[57] People who experience tension headaches 15 or more times per month are deemed to have chronic tension headaches.[63] These headaches are more painful than episodic tension headaches and can be debilitating.[57]

Trigeminal Autonomic Cephalalgias

Trigeminal autonomic cephalalgias are headaches that present along the trigeminal nerve and result in autonomic nervous system symptoms, such as pain in the face, eye watering, or eye redness.[65] The pain associated with the attacks is moderate to severe. Cluster headaches are the most common type of trigeminal autonomic cephalalgia and affect men more than women. Cluster headaches typically begin to develop in 20- to 40-year-olds, and they can be immediately stimulated by substances such as alcohol, nitroglycerin, and histamine. During physical activity, the release of histamine may result in a cluster headache. Similarly, perfumes and other strong scents may also trigger an attack.[57] Two other trigeminal autonomic cephalalgias include short-lasting unilateral neuralgiform headaches and hemicrania continua. Patients describe hemicrania continua as a constant pain in the background that has peaks of severe pain.[65] People with trigeminal autonomic cephalalgia, in particular hemicrania continua, may experience photophobia or phonophobia.[57,65]

Migraines

Similar to general headache statistics, migraine prevalence is more than double in women compared to men.[60,61] The age group most likely to experience migraines is 30- to 39-year-olds.[60,61] The societal impact of migraines is greater than that of tension headaches; people with migraines miss work or activities of daily living at a greater rate.[63]

The 3 main categories for migraines are migraines without **aura**, migraines with aura, and chronic migraines. Phonophobia is the most commonly reported concomitant symptom in people who experience migraines.[63] Migraine

Sinus	Cluster	Tension	Migraine
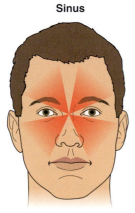	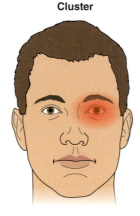	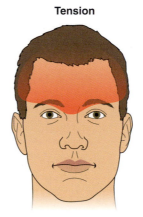	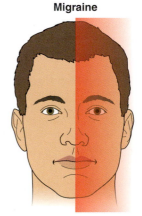
Pain is usually behind the forehead or cheekbones	Pain is in and around one eye	Pain is like a band squeezing the head	Pain, nausea, and visual changes are typical of classic form

FIGURE 8.7   Location of pain in the head for certain types of headaches.

without aura is a neurobiological disorder. For women, the onset is often related to menstruation. Migraines with aura affect 90% of people with migraines. Understanding the development of the migraine can help identify the optimal time to treat the migraine. Visual disturbances are the most common aura, followed by sensory, then speech disturbances. Medication overuse is the most common cause of chronic migraines. However, once the overmedication is ceased, the migraine conditions may continue as chronic or become episodic in nature.[57]

Other Headache Disorders

Some primary headaches do not fall under the main categories of primary headaches but are causes of complaint in physically active people. Primary exercise headache was previously termed *primary exertional headache*. Strenuous activity is the precursor to primary exercise headaches; the headache may develop during or after continuous strenuous activity,[57] and it may develop as neck pain before beginning to pulsate.[66] High altitudes and other environmental conditions can exacerbate the headache. Due to the seriousness of conditions that may be missed if the headache is treated as the sole complaint, all patients who report an initial severe headache associated with strenuous activity should be evaluated with possible imaging for subarachnoid hemorrhage, arterial dissection, and reversible cerebral vasoconstriction syndrome.[57]

Cold exposure and tight-fitting equipment can result in headaches. Cold-stimulus headaches are triggered by severely low temperatures applied to the head through ingestion, direct application, or inhalation. The headache will resolve with the removal of the trigger, typically within 30 minutes. Similar to the direct onset of a cold-stimulus headache after exposure to cold, the onset of external pressure headaches are directly associated with tight-fitting helmets, goggles, or hats, which result in localized pain on pericranial soft tissue. Once the external compression is removed, the headache ceases within an hour.[57]

Secondary Headaches

Numerous primary conditions may cause a secondary headache. Beyond injury to the head and neck, whiplash is also a primary condition that can result in secondary headaches. The excessive movement of the head during a whiplash event may cause muscular damage, tightness, and tension along the structures supporting the neck and head. Headaches attributed to trauma or injury to the brain are either acute or persistent. Acute headaches are those that occur within the first 3 months of the trauma. *Persistent* (previously referred to as *chronic*) is the term for headaches that continue beyond the 3-month mark. A concern for patient with a headache following a traumatic incident to the head or neck is post-concussive

syndrome.[57] Symptoms beyond that of the headache should be assessed to rule out post-concussive syndrome or other more serious conditions.

Patients who sustained a concussion and have a post-traumatic headache are likely to have significantly higher symptom severity scores and symptom scores, as measured by SCAT-5, than those who sustained a concussion but do not have a headache, even when headache items are removed from the SCAT-5. Furthermore, patients who sustain a concussion and have a post-traumatic headache may also have motor deficits, such as balance error scoring system (BESS) scores more than double that of those who sustain a concussion but do not have a headache.[67]

Risk Factors

If a person has a known headache disorder and can identify a trigger, avoiding the trigger is the best way to lower the risk of experiencing a headache. However, not all headaches have known triggers. One known major risk factor for secondary headache associated with exercise is inadequate respiration. The reduced respiration may lead to **hypoxia** or **hypercapnia** in the tissues surrounding the brain resulting in a headache attributed to hypoxia or hypercapnia (a secondary headache). People with low $\dot{V}O_{2max}$ are at a greater risk of experiencing a hypoxic headache.[68] When the hypoxic condition is due to high altitudes, the headache is referred to as a high-altitude headache. Beyond a lack of oxygen, other risk factors for high-altitude headaches include decreased fluid intake and intense exertion. Preventive measures for avoiding high-altitude headaches include multiday acclimatization, moderate to aggressive fluid intake, and avoidance of alcohol.[57] The best example of hypercapnia is a diving headache. Divers who are most likely to sustain a diving headache are those that attempt skip breathing or hypoventilate due to strenuous swimming.[69] The pain of a diving headache intensifies during decompression and resurfacing.[57,69] Following proper diving procedures and resurfacing recommendations will reduce the risk of a diving headache.

Signs and Symptoms

A headache may result from TBI, seizure, or other medical condition. Understanding the headache development and progression is critical to determining whether the headache is primary or secondary, or a warning of a medical emergency. For patients with chronic headache disorders, assessment of auras and symptoms is difficult due to inaccurate patient reporting and recall; therefore they should keep a headache or symptom diary. The diary should include frequency, symptoms, duration of symptoms, and location of symptoms.[57] The headache diary will aid the patient and the medical personnel in diagnosing the headache and providing proper and effective care. A headache diary can also be beneficial in the management of headaches after a head or neck injury. While headaches are not adequate predictors of concussion severity or sole determinants of return-to-play status, the presence or absence and frequency of headaches does play a role in concussion management (see Concussion section).

Field Assessment Techniques

A complete medical history is essential, including questions pertaining to illnesses or health conditions, medication and drug use, and recent physical activity. The evaluation should also include questions regarding additional signs and symptoms. It is important to determine whether the headache is primary or secondary in order to determine the best route of care. Headaches can have a variety of comorbidities that may need to be addressed. Some comorbidities include recurrent gastrointestinal disturbance with nonremarkable clinical exam of abdomen, cyclical vomiting syndrome, and benign paroxysmal vertigo.[57] The diagnosis of the headache is based on the medical history and clinical presentation.

Immediate Management Techniques

Immediate management of headaches is symptom based. However, if the individual presents with any of the symptoms included in the acronym SSNOOP (presented in the Red Flag),[70] they are in need of advanced medical care. Pain management of acute headaches is primarily achieved through oral medication. Nonsteroidal anti-inflammatory drugs (NSAIDs) and over-the-counter analgesic medications are effective in treating infrequent tension headaches. However, frequent tension headaches or cluster headaches may require more potent medication.[71] Due to the intense symptoms of migraines, patients often self-treat with bed rest; on average, women spend 6 hours in bed and men spend 4.5 hours in bed during migraine attacks.[72] If medication is selected, most people with migraines treat their symptoms with over-the-counter medication, while a few use prescription medication.[73] Some get relief from ibuprofen or aspirin if taken at the onset of the migraine; however, patients should be advised to follow the medication directions as listed on the bottle and contact a pharmacist for additional clarification and information.[71] If over-the-counter medication does not reduce the symptoms of the migraine, triptans may be prescribed. Preventive therapy, such as beta blockers, antidepressants, and anticonvulsants,[71] would help approximately 26% of people who experience migraines.[61]

RED FLAG

To determine whether a headache warrants further evaluation of a primary condition or possible primary condition, use the pneumonic SSNOOP as follows:[75]

- **S**ystematic signs/symptoms: Present with fever, malaise, lethargy—possible meningitis, encephalitis.
- **S**ystemic disease: Comorbidity of autoimmune disease—possible meningitis.
- **N**eurological signs/symptoms: Present with decreased myotomes or dermatomes—possible transient ischemic attack, stroke, central nervous system infection.
- **O**nset sudden: Complains of **thunderclap** headache—possible hemorrhage or epidural/subdural hematoma.
- **O**nset in people aged over 40 years: Present with pain local to temples—possible temporal arteritis.
- **P**revious headache pattern: More/less frequent—possible change in primary condition, medical overuse headache.

Secondary headaches resolve with the removal of the primary condition. NSAIDs help decrease the pain from a high-altitude headache.[57] However, NSAIDs are not likely to help a patient with a diving headache.[71] Treatment of high-altitude headaches should also include ruling out mountain sickness, which can be multisymptomatic.[57]

Stroke

Globally, strokes are one of the leading causes of death. A stroke is a neurovascular injury, the result of a cerebrovascular accident (commonly abbreviated as CVA), where the brain cannot function due to a sudden vascular deficit.

Incidence and Epidemiology

Statistically, women and African Americans are more likely to experience a stroke. The top causes of disrupted cerebral blood flow are thrombosis, arterial rupture, and cerebral embolisms. Lifestyle factors, specifically those pertaining to diet and exercise, play a significant role in the risk of experiencing a stroke. Atherosclerosis, hypertension, and diabetes mellitus are the highest concomitant diseases in patients who experience a stroke.[76,77] Psychosocial stress and depression are also risk factors for strokes.[76]

Cerebral strokes, often abbreviated CVA for cerebrovascular accident, are divided into two types, ischemic and hemorrhagic (figure 8.8). Ischemic strokes have a gradual onset, while hemorrhagic strokes occur suddenly. Less than 15% of all strokes are hemorrhagic. Hemorrhagic stroke patients initially have a more severe condition, but they recover more quickly because of the mechanical nature of the condition. Once the pressure is removed, the brain cells are able to function. Ischemic stroke patients present less severely on initial evaluation; however, the damage to the cells remains after treatment.[78]

Ischemic Strokes

Embolisms and thrombosis are two main mechanisms for an ischemic stroke. When a person experiences a reduction of cerebral blood flow, a cerebral **infarction** occurs.[78] The infarction causes the brain to be deprived of oxygen and glucose, the brain's energy source. The reduction in blood flow also results in a lack of removal of lactic acid, a waste product. The imbalance in metabolites results in cerebral dysfunction. A prolonged period of reduced blood flow in the brain results in irreversible ischemic necrosis; even after reperfusion, necrotic tissue remains nonfunctional.[78]

Hemorrhagic Strokes

Weakened arterial vessels due to cardiovascular disease, most frequently hypertension, are the leading cause of an intracerebral hemorrhagic stroke. Increased intracranial pressure due to a ruptured blood vessel in the brain results in neural injury.[78] After the vessel ruptures, the patient will likely experience a severe thunderclap headache.[70,75]

Risk Factors

Factors pertaining to ischemic strokes are almost all modifiable. The relationship between body mass index (BMI) and ischemic stroke is not universally accepted. Some evidence shows that people with high BMIs are more likely to experience an ischemic stroke than hemorrhagic stroke.[79] The exact cause for this relationship is unknown; it is likely due to the relationship between obesity and hypertension, dyslipidemia, and diabetes. Dyslipidemia and diabetes are greater risk factors for ischemic stroke compared to hemorrhagic stroke.[76] The most evident social modifiable risk factor for ischemic stroke is cigarette smoking; the greater the number of cigarettes smoked, the greater the risk.[76] Socioeconomic status also plays a part in incidence of stroke; men of lower socioeconomic status who smoke are of greatest concern.[80]

Drug use and exercise may lead to hemorrhagic strokes in relatively healthy and physically active people. Those who have ingested stimulants such as synthetic marijuana[81] or performance aids such as beta-methylphenethylamine (BMPEA, an isomer of amphetamine),[82,83] dimethylamylamine (DMAA or geranium extract), and caffeine have experienced hemorrhagic strokes.[84] While the relationship between performance aids and hemorrhagic strokes has not been established, determining whether the patient with a stroke has a history of using such substances can provide the advanced medical staff a point of consideration during the evaluation.

Field Assessment Techniques

Through the use of screening tools, recognizing the signs and symptoms of a stroke is made easy. When a standardized screening tool such as the Cincinnati Prehospital Stroke Scale (table 8.4) is used, nonmedical[85] and medically trained personnel[86] can accurately identify and relay the signs and symptoms to an emergency dispatcher or physician. The Cincinnati Prehospital Stroke Scale can be performed in approximately 1 minute and

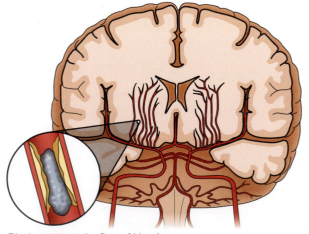

Blockage stops the flow of blood to an area of the brain

a

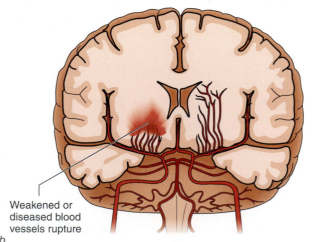

Weakened or diseased blood vessels rupture

b

FIGURE 8.8 *(a)* Ischemic stroke and *(b)* hemorrhagic stroke.

is a valid tool in identifying patients with a stroke.[86] If a patient is experiencing any of the symptoms identified in the stroke scale, emergency dispatch should be contacted immediately. With the addition of time to call 9-1-1, the components of the Cincinnati Prehospital Stroke Scale are combined into the acronym FAST as follows:

Facial drop

Arm weakness

Speech difficulty

Time to call 9-1-1

Immediate Management Techniques

Once a stroke is suspected, proper and detailed information should be reported to emergency medical providers. The American Heart Association and American Stroke Association recommend that all people suspected of experiencing a stroke be screened using a standardized instrument, such as the Cincinnati Prehospital Stroke Scale (see table 8.4) and transported to a medical facility that can administer appropriate medications, such as alteplase, intravenously.[87]

Indications

HCPs should address comorbidities if they pose an additional risk to survival or can exacerbate the stroke severity. If the patient is experiencing difficulty breathing or reduced consciousness, the responding medical staff should support and provide airway assistance before, during, and after transport; for patients with less than 94% oxygen saturation, supplemental oxygen should be administered.[87] In stroke patients with hyperthermia, the core body temperature should be continuously monitored and lowered below 38°C. If antipyretic medication is available, it should be administered to help reduce the in-hospital death associated with elevated core temperature and stroke.[87] The American Stroke Association also recommends treating the patient for hypoglycemia if the serum glucose levels are under 60 mg/dL.

Procedures and Protocols

To optimize patient outcomes, stroke patients should be transported to a hospital that provides advanced stroke care, specifically a Joint Commission primary stroke center.[88] When a primary stroke center is not within a drivable distance, the options are to transport the patient to an acute stroke–ready hospital or to helicopter transport the patient from a nonspecialized stroke hospital to one that is. Optimal stroke care should be provided within an hour to a few hours of stroke onset. Primary stroke centers have hospital beds or a medical unit that specializes in stroke care. If more advanced care is needed, the patient may be transported to a thrombectomy-capable stroke center or a comprehensive stroke center. Both of these facilities have medical staff with extensive and continual training in the management and treatment of strokes.

Seizures

Historically, people with epilepsy were discouraged from participating in athletic events or adhering to rigorous exercise routines. This avoidance is no longer recommended. In fact, people with epilepsy are encouraged to participate in sports, because exercise may reduce the recovery time for a seizure and provides health benefits.[89] Safe participation depends on each person's seizure type and control of seizures, including recurrence rates and medication effectiveness.

TABLE 8.4   **Tasks and Responses to Identify a Stroke Before Transport**

Task/Instructions	Normal	Abnormal
Facial drop Have the patient smile.	Both sides of the face move symmetrically.	Movement is asymmetric.
Arm weakness Have the patient close the eyes and raise both arms straight out in front, and hold the position for 10 seconds.	Both arms move at the same time; or both arms do not move.	Movement is asymmetric.
Speech difficulty Have the patient say, "The sky is blue in Cincinnati" or another phrase that requires the patient to vocalize multiple sounds.	Correct words are said without slurring.	Patient says incorrect or slurred words; or patient is unable to speak.
Timeliness Recognition and treatment within 2 h of incident.		Promptly refer to primary stroke center.

Diagnostic values for the Cincinnati Prehospital Stroke Scale: sensitivity 59%-66%; specificity 87%-89%[86]

Incidence and Epidemiology

Seizures do not affect many people, and they account for 1% of ED visits.[90] Seizures are divided into 3 groups—general, focal, and unknown onset—described as follows:

- *General seizures,* including tonic-clonic, absence, and atonic seizures, affect both cerebral hemispheres and cause loss of awareness.[91,93]
- *Focal onset seizures* start in a specific area of the brain and can either occur with or without convulsions.
- *Unknown onset seizures* are unknown because they are not witnessed, they occur during sleep, or the part of the brain involved is not known.

Typically seizures last around 3 minutes, and they may occur in multiples referred to as clusters. Clusters of seizures may last minutes to an hour; the longer durations result in poor outcomes for the patient.

Seizures have numerous causes:

- Congenital seizure disorder, commonly referred to as epilepsy, can be controlled medicinally. If the patient skips a dose or stops taking the medicine, or if the dosage is not strong enough, the seizures may reappear.
- Provoked seizures have a direct trigger, which may be a variety of intrinsic or extrinsic mechanisms such as metabolic abnormalities, ingested toxins, infectious conditions, and inflammatory conditions.
- Metabolic abnormalities include hypoxia and **hypoglycemia**, which are the two leading reversible metabolic causes of seizures. The brain requires both glycogen and oxygen to function. When one or both are lacking, the brain is unable to function, resulting in impaired cognition. Hypoxia and hypoglycemia are often the result of other serious health conditions, therefore a thorough medical history and evaluation are essential to proper treatment and prevention strategies.
- Electrolyte abnormalities may also result in seizures. Severely deficient serum sodium concentrations, **hyponatremia**, can lead to confusion, lethargy, and gastrointestinal upset. If the imbalance goes untreated, seizures, altered mental status, or death may result. On the opposite end of serum sodium concentrations, **hypernatremia** can also lead to seizures.[91]
- Recreational, herbal, and prescription drugs can provoke seizures. Drug-induced seizures can result from inhibitory or excitatory pathways. Alcohol and benzodiazepine withdrawal have inhibitory effects on gamma-aminobutyric acid (GABA) receptors, while alcohol withdrawal has an excitatory effect on norepinephrine receptors, all of which can result in seizures. When taken in excess or abused, stimulants can initially cause mood changes, elevated blood pressure, and increased temperature. When the drug is continued or the symptoms not treated, seizures, altered mental status, and death may occur. Drug abuse and withdrawal are not the only causes of drug-associated seizures; antibiotics and analgesics may cause seizures as well. Penicillin, opiates, and salicylates in high doses can cause seizures, while tramadol can result in seizures in therapeutic doses.[91]
- While not common in adolescents or adults, **febrile** seizures are the result of abnormally high body temperatures. This condition is most often present in young children and infants. The seizure is not a medical emergency but warrants evaluation to determine the cause of the excessive body temperature. In athletic events, the body may also experience excessive body temperatures that may trigger a seizure in a person with epilepsy.[91] People with epilepsy who are exercising in hot and humid environments benefit from technological support such as heart rate monitors and ingestible thermistors.[89]

Risk Factors

Physical activities that have the greatest risk of serious injury or death related to a seizure event are nontraditional sporting events such as motorsports, surfing, and scuba diving. Platform and springboard diving, ski jumping, and rodeo are also high-risk events. Sports of low risk are most traditional athletic events such as softball or baseball, basketball, track and field (except pole vaulting), volleyball, and golf. Moderate-risk sports include weightlifting, swimming, cycling, and gymnastics.[92]

Signs and Symptoms

Depending on the type of seizure, the person will have various signs and symptoms as illustrated in table 8.5. Following a seizure, the patient will have a recovery period. The postictal state (state of altered consciousness) may include mental confusion, labored breathing, relaxed muscles, migraines, and emotional changes. More medically troubling presentations may include **hemiparesis**, postictal delirium, and postictal psychosis.[95] During the postictal state, the patient may become aggressive and irritated; the patient is unaware of the seizure event. Depending on the type of seizure, identifying the start and end of the ictal phase is difficult; symptoms may last longer than the electroencephalography (EEG) recording

TABLE 8.5   **Symptom Presentation for General, Focal, and Unknown-Onset Seizures**

	Motor symptoms	Nonmotor symptoms
Generalized onset	Rhythmic jerking (clonic) Limp or weak muscles (atonic) Rigid muscles (tonic) Twitching of muscles (myoclonic) Epileptic spasms	Typical absence Atypical absence Myoclonic
Focal onset	Rhythmic jerking (clonic) Limp or weak muscles (atonic) Rigid muscles (tonic) Twitching of muscles (myoclonic) Epileptic spasms Repeated movements (automatisms)	Change in sensations Change in emotions Change in cognition Hot/cold flashes Lack of movement (behavior arrest)
Unknown onset	Tonic-clonic Epileptic spasms	Behavior arrest

Based on Fisher et al. (2017); Epilepsy Foundation (2018).

of ictal activity, and some postictal symptoms last beyond the postictal state.[96]

Immediate Management Techniques

Initial emergency care for a seizure includes a primary survey of the scene and a secondary survey of the patient. The care for the patient will be determined by the patient's presentation. If the patient is choking, the appropriate steps should be taken to dislodge the obstruction. The patient may have elevated respiration and heart rates due to the stress response of the seizure. The body responds to the stress similar to other stressful physical events, such as an intense run. The patient's breathing and heart rate should return to a normal level within minutes. If the patient presents with convulsions, care should be provided to protect and support the airway and cervical spine, without bracing or restricting the movements. Recording the duration of the convulsions can help the advanced medical providers. If underlying conditions are noted, the treatment plan should address the conditions along with protecting the patient from seizure symptoms. The seizure presentation provides indications and contraindications to further treatment.

Indications

If the patient has epilepsy and the seizure presents in the expected pattern, no advanced medical care is required. However, if the patient does not have epilepsy, the seizures are long in duration or frequent, or if the seizure presentation has changed, advanced medical care is warranted.[97]

For some people, the advanced treatment may start with an emergency dose of diazepam, a muscle relaxer, administered rectally. Suppository diazepam prescriptions come with detailed and illustrated instructions, which should be reviewed by caregivers and responsible medical personnel upon filling the prescription to avoid confusion at the time of the emergency. A medical provider may give a second dose of diazepam suppository as prescribed 4 to 12 hours following the initial dose if deemed necessary.[98] Beyond the suppository form, a slow drip intravenous (IV) administration of diazepam may be prescribed.[99]

Contraindications

People with known drug allergies or responses to diazepam should not be given the suppository or the IV form of diazepam. Similarly, those with acute angle glaucoma should not be given diazepam.[98]

Procedures and Protocols

People with epilepsy who have long-duration or frequent seizures or seizures that change in presentation, or people who experience a seizure and do not have epilepsy should be transported for advanced medical care. If anticonvulsant or other medication is administered, the time, dose, and method of administration should be documented and provided to the advanced medical provider.

In the event that the seizure is long in duration, the patient may have decreased oxygen available to the lungs and body tissues, resulting in cyanosis. The longer the duration of the seizure, the worse the outcome; however, seizure duration can be reduced with prompt and appropriate care.[100] If the patient is hypoglycemic or hypoxic, the post-incident treatment should include a simple carbohydrate or oxygen administration, respectively. Hyponatremia-induced seizures should be treated with slow and controlled infusion of saline solution.[91] If sodium levels rise too quickly, a separate medical condition called **osmotic demyelination syndrome** may result.[91] In the event of exertional hyponatremia (discussed in chapter

15), intravenous fluids should not be administered so as to prevent further fluid/electrolyte imbalance.

Altered Mental Status

A person might experience altered mental status separate from a stroke or a seizure and require advanced medical care. Common causes and presentations of altered mental status are shown in table 8.6.

Incidence and Epidemiology

Cardiovascular and endocrine system abnormalities are two common causes of altered mental status. Recognizing the signs and symptoms of altered mental status and taking a thorough medical history can allow for adequate medical care. The causes of altered mental status vary, and not all are well understood. Patients may be irritable, disoriented, or have an inability to concentrate.

Syncope can occur due to various medical conditions. Syncope can be cardiac or neutrally mediated. When a person is hypotensive and the brain cannot get enough oxygen, the brain protects itself by causing loss of consciousness.[107] A change in body position can result in hypotension, specifically orthostatic hypotension, which typically occurs in people aged over 65 years.[108] Neurally mediated syncope can result from the body's mismanagement of stress. Neurally mediated syncope is the most common and does not typically warrant immediate medical attention.[109] The 3 types of neurally mediated syncope are vasovagal, situation-related, and carotid sinus syncope.[107,109]

Risk Factors

Cardiovascular syncope may present in people who have heart failure or abnormal sinus rhythms.[107] Cardiovascular syncopes have a 50% mortality and morbidity rate within 3 years after the initial event. The most common presyncopal symptoms mimic those of cardiovascular disease, such as chest pain, shortness of breath, and fatigue. Intense activity and stress along with a cardiovascular disruption precede the syncopal event.[109] Immediate medical attention is needed for a person who has a known cardiovascular condition and a syncopal event.

Field Assessment Techniques

Body temperature, blood glucose, and blood pressure measures are quick and effective assessments that can aid in the differential diagnosis of what is causing the altered mental status.

Immediate Management Techniques

Monitoring of vitals and referral to advanced medical personnel are essential for most incidences of altered mental status; some specific management techniques are presented in table 8.7.

Overview of Facial Injuries

Current estimates place facial injury representation in sport anywhere from 4% to 41% of injuries seen in

TABLE 8.6   Descriptions and Patient Presentation for Causes of Altered Mental Status

Cause	Description	Patient presentation
Adrenal insufficiency[101]	Decreased cortisol and aldosterone	Drastic change from depression to psychosis/coma, salt craving, hyperpigmentation, hyponatremia, hypercalcemia, GI distress, fatigue
Diabetic ketoacidosis [101]	Blood glucose levels >250 mg/dL Blood pH <7.35 Ketonemia/heavy ketonuria[102]	Dehydration, tachycardia, hypotension, Kussmaul respirations, lethargy, coma
Hypertensive emergency [103]	Systolic pressure >180 mm Hg Diastolic pressure >120 mm Hg	Chest pain, shortness of breath, vision changes, weakness/lack of coordination
Hypoglycemia [101]	Decreased blood glucose levels (<70 mg/dL)[104]	Diaphoresis, irritability, tremors, paralysis, seizure, coma
Hypothermia [105]	Body temperature <35°C	Cyanotic, shivering, abnormal respirations, slurred speech
Myxedema coma [101]	Severe hypothyroidism	Thyroidectomy scar, hypothermia, minimal deep tendon reflexes, dry skin, signs of heart failure
Orthostatic hypotension[106]	Rapid decrease in blood pressure upon sitting or standing	Syncope or near syncope

TABLE 8.7 **Management of Altered Mental Status**

Condition	Acute/emergent care	Clinical and laboratory tests	Referral
Adrenal insufficiency[110,111]	Hydrocortisone 100 mg injection Intravenous infusion of 1,000 mL isotonic saline	Corticotropin test, blood tests	Immediately to endocrinologist
Diabetic ketoacidosis[106]	500 mL/h of 0.9% saline for 4 h 0.1 unit/kg/h of insulin followed by potassium supplementation	Blood glucose, urinalysis, blood potassium	Immediately to diabetic specialist
Hypertensive emergency[112]	Dependent on the comorbidities: • Acute aortic dissection—beta blocker • Acute pulmonary edema—nitroglycerin • Myocardial infarction—beta blocker or nitroglycerin • Unstable angina pectoris—beta blocker or nitroglycerin	Electrocardiogram, complete blood count, urinalysis, radiographs	Immediately to cardiologist
Hypoglycemia[113]	15-20 g glucose	Blood glucose	If blood glucose level fails to rise after initial glucose treatment or the individual is unconscious
Hypothermia[114]	15-20 g glucose Thiamine Removal of wet clothing 30- to 45-sec minimum pulse assessment Passive or active rewarming dependent on level of thermoregulatory function	Renal function, blood glucose, Doppler ultrasound, electrocardiogram (ECG)	If cardiac or other complications exist
Myxedema coma[115]	Ventilatory support	ECG, renal function, thyroid function	Immediately to critical care specialist, cardiologist, and endocrinologist
Orthostatic hypotension[108]	Basic body movements (supervised): Stand with legs crossed Squat Upper-body isometrics	Metabolic profile, complete blood count, echocardiogram, ECG	Refer to cardiologist (nonemergent)

emergency facilities. However, a small number of epidemiological studies exist related to facial injury in sport, and injury rate estimates are complicated by inconsistent reporting on specific injury types, differing reporting levels within each study, and the varied types of injuries that exist.[115] In addition, facial injury definitions vary greatly across studies, highlighting the need for consistency in order to better understand the epidemiology and prevention effectiveness.

Much like head injuries, injuries to the face can range from mild to severe. Traumatic assessment of the face follows the same pattern as with other injuries. An assessment of mental status, including alertness and level of responsiveness, should begin the evaluation. Unconsciousness, unresponsiveness, or mental status changes may indicate the presence of TBI. Checking for an adequate airway, breathing, and circulation follows the mental status assessment. In some instances, an oral airway may be necessary to ensure maintenance of a patent airway (see chapter 10). Controlling facial hemorrhage with direct pressure and dressings is considered mainstay treatment.[117] A secondary survey to determine the presence of underlying injuries should follow the primary survey.

Corneal Abrasion and Foreign Objects in the Eye

Corneal abrasions (scratches on the eye) occur when the epithelium of the eye's surface is injured. Foreign objects can cause a significant amount of damage to the eye. Once an object enters the eye, the conjunctiva becomes inflamed and red (conjunctivitis), and tear production begins as a means of flushing the eye of the object. If the object is irritating enough to cause corneal abrasion, intense pain can occur, making it challenging for patients to keep the eyelid open.

Following blunt trauma to the head, the eye may exhibit signs indicative of a closed head injury. If any signs are observed, the time should be recorded in addition to the sign itself. If the patient is unconscious, cover the eyelids with moist gauze or hold them closed with clear tape to limit the amount of dryness.

Blunt trauma may cause movement of a contact lens. In such cases, avoid manipulating or removing the lens, because additional damage could result. An exception is in cases of chemical burns. In such cases, the contact lens can trap the chemical and make irrigation of the eye difficult. Any suspected chemical burns should be irrigated immediately, preferably with sterile saline, for a minimum of 5 minutes. An irrigation syringe should be used; if one is not available, you may pour water directly into the eye.

Incidence and Epidemiology

In the United States, baseball produces the most eye injuries,[118,119] while soccer tops the list in England.[120] Other sports with the potential for serious eye injury include softball, basketball, ice hockey, field hockey, and lacrosse. Epidemiological data indicate more than 120,000 patients in the United States were treated for sports-related ocular trauma in EDs from 2011 to 2013.[121] Regardless of the type of sport played, blunt trauma, penetrating trauma, and corneal abrasions represent the most common types of ocular injuries.

Risk Factors

Corneal abrasion risk factors include decreased tear production, inability to adequately close the eye, extended wear of contact lenses, and occupational exposure to foreign objects, such as is encountered in a sports environment. Prevention efforts are aimed at educating the patient regarding protective eyewear, which is composed of a polycarbonate, high-impact–resistant plastic lens and is available with or without a prescription.[122]

Signs and Symptoms

Because of the abundance of sensory nerve fibers located on the surface of the eye, corneal abrasions are an exceptionally painful ocular injury. Other symptomology includes blurred vision, sensation of a foreign body in the eye (absent a foreign body as the MOI), and tearing. Photophobia (light sensitivity) may also create difficulty with opening the eye.

Immediate Management Techniques

Irrigate the eye with normal saline, flushing from the nose to the outward edge of the eye to avoid flushing the material into the unaffected eye. Assess extraocular motion, pupillary reaction, and visual acuity. Patients may still experience pain once the debris is removed, usually due to abrasion of the corneal surface. If irrigation is not effective, the foreign body may be stuck to the corneal surface or lodged under the upper eyelid. You should not attempt to remove an object stuck to the cornea. If the foreign object impales the eye it should be left in place, but it needs to be stabilized prior to transport. Bandage the object; cover the eye itself with a moist, sterile dressing, and use a gauze roll to create a ring to place over the eye and the impaled object (figure 8.9). Diagnosis of a corneal abrasion is typically made using a blue-light slit lamp once the eye's surface has been stained with fluorescein, an orange-yellow dye.[123]

Penetrating trauma can cause lacerations to the eye. If a laceration is suspected, no direct pressure should be placed on the eye, because it could interfere with the blood supply to the eye or cause further damage. If a portion of the eyeball is exposed or protruding from the orbit, cover it with a moist, sterile dressing to prevent

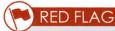
RED FLAG

Possible ocular indicators of closed head injury include the following:

- Anisocoria (unequal pupil size; <3 mm)
- Unequal movement
- Unequal alignment; differing directions
- Inability to follow finger motion
- Bleeding under conjunctiva that obscures the sclera (white portion)
- Protrusion or bulging

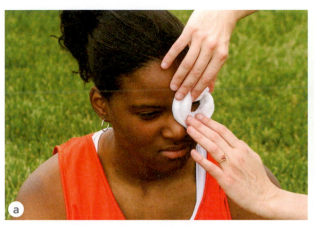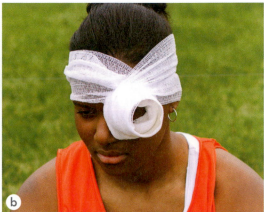

FIGURE 8.9   First aid care for embedded objects in the eye includes *(a)* loosely applying donut-shaped gauze padding around the eye and *(b)* putting a paper cup securely in place with roller gauze and tape.

dryness. Encourage the patient to lie supine during transport and consider covering both eyes so as to avoid unnecessary movement.

Retinal Detachment

The retina is a thin layer of tissue lining the back of the eye. As light enters the eye, it is focused on the retina by the cornea and lens and then transmitted to the brain via the optic nerve. Although retinal trauma does not occur as often in sport when compared with other eye injuries, it is still considered a consequence of sport-related injury.[119]

Incidence and Epidemiology

History of traumatic retinal detachment in children and adolescents has been reported at 61.5%, with age-related annual incidence of 2.9 per 100,000 in those aged 10 to 19.[124] The etiology of retinal detachment may be related to the structure of the eye. Nontraumatic detachment is attributable to myopia in the majority of cases (55%).[125]

Signs and Symptoms

Signs and symptoms of retinal detachment include the appearance of a shadow or curtain falling over the visual

CLINICAL SKILLS

Removal of Foreign Object Under the Upper Eyelid

1. Instruct the patient to look down.
2. Place a cotton-tipped applicator across the outer surface of the eyelid *(a)*.
3. Gently pull the eyelid forward and up, causing it to fold back over applicator and exposing the underside of the eyelid *(b)*.
4. Upon visualization, if an object is seen, remove it with a moistened (using sterile saline solution), sterile, cotton-tipped applicator or gauze pad *(c)*.

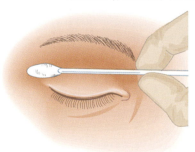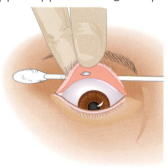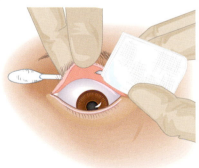

a   *b*   *c*

FIGURE 8.10

field, an increase in the number of floaters in the visual field (e.g., dark spots or strands), and abnormal flashes of light in the peripheral vision. Floaters are caused by solidifications in the vitreous humor, a gel-like substance attached to the retina. Flashes of light are caused by the vitreous humor pulling on the retina. Although retinal detachment can occur spontaneously, in the case of sport-related retinal detachment, a blunt traumatic MOI is common.

Immediate Management Techniques

A patient experiencing symptoms of retinal detachment should be immediately referred to an ophthalmologist for further evaluation. Due to the likelihood of retinal surgery, patients should not consume fluids or solid foods. Avoid pressure and minimize eye movement; the globe of the eye can be protected as previously mentioned in cases with associated trauma.

Hyphema

Blunt trauma to the eye can cause several injuries. Hyphema, or bleeding into the anterior chamber of the eye (figure 8.11), can cause difficulty with visualizing the iris. Hyphema may indicate more serious globe (eye) injury. Blunt trauma can also cause orbital fractures, discussed in further detail later in the chapter. Associated causes of hyphema are attributable to sports-related trauma, falls, eye infection, blood clotting disorders (including sickle cell anemia), artificial lens implants, and cancers of the eye.[126]

Signs and Symptoms

Hyphemas present with pain and discomfort. The obvious sign of hyphema is the visualization of blood in the anterior chamber, although it may not be possible if the

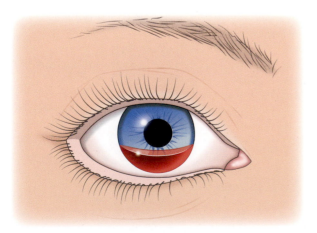

FIGURE 8.11 Hyphema.

hyphema is small. Patients may also struggle with vision impairment (cloudiness or blurriness) and photophobia.

Immediate Management Techniques

An eye shield can be placed over the injured eye to avoid further damage. If the patient is comfortable, the other eye should be covered to minimize movement of the injured eye. Upon referral, visual acuity, eye pressure checks, and examination of the eye using a slit lamp are generally performed.

Tympanic Membrane Rupture

Blunt, traumatic soft tissue injuries of the ear occur during participation in sports such as boxing and wrestling. One such injury is ruptured tympanic membrane, or a perforated eardrum. A tympanic membrane rupture occurs when the thin tissue separating the ear canal from the eardrum is torn.

Incidence and Epidemiology

Potential causes and associated risk factors for tympanic membrane rupture include current ear infection, previous history of rupture, ear surgery (commonly for tubes in the canal), scuba diving (due to increased pressure), traumatic ear injury, and insertion of objects (e.g., cotton swab) into the ear. Incidence of tympanic membrane perforation in the general population is unknown as of this writing.

Signs and Symptoms

Symptomology of tympanic membrane rupture includes pain following popping of the ear, loss of hearing, tinnitus, dizziness, and presence of fluid (e.g., watery pus or blood) in the canal. A patient with a suspected tympanic membrane rupture should be immediately referred to a physician.[127] In some cases, the wound may heal on its own. In others, surgical intervention is indicated. Antibiotics may be used to clear up any preexisting infections that may have initially led to the rupture. In the military patient, tympanic membrane perforation may be indicative of mild TBI or concussion.[128]

Immediate Management Techniques

The pinna and auricle of the ear should be visually inspected with an otoscope for defect, hemorrhage, swelling, and ecchymosis. Performing an assessment of auditory and vestibular function is also indicated. Excessive pain and swelling, significant auditory disturbances, uncontrolled hemorrhage, and suspected tympanic membrane ruptures require referral for additional treatment.

Patients should be instructed to avoid over-the-counter eardrops and to avoid blowing the nose as much as possible to limit pressure buildup.

Facial Fractures

The facial orbit consists of 7 bones: frontal, sphenoid, palatine, zygoma, maxilla, lacrimal, and ethmoid (see figure 8.1). Due to its thinness, the most frequent site of orbital fracture is the inferior margin, formed by the zygoma and maxilla. These combination fractures are known as tripod fractures. Orbital floor fractures, also known as **blowout fractures**, may result in entrapment of the inferior rectus muscle, leading to an inability of the eye to look upward (figure 8.12).

Maxillary fractures are were first described by René Le Fort and thus are termed Le Fort fractures.[129] Le Fort fractures are classified from I to III based on the location of the fracture site (figure 8.13).

- *Type I* fractures occur in the maxilla and separate the teeth from the upper face.

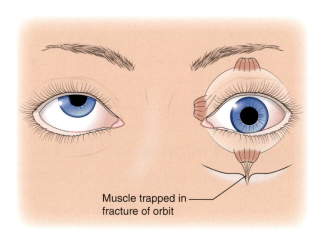

FIGURE 8.12 Blowout fracture.

- *Type II* fractures are pyramidal in nature, affecting the upper teeth, maxillary sinuses, inferior orbital rim, and nasal bones.
- *Type III* fractures include the nasofrontal suture, maxillofrontal suture, orbital wall, and zygomatic arch.

Mandibular fractures occur most commonly at or just below the condyle and can present with **malocclusion**. In addition, 50% of mandible fractures are multiple; therefore, the presence of one fracture necessitates evaluation for additional fracture sites.[130]

Incidence and Epidemiology

Facial fractures in sport can occur for a variety of reasons, including contact with equipment, contact with other participants, and contact with the environment. It is estimated that approximately 4% to 18% of all sports injuries are related to facial fracture.[130] Facial fractures may be associated with head and cervical spine injuries, necessitating a proper assessment. Blowout fractures are common in sports such as baseball, softball, hockey, and lacrosse, where the likelihood of a high-impact injury to the orbital rim is likely.[131]

Risk Factors

The main risk factor for mandibular fractures and multiple facial bone fractures is participation in sports, followed by motorcycle accident. Zygomatic and nasal fractures are predominantly associated with animal accidents and sports trauma.[132] Although medical literature indicates that nasal fractures represent the most common type of facial fracture, the statistics may or may not be accurate given lack of patient reporting. It is likely that the thinness of the nasal area contributes to the ease of fracture at that site. Sports that represent a higher associated risk include those with high-velocity smaller projectiles.

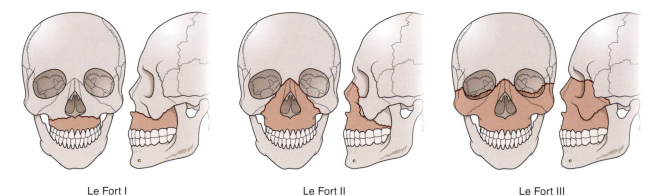

Le Fort I   Le Fort II   Le Fort III

FIGURE 8.13 Le Fort fractures.

Signs and Symptoms

Common signs and symptoms of facial fractures may differ based on location. General signs and symptoms include difficulty breathing or speaking, blurred or double vision, numbness, pain, and malocclusion. With a blowout fracture, patients may have a difficulty or inability to look upward when ocular motion is assessed.

Immediate Management Techniques

First, protect the airway by removing any foreign bodies and by placing the patient in a sitting position. If severe maxillofacial trauma is present, the athlete is at risk for airway obstruction because of a lack of tongue support from the mandibular structures. Second, assess the athlete for breathing and circulation. Lastly, consider immobilization of the cervical spine. Following initial stabilization, address symptomology and transport.

Temporomandibular Joint Dislocation

Temporomandibular joint (TMJ) dislocation can be unilateral or bilateral as well as chronic or acute. Dislocation involves the disarticulation of the mandibular condyle and the temporal bone. Anterior dislocation is most common; others, including posterior, are mostly associated with trauma.[133]

Incidence and Epidemiology

Dislocation of the TMJ is related to structural deficits (e.g., arthritis, dental age) or neuromuscular dysfunction (e.g., capsular or ligamentous laxity, muscle spasm).[133] Other causes include forceful yawning or laughing, excessive or prolonged vomiting, seizures, and dental work. The condition has also been associated with facial dystonia and Marfan syndrome.

Signs and Symptoms

The most common clinical sign of TMJ is an inability to close the mouth, often called open lock. Other symptoms include pain, speech difficulty, and drooling. TMJ dislocation can present with malocclusion, as can a mandibular fracture.

Immediate Management Techniques

To differentiate between a true TMJ injury and a mandibular injury, the HCP should insert both index fingers into the mouth, place them on the interior border of the mandible, and press outward. Pain and movement of the mandible itself may indicate the presence of a fracture. Pain only at the TMJ may indicate the presence of a dislocation. Lateral movement of the jaw may reduce the dislocation, but referral to a physician is still indicated. Depending on severity, return to activity with the protection of a mouth guard could take place within 2 to 4 weeks.[134]

Dental Injuries

Contact with other players, sports equipment, and surfaces, as well as falls and collisions, often result in traumatic dental injuries in sport. If properly fitted, mouth guards and protective equipment may help minimize injury incidence. However, such incidences cannot be eliminated, so it is important for HCPs to understand what injuries might occur and how to manage such injuries.

Immediate Management Techniques

The incorporation of management guidelines into an EAP is recommended in the position statement as well due to the time-critical nature and prognosis of dental injuries. The NATA provides recommendations regarding acute management of dental trauma (table 8.8).[135] In addition to traditional first aid items such as a Save-A-Tooth kit, a dental diagnostic aid such as an emergency treatment card should be included in a field kit.[138]

Laryngeal Injuries

Laryngeal injuries occur to the voice box (larynx), the upper portion of the airway. The range of laryngeal trauma can include minor injury such as vocal cord weakness, and major injury such as cartilaginous fracture of the larynx or trachea. Sports-related laryngeal injuries can occur even in the presence of protective equipment. Although they are relatively uncommon, life-threatening conditions can result.

Incidence and Epidemiology

The incidence of laryngeal fracture is rare, occurring only in 1 in 30,000 patients.[136] Consequently, many laryngeal fractures are undiagnosed or poorly managed.[136] The mortality rate for laryngeal trauma is approximately 17.9%.[137]

Risk Factors

Because of the position of the larynx in children, younger patients are more susceptible to soft tissue–related injuries than fractures. Blunt or penetrating neck trauma is

TABLE 8.8 Dental and Oral Injury Classification and Acute Care

Injury classification	Injury name	Signs and symptoms	Dental emergency?	Referral and return to activity (RTA)	Immediate treatment
Tooth fractures	Crown infraction	Craze lines (small enamel cracks)	No	Delayed referral; immediate RTA with mouth guard	Craze lines may be identified via transillumination.
	Enamel-only crown fracture	Roughness along crown	No	Delayed referral; immediate RTA with mouth guard	N/A
	Enamel-dentin crown fracture	Air, cold, touch sensitivity	No	Referral within 24 h; RTA as pain permits with mouth guard	If located, place tooth in water, saline, or milk, and send with patient to dentist.
	Enamel-dentin pulp fracture	Pulp is vital: focal bleeding in yellow dentin; constant, piercing, or throbbing pain Pulp not vital: foul odor; pus; no pain	No	If acute pain and hemorrhage, immediate referral to trauma dentist. If not present, refer within 24 h and RTA as pain permits with mouth guard.	If located, place tooth in water, saline, or milk, and send with patient to dentist.
Root fractures—verified only with X-ray	Apical third	Not definitive	No	Referral can be postponed; immediate RTA with mouth guard.	Frequently undetected due to minimal mobility and absence of pain.
	Middle third	Elongated appearance when compared to adjacent teeth	No	Referral within 24 h; RTA as pain permits with mouth guard; discontinue play if tooth is loose.	If displaced, may reposition with finger pressure. Patient may bite down on sterile gauze to prevent further displacement.
	Cervical third	Crown dangling from lacerated gingival tissue	No	Referral within 24 h; RTA as pain permits with mouth guard; discontinue play if tooth is loose.	Clean area with water or saline; reposition tooth. Patient should bite down on sterile gauze to prevent further displacement.
Tooth displacement	Tooth concussion and subluxation	Concussion: no fracture or displacement Subluxation: minimal blood around gingival sulcus	No	Referral can be postponed for up to 24 h; immediate RTA.	Concussion: dentist should observe for any clinical/radiographic changes periodically. Subluxation: warm salt water rinses if tender.
	Lateral and extrusive lacerations	Marked displacement and misalignment	Yes	Immediate removal from participation and referral to trauma dentist or emergency facility	Reposition within socket using finger pressure. Patient should bite down on sterile gauze to stabilize tooth for transport.

> continued

Table 8.8   > *continued*

Injury classification	Injury name	Signs and symptoms	Dental emergency?	Referral and return to activity (RTA)	Immediate treatment
	Intrusive luxation	Forced into socket in an axial direction	Yes	Immediate removal from participation and referral to trauma dentist or emergency facility	Depending on root maturity (requires X-ray), patient may require root canal.
	Avulsion-exarticulated	Complete removal from socket	Yes	Immediate removal from participation and referral to trauma dentist or emergency facility	If patient is alert and oriented and sterility is not an issue, attempt replantation by inserting root end into cavity and orient by comparing with adjacent teeth; should occur within 5 minutes. Do not handle root, brush or scrub away debris, or sterilize. If visible debris, gently rinse with cold water, milk, or saline for 10 seconds. Once replanted, patient should bite down on sterile gauze to stabilize for transport. If unable to replant, submerge tooth in Hanks' Balanced Salt Solution, a Save-A-Tooth kit, or cold low-fat milk. Do not wrap in dry gauze or paper towel.

Adapted from Gould et al. (2016).

the typical MOI; and the voice, airway, and esophagus are potential at-risk areas. Low-impact trauma may cause abrasions, edema, or contusion.[1]

Signs and Symptoms

Common symptoms and signs of laryngeal trauma include hoarseness, stridor, dyspnea, **hemoptysis**, **dysphonia**, respiratory distress, anterior neck tenderness, and **subcutaneous emphysema**.[1] Symptoms may not manifest right away; patients should undergo serial assessment to ensure continued monitoring post-injury. The most common long-term complication of laryngeal injury is dysphonia with hoarseness, poor vocal control, and voice fatigue.[139]

Immediate Management Techniques

The initial goal of injury management should be the maintenance of a patent airway. The jaw-thrust maneuver should be used in caring for the cervical spine (see figure 9.9).

Cervical spine tenderness and pain should be treated as a cervical spinal injury, with manual in-line stabilization while the patient is supine. Patients with significant trauma should be immediately referred to an emergency facility. Depending on the injury, typical treatment may include observation for signs of airway compromise, the application of ice if soft-tissue injury is sustained, vocal rest to minimize hoarseness and bleeding, the use of humidified air, and a clear liquid diet.[1]

Summary

Traumatic injuries to the head and face are often associated with sport-related activities. Because these injuries are potentially serious, patients often need immediate medical care. Presented in this chapter were common traumatic conditions in sport (e.g., concussions and lacerations), rare conditions (e.g., strokes and laryngeal injuries), as well as recommendations for acute care and management to assist HCPs in making treatment decisions.

 Go to the web study guide to complete the case studies for this chapter.

CHAPTER 9

Traumatic Injuries to the Spine

Laura Zdziarski-Horodyski, PhD, LAT, ATC
Dewayne DuBose, PhD, ATC, LAT, NCPT

OBJECTIVES

After reading this chapter, you will be able to do the following:

- Identify signs and symptoms indicative of a spine injury.

- Assess and determine when it is appropriate to use spinal motion restriction procedures.

- Explain the importance of collaborating with other emergency medical personnel prior to an emergency occurring.

- Design a spinal motion restriction protocol based on your institution's setting and resources.

- Implement the proper care procedures for a patient with a spine injury based on signs, symptoms, and current research evidence.

The incidence of spinal cord injury (SCI) in the United States between 2014 and 2017 rose from 12,500 new cases to about 17,500 annually.[1,2] The percentage attributed to sports participation has remained consistent at 9% of all new SCIs.[1] More than 460,000 NCAA student athletes and 7.96 million high school athletes participate in sports, and it is unclear exactly how many youth (younger than high school or participating outside of varsity athletics) athletes participate annually.[3,4] Proper prehospital management and care of SCIs is critical in reducing and preventing further injury to the patient. It is the responsibility of the sports medicine team, athletic trainer (AT), team physician, paramedics, emergency medical technicians, and other specialty health care providers (HCPs) to be prepared when a spine injury occurs.

Anatomy and Physiology of the Spine

The human spine is a fascinating and elaborate central communication channel to one of the most important organs in the body, the brain. In fact, with all of the ancillary nerves, the spine serves as the main communication pathway between the central and peripheral nervous systems. Protection of this communication channel is critical to survival. Fortunately, the human body has several defense mechanisms in place to mitigate the impact of injury. The next section discusses these systems as well as scenarios of when protective mechanisms fail and injury may result.

Skeletal System

The vertebral column functions as axial support for the body from the occiput to the pelvis, and as protection for the spinal cord. When a fetus is forming, the body initially has 33 individual vertebrae. Throughout gestation, 8 or 9 vertebrae begin to fuse to form the sacrum and coccyx; the sacrum and coccyx do not become fully fused until later in life. Once adulthood is reached, 24 individual vertebrae remain, 5 fused vertebrae at the sacrum and 5 fused vertebrae at the coccyx.[5]

Regions of the Vertebral Column

The vertebral column has 5 distinct regions—cervical, thoracic, lumbar, sacral, and the coccyx (figure 9.1). The cervical region is made up of 7 vertebrae (C1-C7). Cervical vertebrae 1 and 2 have specialized names, the **atlas** and **dens** (figure 9.2), respectively. The cervical region has a concave curve (cervical lordosis) from C1-C7. Cervical lordosis allows the cervical spine to properly absorb forces during locomotion and other activities. The thoracic region consists of 12 vertebrae (T1-T12). The thoracic vertebrae align to form a kyphotic curve. The third region of the vertebral column is the lumbar region, which contains 5 vertebrae (L1-L5) in a concave S-shaped curve.[5] As stated previously, the sacrum and coccyx are regions of the vertebral column that contain fused vertebrae, making these 2 regions distinct from the 3 previously described regions. Furthermore, the sacrum

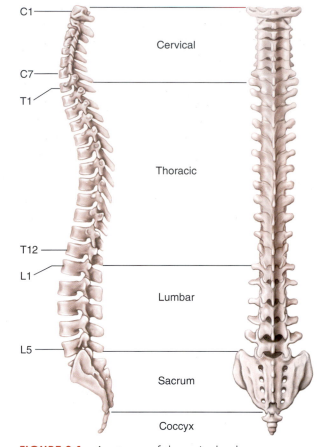

FIGURE 9.1   Anatomy of the spinal column.

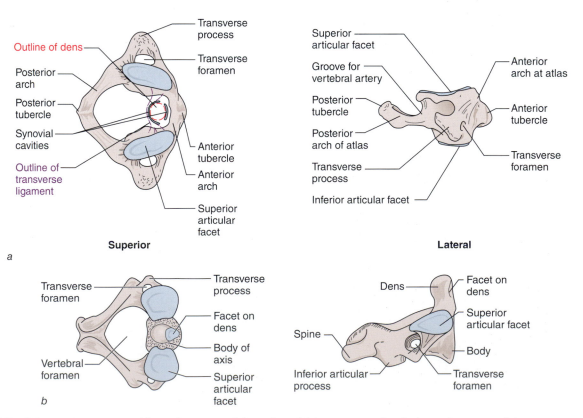

FIGURE 9.2   (a) Superior and lateral aspect of the atlas. (b) Superior and right lateral aspect of the axis.

and coccyx are equally different. The sacrum typically contains 5 vertebrae that begin to fuse at 4 years and are not completely fused and ossified until ages 14 to 25. The number of vertebral segments in the coccyx is much more varied within the population, with around 54% having 3 segments. Unlike the sacrum, the coccyx does not initiate the fusing process until just after birth and may not fully become fused until age 30.[6]

General Structure of Vertebrae

The anterior portion of a vertebra is disc shaped and referred to as the body. The exception to this description

is C1 and C2, which do not have a true vertebral body.[5] The bodies of all other vertebrae increase in size as you move down the spinal column; L5 has the largest vertebral body. On the posterior side of each vertebra, 2 laminae come together to form a spinous process. The spinous process is the attachment site for various muscles and ligaments.[5,7] One transverse process protrudes laterally on each side of the vertebra and is also an attachment site for muscles and ligaments. Also on the lateral side of the vertebra are the inferior and superior vertebral notches (figure 9.3). When viewing the entire spinal column, the inferior vertebral notch of a superior vertebra and the

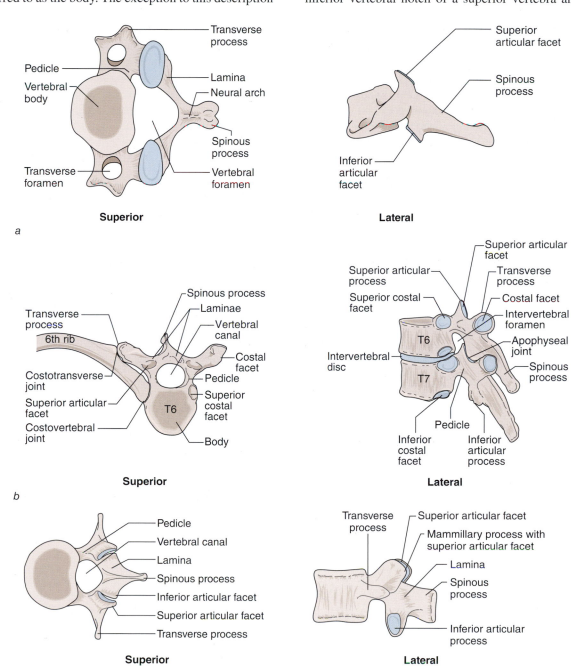

FIGURE 9.3   (a) Cervical, (b) thoracic, and (c) lumbar vertebrae.

superior vertebral notch of an inferior vertebra form an intervertebral foramen, through which spinal nerves exit the vertebral column. Articular facets on the superior and inferior aspects of each vertebra serve as joining points for the vertebra above and below an individual vertebra. In the center of each vertebra is the vertebral foramen, which is the canal for the spinal cord to traverse the spinal column.[5,7] The transverse foramina of C1-C7 contain the vertebral arteries.[5]

The atlas (C1) is ring shaped and does not have a vertebral body. It is the widest of the cervical vertebrae, because it has to distribute the weight of the head. The occipital condyles (occipital bone) articulate with the superior articular facets on the lateral sides of the atlas. C1 also lacks a spinous process. The atlas articulates with the odontoid processes (dens) of the **axis** (C2), allowing for rotational and pivoting movement of the skull.[5,7]

While they have vertebrae, the sacrum and coccyx do not fit the description of the general vertebral structure. The 5 fused vertebrae within the sacrum can be palpated based on median sacral crest. The median sacral crest is formed by the spinous processes aligning when the sacral vertebrae fuse. The sacrum itself is triangular in shape and provides the main articulation points for the pelvic

bones to the axial skeleton. Similar to the vertebral canal, the sacrum contains the sacral canal, and it provides bony protection to the sacral nerves. The coccygeal vertebrae form a triangular shape, and only the first vertebra is considered to have defined bony landmarks. The size, shape, and position of both the sacrum and coccyx are distinct between sexes. Differences in other segments of the vertebral column are not as prominent but can be observed.

Soft Tissue Structures

Several soft tissue structures provide stability to the vertebral column (figure 9.4). The anterior longitudinal ligament is a wide, broad band that originates on the pelvis and inserts at the anterior tubercle of C1 and the occipital bone anterior to the foramen magnum. The ligament attaches the anterior aspects of the vertebral bodies together and prevents hyperextension of the vertebral column. The posterior longitudinal ligament is narrower and weaker than the anterior longitudinal ligament. The posterior longitudinal ligament is located inside the vertebral canal along the vertebral bodies. The ligament originates at C2, inserts at the sacrum, and attaches the posterior edges of the vertebral bodies and discs together.

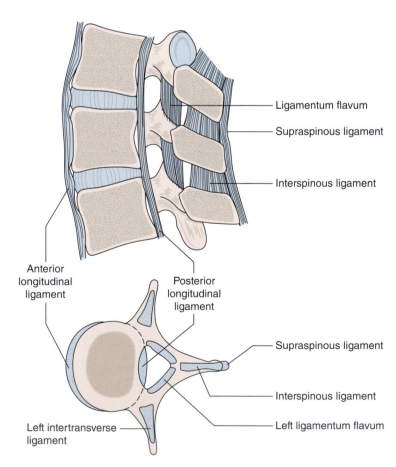

FIGURE 9.4 Ligaments of the vertebral column.

The function of the posterior longitudinal ligament is to prevent hyperflexion.[5,7]

Other accessory ligaments include the ligamentum flavum, a yellow band that attaches the lamina of a superior vertebra to the lamina of an inferior vertebra. It is elastic, preserves the natural curvature of the vertebral column, and assists with extension after flexion occurs. The interspinous ligaments connect adjoining spinous processes. The supraspinous ligaments attach the spinous processes from C7 to the sacrum.

Intervertebral discs are located between every unfused vertebra and act as a cushion and shock absorber during walking, running and jumping.[5,7] The C1-C2 segment is the only unfused vertebral interface that is not separated by a vertebral disc. The intervertebral discs are composed of 2 parts, the annulus fibrosus and nucleus pulposus (figure 9.5). The annulus fibrosus is a fibrocartilage structure forming a ring around the nucleus pulposus. The annulus fibrosus functions to limit the expansion of the nucleus pulposus when the vertebral column is compressed.[7] The nucleus pulposus is a soft, gelatinous core composed of elastic fibers. Throughout the day and with aging, the nucleus pulposus loses some of its water content and gradually becomes harder. The structural composition of the intervertebral discs plays an important role in the biomechanics of the spine and can become more of hindrance to movement and function as people age.

Nervous System

The nervous system can be divided into 2 subunits, the central and peripheral nervous systems. The central nervous system (CNS) contains the brain and the spinal cord, while peripheral nervous system (PNS) encompasses everything outside of the brain and spinal cord. The nervous system is a 2-way conduction pathway that sends sensory information from the periphery to the brain or spinal cord; then in return, the CNS sends motor response information from the center to the periphery.[5,7] Many of the neural responses or actions that occur within the human body occur without conscious thought or awareness. The nervous system is a complex and highly sophisticated network of tissue that requires the utmost care and protection.

The spinal cord travels through the spinal canal of the vertebral column from the foramen magnum to L1 or L2 (figure 9.6). The end of the actual cordlike structure is called the **conus medullaris**. Once past L1 or L2, the spinal cord branches out into the **cauda equina**, which is a collection of lumbar and sacral nerve roots that travel within the canal to reach the corresponding intervertebral foramina. Thirty-one pairs of spinal nerves branch off the spinal cord and travel out of the vertebral column by way of the intervertebral foramina (cervical—8 pairs, thoracic—12 pairs, lumbar—5 pairs, sacral—5 pairs, coccygeal—1 pair). The spinal nerves branch from the spinal cord by a **ventral root** and **dorsal root**. The dorsal

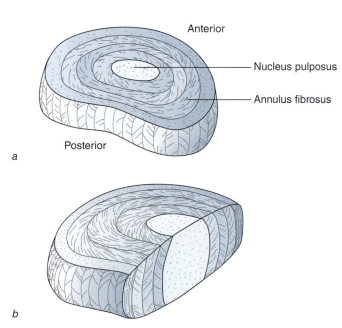

a

b

FIGURE 9.5 Intervertebral disc.

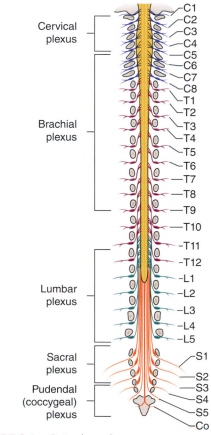

FIGURE 9.6 Spinal cord.

root is responsible for carrying the sensory nerve signal to the spinal cord, while the ventral root carries the motor nerve signal away from the spinal cord. The cervical and lumbar enlargements in the spinal cord give rise to upper- and lower-limb neurological functions, respectively.[5,7]

The spinal cord has distinct features as it descends from the cervical region to the sacral region. In the cervical and lumbar regions, the spinal cord has enlargements. The cervical enlargement contains nerves that control the upper limbs, while the lumbar enlargement contains nerves that control the lower limbs. Another feature of the spinal cord is the network of nerves called nerve plexuses. Originating off the ventral rami, these plexuses can be found in the cervical, brachial, lumbar, and sacral regions and serve the limbs of the body in those regions. Muscles in the limbs can be innervated by multiple branches of a specific plexus, which decreases the chance of paralysis if a single nerve is destroyed.[7]

Pathophysiology

Although infrequent, injuries to the spine are often catastrophic. As of 2017, 46% of all people who sustained a SCI (irrespective of injury mechanism) had a neurologic injury of incomplete **tetraplegia**.[1] Multiple biomechanical forces can lead to an injury of the spinal cord. While people typically associate spine injuries with American football during tackling, similar biomechanical forces can occur in other sports such as gymnastics, cheerleading, lacrosse, wrestling, diving, cycling or motocross, and any other sport with the potential for forceful contact.[8] These biomechanical forces can disrupt bony and soft tissue structures in the spine, which can lead to a decrease in space available for the cord (**SAC**). The decreased SAC can result in neurologic injury as well as other vascular responses.

Common Mechanisms of Spine Injury

One of the most frequently studied mechanisms of injury (MOIs) is the compression force caused by axial loading, which leads to buckling or burst fractures of the vertebrae.[9] Forced flexion caused by a decelerating force can cause fractures and subluxations of the vertebrae.[10] Tension-loading forces on the spine may lead to damaged intervertebral discs, joint capsule tears, and fractures to the vertebral column. Horizontal shearing forces are known to cause injuries to transverse ligaments and odontoid fractures.[9]

Compression forces usually occur during axial loading through the crown of the head, such as when a football player leads with the head while making a tackle (spearing) or a diver dives into the water.[8,10-12] During these activities, the head moves from the neutral position to a slightly flexed position that decreases the natural cervical lordosis (figure 9.7). In the slightly flexed position, the spine becomes a rigid segmented column, which causes the compression force to be transmitted down the vertical axis of the spine.[11] Once the musculature and intervertebral disc absorb the their maximum forces, the continued axial loading causes a buckling of the bony structures in the spine.[10] This action is known as the **buckling effect**, which can lead to cervical spine injuries. Another way to describe the buckling effect is when the axial loading

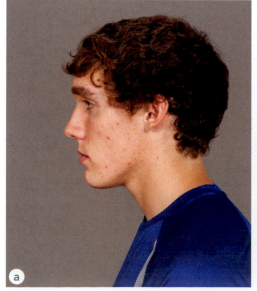
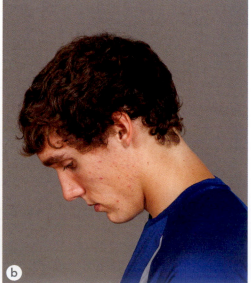

FIGURE 9.7   Axial loading: *(a)* neutral position and *(b)* cervical flexion.

forces the superior vertebra into either flexion or extension, then the inferior vertebra moves in the opposite direction of the superior vertebra. That buckling occurs down the spinal column until the axial forces dissipate.[13,14] When this buckling occurs, the bone structures in the spine go through large angulations in order to reduce the extra strain on the vertebrae caused by the axial loading, ultimately ending with structural failure at the weakest point. The National Football League, National Collegiate Athletic Association, and National High School Federation all made spearing an illegal maneuver as a result of a significant number of spine injuries. The 25-year period following these rule changes saw a 270% decrease in the number of spine injuries resulting in long-term neurologic injury.[15]

Spinal Column Versus Spinal Cord

The biomechanical forces that cause SCI can disrupt both the soft tissue and bony structures that comprise the spine. SCIs often represent disruption of the ligamentous and bony structures that surround and support the spinal cord. It is possible to have an injury to the spinal *column* with no apparent spinal *cord* injury.

• *Spinal column.* The posterior ligamentous complex, posterior longitudinal ligament, and anterior longitudinal ligament are soft tissue structures that can be disrupted.[16,17] Disrupting these structures can lead to instability in the spinal column. When the vertebral column becomes unstable, vertebrae can move independently of one another. The SAC can become compromised, leading to an increased risk of secondary injury when the spinal column becomes unstable.[18-21] The decrease in SAC can lead to impingement on the spinal cord and spinal nerves, which can result in a decrease in sensory and motor function. The impingement can cause tissue damage that leads to vasospasm and edema, which leads to hemorrhagic necrosis and a decrease in perfusion of the spinal cord.[22,23]

• *Spinal cord.* Isolated injuries to the cord are rare, and they are typically associated with an underlying medical condition such as meningitis, aneurysm,[24] or transverse myelitis,[25] as well as many others. Mechanical

insult to the spinal column with sufficient force is more commonly associated with SCI. The term *secondary injury* refers to injury as a result of an additional mechanism. SCI is often associated with secondary injury, which either induces or exacerbates the initial spine injury. The cascading physiologic responses to injury and the HCP's actions during the prehospital and hospital management may lead to secondary injury. As with any soft tissue injury, hemorrhage precipitates an ischemic event. This occlusion of blood supply to the spinal cord may be unavoidable but illustrates the need for timely intervention.

All HCPs caring for traumatic spine injuries should be aware of the differences in spinal column versus spinal cord injuries. When caring for a suspected spine injury, any and all excessive motion should be avoided to reduce the possibilities of HCP-induced secondary injury. Extension of the spinal column is the most important motion to limit. Compared to other motions such as flexion, lateral bending, and lateral rotation, extension may elicit the greatest decrease in SAC for a patient with a suspected cervical spine injury.[18-21] Therefore, once a possible SCI has occurred, it is important to limit the amount of motion occurring to the patient's cervical spine.

 RED FLAG

Several indicators show a suspected traumatic spine injury. If the patient exhibits any of the following signs or symptoms, medical personnel must provide the appropriate spine management.[8]

- Altered level of consciousness or bilateral neurological findings or neurologic complaints by the patient
- Reported pain along the spine with or without palpation
- Obvious deformity along the spine that is a result of a dislocated or damaged/fractured vertebra

Clinical Note

- *Spinal column:* Not all injuries to the spinal column present with neurologic symptoms; therefore, they may be missed. Careful palpation of the bony spinous structures can identify these injuries. The unstable spinal segment may move if the patient is allowed to return to activity, which compresses spinal nerve roots or the spinal cord.

- *Spinal cord:* Spinal cord injuries present with bilateral neurologic symptoms. In almost all spinal cord injuries, an injury to the column is also present.

Palpating Bony Spinous Structures

To assess for vertebral fracture, the emergency responder should begin the exam at the base of the skull (occiput) and progress down the vertebral column 1 vertebra at a time. Cervical vertebrae 1 and 2 are the most difficult to palpate, because their spinous processes are either nonexistent or very small. The spinous process of cervical vertebrae 3 through 7 become more prominent as you palpate down the spine.

The transverse processes of each vertebra should also be examined during palpation. When palpating, the HCP should be feeling for a step-off deformity, swelling, crepitus, or increased pain (as reported by the patient). In the presence of ligamentous injury, there may be increased translation of a vertebra on the vertebrae above or below.

The patient can be either supine or prone. If you suspect a thoracic or lumbar spine injury, it may be easier to examine the patient in the prone position. However, if rolling or moving the patient is required to examine her in the prone position, all possible consequences should be considered.

Emergency Medical Care of Injuries to the Spine

When initially assessing a patient, the AT and sports medicine team should first conduct a primary survey (see chapter 4). The primary survey allows the sports medicine team to establish the patient's airway, breathing, circulation, disability, and exposure (ABCDE). For detailed processes and procedures of the musculoskeletal primary survey, refer to chapter 7. Based on observation of MOI, the patient's current physical or mental status, body position (**decorticate** or **decerebrate**), complaints of neurologic symptoms, and midline spine tenderness, the **spinal motion restriction (SMR)** protocol and emergency action plan (EAP) should be initiated. This information is gathered through the secondary survey of the patient. The decision to use SMR is in an effort to prevent further neurologic damage during transportation.

Some states and counties across the United States have witnessed the removal of the traditional long spine board from emergency medical vehicles. This movement is in an effort to significantly reduce the number of unnecessary SMR applications. However, the National Association of State EMS Officials, the National Association of EMS Physicians, and the American College of Surgeons Committee on Trauma have indicated that there are circumstances or specific patients in which the use of spinal motion restriction is appropriate.[26,27] The position statements published by these organizations have indicated that patients meeting the criteria of the Canadian C-Spine Rule or the NEXUS criteria should receive SMR.

When making a decision to activate the SMR protocol, sports medicine teams should use the **Canadian C-Spine Rule** and the National Emergency X-Radiography Utilization Study (**NEXUS criteria**) in conjunction with the information gathered from their primary and secondary surveys. Furthermore, sports medicine teams should preemptively discuss SMR protocols with their local EMS or paramedic groups that would be working with them in the event a patient is suspected to have a spine injury. Emergency medical personnel use the Canadian C-Spine Rule and NEXUS criteria to aid them in their decisions to use SMR.[26] Familiarity with these criteria can facilitate effective communication between all parties in establishing the necessary criteria to accurately activate SMR protocols. Appropriate patients based on the EMS spinal precautions and use of the long spine board[26,27] as well as the Canadian C-Spine Rule[28,29] and NEXUS criteria[30] meet any of the following 5 conditions:

1. MOI via blunt trauma
   - With an altered level of consciousness
2. MOI via high energy in conjunction with any of the following:
   - Drug or alcohol intoxication
   - Inability to communicate
   - **Distracting injury**
3. Spinal pain or tenderness
4. Neurologic symptoms
   - Numbness or tingling
   - Motor deficits
5. Anatomic deformity of the spine

Figure 9.8 provides the Canadian C-Spine Rule; it is a decision-making protocol (algorithm) for implementing SMR procedures for dangerous MOIs, including motor vehicle collisions (MVCs). The idea of systematic selective determination of SMR use is supported by almost all of the opponents to widespread SMR use.[26,27,31-33]

Please check off all choices within applicable boxes:

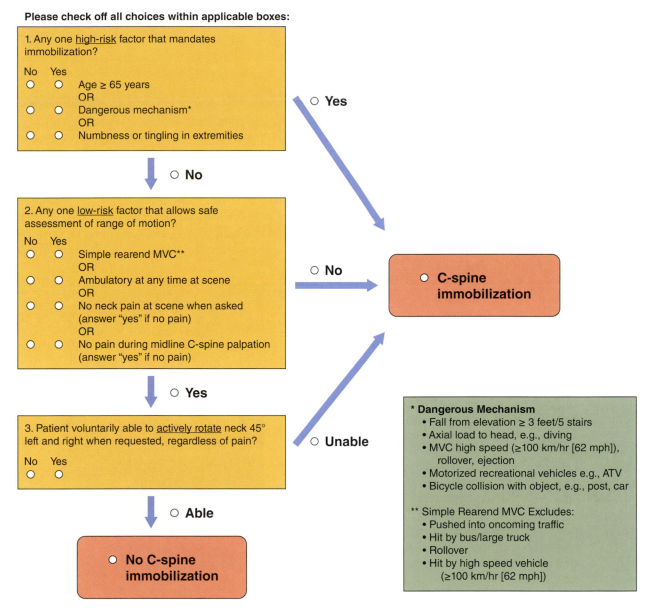

FIGURE 9.8   Canadian C-Spine Rule for immobilization.

Reprinted by permission from C. Vaillancourt et al. "The Out-of-Hospital Validation of the Canadian C-Spine Rule by Paramedics," *Annals of Emergency Medicine* 54, no. 5 (2009):663-671.

This paradigm shift in EMS practices of SMR is based on research that suggests many trauma patients are spine boarded unnecessarily and too frequently.[31,32] Furthermore, some studies indicate that an increased cranial pressure,[34] restricted breathing, and increased risk for sacral pressure sores result from spine boarding.[31,32,35] While these complications should be considered, so too should be the risk of further neurologic complication. Many of the studies referencing negative implications of SMR are case series, case reports, or retrospective cohorts. To date, no randomized controlled trials exist comparing the use of SMR techniques and self-immobilization or the lack of SMR on neurologic outcomes with

cervical spine–injured patients. These studies pose a great ethical concern. Therefore, based on available evidence it is recommended that the clinical assessment (primary and secondary survey) in conjunction with knowledge from the Canadian C-Spine Rule or the NEXUS criteria inform the sports medicine team's decision to use SMR procedures.

The NEXUS criteria are widely used by EMS and emergency physicians when determining the need for SMR and use of the long spine board. If a patient meets the NEXUS criteria, little disagreement should occur. As previously stated, the governing bodies for EMS and trauma physicians support the use of SMR and the long spine board when a patient meets any one of the NEXUS criteria. Therefore, all sports medicine personnel should become familiar with both the Canadian C-Spine Rule and the NEXUS criteria in an effort to effectively communicate with all emergency personnel in the event that a disagreement occurs as to how the patient should be transported. In addition, as discussed in chapter 3 and previously within this chapter, meeting with the local EMS prior to the athletic competition season can help avoid any disagreements or complications at the scene.

Once the decision has been made to activate the SMR protocol, the patient's vital processes must be maintained and monitored. Before moving the patient, a survey of the patient's airway, breathing, blood pressure, circulation, and neurologic condition should be assessed. As in any situation where you are delivering care, these vital signs should be reevaluated and monitored after you have moved or provided care to the patient. The following section discusses managing and maintaining access to areas of vital organs when caring for a spine injury.

Managing the Airway

When caring for a possible spine injury, access to the airway of the patient should be exposed immediately. Barriers such as protective face masks or plastic face shields should be removed; proper removal techniques are discussed later in the chapter.[8] In the event rescue breathing must be performed (see chapter 10), the face mask can prohibit a bag-valve mask from sealing or limiting intubation tools. The airway should be opened and maintained in the safest method possible, creating the least amount of motion.[36,37] Regardless of the patient's breathing status, at minimum, the face mask must be removed in anticipation of status changes during transport.[8]

Two methods are possible to establish the airway, the jaw-thrust and head-tilt–chin-lift maneuver. However,

---

🚩 **RED FLAG**

In the event the face mask cannot be removed in a timely manner, the helmet and shoulder pads should be removed to allow access to the airway and chest (should CPR need to be administered). Football helmets and shoulder pads should be considered a single unit; if one needs to be removed, the other should be removed as well. In other sports such as baseball (catchers), hockey, and lacrosse, the protective equipment may place the head and neck in a flexed or extended position depending on the thickness of the helmet or pads. Therefore, just removing the face mask may not be an option.

---

in the presence of a suspected cervical spine injury, all trained medical personnel are expected to use the jaw-thrust or modified jaw-thrust maneuver. The jaw-thrust is the safest method of establishing an airway of a person with a suspected cervical spine injury.[38] This maneuver creates less extension and therefore limits the decrease in SAC, reducing the chance for a secondary injury.[18,38] The jaw-thrust maneuver is performed with the rescuer positioned at the head of the patient, grasping and lifting angles of the jaw with both hands (figure 9.9).[38]

If the airway cannot be opened with the jaw-thrust maneuver or modified jaw-thrust maneuver, you should try the head-tilt–chin-lift maneuver. The head-tilt–chin-lift maneuver is a last option when caring for a patient with an injured cervical spine (figure 9.10). The maneuver

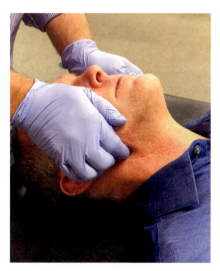

FIGURE 9.9 Jaw-thrust maneuver.
Courtesy of Laura A. Zdziarski-Horodyski.

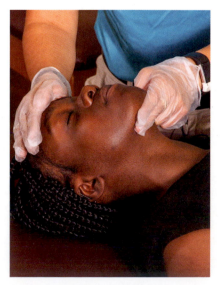

FIGURE 9.10 Head-tilt–chin-lift maneuver.

is performed with the rescuer positioned at the side of the patient. Backward pressure is applied on the patient's forehead with the palm of one hand, and the rescuer places two fingers of the other hand under the patient's chin and lifts the chin forward.[38]

When the airway cannot be maintained with either maneuver, devices such as an oropharyngeal or nasopharyngeal airway adjunct should be used. The oropharyngeal and nasopharyngeal devices are considered basic airway adjuncts and are often the easiest to insert.[39] In the unconscious patient, the muscles of the pharyngeal wall and tongue become relaxed and can obstruct the airway. In addition, body habitus of the patient can impact the rescuer's ability to open and maintain the airway. Chapter 10 discusses airway maintenance in greater detail.

Cardiac Arrest

When managing a traumatic spine injury, cardiovascular complications are possible sequelae and cardiopulmonary resuscitation (CPR) becomes necessary. Immediate access to and exposure of the chest is pertinent to facilitate adequate chest compressions and automated external defibrillator (AED) application (as described in chapter 11). Manual inline stabilization should be maintained; however, the heart is now the main concern.

The jersey and shoulder pads must be cut anteriorly to expose the chest for chest compressions (see the section Shoulder Pad Removal later in this chapter). Research indicates that complete removal of the shoulder pads allows for improved quality of chest compressions.[49] While completely removing the pads may increase the risk of generating more motion in the injured spine region, leaving the pads in place may compromise the efficacy of CPR efforts. These considerations must be evaluated in every scenario, and the decision depends on individual settings and resources.

Spinal Motion Restriction

Medical personnel must always be prepared to care for and transport an injured patient from the scene to the definitive care facility when an injury to the spine is suspected. Historically in the prehospital setting, the steps to prepare the patient for transport have been referred to as *spinal immobilization;* however, authors from 3 decades preceding modern research techniques have debated the feasibility of achieving true immobilization.[50,51] Present investigators of spine boarding techniques assess the amount of motion generated with the use of various techniques. Therefore, the techniques used to prepare a patient for transport with a suspected spine injury are *restricting motion* of the spinal column. The steps discussed in the following sections should be observed regardless of the patient's sport or activity participation. In later sections of this chapter, equipment removal and other considerations are addressed. The authors recognize that not all scenarios can be specifically addressed, but the steps, information, references, and images provided will assist all medical professionals in making the best decisions based on their sport environment and access to resources.

Cervical Inline Stabilization

The first step in achieving cervical inline stabilization is applying manual cervical inline stabilization to the patient's head and cervical spine as soon as a spine injury is suspected.[8] This principle applies to all injuries to the spine—cervical, thoracic, and lumbar. Remember that the cervical spine should be aligned in a neutral position to reduce chances of secondary injury to the spinal cord and provide proper access to the airway. However, if resistance is met, if neurologic symptoms worsen or pain increases, or if the airway becomes compromised, the attempt for a neutral position should cease.[8]

The two hand positions recognized for achieving manual cervical inline stabilization in a supine patient are the traditional handhold and trap squeeze method. They are described as follows:

- *Traditional handhold.* First, position yourself at the head of the patient. Grasp the mastoid processes bilaterally while cupping the occiput of the skull with both hands; your thumbs should be pointing upward toward the patient's face. This position allows you to keep your hands in the same place without having to reposition them if the patient is to be moved (figure 9.11*a*).[8]

- *Trap squeeze method.* Position yourself at the head of the injured patient. Grab the trapezius muscles on both sides of the head with the thumbs facing anteriorly. Then use your forearms to firmly squeeze the patient's head at the ears in order to reduce motion of the cervical spine (figure 9.11*b*).[52,53]

If you are alone, an alternate method of inline stabilization is available (figure 9.11*c*). This method allows for use of your hands to call EMS and monitor vitals while providing inline stabilization.

In the event that the patient is in the prone position, you will have to cross your arms so the patient can be log-rolled into the supine position (figure 9.12).[8] When the log-roll is completed the rescuer's hands will have uncrossed during the maneuver, without releasing hold of the head. If this does not happen, then the hand placement was incorrect. The patient should be log-rolled in congruence with the direction her head is already facing. The patient's face should not be rolled into the ground.

Do not apply traction with inline stabilization.[44,46] The application of traction can increase the chance of ligamentous instability[54,55] and posterior dislocations, which can lead to an impingement due to the decrease

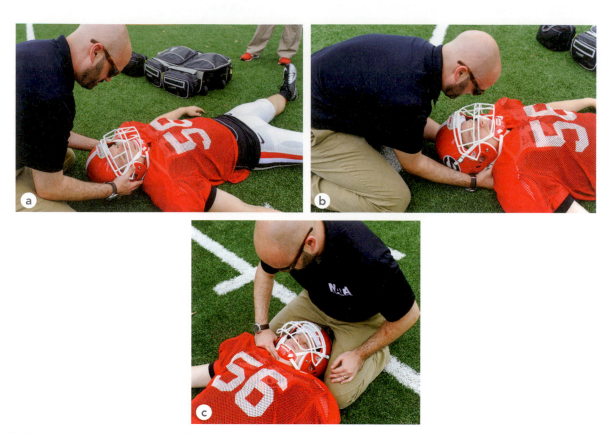

FIGURE 9.11 Cervical spine stabilization: *(a)* traditional handhold, *(b)* trap squeeze method, and *(c)* alternate inline stabilization.

Courtesy of University of Georgia.

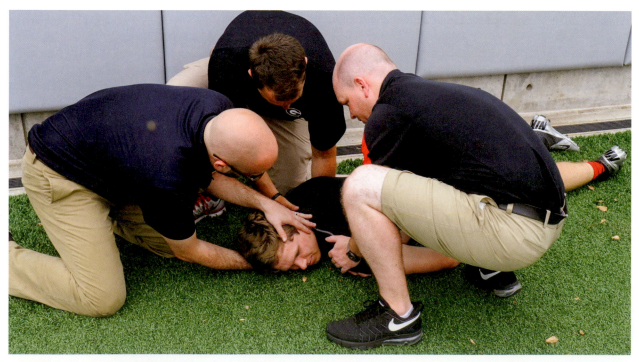

FIGURE 9.12 Inline stabilization in the prone position.

Courtesy of University of Georgia.

CLINICAL SKILLS

Hand Positions for Inline Stabilization

During inline stabilization in the prone position, your top hand (the hand on the side of the head more exposed to the sky) should be the hand opposite in direction of which the patient's head is facing. For example, if the patient is prone and her face is pointed toward your right knee, then your left hand will be on top and cross over her right arm. When the patient is log-rolled toward your left, your arms should uncross.

in space available for the spinal cord. Along with inline stabilization, the spine should be returned to the neutral position for better airway management.[44] Returning to the neutral position gives the spinal cord optimal space within the spinal canal.[56] However, some contraindications exist for returning the spine to the neutral position:

- The movement causes or increases pain.
- The movement compromises the airway.[57]
- Resistance is encountered during the return to neutral.[51]
- The patient expresses apprehension.

Manual cervical inline stabilization should not be released until the patient's body and head are secured to a rigid SMR device (see SMR for Supine Patients later in this chapter). Application of foam head blocks or rolled towels should be fashioned to either side of the patient's head, so as to simulate the position of your hands or forearms when applying manual inline stabilization. Once the foam blocks or towels are in place, use prefabricated straps or tape to anchor the head and blocks or towels to the rigid device. This is the final step in securing the patient to the SMR device before transport; therefore, manual cervical inline stabilization should not be released until the very last moment.

Application of Cervical Collars

To minimize motion during transportation, a rigid cervical collar should be applied to patients with suspected cervical spine injuries. The type of cervical collar should be selected in advance, and the medical staff should be familiar with fitting the collar. The collar should be adjustable, or medical staff should have varying sizes available to fit different patients. Research has shown that cervical collars are not able to limit all ranges of motion.[58,59] Cervical collars, especially poorly fitted collars, may cause distraction in the cervical spine, which can lead

to creation of a pivot point between the head and the shoulders.[60,61] This pivot point can lead to intervertebral motion in the cervical spine. Therefore, manual inline stabilization should be applied until the patient is placed on a spinal motion restriction device (e.g., spine board, stretcher, vacuum mattress) and head immobilizer devices are applied, even after a cervical collar is applied. Only patients with suspected cervical spine injuries should have collars applied before transportation to the hospital, and the cervical collar should be applied to the patient before any spine boarding techniques are performed.

Research has indicated that continued use of manual inline cervical stabilization restricts motion more effectively than cervical collars during intubation.[62] In addition, the cervical collar can limit or prevent access to the airway.[37] HCPs should reassess the patient's condition and airway prior to collar application. While manual inline stabilization is not currently recommended during transport, it may be necessary if the patient's condition deteriorates during transport and the collar blocks advanced airway access.

SMR for Supine Patients

Once the supine patient is ready to be placed on the rigid spinal motion restriction device, one or more HCPs (rescuers) can move the supine patient onto the SMR device using one of these recognized techniques:

1. Multiperson lift and slide
2. Straddle lift and slide
3. Log-roll

Each technique has benefits and disadvantages, so HCPs should review and practice all techniques and determine which is best for their individual setting and sports.

When possible, you should use the multiperson lift and slide and straddle lift and slide techniques instead of the log-roll. These techniques cause less motion than

Clinical Tip

When caring for large patients, rescuers should position themselves so that the stronger rescuers are at the hips and shoulders of the patient. The hips and chest are typically heavier and thus more difficult to lift. Additional rescuers can also be added to aid in elevating the patient.

Multiperson Lift and Slide

The **multiperson lift and slide** technique typically uses a minimum of 8 rescuers. The number of rescuers can be adjusted based on the size of the patient; smaller patients could need fewer, whereas a larger patient would need additional personnel.[63]

Step 1: Position

- Rescuer 1: Provides manual inline stabilization and gives instructions to the other rescuers.
- Rescuers 2 and 3: Positioned at the shoulders on opposite sides.
- Rescuers 4 and 5: Positioned at the hips on opposite sides.
- Rescuers 6 and 7: Positioned at the legs on opposite sides.
- Rescuers 2-7: Gently slide their hands under the patient in preparation to lift.
  - Rescuers stay mindful to not crisscross their hands or forearms with the rescuer adjacent to them.
  - Rescuers should also be cautious not to cause lateral spinal motion when placing their hands under the patient.
- Rescuer 8: Positions the rigid SMR device (typically long spine board) at the feet of the patient in preparation to slide the device underneath the patient.

Step 2: Lift

- Rescuer 1: Instructs rescuers 2-7 to lift the patient 4-6 inches (10-15 cm) off the ground in unison.

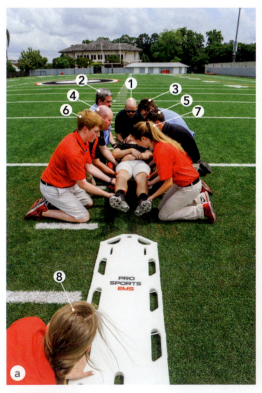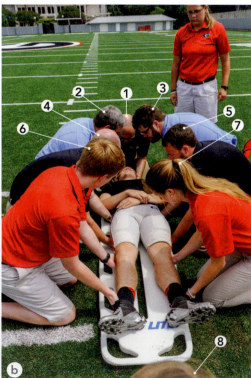

FIGURE 9.13
Courtesy of University of Georgia.

- Rescuer 8: Slides the long spine board along the ground underneath the patient in a cephalic (toward the top of the board) direction *(a)*.

Step 3: Communicate

- Rescuer 1: Communicates with rescuer 8 if the long spine board needs any adjustments in alignment and indicates when rescuer 8 can stop moving the board.

Step 4: Lower

- Rescuer 1: Gives the command to lower the patient onto the long spine board in unison *(b)*.[64]

Step 6: Secure and Prepare for Transport

- Apply appropriate strapping techniques. Rescuers 2-7 should work together to apply the straps nearest them with similar tension and in unison.

Note: Rescuer 1 should not release manual inline stabilization until the patient's body and head have been secured to the board with straps and head blocks.

Straddle Lift and Slide

The **straddle lift and slide** is performed with 5 rescuers.[64]

1. Rescuer 1: Positioned at the head, holds manual inline stabilization, and gives commands to the other rescuers.
2. Rescuers 2-4: Straddle the patient and prepare to lift the upper torso, hips, pelvis and lower extremities.
3. Rescuer 5: Positioned to slide the spine board under the patient when rescuer 1 gives the command to lift.
4. The patient is then lowered on the spine board when rescuer 1 gives the command.

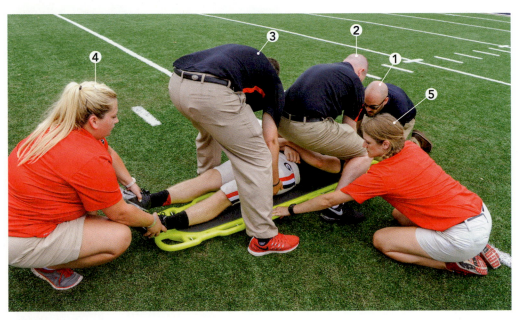

FIGURE 9.14

Courtesy of University of Georgia.

Log-Roll

The **log-roll** method uses 5 rescuers. Depending on the patient's location (against some immovable object, preventing rescuers from accessing the body on both sides) either the log-roll push or log-roll pull should be used.

Step 1: Position

- Rescuer 1: Positioned at the head, maintains manual inline stabilization and gives instructions to the other rescuers.
- Rescuer 2: Positioned at the side of the patient near the shoulders and thorax.
- Rescuers 3 and 4: Align themselves at the hips and legs on the same side as rescuer 2.
- Rescuer 5: Prepares to place the spine board behind the patient (a).

Step 2: Roll

- Rescuer 1: Gives the command to roll the patient either right or left to a 45° angle. The patient may be log-rolled in a pushing or pulling motion depending on the situation (e.g., patient against a wall).
- Rescuers 2-4: Simultaneously roll the patient.
- Rescuer 5: Places the spine board under the patient at the same angle the patient has been rolled (b).

Note: Rescuer 1 should clarify right and left prior to moving the patient. Rescuers 2-5 can become confused as to whose right or left—the patient's or rescuer 1's or their own. This communication becomes imperative when the patient is prone.

Step 3: Lower and Center

- Rescuer 1: Gives the command to lower the patient and board to the ground as a single unit, with no pauses.[8] The patient may then have to be centered on the spine board.

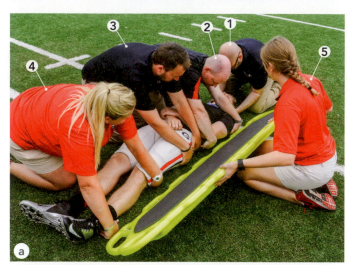

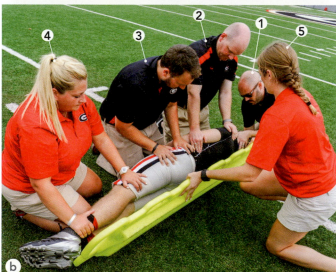

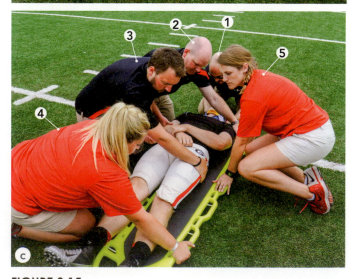

FIGURE 9.15

Courtesy of University of Georgia.

- Horizontal adjustment: Rescuer 1 instructs all rescuers (1-4) to move the patient to the right or left (depends on patient's position on the board).
- V adjustment or diagonal: Rescuer 1 instructs all rescuers (1-4) to move the patient in a caudal leftward or rightward diagonal. Then rescuer 1 instructs all rescuers (1-4) to move the patient in a cephalic direction (c).

Step 4: Secure and Prepare for Transport

- Apply appropriate strapping techniques.
- Rescuers 2-4 should work together to apply the straps nearest them with similar tension and in unison.

Note: Research suggests that the horizontal slide adjustment creates less motion compared to the V adjustment and diagonal slide adjustment.[65] However, HCPs should be familiar with all techniques.

the log-roll, which minimizes the chance for causing further injury to the patient. However, the spine boarding technique should be chosen based on the level of familiarity with the various techniques, the number of rescuers available to help place the patient on the spine board, and the ability of the rescuers to properly position the patient.

SMR for Prone Patients

In the prone patient scenario, it is crucial that all equipment be on the scene prior to moving the patient to reduce the amount or number of times the patient is log-rolled or moved. However, if an initial assessment for airway, breathing, and circulation cannot be achieved with the patient in the prone position or suspicion is high for cardiac arrest, the log-roll must be performed to provide further care prior to retrieving all SMR equipment.

When a patient with a suspected spine injury is in the prone position, the log-roll maneuver is the only technique that can be used to position the patient on the SMR device safely. As discussed in the previous section, the patient can be log-rolled using the push or the pull method.[8] The rescuer applies manual inline stabilization in a crossed-hand position in order to return the patient's cervical spine to the neutral position.[66] The patient should never be log-rolled across the face. For example, if the patient is prone and with the head facing toward the left shoulder, rescuers should log-roll push or pull in a counterclockwise direction (if patient is facing toward the right shoulder, rotate in a clockwise direction) so that the shoulder to which the patient's head is facing moves up toward the sky. If the patient is facedown, then the direction should be chosen based on the situation.

CLINICAL SKILLS

Log-Roll Pull

Step 1: Position

- Rescuer 1: Positioned at the head maintaining manual inline stabilization, gives instructions to the other rescuers.
- Rescuer 2: Positioned at the side of the patient near the shoulders and thorax.
- Rescuers 3 and 4: Align themselves at the hips and legs on the same side as rescuer 2.
- Rescuer 5: Places the spine board against the legs (thighs) of rescuers 2-4 and behind the patient; same side as rescuers 2-4.

Step 2: Roll

- Rescuer 1: Gives the command to pull the patient either right or left to a 45° angle.
- Rescuers 2-4: Simultaneously pull the patient toward them and onto the board.
- Rescuer 5: Helps to stabilize the board so that it does not move.

> continued

Step 3: Lower and Center

- Rescuer 1: Gives the command to lower the patient and board to the ground as a single unit, with no pauses;[8] the patient may then have to be centered on the spine board.

  - Horizontal adjustment: Rescuer 1 instructs all rescuers (1-4) to move the patient to the right or left (depends on patient's position on the board).

  - V adjustment or diagonal: Rescuer 1 instructs all rescuers (1-4) to move the patient in a caudal leftward or rightward diagonal. Then rescuer 1 instructs all rescuers (1-4) to move the patient in a cephalic direction.

Step 4: Secure and Prepare for Transport

- Apply appropriate strapping techniques.
- Rescuers 2-4 should work together to apply the straps nearest them with similar tension and in unison.

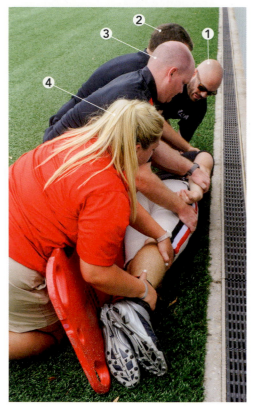

FIGURE 9.16
Courtesy of University of Georgia.

Log-Roll Push

Step 1: Position

- Rescuer 1: Positioned at the head maintaining manual inline stabilization, gives instructions to the other rescuers.

- Rescuer 2: Positioned at the side of the patient near the shoulders and thorax.

- Rescuers 3 and 4: Align themselves at the hips and legs on the same side as rescuer 2.

- Rescuer 5: Prepares to place the spine board behind the patient, opposite side from rescuers 2-4.

Step 2: Roll

- Rescuer 1: Gives the command to push the patient either right or left to a 45° angle.

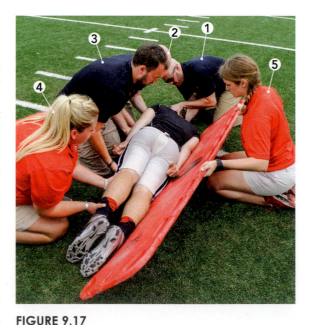

FIGURE 9.17
Courtesy of University of Georgia.

- Rescuers 2-4: Simultaneously roll the patient.
- Rescuer 5: Places the spine board under the patient at the same angle the patient has been pushed (opposite side from rescuers pushing).

Step 3: Lower and Center

- Rescuer 1: Gives the command to lower the patient and board to the ground as a single unit, with no pauses.[8]
- Rescuers 2-5: Aid in lowering the patient and the board back to the ground. The patient may then have to be centered on the spine board.
  - Horizontal adjustment: Rescuer 1 instructs all rescuers (1-4) to move the patient to the right or left (depends on patient's position on the board).
  - V adjustment or diagonal: Rescuer 1 instructs all rescuers (1-4) to move the patient in a caudal leftward or rightward diagonal. Then rescuer 1 instructs all rescuers (1-4) to move the patient in a cephalic direction.

Step 4: Secure and Prepare for Transport

- Apply appropriate strapping techniques.
- Rescuers 2-4 should work together to apply the straps nearest them with similar tension and in unison.

During the log-roll pull, the spine board must be placed between the rescuers and the patient, which can be a difficult task. To address this issue the log-roll push is recommended to place a prone patient on a rigid spine board. Research shows that the log-roll push limits the amount of motion when compared to the log-roll pull when performed in one smooth motion.[66]

SMR for Standing or Seated Patients

Sports such as gymnastics, pole vaulting, various aerial sports, and some winter sports where the athlete has the potential to be found injured in an upright or erect position may require specialized SMR devices. The **Kendrick Extrication Device (K.E.D.)** (figure 9.18)[67] is a device specifically used to achieve SMR where a traditional long spine board or other rigid device cannot fit.[68,69] The K.E.D.

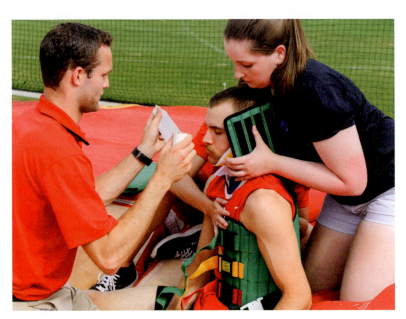

FIGURE 9.18 K.E.D.
Courtesy of University of Georgia.

K.E.D. Application

The K.E.D. is applied with 4 rescuers, and additional rescuers may be needed to remove the patient from the scene.[63]

Step 1: Position

- Rescuer 1: Positioned behind the patient, and stabilizes the cervical spine.
- Rescuers 2-4: Get cervical collar and K.E.D. ready to be applied.

Step 2: Application—Cervical Collar

- Rescuer 2: Ensures proper size and fit of the cervical collar and places it on the patient.
- Rescuers 2 and 3: Positioned on opposite sides of the patient.

Step 3: Application—K.E.D.

- Rescuer 4: Prepares the K.E.D. to be placed behind the patient.[63]
  - The patient's position in space or the surroundings (gymnastics pit or upright against a wall or rocks) will determine whether the patient has to be tilted forward to insert the K.E.D. against the dorsal side or not.
- Rescuers 2 and 3: Should slightly lean the patient forward (if necessary).
- Meanwhile, Rescuer 1: Maintains inline stabilization.
- Rescuer 4: Slides the K.E.D. between the patient's back and rescuer 1.

Step 4: Secure and Prepare for Transport

- The K.E.D. should then be secured based on the manufacturer's specifications via securing the 2 leg straps, the 3 torso straps, and then applying the head motion restriction straps.[67]
- Once the head has been secured to the K.E.D. rescuer 1 may then release manual inline stabilization.

---

restricts motion at the head, neck, and torso, which are the 3 key areas for SMR.[70] The same general principles for applying SMR should be followed when using this device. It includes manual inline stabilization, cervical collar application, and securing the patient to the device with the proper strapping technique.

SMR Equipment

The basic equipment needed for SMR is a rigid cervical collar, a rigid board (options discussed next), specific straps to secure patient to the SMR device, an AED, a pocket mask (or other airway device), a cell phone, and personnel. Other equipment may be necessary depending on the sport, your location, and the SMR device you are using. Specifics to each of these variations are discussed in this section or the subsequent section titled Equipment Removal.

Various devices are available for SMR (figure 9.19). They vary based on size, cost, and functionality within specific athletic settings. In addition, individual sports

medicine teams should identify the device that best suits their needs, patient population, and budget. The most commonly recognized and used SMR device is the long spine board. This device is the traditional hard plastic board in varying colors with handholds along the sides of the board. These devices are most commonly found in the standard size, but they can be found in pediatric or bariatric sizes. The bariatric long spine boards may need to be considered for sports teams with larger athletes. Another consideration for selecting board size is height of the patient. Some volleyball, basketball, or other tall athletes will not fit on the standard long spine board.

A scoop stretcher is to be used in conjunction with the previously mentioned devices. The scoop device is not intended as a primary SMR device and can only be used with supine patients. Patients can be transported on the scoop stretcher once they have been secured to the device. Scoop stretchers may be an ideal option based on ease of use and potential for fewer rescuers needed, depending on the size of the patient. Most scoop stretchers are fairly lightweight and are height adjustable. This device is not

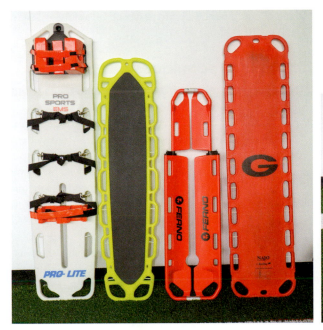 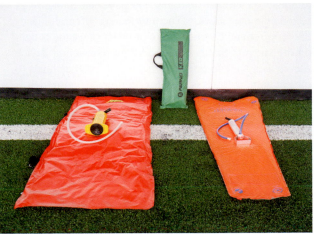

FIGURE 9.19 Spinal motion restriction devices: spine boards, scoop stretcher, and vacuum mattresses.
Courtesy of University of Georgia.

ideal for very large or wide patients because of the nature of its construction. Before using the device, consider the height and weight limitations of the device and ensure the clips are in proper working order.

To properly operate the scoop stretcher, the two halves are unlocked and readied on either side of the patient. On the command of rescuer 1 (who is providing manual inline stabilization), rescuers 2 through 5 begin to slide the halves under the right and left side of the patient (see figure 9.20a) until the hinges are locked.[71] Manual inline stabilization must be maintained until the patient is either transferred and properly secured to another SMR device or secured to the scoop stretcher.

An alternative to the long spine board is the vacuum mattress (figure 9.20b). Many research studies have indicated that the vacuum mattress is very effective in restricting spinal motion in the injured and uninjured patient.[72,73] An additional benefit to using the vacuum mattress is that

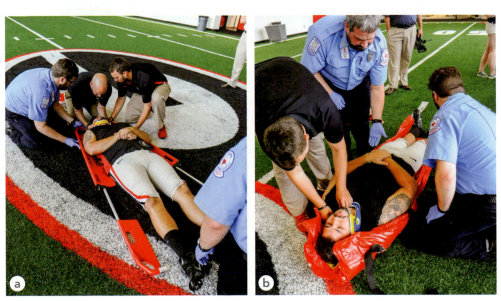

FIGURE 9.20 (a) Scoop stretcher and (b) vacuum mattress.
Courtesy of University of Georgia.

the sacral and cranial pressure that can become uncomfortable for patients are often reduced.[35,74,75] If choosing to use the vacuum mattress, a few considerations should be recognized prior to purchasing and using. First, a second device, such as a scoop stretcher, is recommended in conjunction with the mattress. The patient cannot be logrolled onto the mattress. The multiperson lift and slide or the scoop stretcher is needed to properly place the patient on the vacuum mattress. In addition, the second device serves as a backup device. One of the disadvantages to the vacuum mattress is that if it becomes punctured, it is no longer effective. Therefore, having a second device available is recommended in the event the mattress becomes defective. Another disadvantage is the high cost associated with a vacuum mattress. Many devices cost upwards of $400 and do not include the cost of a scoop stretcher or alternate method. Scoop stretchers can range in price from half the cost of a vacuum mattress to almost three times more; thus, the total cost for using a vacuum mattress is between $600 and $1600 depending on the

brand of equipment. Put into perspective, a standard rigid spine board is about $100.

Strapping Techniques

The emergency medical community employs several strapping techniques. The more frequently used are Spider Straps,[76] Speed Clips,[77] or the 7-strap system. The Spider-Straps (figure 9.21a) and the 7-strap system (figure 9.21b) are similar in strap placement, whereas the traditional Speed Clips are the 3-strap system. Some 7-strap systems come equipped with the speed clip mechanism. The speed clip mechanism allows for the strap to be quickly locked onto the special horizontal pin located within the handholds along the long spine board. These straps can only be used on boards equipped with the pins. Present data support the use of more straps when securing a patient to the SMR device as compared to the traditional 3-strap method. for strapping techniques. Mazolewski and Manix[78] describe the importance of securing the torso

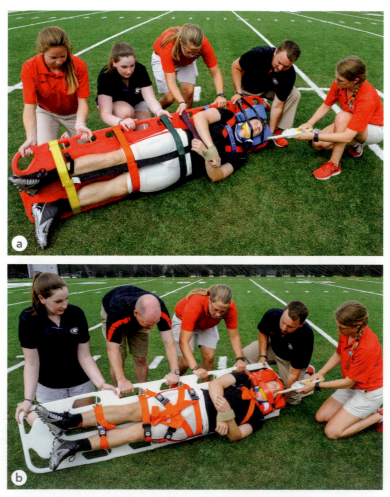

FIGURE 9.21   Strapping techniques: *(a)* Spider-Straps and *(b)* 7-strap system.
Courtesy of University of Georgia.

with additional straps due to the increase in body weight compared to the lower extremities.

Guidelines and Recommendations

All HCPs should examine their state practice acts, review and discuss their institution's standard operating procedures, and adhere to the guidelines and recommendations set forth by the National Athletic Trainers' Association (NATA) and any other governing bodies for their specific practice of medicine or emergency medical care. The guidelines and recommendations discussed and presented in this chapter are based on current published and available literature or data. In addition, all emergency care provided to an injured patient should be undertaken with the primary goal to prevent or reduce the risk of secondary injury.

When rescuers initially arrive on the scene, it is their responsibility to ensure the scene is safe and conduct a primary and secondary survey of the patient (described in chapter 4).[8,63,79] As discussed previously, the SMR protocol should be immediately activated when a spine injury is suspected. Routine rehearsal of these protocols and the medical time-out[80] prior to every athletic event allow for efficient activation and successful packaging and transport of the injured patient (described in chapter 3). The decision to remove the athletic equipment prior to transport should be made prior to the commencement of any athletic event, specifically within the EAP or medical time-out. Specific details of these procedures are discussed in the section titled Equipment Removal.

The patient should not be removed from the scene or moved until fully secured to an SMR device. If a situation arises in which the patient's airway, breathing, or circulation cannot be preserved without moving the patient prior to deploying all SMR procedures, then the patient can be moved.[8] Manual inline stabilization should immediately commence while EMS and other personnel are activated. A properly sized and rigid cervical collar should be applied.

In situations where the patient is supine and adequate personnel are available, the multiperson lift and slide is recommended.[8,81,82] The number of personnel can be adjusted based on size of the patient. In some circumstances, the log-roll is recommended for a supine patient. For example, one such scenario is when the patient is against a wall and it is not physically possible for rescuers to position themselves on both sides. In the scenario of a prone patient, the log-roll is the only option. The log-roll push is recommended over the pull technique.[83]

When securing a patient for transport, a rigid SMR device is recommended. Any of the devices previously described are acceptable; selection depends on the athletic environment, personnel, and budget. As it relates to strapping techniques, based on current literature, using more than 3 straps is recommended. Emphasize securing

the torso due to the increased mass.[78] The last step should be to secure the head to the board. Foam blocks or towels can be used on either side to provide inline stabilization with the application of straps or tape. Once all of these steps have been accomplished, the patient's neurologic status should be reassessed prior to transport.[79] The patient should then be transported to the most appropriate hospital for definitive care treatment with the accompaniment of a sports medicine team member (if possible).

In some athletic settings, it may not be feasible for the sports medicine team to secure an athlete to an SMR device on-site preceding EMS arrival. In these situations, minimum manual inline stabilization should be maintained until EMS arrives. In addition, airway, breathing, and circulation should be sustained and monitored while a more thorough secondary assessment is completed in preparation for EMS arrival.[8,79]

Equipment Removal

In the event of a suspected spine injury, protective equipment such as football helmets and shoulder pads (e.g., catcher's helmet and chest protector; lacrosse helmets and chest protectors) may need to be removed from the athlete prior to transport and must be removed for definitive treatment of the injury. The decision to remove the equipment should be based on the following:

- Type of equipment the athlete is wearing (helmet, shoulder pads)
- Status of the patient (airway and cardiovascular needs)
- Rescuers' experience (on-site) versus hospital staff experience[70]

Advantages to removing equipment are as follows:

- Better airway management is achieved when the helmet is removed. The jaw-thrust maneuver and bag-valve mask use can be impeded by the helmet and chin strap.[49,84,85]
- Removal of the shoulder pads allows for access to the chest in the event that an AED must be used on the patient.
- In the event that chest compressions need to be started before an AED is available, having access to the chest immediately allows for rapid activation of CPR protocol. In addition, the quality of chest compressions is higher when the shoulder pads are removed.[49,84,85]

When the equipment is removed in the prehospital setting, it is typically removed by HCPs with the most training and experience with that protective equipment. Furthermore, it is vital that all HCPs involved or with the potential to care for patients laden with equipment be trained in equipment removal procedures routinely. Standards of care may change with respect to techniques for equipment removal, so all providers should continually stay abreast of current recommendations.

These considerations should be acknowledged prior to removing equipment from a patient with a suspected spine injury:

- Number of personnel
- Training of people at the scene
- Physiologic status of the patient

Research suggests that removing the equipment prior to transport may delay care and treatment for the patient.[86] Other research suggests that removing the equipment prior to transport can place the cervical spine in a slightly flexed position, decreasing the SAC.[87-89] While some argue that removal of equipment causes more motion at the injured segment, at some point in the care process the equipment must be fully removed. Diagnostic imaging is impeded or impossible with equipment in place, and definitive care cannot be provided until all protective equipment has been removed. Each institution, athletic setting, and workplace environment will have varying circumstances, and the decision to remove equipment prior to transport should be discussed with all involved parties preceding the start of athletic season competitions or activities.

Face Mask Removal

If the decision has been made to transport the patient with equipment in place, the face mask should always be removed prior to transport.[8,90] Removing the face mask facilitates improved airway access and makes removal of the helmet easier in the event the patient's

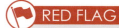

condition declines.[8] Proper tools and methods for face mask removal are discussed in this section.

Football Helmets

Several methods are useful for removing the face mask from a football helmet of a patient with a suspected spine injury. The combined-tool approach is best practice for removing a face mask and involves using screwdrivers and a cutting device. An electric screwdriver (figure 9.22a) or a handheld screwdriver are the fastest[86,91,92] and easiest[86] methods for removing a face mask. The electric screwdriver method creates less torque[92] and less motion,[86] which reduces the chance of causing further injury to the patient. The handheld screwdriver should be used in the event that the electric screwdriver fails. However, a screwdriver may not be an effective tool because the screws may be rusted or stripped. If this occurs, angle shears (figure 9.22b) or other cutting devices should be used to cut the plastic loop that holds the screw in place on the helmet.[93]

Riddell makes the Revolution helmet that is equipped with a quick-release system for the side loop straps (figure 9.23a). A small pin-shaped device is used to press the quick-release mechanism, and the screw comes out of the helmet to release the face mask. Schutt helmets are also equipped with a similar fast-releasing mechanism for

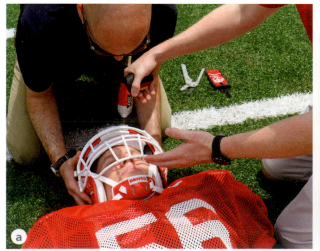
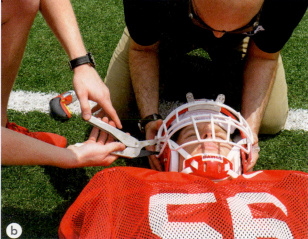

FIGURE 9.22 Face mask removal: *(a)* electric screwdriver and *(b)* angle shears.

Courtesy of University of Georgia.

the face mask. The Schutt Twist Release Retainer allows for the use of a Phillips or flat-head screwdriver to make a one-quarter turn of the screw at the side clips that then allows the face mask to be rotated and removed (figure 9.23*b*). If the face mask cannot be quickly released (30-45 seconds) and an emergent need to access the airway arises, rescuers should proceed to remove the helmet to gain access to the airway.[94]

Baseball, Hockey, and Lacrosse Helmets

Baseball, hockey, and lacrosse and any other sports requiring protective equipment pose different considerations for removal. For example, many catcher's helmets are not continuous, and the posterior portion of the helmet is thinner and secured by elastic straps. Other helmets have numerous screws that must be removed or have a neck guard that is contiguous. Lacrosse goalie helmets have an additional neck guard. Male lacrosse field players wear helmets with a face mask but no neck guard. Hockey goalies have similar helmets to lacrosse goalies, while other hockey players wear very different helmets.

Removal techniques for these face masks are similar to football helmets but have varying subtleties based on the screw placement and design.

Step 1: Stabilization and Preparation

- Rescuer 1: Provides manual inline stabilization.
- Rescuer 2: Gathers appropriate equipment (cordless electric screwdriver, shears, or special tools for quick release).

Step 2: Removal

- Rescuer 2: Unscrews the screws holding the face mask to the helmet, beginning with the top screws and working laterally.

- Rescuer 2: Once all screws have been removed, the face mask can be lifted off the helmet.

Note: In baseball and softball, hockey, and lacrosse the chest protector or shoulder pads may place the cervical spine into flexion or extension (not neutral) based on the thickness of the torso protective equipment and helmet. This discrepancy should be considered when making the decision whether to remove equipment or not.

Helmet Removal

If the decision has been made to remove the athlete's equipment, the helmet and shoulder pads should be considered a unit and both be removed. Once the face mask has been removed, the helmet can be removed from the injured patient. Less motion in the cervical spine is generated when the face mask is removed from the football helmet prior to removing the helmet.[95] Removal of the face mask allows for easier access to stabilize the cervical spine. However, circumstances may arise where the face mask cannot be removed. The sports medicine team should be prepared to remove the helmet under both conditions. Figures 9.24 and 9.25 demonstrate helmet removal with the face mask off and on, respectively. When working with lacrosse, hockey, or other types of helmets, different considerations may need to be made.[96-98] If time is of the essence, consider leaving the face mask on and simply removing the helmet with the face mask attached.

Here are some tips for helmet removal:

- The chin strap should be cut away, because unsnapping the helmet may create unnecessary movement.
- Cheek pads should be removed from the helmet using a tongue depressor (or something similar) to

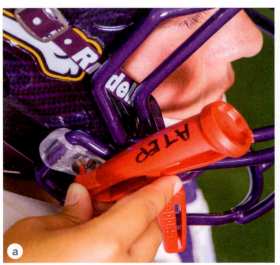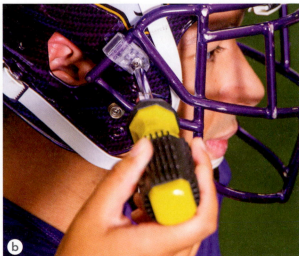

FIGURE 9.23 *(a)* Riddell quick-release pin system; and *(b)* Schutt Twist Release Retainer.

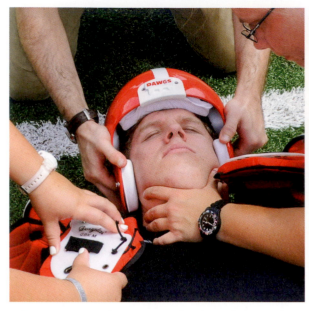
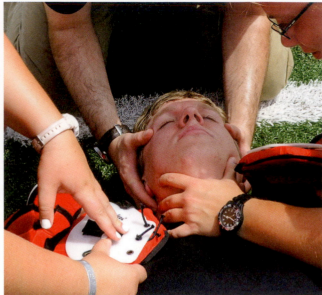

FIGURE 9.24   Helmet removal with no face mask.
Courtesy of University of Georgia.

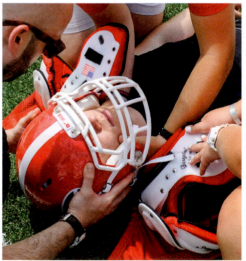
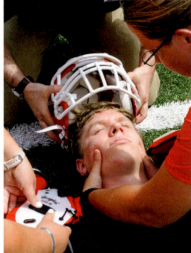
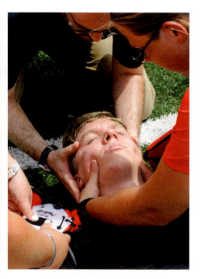

FIGURE 9.25   Helmet removal with face mask.
Courtesy of University of Georgia.

snap the pad away from the inside of the helmet. However, the ability to remove the cheek pads varies based on the model of the helmet.

- If possible, air bladders in the helmet should be deflated to loosen the fit on the helmet on the patient's head.

- Before the removing the helmet:
  - Manual inline stabilization should be transferred from the rescuer at the patient's head (rescuer 1) to rescuer 2, who can provide inline stabilization from the front of the patient.

- Rescuer 2 places 1 hand on the chin and the other hand on the posterior side of the patient's neck (or as depicted in figure 9.26, on either side of the patient's head).

- Rescuer 1, located at the head, grasps the side of the helmet while slightly spreading the cheek pad area on the helmet.

- Rescuer 1 then rotates the helmet forward while sliding the helmet off the patient's head, being mindful to not place the head into flexion or extension.

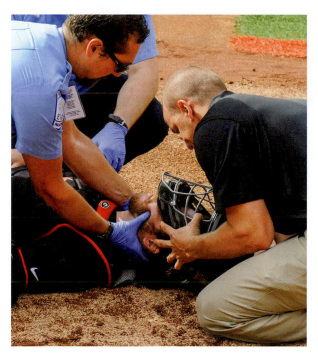

FIGURE 9.26 Helmet removal: baseball catcher.

Courtesy of University of Georgia.

- Once the helmet is removed, manual inline stabilization should be returned to rescuer 1 and padding (such as a folded towel) should be placed under the patient's head.[8] This padding will offset the height of the shoulder pads and prevent hyperextension, which can decrease space available for the cord.
- ATs and other rescue personnel should practice helmet removal with all types of helmets used at their venue.

Shoulder Pad Removal

The shoulder pads can be removed only after the helmet has been removed. Many techniques are available, and rescuers should select the best technique based on the situation and training of those involved. Shoulder pad removal techniques should be incorporated into the SMR techniques based on patient position, technique selected, equipment, and injury type. In cases where a lumbar or thoracic spine injury is suspected, the tilt technique (also called elevated torso) should not be used. It is also important for the AT and all medical staff to know and be familiar with the equipment their athletes are wearing. If athletes are wearing shoulder pads with the solid breast or back plate, only one option exists for removal. Conversely, if the athlete has bivalve or quick-release (Ripkord) pads, only one technique should be used even though others are possible.

With the supine patient, shoulder pad removal techniques include the following:

- Multiperson lift
- Straddle
- Tilt technique
- Over the head
- Flat torso
- Log-roll techniques
- Quick-release shoulder pads

The goal in caring for the spine-injured patient is to move the patient the lowest number of times; therefore, the steps described for each of the removal techniques may include a step or two from the SMR process. Before beginning the removal process, ensure that adequate personnel are available and proper cutting tools are on-site.[99]

CLINICAL SKILLS

Multiperson Lift

1. Rescuer 1: Provides manual inline stabilization.
2. Rescuer 2: Cuts the jersey (T shape, right to left arm, cephalic to caudal) and breast-plate strings, and releases or cuts the axilla straps.
3. From this point, the multiperson lift and slide SMR technique is carried out with the addition of a ninth rescuer (a).
4. Rescuer 9: Positioned near rescuer 1 near the shoulders and carefully pulls the shoulder pads away from the patient when the patient is elevated and the board is slid under (b-c).

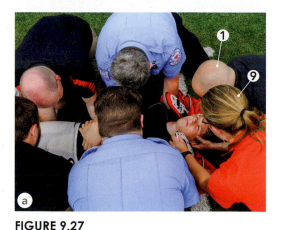

FIGURE 9.27

Courtesy of University of Georgia.

> *continued*

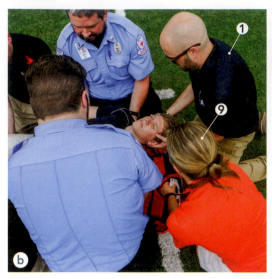
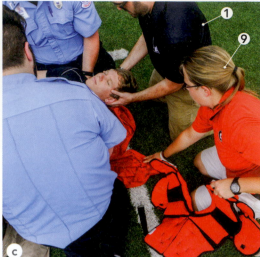

FIGURE 9.27 > *continued*
Courtesy of University of Georgia.

When using this technique, the patient may have to be lifted a bit higher to allow the shoulder pads clearance. After the pads are removed, the patient is lowered to the SMR device on rescuer 1's command.[100]

CLINICAL SKILLS

Straddle Technique

This technique is recommended for use on smaller patients.

1. Rescuers 1 and 2: Perform the same duties as they did in the multiperson lift.

2. Once the jersey and equipment have been released, rescuers 2-5 straddle the patient, while rescuer 6 is positioned by rescuer 1 near the patient's shoulders.

3. Rescuer 1: Gives the command when all are ready and proceeds to lift the patient about 4-6 inches (10-15 cm) from the ground, and rescuer 5 carefully removes the pads.

4. Simultaneously, rescuer 7 (not shown) slides the long spine board in under the patient and between the rescuers' legs.

5. When all equipment is removed and properly placed, the patient is lowered on the command of rescuer 1.

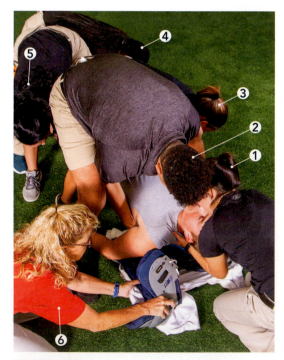

FIGURE 9.28

Tilt Technique

1. Rescuers 1 and 2: Complete same roles of stabilization and cutting equipment as in the multiperson technique.
2. At the direction of rescuer 1, rescuers 2 and 3 hinge the patient forward about 30° to 50° (bending at the waist).
3. Rescuer 4: Removes the shoulder pads by sliding them out along the ground, moving in a cephalic and either right or left direction.
4. The patient is then lowered to the ground.[101]

Three-Rescuer Modification

1. Rescuers 1 and 2: Complete same roles of stabilization and cutting equipment as in the multiperson technique.
2. Rescuer 2: Straddles the patient to lift the torso (a) while rescuer 3 removes the pads (b).

If using this method, ensure that rescuer 2 feels completely comfortable lifting the patient's torso, as it can be deceptively heavy. When performing this technique, the person at the head has to be sure not to apply traction.

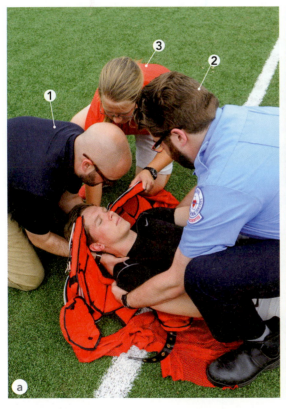
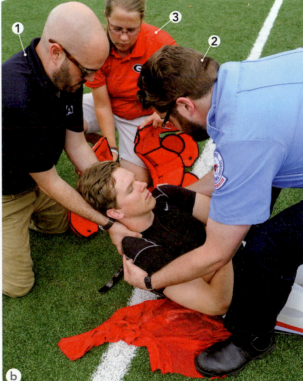

FIGURE 9.29

Courtesy of University of Georgia.

Over-the-Head Technique

Follow similar steps from the tilt technique, except in this scenario rescuer 2 has not cut the breast plate, because the plate is solid and therefore no shears can penetrate. The jersey and side straps should still be released.

1. Rescuer 2: Positions himself to the side of the patient, slides his hands under the shoulder pads, and assumes cervical spine stabilization from rescuer 1 from the front (a).
2. Rescuers 3 and 4: Help to elevate the torso on rescuer 2's command.
3. Once the patient is elevated, rescuer 1 removes the shoulder pads over the patient's head (b).
4. After the pads are removed and the patient is lowered to the ground, rescuer 1 reassumes inline stabilization (c).

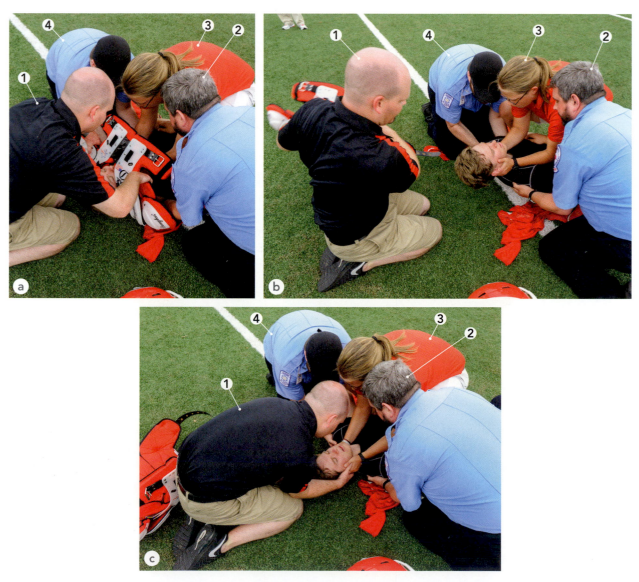

FIGURE 9.30

Courtesy of University of Georgia.

Flat Torso Technique

The same steps and roles are completed for rescuers 1 and 2 for stabilization and releasing the jersey and shoulder pads from the multiperson lift.

1. Rescuer 2: Reaches up through the cut jersey and pads to assume manual inline stabilization of cervical spine from rescuer 1.
2. Rescuers 1 and 3: Pull the shoulder pads in an axial direction on either side of the patient, ensuring to move succinctly and carefully over the patient's head.[101]
3. Once the pads are removed, then rescuer 1 reassumes inline stabilization.

This technique is used when a thoracic or lumbar injury is suspected and it would not be recommended to use the tilt or over-the-head techniques.

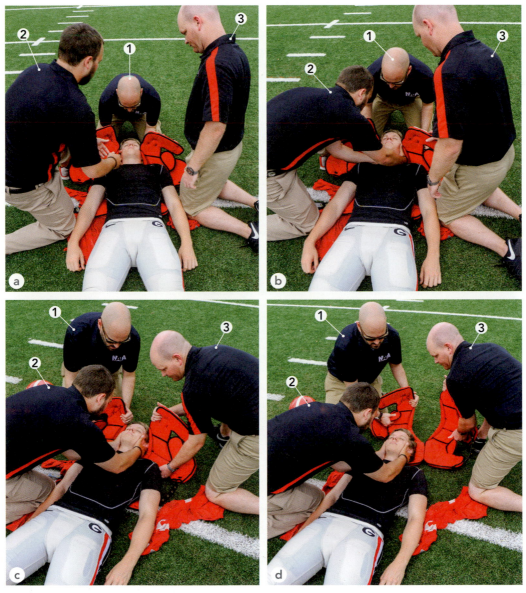

FIGURE 9.31

Courtesy of University of Georgia.

Log-Roll Technique

1. Rescuer 1: Maintains inline stabilization while a traditional log-roll maneuver is completed (Note: The shoulder pads should not be released in the front prior to log-rolling).

2. Rescuer 5: Cuts the jersey and shoulder pads posteriorly when the patient is log-rolled off the ground.

3. Once all equipment has been cut posteriorly, the long spine board is put in place and the patient is log-rolled down on rescuer 1's command.

4. Rescuer 2: Cuts the jersey and shoulder pads anteriorly and releases the side straps.

5. These steps have now created bivalve shoulder pads which can be removed like the quick-release pads. Rescuers 2 and 3 can now pull their respective halves of the pads out from the side of the patient.

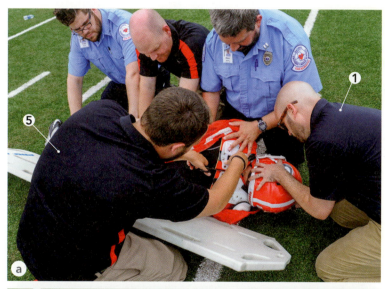

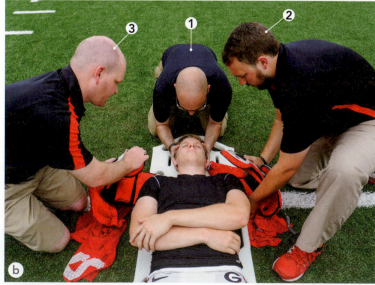

FIGURE 9.32
Courtesy of University of Georgia.

Quick-Release Shoulder Pads

1. Rescuer 1: Provides manual inline stabilization.
2. Rescuer 2: Cuts the jersey, breast plate strings, axilla straps, and the emergency quick-release tab.
3. Once all equipment is cut, the quick-release cable is pulled, fully releasing the shoulder pads in the front and back.
4. The pads are now able to be removed in the bivalve process described earlier (rescuers 2 and 3 pull pads out from either side.[94]

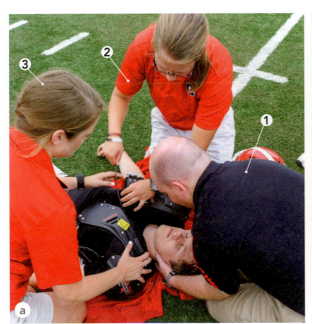
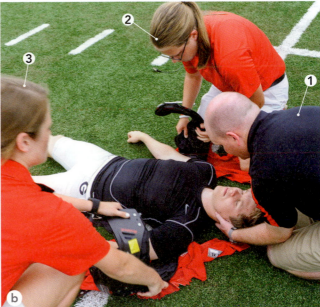

FIGURE 9.33
Courtesy of University of Georgia.

Guidelines and Recommendations

When preparing to transport a patient with an injured spine, regardless of equipment removal decisions, the face mask should *always* be completely removed prior to transport.[8,49] A cordless screwdriver produces less motion when removing a face mask that is not quick-release.[86,93,102] All sports medicine team members should have immediate access to and be familiar with an alternate removal tool, in case of primary device failure.[86,103,104]

Before the shoulder pads can be removed, the chin strap must be cut and helmet removed. Presently, sufficient data do not exist to support one shoulder pad removal technique more strongly than any other. One study by Horodyski and colleagues[101] suggests that the tilt technique created less motion in the injured C5-C6 spinal segment when compared to the flat torso technique.

Quick-release shoulder pads show extreme promise for reducing the amount of motion generated compared to removing traditional shoulder pads. This pad construction is not yet widely used. Therefore, having an understanding and experience with multiple removal techniques is strongly recommended.

Summary

The spinal motion restriction techniques, devices, and equipment removal steps discussed in this chapter should be reviewed frequently and clearly described in an EAP. Every institution, setting, and sport will have different resources and abilities. Therefore, an absolute statement regarding recommendations for treatment and care would not be appropriate. The items discussed in this chapter should be referred to in conjunction with state practice acts, individual standard operating procedures, and the NATA position statements and guidelines to select what is most appropriate for each situation and institution.

All sports medicine personnel should reach out to their local EMS or paramedic crews that would be assisting them in any emergency situations prior to having to rely on their services. Communicating with all parties involved in the care of athletes (or any patient population) is critical to ensuring the best possible medical care delivered. In recent years many state EMS or paramedic services have completely removed the rigid long spine board from their emergency vehicles or will not transport a patient if she is already secured to a rigid long spine board. Therefore, communicating with local emergency personnel prior to any situations can help avoid any conflicts when a patient is involved.

Just as in any emergent medical scenario, events may not always go as rehearsed. However, repeated rehearsal ensures that all staff involved will know the proper steps and feel comfortable adapting to the situation or environment. The rehearsal will also give each rescuer a chance to know and understand his role during on the field management of a spinal cord injury. Communication and collaboration with all medical personnel involved in the care and treatment of the athlete with a spine injury is essential for optimal outcomes. No one hopes for these emergencies to arise, but ATs and other sports medicine team members must be prepared for any situation.

 Go to the web study guide to complete the case studies for this chapter.

CHAPTER 10

Injuries of the Thorax and Lungs

OBJECTIVES

After reading this chapter, you will be able to do the following:

- Choose an appropriate airway when an urgent situation justifies it.

- Describe the anatomical components of the thorax.

- Evaluate emergent conditions of the thorax.

- Manage emergent conditions of the thorax.

- Determine appropriate care and disposition of acute conditions of the thorax.

- Justify if an emergent condition of the thorax requires transportation via ambulance to a hospital or trauma center.

Trauma to the thorax is particularly alarming, because patients can face life-threatening sequelae. Knowing relevant anatomy, in conjunction with understanding mechanisms of injury (MOIs) to structures in the thorax, can alert the health care provider (HCP) to be diligent in assessing injuries to the trunk. This chapter discusses use of airways and supplemental oxygen in terms of providing respiratory support while waiting for emergent transportation to a trauma center. Some conditions relevant to this chapter that are also related to cardiac conditions (e.g., commotio cordis) are discussed in chapter 11.

Overview of Anatomical Structures in the Thorax

The heart is one of the most protected organs in the body. Together with the lungs, it is surrounded on all four sides by the bony structure of the rib cage. The rib cage attaches to the thoracic spine posteriorly, and sternum anteriorly, to provide a sturdy frame that shelters the heart and lungs. Cartilaginous tissue joins ribs to the costal cartilage and the sternum, allowing for some freedom of the rigid rib cage, which moves with respiratory inhalation and exhalation. Because of its flexibility and ability to allow movement, the costal cartilage junctions are susceptible to injury and therefore can affect underlying structures.

Bones

The human body has 12 pairs of ribs, but only pairs 1 through 7 are considered true ribs. They are named *true ribs* because they attach directly from each of the thoracic vertebrae posteriorly via costal cartilage to the sternum anteriorly. Each of ribs 1 through 7 projects laterally farther than the rib above it. Each rib has a costochondral joint that is the articulation between the bony rib and cartilage that articulates with the sternum. Ribs 8, 9, and 10 attach via cartilage with each other anteriorly, then to the sternum. These 3 pairs are often called *false ribs*. The final two pairs are termed *floating ribs,* because they arise from thoracic vertebrae and have no other attachment (figure 10.1). These last ribs provide bony protection for the kidneys, which are discussed in chapter 12. The lack of anterior attachment of the floating ribs also makes a blow to this area more concerning; they can fracture and injure the kidney.

The sternum is a bony plate anterior to the heart, aorta, and bronchi. It has 3 distinct parts—the manubrium, which is most superior; the body; and the xiphoid process, which is most inferior (figure 10.2). The manubrium has a central sternal (sometimes called jugular) notch and 2 (lateral) articulating facets for each clavicle. The clavicle is a thin, anterior visible bone that offers another protective layer over the thorax. It attaches medially to the manubrium and laterally to the scapula via the acromion. Two interesting facts about the clavicle are that the first rib is above the clavicle and that the articulation of the clavicle and manubrium is the only bony attachment of the upper extremity to the body.

On the posterior aspect of the thorax are 2 bony protectors, the vertebral spine and the scapula. The vertebral spinous and transverse processes provide for muscular attachments and movement of the spine. The thin plate of the scapula offers not only bony protection of the thorax but also musculature to facilitate movement of the humerus. The posterior aspect of the scapula has a spine, which begins medially and continues to become the most lateral aspect of the scapula, the acromion. Both the spine of the scapula and acromion provide bony attachments for muscles. Under the scapula, atop the posterior trunk, lies the subscapularis muscle, which does not attach to the trunk but to the humerus.

Ligaments

Ligaments critical to the thorax are the sternoclavicular (SC) and costoclavicular (CC) ligaments. Injury to the SC ligaments can cause the clavicle to move posteriorly, which is a life-threatening condition because the trachea and common carotid arteries lie directly underneath. The CC ligaments hold the clavicle down to the first rib, maintaining the stability of the SC joint as well as protection of the ribs by the clavicle (figure 10.3).

Muscles

The major anterior muscles to the trunk include the pectoralis major (sternum to anterior humerus) and pectoralis minor (ribs to coracoid of the scapula; figure 10.4). Also of note is the sternocleidomastoid, which is not really a thoracic muscle; its origin is at the medial clavicle and sternum junction, and it moves superiorly along the neck to insert behind the ear at the mastoid of the skull. The long rectus abdominis begins at the pubic crest, supports the abdomen, and inserts at the costal cartilage of ribs 5 through 7 and the xiphoid process. The rectus abdominis assists with breathing, as do the intercostal muscles.

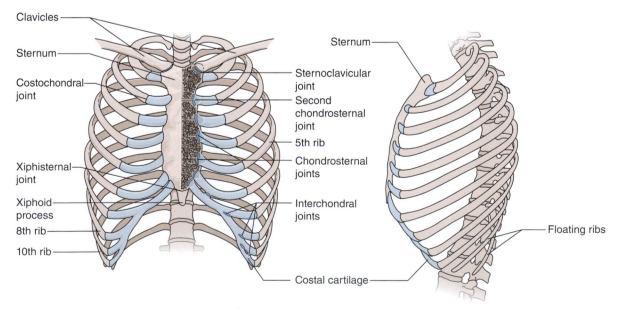

FIGURE 10.1   Anterior and lateral view of the ribs.

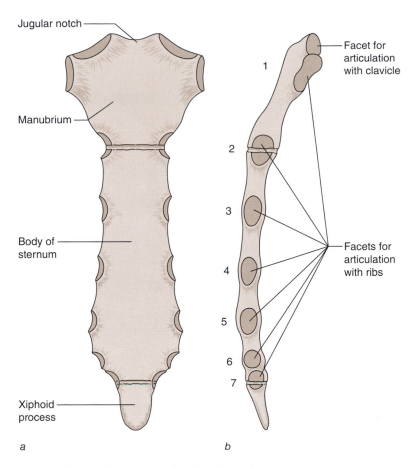

FIGURE 10.2   The sternum: *(a)* anterior view and *(b)* left lateral view.

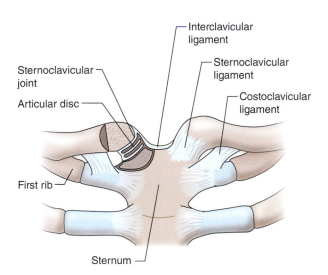

FIGURE 10.3   The sternoclavicular (SC) joint.

In addition to the major musculature of the thorax, small interossei muscles (intercostals) attach each rib to the one superior and inferior to it and allow for breathing

as well as movement. Injury to these muscles can create pain or difficulty with normal breathing.

Lateral to the trunk lie the serratus muscles. These protected muscles assist with breathing.

Major posterior muscles covering the thorax are the trapezius muscles, latissimus dorsi, and spinal muscles (figure 10.4). The upper trapezius begins on the posterior skull, attaching to the lateral clavicle and acromion of the scapula. The middle trapezius originates from the spinous processes of the last cervical vertebra and first 5 thoracic vertebrae, and its insertion is on the lateral aspect of the spine of the scapula, posteriorly; whereas the lower trapezius originates below the middle trapezius, on the spinous processes of the last 5 thoracic vertebral spinous processes, and also inserts on the spine of the scapula (medial portion). The latissimus dorsi extends from the posterior pelvic crest, lumbar vertebra, and lower 6 thoracic spinous processes, and moves along the lateral trunk inserting on the anterior humerus. Providing coverage over the ribs on the lateral posterior aspect of the trunk are the infraspinatus and teres muscles (major and minor), all of which originate on the posterior scapula and insert on the humerus.

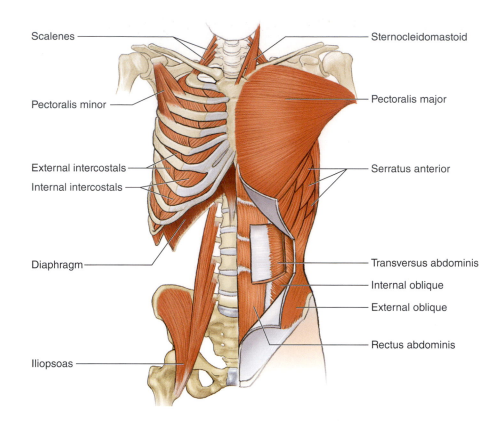

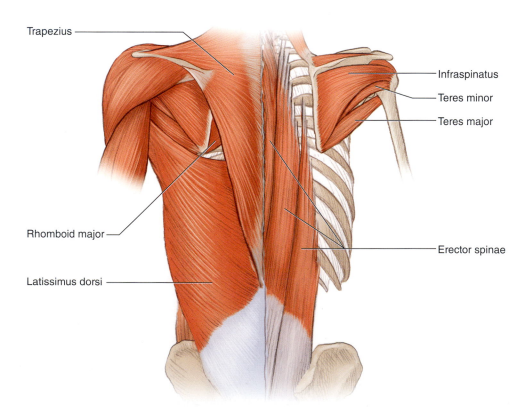

FIGURE 10.4 *(top)* Anterior muscles of the chest. *(bottom)* Posterior muscles of the chest.

Cavities

Within the thorax lie several cavities that protect internal structures (figure 10.5). The mediastinum is a fascia that extends from the sternum to the thoracic vertebrae and contains the heart, thymus, and several other key structures (e.g., bronchi, aorta). The heart has its own layer of protection with the pericardium. In addition, pleural cavities form the space containing each lung. The visceral pleura adheres directly to the lungs and the parietal pleura lines the outer wall of the thorax. Between the 2 pleurae is a pleural space, which contains a small amount of lubricant, which facilitates the lungs' easy movement on the parietal pleura, allowing respiration to occur. During injury, blood can accumulate in this pleural space, causing pneumothorax and hemothorax conditions (described in the Pneumothorax, Hemothorax, and Hemopneumothorax section). All of these cavities and spaces have potential for fluid to accumulate and thereby apply pressure on the very structures they protect.

Organs

The heart and lungs are the primary organs in the thorax. In children (and less so in adolescents) the thymus gland is present superficial to the heart beneath the sternum, but it diminishes in size and endocrine function as a person grows into adulthood. Whereas humans can survive without some organs (e.g., a kidney), a person cannot survive without these two critical organs of the thorax.

Heart

Anatomy and physiology of the heart is carefully described in chapter 11, so this brief overview includes some vessels germane to the thorax. The heart is a four-chambered muscular organ. Its movement is controlled by electrical impulses within the right atrium and intraventricular septum, which engage the cardiac muscles to propel the blood from the atrium and ventricles, to the lungs, and through the aorta into the body proper (see figure 11.2). Surrounding the heart is a pericardium, a tough, protective membrane that also separates the heart from any external fluid and other structures. The aorta is the primary vessel carrying oxygenated blood to the remainder of the body. It arises from the left ventricle and, as it arches external to the heart, it delivers oxygenated blood inferior to the abdomen and lower extremity and superior to the carotid and subclavian arteries. These arteries are critical to know in evaluation of injuries to the sternoclavicular joint, because they pass close to its junction and could be compromised in injuries to this area.

Lungs

The two lungs differ in size. The right lung has 3 lobes; and the left has one fewer, accommodating the heart, which lies largely left of the sternum. The lungs function as the physiological transportation of oxygen to the blood, and they remove carbon dioxide from the blood. This exchange occurs at the smallest unit of the respiratory system, the alveoli. After inhaling air into the nares (nostrils), it passes through the pharynx (throat), past the epiglottis which, when closed, prevents food and liquid from entering the trachea. Air continues through the trachea (windpipe) at the anterior aspect of the throat, and it is divided into 2 smaller pathways, the bronchi, each entering a separate lung. Each bronchus continues to divide into smaller units (bronchioles), ending at the alveoli (figure 10.6).

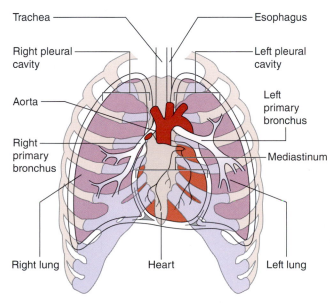

FIGURE 10.5 Cavities of the thorax.

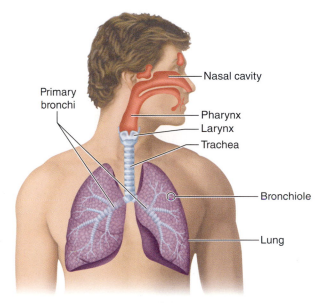

FIGURE 10.6 Anatomy of the lungs.

An important, often forgotten aspect of lung anatomy is that they extend above the first rib and thereby also above the clavicle, about 1-1/2 inch (4 cm). Respiration is active; it requires work from the diaphragm, ribs, and musculature, whereas expiration is a primarily passive event. The chest rises and falls with breathing, which is a good sign if an underlying issue exists with respiration. With a stethoscope, you can hear the *whoosh* of healthy breathing in each lung.

Respiratory Assessment

Respiration is measured based on rate and quality. Rate is the number of breaths per minute. Quality is the sound of air exchange; the *whoosh* sound is the audible quality of respiration. Quality can sometimes be determined without a stethoscope and auscultation, but it is more effective with the stethoscope. For respiration quality, assess for regular, smooth, and noiseless breathing. This section does not cover the various deviants from typical respiration, because they are more medical in nature. The purpose of this section is to review healthy breathing patterns and sounds.

Respiratory Rate

Respiratory rate depends on a person's age, fitness, and overall health. Healthy people have steady, regular breathing without sounds or breaks (**apnea**). Absent any lung diseases, typical adult respiration is 12 to 20 breaths/min. The HCP evaluates for bilateral symmetry in chest movement and a relatively silent exchange of air. Patients with noisy breathing or who use accessory musculature to assist breathing are not within normal definitions of healthy breathing. Tachypnea is defined as more than 20 breaths/min; it is normal when people are exercising but not at rest. Different from tachypnea is hyperventilation, or hyperpnea. This fast, deep breathing does not allow for full exchange of oxygen and carbon dioxide, and it is ineffective breathing. Anxiety and post-exercise deep breathing are more common reasons for hyperventilation than is injury, but it can occur in response to trauma.

Normal Respiratory Sounds

Healthy people make these 3 types of respiratory sounds:

1. *Bronchial sounds* occur when air moves freely through the larger passageways of the lungs and are heard over the anterior chest in the trachea and bronchi.

2. *Bronchovesicular sounds* are heard both anteriorly and posteriorly toward the midline of the thorax. They are the sounds made as air moves through medium-sized air passages.

3. *Vesicular sounds* are lower-pitched noises that are heard anteriorly and posteriorly away from the midline, in all other areas of the lungs, especially the bronchioles.

All of these sounds represent free, unobstructed movement through airways of varying sizes, and they are not accompanied by extraneous noises. These sounds can be clearly heard and distinguished by auscultation using a stethoscope.

Using Supplemental Oxygen

When a person's normal breathing is challenged, the usual amount of oxygen is not provided to tissues. A pulse oximeter is an easy and effective means of determining the percent of oxygen saturation (hemoglobin) in blood and is listed as SpO_2. The pulse oximeter is applied to any unpainted digit (finger or toe) or the earlobe (see figure 4.7). The unit is nearly spontaneous in delivering a number, which is the percent oxygen in the blood (SpO_2), and most oximeters also relate heart rate. The American Red Cross provides guidelines with ranges of SpO_2 levels. They are listed in table 10.1.

TABLE 10.1   **Patient Pulse Oximeter Ranges and Recommended Delivery Device**

Range	Patient % oxygen saturation (SpO_2)	Common flow rate (in L/min)	Best device to deliver supplemental oxygen
Normal	95%-100%	None needed	None needed
Mild hypoxia	91%-94%	1-6 L\min	Nasal cannula
Mild-moderate hypoxia	88%-92%	6-10 L\min	Simple oxygen mask
Moderate hypoxia	86%-90%	10-15 L/min	Non-rebreather mask or bag-valve mask
Severe hypoxia	<85%	15 L/min or higher	Non-rebreather mask or bag-valve mask

Data from Miller (2015, 2017); EMS Safety (2012); American Red Cross (2011).

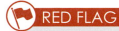

For the purposes of this textbook, any condition requiring *low-flow* supplemental oxygen refers to applying a nasal cannula or simple oxygen mask and administering 2 to 10 L/min of oxygen; whereas administering *high-flow* oxygen uses a non-rebreather mask and delivers oxygen over 10 L/min. As a HCP you should use these references as a guide, and consult with local regulations and the medical protocols for your worksite.

External airways use a human rescuer or oxygen and are the only means of oxygen delivery to a person who cannot breathe independently. External airways are used on unconscious or unresponsive patients in respiratory failure; they are discussed in the next section. Supplemental oxygen assists breathing effectiveness in a person who is breathing independently but not efficiently. Emergency oxygen cylinders are available without a prescription as long as the tank provides at least 15 minutes of oxygen at a preset level.

Oxygen cylinders are high-pressure devices and come in various sizes (e.g., see figure 5.6). They are to be handled carefully, because if dropped or knocked over, these tanks can cause serious injury due to the high pressure they are under. Because oxygen cylinders are used for many purposes, including welding, a metal tank of oxygen that is approved for human consumption is required to be labeled as such. The Occupational Health and Safety Administration (**OSHA**) mandates that every metal container have a yellow diamond symbol on it denoting the oxygen is medical-grade oxygen and is safe for human use. An affixed label stating U.S.P (United States Pharmacopeia) also confirms the medical grade of the oxygen.

Separate from the metal container is a pressure regulator with a flow meter dial that attaches to the oxygen tank. The flow meter adjusts the flow of oxygen and controls the pressure of oxygen output in pounds per square inch (psi). The regulator is fitted by aligning the 2 holes of the regulator with the 2 similar holes on the oxygen tank, then it is tightened by turning the knob on the regulator. After applying the regulator to the tank, the oxygen is ready for use but needs to be delivered through a tube to a mask and person. Typically, the oxygen tank has the regulator attached when being stored, but not the long tube. To deliver oxygen to a person, a tube needs to be attached to the proper receptacle on the regulator, and the regulator needs to be turned on with a metal key, which allows oxygen to flow into the tube.

Supplemental oxygen delivery can occur using the following methods:

• A *nasal cannula* (figure 10.7*a*) is used when a person can breathe independently but needs more oxygen saturation than is delivered in the typical environment (which is about 21%). This device is attached to an oxygen tank by a long tube, and it is secured by a loop over the patient's ears. It delivers oxygen through 2 small openings in the tube that is in each nostril.

• A *simple oxygen mask* (figure 10.7*b*) delivers low-flow oxygen to both the nose and mouth, unlike the nasal cannula, which provides oxygen through the nares only. As with the cannula, it is likewise attached by a tube to an oxygen tank. The patient can either hold the mask on her face or use a strap to hold it around her head. Oxygen delivery differs with the seal on the face; the tighter the seal, the higher the oxygen concentration delivered.

• A *non-rebreather mask* (figure 10.7*c*) allows a patient to inhale oxygen from the bag, which is connected to oxygen, and exhale the carbon dioxide into the atmosphere. When it is apparent that supplemental oxygen is required, most patients with thorax injuries who can

CLINICAL SKILLS

Administration of Supplemental Oxygen

1. Ensure the regulator is firmly connected to the oxygen tank.
2. Ensure the oxygen tank is secure and not in danger of tipping over.
3. Check the oxygen tank level by validating that at least 1,500 psi remains in the tank.
4. Attach tube to the regulator.
5. Turn on the oxygen tank, and adjust the knob on the regulator.
6. Adjust the flow meter to the desired oxygen flow rate.
7. Attach the appropriate device to the tube (nasal cannula, non-rebreather mask, bag-valve mask).
8. Monitor oxygen levels using a pulse oximeter, and adjust oxygen flow as necessary.

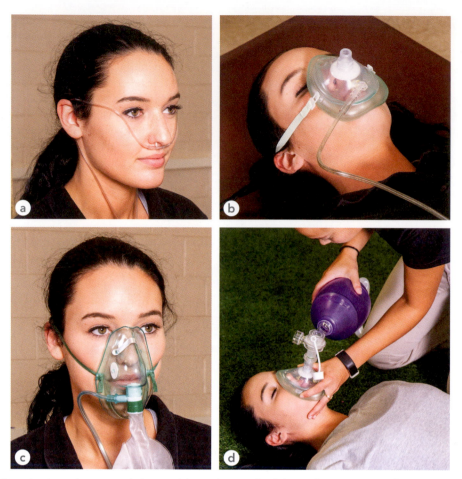

FIGURE 10.7 Supplemental oxygen delivery: *(a)* nasal cannula, *(b)* simple oxygen mask, *(c)* non-rebreather mask, and *(d)* bag-valve mask.

breathe on their own can be given 100% oxygen with a non-rebreather mask. This method delivers a higher percentage of oxygen than does the nasal cannula (see table 5.6).

• The *bag-valve method* (figure 10.7d) typically is used with at least one HCP and may be used in conjunction with an external airway (see next section). A bag-valve mask is used when a patient is unable to breathe on his own. The HCP introduces positive pressure by squeezing the bag. The bag is attached to oxygen on one end, and the mask on the other end, which is held in place with a tight seal over the patient's nose and mouth. This situation is used in respiratory arrest situations and provides 100% oxygen. Typical delivery is one "breath" (bag squeeze) every 5 to 6 seconds for an adult or child.

Airway Maintenance

It is rare that thorax trauma will elicit airway maintenance, but it is wise to review the procedures should they be necessary. After determining respiratory instability, one of these types of airway is used:

1. Nose to throat—nasopharyngeal airway (NPA)

2. Mouth to throat—oropharyngeal airway (OPA)

Both are used in union with external air, be it cardiopulmonary resuscitation (CPR; see chapter 11) or supplemental oxygen (previous section). Both the NPA and OPA are used in unresponsive patients who need oxygen delivered, be it for respiratory arrest or supplemental air (table 10.2). The NPA can also be used on semiconscious patients, because it does not elicit a gag reflex and can be tolerated.

In order for external airways to be effective, the patient must be positioned properly, and the person's airway must be clear of any obstructions. Obstructions can be external (e.g., a mouth guard or removable retainer) or internal (e.g., loose teeth, tissue damage). In addition, the airway must be opened as demonstrated in CPR—with a head-tilt–chin-lift maneuver or a jaw-thrust if cervical spine trauma cannot be ruled out (as described in chapter 9). As always, maintaining proper sanitation is a must, and gloves and other OSHA-approved measures are in effect.

TABLE 10.2   **Comparison of Nasopharyngeal and Oropharyngeal Airways**

Airway	Indications	Contraindications
Nasopharyngeal airway	• Unresponsive patients • Patients with altered mental status • Patients with intact gag reflex • Oral trauma preventing OPA	• Patient intolerance • Caution with presence of facial fractures • Nasal obstruction, including uncontrolled epistaxis • Caution with presence of skull fracture
Oropharyngeal airway	• Unresponsive patients • Absent gag reflex	• Conscious patients • Patients with a gag reflex • Trauma to the mandible and teeth

Nasopharyngeal Airway

A nasopharyngeal airway (NPA) is a soft, pliable tube that inserts into the nostril and provides a valid airway to the patient (figure 10.8). It is a useful technique if the mouth has damage (e.g., broken teeth, laceration to the cheek), if the mouth cannot be opened, or if the patient has a gag reflex that would prohibit use of the oropharyngeal airway.

Suction can be used through the NPA. Sizes of NPA are specific to patient size. They are measured from the patient's earlobe to tip of the nostril. After selecting the correct size, apply a lubricant to the slanted opening of the NPA. Gently advance the NPA with slight rotating (only 10°-25° each turn) to maintain the slanted opening toward the midline of the nose. When the flared end (flange) rests at the opening of the nostril, the NPA is in place. You can use this airway with suction or with a bag-valve mask. The NPA remains in place until it is decided that a different airway is necessary or the NPA is no longer needed.

Oropharyngeal Airway

The oropharyngeal airway (OPA) is used on unconscious or unresponsive patients. The rigid, curved instrument holds the tongue in place, thereby preventing it from blocking the glottis, which would not allow air to reach the lungs. The OPA also comes in different sizes, which also relate to the size of the patient. To choose the appropriate size, place the opening lateral to the patient's lips. If the end reaches the angle of the mandible, the size is appropriate.

Insert the airway into the mouth upside down, and the tip is run along the roof of the mouth (figure 10.9). Use a tongue depressor to hold the tongue down, if necessary. When the hard palate is cleared, rotate the OPA 180° so that the curve of the airway rests on the natural curve of the patient's tongue. The OPA is in place when the flared opening rests at the lips. If a patient begins to gag, remove the OPA by gently following the anatomy of the tongue, and be prepared to use suction and roll the patient to her side to prevent **aspiration**.

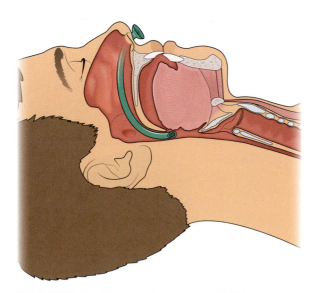

FIGURE 10.8   Correct placement of NPA.

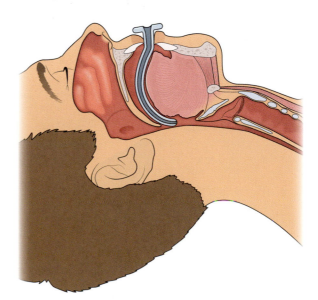

FIGURE 10.9   Correct placement of OPA.

Inserting an OPA

1. Size the airway by placing the OPA flared opening lateral to the patient's lips and the end at the angle of the mandible.
2. Insert the OPA upside down along the roof of the patient's mouth.
3. Alternatively, insert the OPA at a 90° angle to the roof of the mouth.
4. After passing the hard palate, rotate the OPA 180° (to right-side up) and complete inserting the OPA until the flared opening rests on the lips of the patient.
5. Attach an oxygen source, such as a bag-valve mask, and ensure the chest rises with administration of oxygen.

Advanced Airway Management: Blind Airways

Emergency medical personnel commonly use *blind airways*, which are called such because the provider inserting the airway cannot visualize the internal structures of the throat. These airways are only used in deeply unresponsive patients who do not have a gag reflex. Blind airways are also called extraglottic devices, because they are inserted into the trachea and are typically single-use tools that are used in airway management on unconscious patients. These devices come in 2 main categories, those that rest above the larynx (supraglottic) and those that are blindly inserted into the upper esophagus (retroglottic and infraglottic). Most of these devices have bladders or balloons that inflate with the purpose of keeping air going into the trachea and lungs, and preventing air from entering the esophagus. These airways are used in conjunction with bag-valve masks to maintain an efficient airway in an unresponsive person who is getting inadequate oxygen exchange. As with the NPA and OPA, these airways are also lubricated before use for ease of insertion.

Supraglottic Devices

Supraglottic devices are airways inserted into the trachea. They are typically single-use tools that are used in airway management on unconscious patients. They are inserted through the mouth and rest on top of the larynx (*supra* means "superior to"). These devises have bladders that, when inflated, provide a better seal to direct ventilation into the lungs. Common devices in this category are the laryngeal mask airway (LMA) and I-gel (figure 10.10).

- *Laryngeal mask airway (LMA).* LMA has a bladder and is sized by patient weight (22-220 lb; 10-100 kg). Should a patient be between sizes, the larger airway

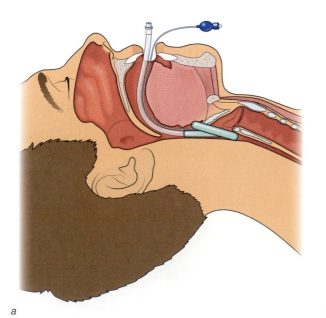
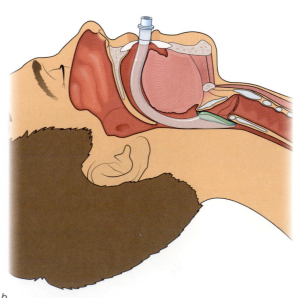

a   *b*

FIGURE 10.10   Correct placement of *(a)* laryngeal mask airway (LMA) and *(b)* I-gel airway.

is used for a better seal.[26] The LMA is easy to use and provides very good ventilation rates, but it does not have a protective bladder that prevents air from entering the stomach or regurgitation, which the retroglottic devices do have.[26,27] The LMA has a bladder that is inflated and then deflated prior to use. This procedure is to ensure it is working and to flatten out the bladder for easier insertion. After insertion, the bladder is reinflated to keep the epiglottis from being trapped between the airway and glottis, and to allow ventilation into the lungs once the airway is in place and oxygen administered.

• *I-gel airway.* The I-gel airway is also a single-use, disposable device that does not require inflation and is easy to use. As such, it is gaining popularity. The I-gel has a pre-shaped, gel-filled distal end, and it is does not require inflation after insertion. It is available in several sizes, from infant to adult. As with the LMA, the patient's weight determines what size I-gel airway is used.

Retroglottic Devices

Retroglottic airway devices are designed to have higher-quality ventilation by preventing air from entering the stomach through the esophagus. They have parts that, when properly inserted, lie behind the glottis and trachea. They use bladders to block entrance to the esophagus that are inflated once the airway is in place. Common airways in this category are the multilumen airway (also known as the Combitube), King airway, and laryngeal mask airway (LMA; figure 10.11).

• *Multilumen/Combitube.* The multilumen airway or Combitube has been in use longer than most of the other blind airways.[28] It is named for the several tubes that are attached to the airway. At the base of the airway are 2 small inflatable bladders that are inflated by 2 tubes external to the mouth. This device is inserted into the esophagus. The distal bladder is then inflated, preventing air from entering the stomach through the esophagus. It comes in 2 sizes—4 feet to 5.5 feet (121-167 cm), and a size for patients over 5.5 feet (167 cm). This airway is not used in pediatric patients and is limited to patients who are between 5 and 7 feet (152-213 cm) tall.

• *King airway.* The King airway is also height based and has 3 sizes—4-5 feet (121-152 cm), 5-6 feet (152-182 cm), and over 6 feet (182 cm); and each size is color coded for quick identification. Similar to the multilumen/Combitube, the King airway has 2 bladders, but only a single tube with 1 port to inflate them.

Rib Fracture

Nearly half of the injuries sustained with a blunt-force blow to the thorax result in a rib fracture.[1] Although a simple rib fracture is rarely life-threatening, the ribs are the outer protection to the lungs and other organs, and an evaluation of respiration as well as underlying organ function is critical. Typically, bones heal within 6 weeks, and many people return to activity sooner with fractured ribs, but some serious potential consequences exist when returning to activity with this injury.

Incidence and Epidemiology

In sports, rib fractures occur from a blow to the chest or pile-up type situation where the affected athlete is

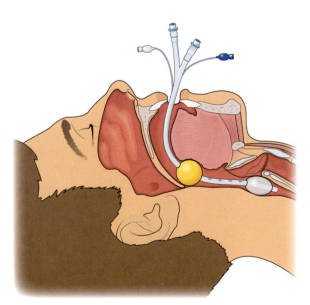
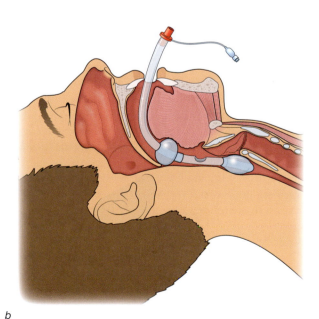

a   b

FIGURE 10.11   Correct placement for *(a)* Combitube and *(b)* King airway.

landed on. In the general population, rib fractures occur most often from motor vehicle accidents, although the most common mechanism for this fracture in the elderly is a fall.[1] Osteoporosis is also a culprit in the elderly; it takes less force to injure the ribs when the bone density is diminished.

Risk Factors

Risk factors for rib fractures in athletes include collision sports and improper protective padding. Stress fractures to the ribs have been known to occur in athletes who have repetitive overhead, high-velocity movements, and coughing has induced rib fractures, though rarely.[1] Outside of the sports arena, motor vehicle accidents, including recreational vehicles, are the primary cause of fractured ribs; osteoporosis is the primary cause in the elderly. Children are less susceptible to rib fractures because of the flexibility in their bones; however, when they do sustain such injuries, they are more likely to have underlying damage.

Signs and Symptoms

Signs and symptoms of simple rib fractures include dyspnea, thorax muscle guarding, and breathing that may be restricted because of pain. Patients often avoid laughing, sneezing, coughing, or any other sudden chest movement. Deep breaths are painful on the affected ribs, but an evaluation of breathing yields normal breathing patterns and sounds. Upon additional physical exam, point tenderness over the affected rib(s), possible crepitus, and visible ecchymosis may occur.

Field Assessment Techniques

On-field evaluation of rib fractures begins with witnessing the incident or determining the mechanism of injury (MOI). Most patients experience shortness of breath immediately following the blow to the thorax, and differentiating between the so-called wind being knocked out of them and a pathological injury may be initially challenging. The clinical suspicion of a fracture is increased if the patient can point to a specific area or spot of pain on the ribs, and the location of the injury is consistent with the MOI for a rib fracture. Challenges are presented if the athlete is wearing protective padding that precludes effective palpation. Removal of such equipment often exacerbates the pain but is necessary.

Respiration rate and quality should be noted, as well as equal and bilateral chest movement with breathing. A pulse oximeter (see figure 4.7) should be applied and the oxygen saturation noted. If oxygen saturation is below 97%, consider supplemental oxygen; if at 95% or lower, administer oxygen.[23-25]

Diagnostic Accuracy

On-field diagnosis of a rib fracture is largely based on clinical presentation and findings. A MOI including a blow to the chest or forcible compression, in addition to dyspnea, deformity or crepitus of the injured rib, is confirmatory for a fracture. However, ecchymosis, pain on respiration, and guarding of trunk movement (which may indicate a fracture) can also denote a contusion or interosseous strain, not a fracture.

Chest radiographs (X-rays) in the anteroposterior (AP) and lateral views are often taken to confirm a fracture, yet early X-rays have low sensitivity (as low as 50%), and often delayed imaging has better, more confirmatory, results.[2,3] Unless there is a reason to suspect pathology beyond a simple rib fracture, radiographs and further imaging are not warranted.

Clinical Prediction Rules

The current guidelines established by the Advanced Trauma Life Support (ATLS) training program recommend chest X-ray and computed tomography (CT) for those who present with blunt chest trauma. However, in a study of nearly 10,000 patients over the age of 14 with blunt chest trauma, a list of 7 clinical criteria was derived that were high predictors of intrathoracic injury.[4] With these data, unnecessary radiation exposure may be avoided for patients with simple fractures.

Immediate Management Techniques

Airway management is of greatest concern with acute rib fractures. Care must be taken to also ensure no underlying trauma exists, including but not limited to lung, spleen, liver, and kidney insult, depending on the location of the rib injury. Damage to each of these organs presents in a different fashion (see other conditions that follow and chapter 12), in addition to the initial contact with the rib. Often the underlying condition is masked by the initial rib injury, so careful supervision and revisiting the patient's signs and symptoms are critical.

On the field, initial airway management entails verifying presence of an open and clear airway and that breathing is within normal ranges. Ineffective breathing is usually apparent with dyspnea, anxiety, potential audible respiratory changes, or unequal chest rising compared to the unaffected side. Adequate respiration can be quickly verified by a pulse oximeter, which displays the amount of oxygen in the blood, as well as heart rate.

The treatments for rib fractures or costochondral injuries are the same, namely, pain management, rest, and actively working on full airway inhalation and exhalation to prevent pneumonia or other sequelae of hypoinhalation. Pain management usually consists of nonsteroidal anti-inflammatory drugs (NSAIDs) and ice; narcotics can diminish normal respiration, which can cause further consequences, including pneumonia.

Indications and Contraindications

When determining return to participation (RTP) status, a rib fracture can have serious complications. It is challenging to truly protect a fractured rib; even a flack-jacket type device will still allow some contact with the injured area if hit directly. Athletes involved in collision sports, including wrestling, judo and rugby, must have physician clearance before RTP with teammates. A blow to healing fractures can injure other tissues, such as the lungs or kidneys, which in turn can further complicate and delay RTP status. Every direct contact with healing rib fractures has a potential for reinjury, additional fractures, and possible organ damage.

Even noncontact sports, such as swimming or cycling, can have potential reactions. Ribs move with respiration, and the increased, forceful breathing will mobilize the ribs as they are trying to heal. Although no finite evidence shows that activity slows rib fracture healing, the act of increased breathing is painful. Binding the ribs with elastic or more rigid devices may protect during practices or events but they should be removed as soon as possible after activity. Binding has been linked to the development of pneumonia because of hypoventilation, and therefore is discouraged.[1]

Criteria for Deciding to Transport for Further Medical Examination

Patients with difficulty breathing, ineffective oxygen exchange, flail chest (multiple rib fractures), or suspected internal organ damage should be transported to an emergency department (ED) for further studies and evaluation. Patients without these criteria should still be observed carefully for worsening signs or symptoms and taken to the ED if conditions deteriorate from first presentation.

Transportation Techniques

A simple rib fracture is not a medical emergency; as long as the patient has usual and effective respiration and has no signs of intrathoracic trauma, no emergency transportation is required. Patients who do have any of the aforementioned signs should be transported to an ED as soon as possible. As with most respiratory conditions, transportation should occur with the patient in a recumbent position. The head should be above the heart, allowing easier breathing. Supine positioning for patients with anterior or lateral rib fractures allows the weight of the chest to negatively affect breathing, because the patient has to counteract his own chest weight with every breath.

Sternoclavicular Joint Injury

The sternoclavicular (SC) joint is the only place on the body where the upper arm attaches via bony articulation to the axial skeleton. This joint is a loose connection between the medial clavicle and manubrium of the superior sternum. It has a joint capsule, disc, and several ligaments in addition to the SC ligament—the intraclavicular ligament (between the two medial aspects of the clavicle, superior to the sternum) and the costoclavicular ligament, which maintains the stability of the clavicle on the ribs below. The SC joint is inherently unstable, and only a portion of the clavicle actually articulates with the manubrium, relying on the SC ligament to provide more stability.

Injury to the SC joint is one of the true medical emergencies in orthopedics. Just posterior to the joint lie the trachea and carotid arteries, and not too lateral from there, the subclavian arteries are located (figure 10.12). A posterior subluxation or dislocation can be a life-threatening emergency with compression on any of these structures.

Because of the SC's importance in connecting the arm to the body proper, the SC joint has many MOIs. One can fall on an outstretched hand or elbow, and the force can transmit along the bones of the arm, acromion of the scapula, and clavicle to the joint, injuring it. Another MOI is a fall on the lateral aspect of the shoulder (humerus or acromion of the scapula), or lying on one side with a pileup on the opposite lateral shoulder. In both of these situations, the force is transmitted along from the humerus/acromion to the clavicle and on to the biomechanically weakest aspect. The athlete could sprain the acromioclavicular joint or fracture the clavicle, or the force could continue medially and injure the SC joint at the sternum.

Incidence and Epidemiology

Injury to the sternoclavicular joint is rare, and posterior dislocations are more unusual. In a study of 251 SC dislocations, only 80 were posterior dislocations. Of the total number of dislocations (both anterior and posterior), the average age of the patient was 29 years old, and 67% of them were male.[5] These data are consistent in other publications, in that younger males are more likely to sustain SC injuries than are other age groups or women.[6]

Risk Factors

Risk factors for injuring the SC joint include falling on an outstretched arm, elbow, or lateral shoulder. As noted, men under 30 years old tend to have higher incidences of SC injuries, so that population is at higher risk. Because high-velocity contact is a MOI, motor vehicle accidents are also a means of sustaining this injury.

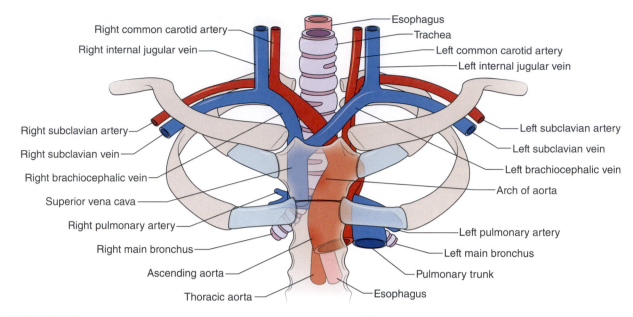

Right common carotid artery

Right internal jugular vein

Esophagus

Trachea

Left common carotid artery

Left internal jugular vein

Right subclavian artery

Right subclavian vein

Right brachiocephalic vein

Superior vena cava

Right pulmonary artery

Right main bronchus

Ascending aorta

Thoracic aorta

Left subclavian artery

Left subclavian vein

Left brachiocephalic vein

Arch of aorta

Left pulmonary artery

Left main bronchus

Pulmonary trunk

Esophagus

FIGURE 10.12   Internal structures behind the sternoclavicular (SC) joint.

Signs and Symptoms

When evaluating an injury to the upper extremity, it is important to be aware of the anatomical connection of the upper extremity and the SC joint. The athlete may initially feel more soreness at the point of impact (e.g., hand, elbow, shoulder) and not recognize the injury to the SC joint. Appreciating the MOI for a potential transmitted force to the medial clavicle and sternum is critical.

On inspection, a deformity may be present over the medial clavicle. It can range from mild swelling to gross deformity. A divot at the SC junction may indicate a posterior dislocation or subluxation, or a posterior fracture of the medial clavicular head (depending on the age of the athlete). Palpation results in a painful SC ligament or joint. Crepitus indicates a fracture, not dislocation or subluxation, but it is equally disconcerting.

Joint stress testing is not recommended, but sometimes the athlete presents with pain away from the SC joint, and that specific injury is not considered at the initial time of testing. The patient will present with an unwillingness to demonstrate full glenohumeral range of motion, because the stress on that joint affects the SC joint.

In a true posterior SC dislocation or subluxation, the patient may have dyspnea or hoarseness and relate difficulty swallowing, because the trachea is pushing posteriorly into the esophagus. If any of these complaints occur, consider it a medical emergency and transport via ambulance as soon as possible. On occasion, the patient will not identify the difficulty swallowing and hoarseness as related to the falling injury, and may not report these conditions. Anecdotal conversations with ATs indicate that athletes sometimes delay reporting issues of the

RED FLAG

The following can indicate a SC injury, if the patient sustained a MOI consistent with this condition:

- Dyspnea*
- Dysphagia*
- Hoarseness*
- Unwillingness to move the affected upper extremity
- Swelling over the SC joint

* Warrants immediate transportation via ambulance to a trauma center.

voice or swallowing because they do not relate it to the SC sprain injury, only to have it be an emergency hours later when swelling increases and the airway begins to be compromised.

Field Assessment Techniques

Always assume a potential SC injury when presented with a mechanism consistent with the biomechanical weakness of the joint. Palpate all aspects of the clavicle, SC joint, and manubrium when evaluating falls resulting in landing on the outstretched hand, olecranon of the elbow, or acromion of scapula. If injury to the SC joint is suspected, assess airway and quality of voice. Ask the athlete to swallow, and query whether that action feels normal. Patients with swelling over the SC joint, who report that it is hard to swallow, or who have altered breath sounds, anxiety, or hoarseness should be removed from activity, have their shoulder pads removed (if wearing them), and be transported to the emergency department via ambulance. While waiting for transport, keep the athlete sitting up to facilitate breathing, and apply a sling to the affected arm. The sling will prevent unnecessary movement of the SC joint.

Reduction of the sternoclavicular joint is not recommended on the field. This procedure is performed under sedation or general anesthesia in an operating room. Open reduction and possible stabilization are necessary in situations of failed closed reduction or ongoing symptoms.[7] Typically, surgical reduction of this injury is performed in conjunction with a cardiothoracic surgeon because of the potential for complications external to orthopedic surgery.

Diagnostic Accuracy

Standard radiographs of the SC joint are ineffective, because the X-rays are poor at viewing relevant anatomy of the joint.[7] One technique that does provide better viewing is the serendipity view, which allows a 40° cephalic tilt.[7] In this technique, an anterior dislocation presents as a superiorly displaced medial clavicle, and a posterior dislocation is represented as an inferiorly displaced medial clavicle.[7] The preferred imaging is CT, which clearly defines the vascular and respiratory features that could be compromised.

Immediate Management Techniques

If the patient reports no difficulty with breathing or swallowing, but has swelling or tenderness over the SC joint, remove the patient from activity, place the affected arm in a sling, and reassess often. In this situation, ice may be held in place by the patient for 15- to 20-minute intervals if it relieves pain and swelling.

Indications

Dyspnea, hoarseness, or dysphagia following a collision or fall on an out stretched arm, elbow, or lateral shoulder are indications to transport the athlete via ambulance to the nearest ED.

Contraindications

Applying ice to the SC region after an acute injury may be contraindicated for a few reasons. The weight of the ice itself could put additional pressure on an unstable joint, further aggravating any dyspnea. Using a wrap to secure the ice to the area provides additional pressure to the area, which can actually worsen an unstable SC joint injury. The anatomical positioning of the trachea and major vessels from the heart immediately under the thin skin of the neck make ice an inappropriate treatment.

Criteria for Deciding to Transport for Further Medical Examination

Dyspnea, hoarseness, and difficulty swallowing following a collision or fall on an outstretched arm, elbow, or lateral shoulder are indications to transport the patient via ambulance to the nearest emergency department.

Transportation Techniques

Patients with a suspected posterior SC sprain should have supplemental oxygen available delivered via a nasal cannula. Transportation should occur in a recumbent position to facilitate easier respiration. A sling should be placed on the affected arm to relieve any traction of the SC joint from the weight of the upper extremity.

Pulmonary Embolism

A pulmonary embolism (PE) is a blockage in a vessel of the lungs caused most commonly by a **thrombus** (figure 10.13), but it can also be attributed to fat, air, or a tumor, which in turn stops blood flow to smaller areas of the lung. When this event occurs, blood gases (oxygen and carbon dioxide) cannot be exchanged in this region, and pulmonary **infarction** will occur without intervention. This section focuses on PEs caused by **thrombi**, although the presentation is the same regardless of the composition of the blockage. PEs can—and often do—arise from **deep vein thrombosis (DVT)**; the risk factors for DVTs are the same risk factors for PEs. Collectively, DVTs and PEs are called venous thromboembolisms. A PE is often fatal and is ranked as the third cause of cardiovascular death in the United States.[8]

Incidence and Epidemiology

Of the common cardiovascular diseases, acute PEs rank third behind coronary artery disease and stroke.[9] Approximately 40% to 50% of patients with DVTs will develop an undiagnosed (called *silent*) PE, and therefore patients with unexplained swelling in distal limbs should be evaluated for DVT. Although most documented cases of PE are found in patients 60 to 70 years old, risk factors for the condition are found in the younger, active population as well.[9] The Centers for Disease Control and Prevention cite that sudden death is the first sign of a PE in 25% of people who have the condition.[10] These data are alarming; 2 of 3 patients with a PE will succumb within 2 hours of presentation. However, if diagnosed and treated acutely, the mortality rate is 8%.[9]

Risk Factors

Certain inherited blood disorders, such as factor V Lieden (a coagulation disorder), are risk factors for both DVT

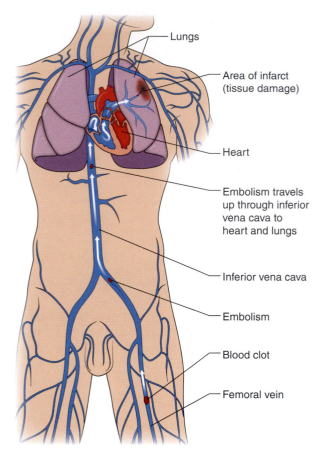

Lungs

Area of infarct (tissue damage)

Heart

Embolism travels up through inferior vena cava to heart and lungs

Inferior vena cava

Embolism

Blood clot

Femoral vein

FIGURE 10.13 How a pulmonary embolism occurs.

and PE. Oral contraceptive birth control has a side effect of blood clots, as do hormone therapy, pregnancy, and childbirth. Immobilization, surgery, trauma, and long-term inactivity such as traveling by bus or long flights on airplanes are also known risk factors for both DVT and PE. The classic Prospective Investigation of Pulmonary Embolism Diagnosis (PIOPED) study has, in addition to chest pain and dyspnea, *travel of 4 hours or more in the past month* as the first indicator of a PE, with recent surgery (in the past 3 months) as the second.[11] In addition,

---

🚩 **RED FLAG**

Patients who have recently had any of the following and also present with lower-leg swelling without a history of trauma should be immediately referred to a hospital for evaluation of a DVT:

- Recent surgery
- Immobilization
- History of sitting for long periods of time (e.g., travel)

---

cancer and obesity are acquired, not genetic risk factors for blood clots.[9,11,12]

Signs and Symptoms

Sudden dyspnea and chest pain are sentinel and alarming precursors to a PE. Anxiety, shock, and cyanosis are also common signs, which are often confused with a **myocardial infarction**. Other notable signs are tachycardia (over 100 bpm), **hemoptysis**, hypotension, **hypoxia**, and **cyanosis**. Symptoms include chest pain worsened by deep breathing, and lightheadedness.[10]

Field Assessment Techniques

Any person who complains of sudden chest pain and difficulty breathing, especially without related trauma, should be immediately evaluated and have respiration thoroughly assessed. A pulse oximeter should be applied to the finger or earlobe and evaluated for an oxygen saturation rate (normal is 95%-100%). Note the anatomical location of the trachea, assessing for deviation, which could indicate a collapsed lung due to either air or blood in the pleural space. Monitor the patient to determine whether respiration is within normal parameters (12-20 breaths/min). Heart rate depends on the person and sport; for example, a resting heart rate of 50 beats per minute (bpm) or lower is common in endurance athletes but can be over 200 when exercising. Check blood pressure for normal range (120/80 mm Hg). Assess skin and mucous membrane color for the usual pinkish color.

A patient who does not quickly recover from dyspnea, who has hemoptysis, a low pulse oximeter reading (indicating low blood oxygen saturation), tachypnea, tachycardia, or low blood pressure should be transported via ambulance to a hospital. An AED should be applied, and supplemental oxygen should be delivered.

Diagnostic Accuracy

The gold standard for diagnosing a PE is pulmonary angiography. However, it has been shown that this tool is not as effective as once thought.[13] Although this imaging method has a high sensitivity for PEs, it also has a high exposure rate to radiation. Less invasive alternatives are pulmonary ventilation-perfusion scan and computed tomographic pulmonary angiogram (CTA or CTPA).[14] These 2 tests may be performed in conjunction with each other. After a radioactive albumin is injected into a vein, the CT will display blood flow through the lungs, using the radioactive dye to illuminate the smallest areas of the lung tissues. The ventilation aspect of the exam is similar, because the patient breathes in radioactive gas through a mask, which in turn displays air movement through the entire lung. The combination of these 2 tests has been used with very high sensitivity and specificity since the 1990s.[11]

An indicator of an acute blood clot is the plasma D-dimer test. Raised levels of D-dimer in the blood could be interpreted as a possible blood clot in the circulatory system but not necessarily the lung. Because the test is most specific for the fibrin aspect of clotting, it could also be a test for other conditions and is therefore not specific to DVT or PE.[9,15] Other laboratory tests, such as blood gases or presence of thrombophilia, are often evaluated for treatment of PEs, but they are not specific for diagnosis.[9]

Clinical Prediction Rules

Neither the modified Wells' criteria/scoring system nor revised Geneva system for clinical prediction of DVT or PE is a good predictor of PE, because they are largely subjective. Yes–no questions in the modified Wells' scoring tool are related to clinical signs (tachycardia, hemoptysis) and patient history (immobilization, prior DVT/PE). The revised Geneva scoring system adds age (over 65), recent surgery, unilateral leg pain, a lower heart rate than the Wells' tachycardia over 100, and leg pain upon palpation, and with edema. Neither tool has been validated to supplant other clinical signs and testing.[9,16] As mentioned earlier, the PIOPED study has high specificity using the ventilation and perfusion scans in determining a PE.

Immediate Management Techniques

An automated external defibrillator (AED) should be applied to the chest to assess cardiac issues (see chapter 11). Concurrently, emergency medical services (EMS) should be notified, and supplemental oxygen should be provided. The patient should remain in a recumbent position to assist with breathing, and the patient should be monitored. On the field, no treatment exists that would reverse a PE, and only anticoagulants provided at a hospital are effective. Using anticoagulants in absence of a thrombus is contraindicated.

Criteria for Deciding to Transport for Further Medical Examination

Any person with sudden chest pain and dyspnea, especially absent any MOI such as a blow to the chest or collision, should immediately raise suspicion of a cardiac or PE event and should be transported via ambulance to an ED as soon as possible. The presence of hemoptysis, cyanosis, or continued dyspnea should increase the urgency of a decision to transport.

Transportation Techniques

As noted previously, the patient should have an AED applied, be delivered supplemental oxygen via nasal cannula or non-rebreather mask to maintain blood oxygenation above 94%, and be transported in a semi-recumbent position to a trauma center via ambulance. Severe hypoxemia or respiratory failure indicates intubation and mechanical ventilation with a bag-valve mask.

Pneumothorax, Hemothorax, and Hemopneumothorax

Pneumothorax is air in the plural cavity, whereas hemothorax is blood in the pleural cavity of the thorax (figure 10.14), either of which impairs respiratory function. This section discusses both, as well as hemopneumothorax, an accumulation of both blood and air in the pleural cavity.

All can occur from an open chest wound that allows entrance of air and blood or from internal insult. With

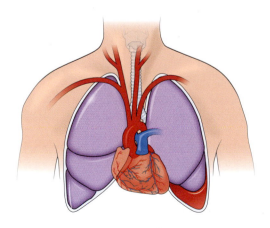

Pneumothorax **Hemothorax**

FIGURE 10.14 Pneumothorax and hemothorax.

any of these conditions, a mass of either air or blood can restrict the lung from fully expanding, which in turn affects respiration. They can be sufficient enough to put pressure on the mediastinum and affect the heart's effectiveness. If untreated, these ailments can lead to respiratory arrest.

Pneumothoraxes can occur for many reasons, ranging from spontaneous, to coughing, to inappropriate medical procedure of the chest (e.g., **iatrogenic pneumothorax**), to onset of a menstrual cycle. This section focuses on the traumatic pneumothorax but briefly discusses spontaneous pneumothoraxes as well. Because pneumothoraxes, hemothoraxes, and hemopneumothoraxes all have the same MOI (in this chapter, traumatic), assessment, and treatment, they are discussed together. If differences exist in a section related to these three conditions, they are noted.

Incidence and Epidemiology

No strong recent studies have been done on the incidence and epidemiology of pneumothorax and hemothorax injuries related to trauma, but robust older data do exist.[16] Traumatic pneumothoraxes occur more often than do spontaneous pneumothoraxes. Spontaneous pneumothoraxes typically occur in the 60- to 65-year-old population, but they are most frequently found in tall, thin men 20 to 40 years of age, which includes the athletic population.[17] For hemothoraxes, the most common MOI is trauma, either external or internal. External trauma consists of penetrating wounds to the chest wall, whereas internal damage may result from blunt chest trauma causing internal bleeding, rib fractures, or laceration of internal vessels.[18] In a classic study involving more than 2,000 children under the age of 15 who were admitted to the hospital for blunt chest trauma, 14 suffered from a hemothorax (which yielded a 57.1% mortality) and 15 had hemopneumothorax (26.7% mortality). This study stated that nontraumatic hemothoraxes carried a much lower mortality rate than did the trauma-associated injury.[19]

Risk Factors

In general, chest trauma has a 10% to 50% risk of pneumothorax associated with the injury.[17] One risk factor for a pneumothorax is previous history of one. Reoccurrence of a pneumothorax typically happens within 6 months to 3 years of the first one with a 5-year recurrence rate of 28% to 32%.[17] A significant risk factor for a spontaneous pneumothorax is smoking, which increases the risk twofold in men and tenfold in women over nonsmokers.[17]

Signs and Symptoms

A patient with a history of a blow to the chest who presents with chest pain, continued dyspnea, gasping for breath, and cyanosis should raise suspicion for possible pneumothorax or hemothorax. Upon inspection, the trachea may appear to be shifted laterally (*tracheal deviation*) away from the injured side (figure 10.15), but that tends to occur later and not at first evaluation. The athlete may have unequal chest motions, with the injured side moving less with inhalation than the healthy side. Other signs include tachypnea (breathing over 20 breaths/min), tachycardia (over 135 bpm), and jugular vein distention.[17] Breath sounds during **auscultation** with a stethoscope may be diminished or absent on the affected side. Use of accessory breathing muscles, including the trapezius, scalenes, sternocleidomastoid, and intercostal muscles, is an indicator of respiratory distress.

Field Assessment Techniques

Athletes who have history of a blow to or compression of the chest who complain of chest pain and dyspnea should be evaluated. Determine and note heart and respiratory rate, and apply a pulse oximeter to a digit or earlobe. Observe for accessory muscle use in breathing, distended jugular veins, and tracheal deviation. If a suitable quiet place is available, auscultation for bilateral and equal respiratory sounds should be performed.

Diagnostic Accuracy

CTs are typically the gold standard for trauma to the thorax, yet they are costly and introduce high levels of radiation. X-rays offer less radiation but are not as conclusive for intrathoracic injuries. A systematic review of the literature revealed that ultrasonography of the chest was more accurate than was a chest X-ray for the diagnosis of a pneumothorax.[20] This conclusion confirms an 18-month

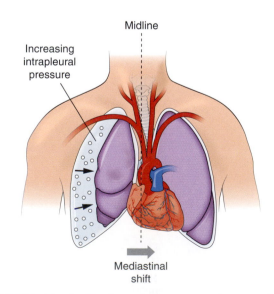

FIGURE 10.15 Trachea shifting away from midline (tracheal deviation).

study in an ED where ultrasonography revealed pneumothoraxes, even **occult** ones, with a 92% sensitivity and 99.4% specificity.[21] Nevertheless, when a patient presents with obvious signs of a pneumothorax, time should not be wasted waiting for confirming diagnostic evaluations to be performed before treating the condition.

In a 4-year study of nearly 1,400 patients with initial minor thorax injuries, about 1 in 10 had a delayed hemothorax 7 to 14 days after discharge from the emergency department. The patients ranged from 43 to 63 years old, and the injuries were not related to athletic activity. Half of those with the late-onset hemothorax had severe chest pain and dyspnea on admission; and 44% had a clinical presentation of a rib fracture at the ED.[22]

Immediate Management Techniques

If it appears that a pneumothorax is possible, the patient is placed on high-flow (above 15 L/min) supplemental oxygen through a non-rebreather mask and transported via ambulance to a hospital. If a physician, physician's assistant, or other HCP trained in emergency decompression is on-site, a needle thoracentesis may be performed while waiting for emergency transport. This decision is based on the situation, patient, and expertise of the HCP performing the skill. In a needle thoracentesis, a large-bore needle is inserted through the chest wall into the pleural space on the collapsed lung side, and a catheter is inserted to relieve the space of air or fluid.

Indications

Pneumothoraxes and other trauma to the thorax have signs and symptoms such as dyspnea and tachycardia. During evaluation of these potential conditions, look for sustained dyspnea, not episodic, brief, or fleeting pain or discomfort with breathing. All athletes have an elevated heart rate during exercise (up to 200 bpm), but a conditioned athlete will rapidly recover at rest to a more normal heart rate (below 90 bpm). Patients who have persistent symptoms, or who worsen, or present additional signs of breathing distress such as use of accessory musculature, jugular vein distention, cyanosis, or hemoptysis must be considered emergent and transported to a hospital as soon as possible.

Contraindications

One thing to keep in mind is that often a pneumothorax can be delayed after trauma. The athlete may sustain a blow to the chest, or complain of chest pain and dyspnea, but have no other discernable signs or symptoms consistent with a pneumothorax. That athlete should be reevaluated prior to leaving the venue for the day, and

given a precautionary warning about symptoms to watch for and when to go to a hospital should pneumothorax present itself later.

Criteria for Deciding to Transport for Further Medical Examination

Any time an athlete sustains a blow to the thorax or a pile-up situation affecting the trunk, that athlete must be assessed for cardiorespiratory illnesses or injuries. If initial assessment is unremarkable, follow up a second time. If the patient presents with any of the aforementioned warnings of a pneumothorax, evaluate cardiorespiratory status, activate the EAP, and arrange emergency transportation to a hospital.

Transportation Techniques

As with all respiratory conditions in this chapter, transportation to a hospital or trauma center is via ambulance. The patient is either seated or in a recumbent position, and has access to supplemental oxygen. If the injury is a hemothorax, internal blood loss may result in shock, and the patient will need to be repositioned and treated accordingly. Depending on the cardiac rate and rhythm, an AED might be applied for transportation. With either pneumothorax or hemothorax injuries, the mediastinum may have pressure exerted upon it, which directly affects cardiac functioning. This condition occurs as the air or fluid continues to build up in the pleural cavity, and it usually presents after initial evaluation.

Asthma

Asthma is a chronic condition caused by a reactive airway triggered by an internal or external irritant. It can be treated by avoiding triggers and by following a medication regimen. Exercise-induced asthma (EIA) and exercise-induced bronchospasm (EIB) are brought on by the histamine release associated with exercise and last several minutes.[30] The terms EIA and EIB are used interchangeably.

Incidence and Epidemiology

Asthma affects approximately 26 million people in the United States, and it is the most common chronic childhood disease, affecting over 7 million children.[29] EIA is attributed to 12% to 15% of the general population, but only 3% to 10% of those with asthma and allergies are not included in the count.[30] In children, asthma is twice as common in boys as in girls, but at puberty they are equally effected. Adult-onset asthma tends to occur mostly in females over 40 years of age.[29]

EIA is more common in the winter and cold-weather sports.[30] One reason is that cold air can dry out airways, leading to an inflammatory response, triggering bronchoconstriction and edema. However, asthma patients with seasonal (environmental) allergies are not only more likely to have EIB, they can have increased asthma symptoms during the allergy season.[31]

Risk Factors

Exposure to allergens, including environmental triggers (e.g., pollutants, smog, smoke, pet dander, dust mites, grasses, pollen, fungi) and smoking, or being around smoke (secondhand smoke) pose a risk to patients with asthma. Gastrointestinal reflux disease, chronic sinusitis or rhinitis, and exercise can also induce asthma.[29] Consuming aspirin or NSAIDs can elicit an asthma response, as can beta-adrenergic receptor blockers.[29] Patients with asthma who take these medicines for pain or inflammation should be cautioned. Chemicals, paint, perfume or cologne, scented candles, and lotions can also create irritants in the airway, which can exacerbate the respiratory hypersensitivity.

Signs and Symptoms

The most common indicators of asthma include shortness of breath, dyspnea, chest congestion, coughing, chest tightness, and the hallmark sign—wheezing.[29] Additional salient signs include respiratory distress, difficulty speaking in complete sentences, and using accessory muscles to breathe (scalenes, sternocleidomastoid, and intercostal muscles). During an asthma attack the patient may have changes in mental status, hypotension, and the unwillingness to lie supine. Sweating, agitation, anxiety or panic, and confusion are not uncommon.[32] Cyanosis is a sign that the respiratory situation is worsening, and immediate emergent action must be undertaken.

Field Assessment Techniques

On the field, determine whether the respiratory response is due to injury, anxiety, blow to the ribs or chest, or asthma (figure 10.16). Pay attention to the sound, quality (deep breaths or not), and rate of breathing. Wheezing is the sound of asthmatic breathing. If available, and the situation warrants it, lung function can be assessed and monitored with a peak flow meter (described in the next section, Diagnostic Accuracy) and compared to the patient's baseline test. If the patient has less than 50% of personal best, supplemental oxygen and transportation to an acute care facility are necessary.

Diagnostic Accuracy

Often asthma is a diagnosis of exclusion; but pulmonary function testing via spirometry assessment is the primary test to determine asthma diagnosis.[29] It should be used as a baseline for all asthmatic patients. In initial testing, people with asthma often perform a peak flow meter test, which provides a baseline of forced peak expiratory flow (PEF).

The peak flow meter is an inexpensive and portable device. It is used by setting the marker on the peak flow meter to zero, then asking the patient to take a deep breath. The patient then places his mouth on the mouthpiece, forming a complete seal with the lips. Forcefully and rapidly, the patient expels all air from the lungs by blowing hard (figure 10.17). The place the maker has moved to is the patient's peak flow number. Typically, this action is repeated 3 times, and the patient's personal best is recorded in the medical record and pre-participation exam. Having knowledge of the asthmatic patient's PEF is instrumental to management, because patients can accurately judge whether their reading is within a stable range (usually indicated in green), a caution (yellow) range (50%-80% of maximum personal best) or danger (red) range (below 50% of personal best).

Immediate Management Techniques

For a patient known to have asthma, administration of the patient's short-acting beta$_2$-agonist (e.g., albuterol) inhaler may provide the highest therapeutic intervention.[30] Usually 2 puffs, properly administered via a metered-dose inhaler (MDI), will result in a desired response (as described in chapter 5). A nebulizer is also effective, but the MDI is usually more readily available. The inhaler may be readministered 1 to 3 times per hour if needed, but if dyspnea continues after multiple treatments, or if it worsens, transport the patient to the nearest acute care facility.[32] If the medication is effective, observe the patient for several hours until respiration sounds, quality, and rate are back to normal before determining RTP status. Patients who continue to have mild reactive respiratory symptoms may have a repeat inhaler dosage, although the recommended interval between deliveries for this situation is 4 hours.[30]

If the inhaler does not ameliorate the asthma attack, check oxygen saturation status with a pulse oximeter. Pulse oximetry is an important assessment in acute asthma reactions, because it can exclude hypoxemia as well as confirm whether supplemental oxygen is necessary. If the patient is not responding adequately to the inhaler, or if the patient does not have access to the inhaler, transport the patient to an acute care facility. If respiratory adequacy deteriorates, subcutaneous epinephrine can be administered.[30]

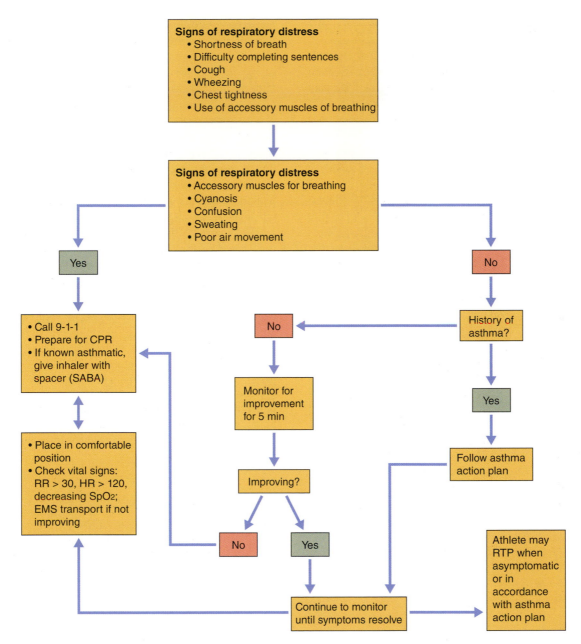

FIGURE 10.16 Asthma decision tree.

Reprinted from Dr. Sharon Rogers Moore.

Criteria for Deciding to Transport for Further Medical Examination

If the inhaled short-acting beta$_2$-agonist is not effective, or vital signs are degrading, administer supplemental oxygen and transport to an acute care center. Vital signs that indicate the situation is worsening include oxygen saturation (measured using pulse oximeter) is decreasing, increased respiratory rate greater than 30 breaths/min, and lowering heart rate (<120 bpm).[32]

Transportation Techniques

Patients experiencing asthma-related difficulty breathing should be transported in a sitting or semi-reclined position, with the head and chest elevated. Depending on

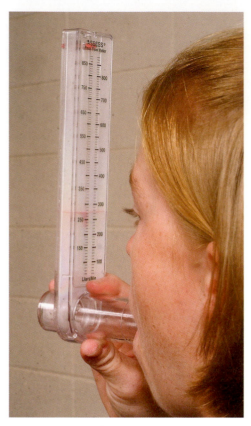

FIGURE 10.17   Peak flow meter.

the oxygen saturation of the patient, oxygen should be delivered using a nasal cannula or non-rebreather mask.

Summary

Emergent conditions of the thorax are often alarming and sometimes life-threatening. It is vital to appreciate the relevant anatomy and to reassess injuries to this area often, because conditions can deteriorate quickly. Patients who display chest pain or dyspnea that does not abates should be thoroughly reevaluated and transported by ambulance to the closest ED. Supplemental oxygen can be an effective treatment for many thorax issues. HCPs must be familiar with setup and use of not only oxygen but with the various airways that can facilitate oxygen transport.

Although rare, SC posterior dislocations are a life-threatening event and must be recognized and managed accordingly. Rib fractures are far more common and rarely require intervention to heal. Pulmonary emboli can occur at any age, have an insidious onset, and are often lethal. Many of the acute conditions of the thorax present with a seemingly benign mechanism but may deteriorate with time. Patients who sustain a blow to the thorax should be carefully monitored for SC dislocations, pneumothorax, and rib fractures, which may not initially present as urgent.

 Go to the web study guide to complete the case studies for this chapter.

CHAPTER 11

Life-Threatening Cardiac Conditions

OBJECTIVES

After reading this chapter, you will be able to do the following:

- Explain how the cardiovascular system supplies the body with oxygen.

- Distinguish between the various causes of sudden cardiac death.

- Interpret the risk factors and incidence of sudden cardiac death.

- Classify the basic types, indications, and contraindications for common medications used to treat acute cardiac conditions.

- Apply a 12-lead electrocardiogram and transmit recordings to an emergency department.

- Demonstrate efficient cardiopulmonary resuscitation and management of sudden cardiac arrest.

- Develop and employ a comprehensive emergency action plan for acute cardiac conditions.

- Appraise the diagnostic accuracy of cardiovascular screening.

Cardiac conditions are the leading causes of nontraumatic death in young, physically active clients and athletes.[1-3] Athletes are considered the healthiest members of society, and their unexpected death during training or competition is a catastrophic event that stimulates debate regarding both pre-participation screening evaluations and appropriate emergency planning for athletic events. Despite pre-participation screening, clients and athletes who appear healthy may harbor unsuspected cardiovascular diseases with the potential to cause sudden death.[4] With the increasing availability of automated external defibrillators (AEDs) at athletic events and other public spaces, potential exists for effective prevention of sudden cardiac death (SCD). The presence of athletic trainers (ATs) and other health care providers (HCPs) trained in cardiopulmonary resuscitation (CPR), and timely access to AEDs at venues, provide a means of early defibrillation in the case of an unexpected sudden cardiac arrest.[5] Early defibrillation is beneficial not only for athletes but also for event spectators, coaches, officials, event staff, and bystanders. Given the unique nature of cardiac conditions and the management of these conditions, this chapter does not follow the structure of previous chapters. This chapter describes the most common causes of SCD in healthy, active people as well as some red flags for recognition of a cardiac event. Also included are emergency life support, medications, and other clinical skills necessary to manage a cardiac emergency.

Overview of the Cardiovascular System

The circulatory system is the transport system of the body that delivers oxygen and nutrients to the tissues and returns the waste products of metabolism (carbon dioxide and cellular waste) to the lungs and kidneys for exhalation and excretion from the body. Body tissues require an adequate oxygen supply for survival. Any compromise in circulation (**ischemia**) can lead to tissue damage or death (necrosis). The most oxygen-dependent tissues of the body are those of the central nervous system and the heart, and a thorough physical examination may reveal the earliest signs of inadequate oxygenation. Therefore, a rapid assessment of the brain and circulatory system function is an essential priority in the early part of the assessment of an emergent patient. The HCP must be able to rapidly recognize signs of cardiovascular distress or failure and promptly administer emergency treatment.[6]

Pulmonary and Systemic Circulations

The cardiovascular system requires proper functioning of the heart and blood vessels, and sufficient volume of blood. The heart provides the driving force to pump blood through the blood vessels to the heart muscle itself (*coronary circulation*), to the lungs for oxygenation (*pulmonary circulation*), and to the body cells (*systemic circulation*; figure 11.1). **Cardiac output** is the volume of blood the heart pumps in 1 minute, and it is related to heart rate and contractility (stroke volume). Cardiac output varies considerably depending on the metabolic demands of body tissue for oxygen and glucose. During exercise, muscles require substantially more blood, which the heart accommodates by increasing both the heart rate and the stroke volume in response to stimulation by the sympathetic nervous system. If heart rate is too slow or the stroke volume is decreased as a result of diminished cardiac output, the patient can experience weakness, lightheadedness, **hypotension**, or other signs of cardiogenic **shock**.[6]

Chambers, Valves, and Vessels of the Heart

The branching network of blood vessels supplying blood to the body is the systemic circulation, and the relatively short vessels delivering and returning blood to and from the lungs comprise the pulmonary circulation. The pulmonary circulation is under relatively low pressure and is the right side of the heart, which receives deoxygenated blood from the inferior vena cava into the right atrium (figure 11.2). The right ventricle pumps blood under relatively low pressure to the lungs through the pulmonary arteries. The systemic circulation is the relatively high-pressure left side of the heart. The pulmonary veins return oxygenated blood from the lungs to the left atrium. The left ventricle pumps blood under very high pressure through the aorta to the rest of the body. In

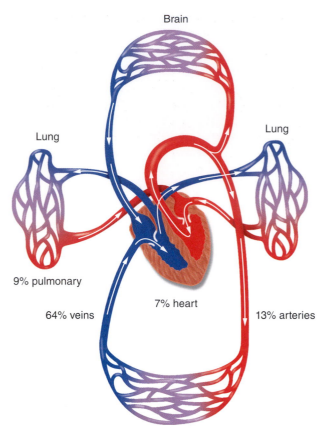

FIGURE 11.1 Systemic and pulmonary circulation. The right side of the heart pumps blood into the pulmonary circuit; the left side of the heart pumps blood into the systemic circuit. Note the percentage of blood found in each area of the circulation; the majority is found in the venous side of the circulation.

general, arteries carry oxygenated blood and veins carry deoxygenated blood, with two exceptions. The pulmonary arteries carry deoxygenated blood from the right ventricle to the lungs, and the pulmonary veins carry oxygenated blood from the lungs to the left atrium. Blood pressure (BP) is measured with the top number (*systolic*) as the pressure in arteries while the ventricles contract, and the bottom number (*diastolic*) as the pressure in vessels when the heart is at rest. **Hypertension** is an abnormal elevation in BP and is a major risk factor for coronary artery disease, stroke, and heart failure (see Normal and Abnormal Blood Pressure).[7,8]

The valves of the heart include 2 atrioventricular (AV) and 2 semilunar valves (figure 11.2). The atrioventricular valves, the tricuspid and bicuspid (mitral) valves, lie between the atria and ventricles of the heart. The semilunar valves, the pulmonary valve and aortic valve, are situated in the arteries leaving the heart. All heart valves are composed of 3 cusps or leaflets, except

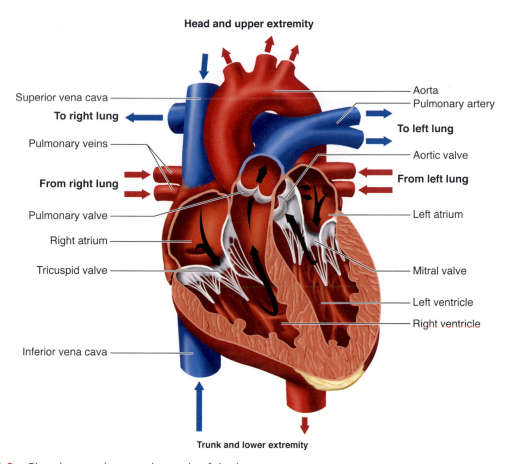

Head and upper extremity

Superior vena cava

Aorta

Pulmonary artery

To right lung

Pulmonary veins

To left lung

Aortic valve

From right lung

From left lung

Pulmonary valve

Left atrium

Right atrium

Tricuspid valve

Mitral valve

Left ventricle

Right ventricle

Inferior vena cava

Trunk and lower extremity

FIGURE 11.2   Chambers, valves, and vessels of the heart.

the mitral valve, which has only 2 cusps. Each cusp is a double layer of endocardium that is attached at its base to the fibrous skeleton of the heart. The margins of the cusps are attached to muscular projections from the ventricles (papillary muscles) through tendinous cords (chordae tendineae). Contraction of the ventricle, and consequently the papillary muscle, results in the opening or closing of the valve depending on its location. During **auscultation**, the closure of the AV valves is heard as *lub,* the first heart sound (S1); the closure of the semilunar valves is heard as *dub,* the second heart sound (S2).[8]

Normal and Abnormal Blood Pressure

Normal BP	<120/80 mm Hg
Hypotension*	<90/60 mm Hg
Prehypertension	120-139/80-89 mm Hg
Stage 1 (mild) hypertension	140-159/90-99 mm Hg
Stage 2 (moderate) hypertension	≥160/≥100 mm Hg
High BP in people over age 60	≥150/90 mm Hg
Emergency severe hypertension	≥180 /110 mm Hg

mm Hg = millimeters of mercury

*Hypotension is normal for many people unless accompanied by symptoms such as lightheadedness, dizziness, or syncope.

Data from Henry and Stapleton (2012); Marx and Rosen (2017); Black et al. (2015).

Electrical Conduction System of the Heart

The heart has its own intrinsic electrical conduction system consisting of specialized cardiac muscle cells that spontaneously depolarize at regular intervals, causing the heart to pump blood on average 60 to 80 bpm at rest. The sinoatrial (SA) node is the area within the walls of the right atrium with the fastest depolarization rate (**sinus rhythm**), effectively making it the primary pacemaker of the heart (see Normal and Abnormal Heart Rates and Rhythms). After initiation of an electrical impulse from the SA node, the depolarization spreads across the right, then left atrium and then down through the ventricles (figure 11.3). The electrical impulses stimulate the atria to contract and fill the ventricles with blood, then the ventricles contract and pump blood through the pulmonary circulation, coronary circulation, and systemic circulation simultaneously.

This movement of electrical activity across the heart is analyzed and recorded on an electrocardiogram (ECG) with each event represented as a wave. The 3 limb leads (right arm, left arm, and left leg) create an imaginary inverted triangle (Einthoven's triangle) with the heart at the center (figure 11.4). When the voltage differences from each lead are summed, the difference in electrical potential is zero. The P wave represents depolarization

of the atria while the QRS wave complex represents depolarization of the ventricles (figure 11.5). The ECG waves can demonstrate abnormal heartbeat patterns (**arrhythmias**), such as ventricular fibrillation, and can be interpreted by a trained professional or by computer analysis in AEDs or other specialized devices.[6]

Sinus bradycardia is a sinus rate under 60 bpm and is common in the athlete and well-trained client. Generally, this heart rhythm is attributed to enhanced vagal tone caused by conditioning and is thus physiological. Occasionally, in the highly conditioned client the heart rate can be as slow as 30 to 40 bpm at rest and decreases to less than 30 bpm during sleep. Sinus pauses or sinus arrest (more than 3 seconds) may be considered clinically significant when accompanied by symptoms, and they require referral.[11]

Ventricular tachycardia (V-tach or VT) is an abnormal rapid heart rhythm resulting from incorrect electrical activity that starts the ventricles, rather than the normal SA node. This potentially life-threatening arrhythmia can cause pathologic hypotension, ventricular fibrillation, asystole, and sudden death. **Ventricular fibrillation (V-fib or VF)** is a medical emergency that requires immediate basic life support or **advanced cardiac life support (ACLS)** interventions. This abnormal rhythm is characterized by chaotic rapid depolarizations and repolarizations, which cause the heart muscle to quiver and

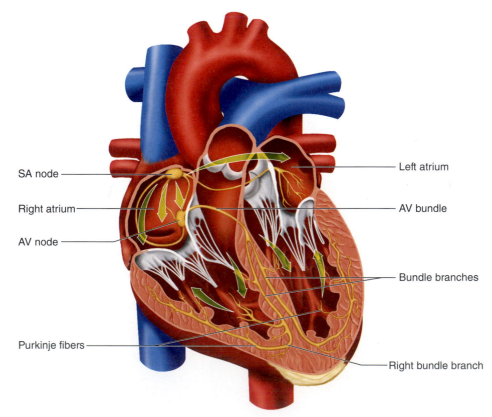

SA node

Right atrium

AV node

Purkinje fibers

Left atrium

AV bundle

Bundle branches

Right bundle branch

FIGURE 11.3   The cardiac conduction system.

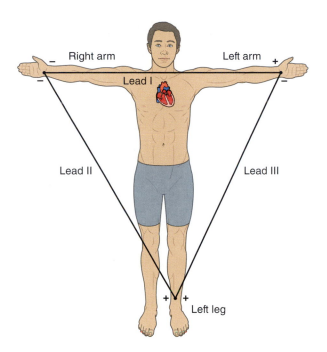

FIGURE 11.4   Einthoven's triangle and leads of the ECG.

lose its ability to pump blood effectively.[5] Sinus rhythm must be restored promptly; within 90 seconds of the onset of VF, the abnormal rhythm may degenerate further into asystole (flatline). **Asystole** represents absence of detectable ventricular electric activity with or without atrial electric activity.[12] VT may result in cardiogenic shock and asystole with SCD in minutes. The patient must have normal sinus rhythm restored within 4 to 5 minutes (at normal body temperature) or sustain irreversible brain damage from cerebral hypoxia.[6,8]

Epidemiology of Sudden Cardiac Death

In the United States, more than 166,000 patients experience an out-of-hospital cardiac arrest annually, and approximately 60% are treated by emergency medical services (EMS).[3] A paradox of sport exists in which despite the undisputed health benefits of physical activity, vigorous exertion may transiently increase the risk of acute cardiac events. Cardiac conditions are the leading medical cause of death during exercise.[1] In the general population, the risk of SCD approximately doubles during physical activity and is twofold to threefold higher in athletes compared to nonathletes. In young athletes, SCD is the leading cause of mortality.[13] The annual incidence (see chapter 3 for epidemiological definitions) of SCD is about 0.7 to 3.0 per 100,000 athletes in young people (<35 years), although a wide range of incidences has been reported.[14] Further, medical causes of sudden death in college student-athletes are most likely (56%) related to SCD with an incident rate of 1 out of 43,770 per year.[15] Basketball by far is the highest-risk sport, with an overall annual death rate of 1 per 11,394; and the highest-risk group of athletes regardless of ethnicity were Division I male basketball athletes, with a risk for SCD of 1 per 3,126. Further, a 3-fold increase in risk of SCD was found for black male basketball athletes compared to white male basketball athletes in all divisions.[15] In military recruits the nontraumatic sudden deaths rate is 13 per 100,000 recruit-years; these deaths were overwhelmingly (86%) related to exercise.[16] The incidence of SCD in older (≥35 years) athletes is higher and may be expected to rise as more and older people take part in organized sports.[14]

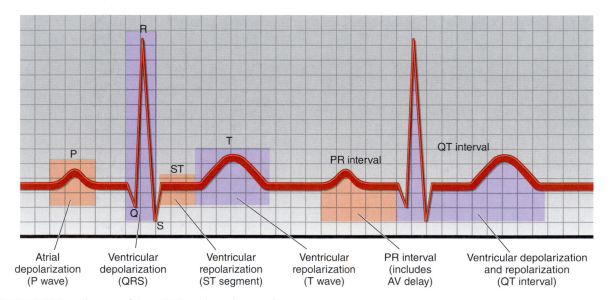

FIGURE 11.5   Phases of the ECG and cardiac cycle.

Normal and Abnormal Heart Rates and Rhythms

Normal heart rate (sinus rhythm)	60-100 bpm
Sinus bradycardia	<60 bpm
Extreme bradycardia	<50 bpm
Tachycardia	>100 bpm
Ventricular tachycardia (V-tach or VT)	Rapid heart rhythm starting in the ventricles; potentially life-threatening arrhythmia
Ventricular fibrillation (V-fib or VF)	Uncoordinated contraction of ventricles and inability to pump blood effectively
Asystole (flatline)	No cardiac electrical activity, no myocardial contractions, and no cardiac output

bpm = beats per minute

Data from Henry and Stapleton (2012); Marx and Rosen (2017); Berg et al. (2010).

Etiology and Pathophysiology of Acute Cardiac Conditions

The most common causes of SCD in physically active people differ depending on population (table 11.1). A critical systematic review of investigations in several populations (athletes, nonathletes, military, national, and international) indicated that the most common finding at autopsy of young people with SCD is actually a structurally normal heart.[1] In younger athletes, SCD is primarily attributed to congenital or inherited cardiac abnormalities; however, in older athletes, coronary artery disease (CAD) is the most common cause.[14] In high school and collegiate football players, the most common cardiac cause of fatalities was cardiac failure (41%).[13] In the military, the most common cause of sudden death was an identifiable cardiac abnormality (51%). However, a substantial number of deaths remained unexplained (35%).[17] Among college student-athletes who died of exertion, 75% were related to cardiac causes; the most common finding at

TABLE 11.1   Causes of Sudden Cardiac Death in Populations of Athletes

Etiology	Prevalence	Population
Identifiable cardiac (structural) abnormality	51%	Military
Coronary artery abnormalities	61%	Military
	14%	NCAA student-athletes
Cardiac failure	41%	High school and collegiate football players
Unexplained cardiac death	35%	Military
Structurally normal heart or autopsy-negative sudden unexplained death	31%	NCAA student-athletes
Myocarditis	20%	Military
	8%	NCAA student–athletes
Hypertrophic cardiomyopathy	13%	Military
	3%	NCAA student-athletes
Idiopathic left ventricular hypertrophy/ possible hypertrophic cardiomyopathy	8%	NCAA student-athletes
Dilated cardiomyopathy	8%	NCAA student-athletes
Aortic dissection	8%	NCAA student-athletes
Commotio cordis	3%	High school and collegiate football players
Embolism/blood clot	2%	Military

Data from Boden et al. (2013); Eckart et al. (2004); Harmon et al. (2014).

death was a structurally normal heart or autopsy-negative unexplained death.[1,18] A more precise understanding of the pathogenesis of cardiovascular deaths in athletes has important implications for finding more effective ways to screen for and prevent SCD.[19] This information is vital for sports medicine clinicians and may ultimately help maximize the ability to detect potentially lethal disease prior to competition.[20]

Structural Causes of Acute Cardiac Conditions

Structural causes of SCD in athletes include genetic **cardiomyopathies** such as hypertrophic cardiomyopathy and arrhythmogenic right ventricular cardiomyopathy or dysplasia, and congenital heart conditions such as coronary artery anomalies and Marfan syndrome (table 11.2). Acquired forms of cardiac abnormalities such as coronary artery disease and viral infection leading to myocarditis, and vascular abnormalities such as aortic dissection, may be responsible for causing SCD.[21]

Acute Coronary Syndromes and Myocardial Infarction

Cardiovascular disease—more specifically, CAD—results from fatty deposits, called plaques, that accumulate in the arterial walls, including the vessels to the heart itself, the coronary arteries. As the deposits accumulate over many years, the internal diameter (lumen) of the artery narrows. Less blood can flow through the narrow artery, resulting in hardening of the arteries, or *arteriosclerosis*. Often the first indication of CAD may occur during emotional or physical stress when the heart rate increases, increasing the need for oxygen to the heart

muscle (myocardium).[6] CAD consists of atherosclerotic coronary arteries with more than 70% lumen occlusion.[19]

Acute coronary syndromes (ACS) include **angina pectoris** and **acute myocardial infarction (AMI)**. When the demand for oxygen from the myocardium outweighs the ability of the obstructed coronary arteries to deliver blood, pain and discomfort in the chest result from myocardial ischemia. Myocardial ischemia can cause chest pain during exertion or stress but no permanent damage to the heart, called angina or *angina pectoris*. When a more severe obstruction of the coronary arteries occurs and not enough oxygen exists to supply the myocardium (heart muscle cells), severe and sustained deprivation of

RED FLAG

A patient with an AMI may present with any of the following signs and symptoms:[24]

- Sudden onset of weakness, nausea, and sweating without an obvious cause
- Chest pain, discomfort, or pressure that is described as crushing or squeezing and that does not change with each breath
- Pain, discomfort, or pressure in the lower jaw, arms, back, abdomen, or neck (referred pain)
- Irregular heartbeat or syncope (fainting)
- Shortness of breath or dyspnea
- Pink, frothy sputum (indicating possible pulmonary edema)
- Sudden death

TABLE 11.2 Categories of Cardiac Conditions in Athletes

Heritability	Structurally abnormal heart	Structurally normal heart
Inherited	Cardiomyopathies • Hypertrophic cardiomyopathy (HCM) • Arrhythmogenic cardiomyopathy • Dilated cardiomyopathy	Channelopathies • Long QT syndrome • Brugada syndrome
	Coronary artery anomalies	Catecholaminergic polymorphic ventricular tachycardia
	Valvular heart disease (e.g., bileaflet mitral valve prolapse syndrome)	Idiopathic ventricular fibrillation
	Aortic disease or aortopathies (e.g., Marfan syndrome and ascending aortic aneurysm)	
Acquired	Coronary artery disease (CAD)/myocardial ischemia	Commotio cordis
	Myocarditis	Substance misuse Electrolyte imbalance

Based on Semsarian, Sweeting, and Ackerman (2015); Chandra et al. (2013); Patel and Elliott (2012).

oxygen to the myocardium results in death of heart cells (AMI). The result of AMI may be a severe failure of the heart to pump blood, life-threatening heart rhythms (dysrhythmias), permanent damage to the heart muscle, and SCD.[6]

Hypertrophic Cardiomyopathy

Hypertrophic cardiomyopathy (HCM) is one of the most common causes of nontraumatic sudden cardiac death in athletes; the estimated prevalence is up to 1 in 200. HCM is a common genetic heart disease, occurring in at least 1 in 500 people in the general population.[25] This condition is characterized by unexplained left ventricular hypertrophy (figure 11.6), which can lead to VF or VT and SCD.[22] This genetic condition is inherited as an autosomal dominant condition that causes structural changes, anterior septal hypertrophy, and left ventricular hypertrophy. This inherited structural disorder is characterized by a heart weight of up to 50% larger than normal weight based on gender, age, and body size for weight or height (using the Mayo nomograms).[19] The highest risk for sudden death in HCM has been associated with any of these noninvasive clinical indications: prior cardiac arrest or spontaneous sustained ventricular tachycardia; or family history of premature HCM-related death, particularly if sudden, in close relatives.[25] Deaths caused by HCM are more common in start–stop sports, such as football and basketball, but they are rare in endurance events such as rowing, long-distance cycling, and running.[22]

People with HCM are often asymptomatic with exercise;[26] however, **premonitory symptoms** may be present and include **syncope**, presyncope, shortness of breath, chest pain, and dizziness during or after exercise.

Physical findings such as systolic ejection heart murmur, loudest at the left lower sternal border,[26] may occur in HCM patients, but most are asymptomatic.[23] The murmur is made louder by the **Valsalva maneuver**. These provocative maneuvers help differentiate a pathological HCM murmur from the common systolic murmur heard in the hearts of clients with physiological hypertrophy of the myocardium.[26] In trained athletes, modest segmental wall thickening (13-15 mm) raises the differential diagnosis between extreme physiologic left ventricular hypertrophy (**athlete's heart**) and mild morphologic expressions of HCM, which can usually be resolved with noninvasive testing.[25]

HCPs use an ECG to identify hypertrophic cardiomyopathy. The ECG pattern is abnormal in 75% to 95% of HCM patients, with diagnostic value in raising a suspicion of HCM. However, not all people harboring the genetic defect will express the clinical features of HCM and have normal findings by echocardiography, ECG, or cardiac symptoms.[26] The most common findings are inverted T waves in multiple ECG leads, as well as left ventricular hypertrophy and Q waves in the lateral or inferior leads. The 2D echocardiogram (echo) is the gold standard for definitive diagnosis of HCM. However, it does have limitations in differentiating between HCM and benign athlete's heart, and even when specifically focusing on potential coronary artery anomalies, the echo does not have the best diagnostic accuracy for detecting these anomalies. The echocardiographic diagnostic criteria include asymmetric interventricular wall thickness more than 15 mm and a left ventricular cavity smaller than 45 mm in thickness. Treatment strategies for HCM depend on appropriate patient selection for drug treat-

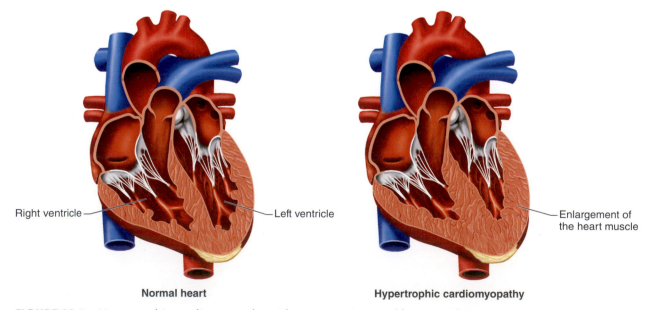

Normal heart   Hypertrophic cardiomyopathy

FIGURE 11.6 Hypertrophic cardiomyopathy with asymmetric septal hypertrophy.

ment, and high-risk patients may be treated effectively for sudden death prevention with an implantable cardioverter defibrillator (ICD).[25]

Coronary Artery Anomalies

Another common cause of SCD is congenital **anomalous coronary arteries**, which may be responsible for 17% of cardiovascular deaths in athletes.[22] Coronary artery abnormalities are usually related to myocardial bridging, tunneled coronary arteries, or coronary artery dissections.[19] Most sudden cardiac deaths related to coronary artery abnormalities in athletes and physically active clients are caused by an anomalous origin of the left coronary artery from the right coronary sinus. The trigger for sudden death is thought to be myocardial ischemia caused by compression of the anomalous coronary artery. Other coronary abnormalities identified in clients who experienced sudden death include coronary **aneurysm**, acute angulation at the coronary insertion, and intussusception (splitting an existing blood vessel in two).[23] The physical exam may be unrevealing in these patients. Many may experience syncope, presyncope, dizziness, or chest pain during exercise but typically have no ECG findings. A 2D echo technique may be modified to detect anomalous coronary arteries, but it requires sophisticated echo equipment with targeted, high-quality imaging.[25]

Arrhythmogenic Right Ventricular Cardiomyopathy or Dysplasia

Arrhythmogenic right ventricular cardiomyopathy or dysplasia (ARVD) is caused by genetic defects in which a fibrofatty replacement of the right ventricular myocardium results in arrhythmias originating in the right ventricle, segmental or diffuse wall thinning, and an association with myocarditis.[25] This condition has an overall prevalence of 1 in 5,000 in the general population and can be exacerbated by intense endurance training with symptoms that are usually related to exercise. This condition is a major cause of ventricular arrhythmias in children and young adults. It is found predominantly in males and is a significant cause of SCD in those aged 1 to 35 years. The majority of people with ARVD present as adolescents with syncope or sudden cardiac death; however, others frequently present with palpitations or other symptoms due to right ventricular tachycardia.[27]

Myocarditis

Myocarditis is an uncommon, potentially life-threatening disease that presents with a wide range of symptoms. Viral infection is the most common cause of myocarditis; adenovirus and enterovirus (including coxsackievirus) are the most frequently identified. Myocarditis commonly presents with disproportionate dyspnea on exertion, chest pain, and arrhythmias. It can also present as an acute myocardial infarction–like syndrome with sudden death.[25] The diagnosis is usually made based on clinical presentation and noninvasive imaging findings. Most patients respond well to standard heart failure therapy, although in severe cases, mechanical circulatory support or heart transplantation is indicated.[28] Patients with acute myocarditis are advised to withdraw from competitive sports and other vigorous exercise for up to 6 months or longer after onset.

Marfan Syndrome and Aortic Aneurysm or Dissection

Marfan syndrome is a systemic connective tissue disorder that can have life-threatening consequences, especially for the athletic population (figure 11.7). This condition crosses several systems, but the cardiovascular consequences are the most lethal. The heritable syndrome is an autosomal dominant disorder caused by a mutation in the gene related to production of fibrillin-1, a glycoprotein complex of the extracellular matrix of connective tissue.[29,30] The mutations in the fibrillin-1 gene lead to aortic root aneurysms, aortic dilation often with aortic regurgitation, and more seriously, left ventricular failure or **aortic dissection**.[29,31,32] Those afflicted are at risk for aortic aneurysm, dissection, or rupture that may be precipitated by the increased hemodynamic stress of exercise. The overall population prevalence is thought to be 1 in 5,000 to 1 in 10,000.[31] In a cohort of 70 patients

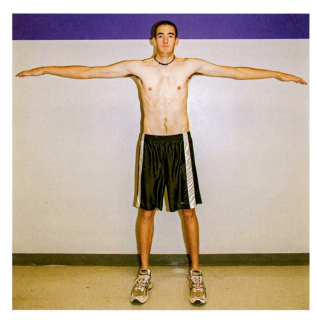

FIGURE 11.7 Physical characteristics of Marfan syndrome include tall, slender build; long, spindly fingers (arachnodactyly); and skeletal abnormalities (pectus excavatum).

Courtesy of Katie Walsh Flanagan.

with Marfan syndrome, no patient died from aortic dissection, while 4% died from arrhythmias. Ventricular arrhythmias were present in 21% and were associated with increased left ventricular size, mitral valve prolapse, and abnormalities of repolarization.[33]

Commonly recognized clinical features include tall stature, **arachnodactyly**, joint hypermobility, skeletal abnormalities including **pectus excavatum**, ocular lens subluxation, and mitral valve prolapse. Athletes with certain physical attributes such as tall stature would be more likely to play sports where being tall is an attribute, such as basketball or volleyball, and they should be carefully screened prior to sport participation. Recognizing the physical signs is the key to identification of Marfan syndrome and early detection of potential cardiovascular involvement. Unfortunately, people with Marfan syndrome are at risk of developing serious cardiovascular complications.[29,34] This risk of SCD emphasizes the importance of the multifaceted approach to the recognition of Marfan patients, specifically the use of personal history, family history, and physical examination.[35] All ATs and HCPs who care for athletes should be familiar with the pertinent physical and historic clues that may lead to a diagnosis of Marfan syndrome, and thus, the early detection of its potential cardiovascular complica-

tions. Although advances have been made in the diagnosis and medical and surgical care of people with Marfan syndrome, substantial morbidity and premature mortality remain associated with this disorder.[30,32]

Arrhythmic Causes of Acute Cardiac Conditions

Despite extensive pathological and toxicological assessment, a large proportion of sudden cardiac deaths in athletes remains unexplained. Sudden cardiac death in athletes under 35 years of age is most commonly caused by an underlying genetic heart disorder, such as hypertrophic cardiomyopathy. However, up to half of all sudden cardiac deaths may be associated with a structurally normal heart at postmortem examination; they are called **autopsy-negative sudden unexplained deaths**.[18,21] Many autopsy-negative sudden unexplained deaths may be caused by a variety of arrhythmias[22] that result in the inability of the heart to generate significant forward blood flow. Any of these 4 arrhythmias can cause cardiac arrest (figure 11.8):

- Ventricular tachycardia: At least 3 consecutive ventricular beats at a rate of at least 120 bpm.[37]

Clinical Features of Marfan Syndrome

People with Marfan syndrome may have one or more of the following clinical features:[29,35,36]

Physical Characteristics Identifiable Through Physical Examination
- Tall and thin body type; overgrowth of the long bones of the arms, legs, and fingers
- Long, spindly fingers ("spider fingers")
- Scoliosis and other skeletal abnormalities
- Chest that sinks in or sticks out
- Flexible joints
- Flat feet
- Crowded teeth
- Stretch marks on skin not related to weight gain or loss

Heart and Blood Vessel Disorders
- Aortic dilation, regurgitation, and dissection
- Left ventricular failure
- Mitral regurgitation
- Sudden lung collapse

Eye Disorders
- Severe nearsightedness, dislocated lens
- Detached retina
- Early glaucoma, early cataracts

- Ventricular fibrillation (VF): Uncoordinated quivering of the ventricle with no useful contractions; it causes immediate syncope and death within minutes if AED is not applied.[38]

- **Pulseless electric activity (PEA)**: Cardiac arrest in which the ECG indicates an electrical activity but the heart does not contract or generate a pulse.[10]

- Asystole: A cardiac arrest rhythm in which electrical activity from the heart completely ceases, and no myocardial contraction or blood flow occurs.[12]

PEA encompasses a heterogeneous group of organized electric rhythms that are associated with either absence of mechanical ventricular activity or mechanical ventricular activity that is insufficient to generate a clinically detectable pulse.[1,12,18]

The pathophysiology of arrhythmogenic disorders relating to sudden cardiac arrest includes **commotio cordis; sudden arrhythmic death syndrome (SADS)**; and **cardiac channelopathies** including **long QT syndrome**, **Brugada syndrome**, and other disorders causing arrhythmias. Unfortunately, the first sign of such disorders may be life-threatening cardiac arrhythmia occurring at rest or during exercise.[23]

Commotio Cordis

Commotio cordis (Latin for "agitation of the heart") is the second most common cause of SCD in athletes.[39] This often fatal condition from spontaneous VF is triggered by a blunt, nonpenetrating blow to the precordial area without structural injury to the ribs, sternum, or heart.[18,40-42] The most common mechanism producing commotio cordis occurs in baseball when balls that have been pitched, batted, or thrown strike players in the chest.[41] This condition has also occurred in hockey,

softball, lacrosse, karate, fistfights, or any situation in which a relatively hard projectile or body part strikes the unprotected chest wall.[40] Youth baseball players are most vulnerable to fatal blows inflicted with a wide range of velocities, but 25% of reported cases were from a pitch that averaged 30 to 50 miles per hour.[39,40,41,43]

Occurrence of commotio cordis is related to time of impact during the cardiac cycle, direct impact over the heart, the hardness and speed of the projectile, and the ineffectiveness of chest barriers. Vulnerability in youth baseball has been attributed to increased chest wall pliability.[39] A variety of experimental models in swine have indicated that if delivered at a particular moment in the cardiac cycle, even innocent-appearing precordial blows to the chest can trigger VF and result in fatal commotio cordis (figure 11.9).[40,41] In juvenile swine, immediately following a 30-mph baseball impact to the chest wall directly over the base of the left ventricle, VF occurred on ECG timed to the upstroke of the T wave.[40] Up to 40% of commotio cordis deaths occurred in young competitive athletes who were wearing commercially available chest barriers with the projectile making direct contact with protective padding (baseball catchers and lacrosse/hockey goalies).[42,43] In swine studies, animals with chest protection had roughly the same likelihood of inducing ventricular fibrillation as that of control impacts, in which animals had no chest protection.[40] A significant proportion of sudden deaths reported in young competitive athletes were related to commotio cordis even while wearing commercially available sports equipment that was generally perceived as protective.[43]

An athlete with a history of trauma to the chest resulting in witnessed sudden collapse should be evaluated for pulse, and it should raise the suspicion of commotio cordis. If no pulse is located, immediate initiation of CPR

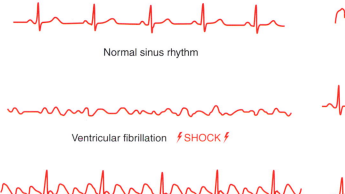

Normal sinus rhythm

Ventricular fibrillation ⚡SHOCK⚡

Atrial flutter

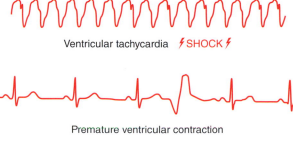

Ventricular tachycardia ⚡SHOCK⚡

Premature ventricular contraction

Atrial fibrillation

FIGURE 11.8 Common ECG rhythm and arrhythmias.

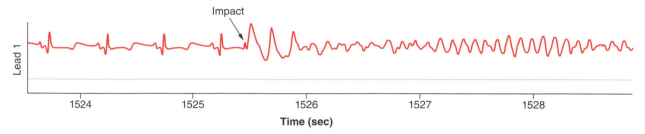

FIGURE 11.9 Six-lead ECG demonstrating VF produced by a 30-mph baseball impact to the chest wall, timed to the upstroke of the T wave.[40] Magnification of the LV pressure tracing obtained at the precise moment of impact; note the marked and immediate pressure rise within the LV, then fall to 0 mm Hg 12 milliseconds later.

Reprinted by permission from M.S. Link et al., "Impact Directly Over the Cardiac Silhouette is Necessary to Produce Ventricular Fibrillation in an Experimental Model of Commotio Cordis," *Journal of the American College of Cardiology* 37, no. 2 (2001): 649-654.

and early defibrillation is critical for survival. In such a situation, only adequate and urgent use of an AED may save an athlete's life.[14] Unfortunately, resuscitation after commotio cordis is often unsuccessful; the survival rate is only 15%.[39,42] Resuscitation within 3 minutes resulted in a 25% survival rate; however, resuscitation delayed beyond 3 minutes decreased survival to 3%.[39] Reduction of commotio cordis morbidity and mortality has resulted from using softer, safety baseballs in youth leagues and making AEDs available at sporting venues. However, further efforts are needed to prevent these largely avoidable deaths by providing more education, better-designed athletic equipment (e.g., effective chest-wall protectors), and wider access to AEDs at organized athletic events. These strategies should result in a safer sports environment for youth.[39,41]

Sudden Arrhythmic Death Syndrome

Also called sudden unexplained death syndrome (SUDS), SADS represents a collection of arrhythmic causes of cardiac arrest. Causes of SADS in young people are primarily cardiac channelopathies (details below) including long-QT syndrome, Brugada syndrome, and catecholaminergic polymorphic ventricular tachycardia (CPVT).[22,44] In addition, **Wolff-Parkinson-White (WPW) syndrome** can cause supraventricular tachycardia, atrial fibrillation, VF, and sudden cardiac death.[22] Activity of adolescents and young adults in sports is associated with an increased risk of SCD; however, sport itself is not a cause of the enhanced mortality. Rather, SCD is triggered in athletes affected by cardiovascular conditions that predispose to life-threatening ventricular arrhythmias during physical exercise.[45]

Long QT syndrome

This channelopathy is a rare inherited or acquired heart condition in which delayed repolarization of the heart following a heartbeat increases the risk of irregular heartbeat originating from the ventricles. The condition is

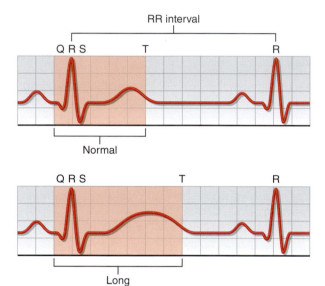

FIGURE 11.10 An ECG of long QT syndrome.

named for the appearance of the ECG where a prolongation of the QT interval occurs (figure 11.10). Symptoms include palpitations, fainting, and sudden death due to VF.[46,47] In addition to medications, this channelopathy can be acquired from malnutrition leading to low blood potassium or low blood magnesium, as in anorexia nervosa.[7]

Brugada Syndrome

This genetic channelopathy is characterized by abnormal ECG findings and an increased risk of sudden cardiac death. The ECG findings of Brugada syndrome were first reported among survivors of cardiac arrest by the Brugada brothers, who recognized it as a distinct clinical entity, causing sudden death by causing VF. Manifestations include syncope, atrial arrhythmias, ventricular arrhythmias, and SCD in the absence of myocardial ischemia or overt heart disease.[48]

Catecholaminergic Polymorphic Ventricular Tachycardia

Catecholamingeric Polymorphic Ventricular Tachycardia (CPVT) is an arrhythmogenic condition characterized by exercise or intense emotional stress, which induces VT and syncope.[22] This condition may affect as many as 1 in 10,000 people and is estimated to cause 15% of all unexplained SCDs in young people.[49] CPVT diagnosis is based on reproducing irregularly shaped ventricular arrhythmias during ECG exercise stress testing, syncope occurring during physical activity or acute emotion, and a history of exercise- or emotion-related palpitations and dizziness with an absence of structural cardiac abnormalities.[50] Syncope during exercise or during sympathetic activation is the key to identifying this disease; 93% of CPVT patients have experienced syncope or cardiac arrest. Most patients with CPVT experience VF during syncope; without treatment it may lead to sudden death[49] unless immediate CPR is applied. Unfortunately, people with CPVT often present with exercise- or emotion-induced syncope, and the first presentation can also be SCD.[50]

Field Assessment Techniques for Emergent Cardiac Conditions

In any athlete who has collapsed and is unresponsive and pulseless, SCA should be suspected and CPR should be provided while waiting for an AED to arrive. It is imperative that HCPs appreciate the causes of SCA in athletes and recognize that SCA can be mistaken for other causes of collapse; they must make an effective differential diagnosis. Potential barriers to appropriately recognizing SCA include inaccurate assessment of pulse or respirations, occasional or **agonal gasping**, and **myoclonic jerking** (seizurelike activity).[5] Although AEDs are safe and do not pose a shock hazard, special situations

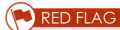
RED FLAG

Special situations that may delay the use of an AED include the following:[13,16,51]

- *Rainy or icy environment:* If a patient is lying on a wet surface or in a puddle, move the patient to a dry location.
- *Metal conducting surface (e.g., stadium bleacher):* Move the patient to a nonmetal surface.
- *Lightning:* If possible, ensure everyone's safety by moving the patient indoors.

can delay prompt recognition of an SCA and use of an AED. When the AED becomes available, the pads and a 12-lead ECG should be quickly applied for rhythm analysis and defibrillation if indicated. ATs or other HCPs must ensure access to an AED and maintain safety during its use.[13,16,51] Interruptions in chest compressions should be minimized and CPR stopped only for rhythm analysis and shock. If normal breathing and pulse are absent, start CPR immediately and activate EMS.

The prehospital ECG is an essential part of emergency cardiac care (ECC) and has the potential to change the management of patients in the emergency department (ED). Early ECGs should be acquired for all patients exhibiting signs and symptoms of acute cardiac conditions. An early, prehospital ECG may enable earlier recognition of abnormal heart function and effectively makes the prehospital professional the first medical contact.[52] In the prehospital setting, AED machines are often equipped with ECG and **biotelemetry** systems that provide data from the patient in the field to the physician at the ED. Cellular phones and radio transmission are also used for both voice communication and biotelemetry.[6] For HCPs not trained to interpret ECGs, field transmission of the ECG or a computer report to the receiving hospital is recommended. Most hospitals have dedicated phones or radio equipment for communication with responders in the field to facilitate and prepare for the patient's arrival by alerting the trauma team or other specialists as necessary.[6] While transmission of the prehospital ECG to the ED physician may improve patient outcomes and therapeutic decision making, if transmission is not performed, it may be reasonable for a trained nonphysician to interpret the ECG in the field for use in decision making, consultation with other HCPs, and selection of destination hospital.[52]

Immediate Management of Sudden Cardiac Arrest

The foundation of ECC is a major component of basic life support (BLS) consisting of immediate recognition of SCA, activation of EMS, early CPR, and rapid defibrillation with an AED. The BLS sequence (see Clinical Skills: Basic Life Support Sequence) should be performed in the order of C-A-B (chest compressions–airway–breathing) while waiting for arrival of the AED and stopped only for AED rhythm analysis and defibrillation. Integrated teams of highly trained providers may use a choreographed approach that accomplishes multiple steps and assessments simultaneously rather than in the sequential manner used by individual providers (e.g., one provider activates EMS while another begins chest compressions, a third either provides ventilation or retrieves the bag-valve-mask

Setting Up the Patient for a 12-Lead ECG

The 12-lead ECG is useful in the diagnosis and treatment of patients with AMI as well as in the documentation of other transient cardiac arrhythmias.[53] When used in the prehospital setting, the 12-lead ECG can be of assistance in diagnosis and treatment decisions once the patient has arrived in the hospital ED. Regardless of the brand or model of ECG used, always carefully read the product manual for warnings and operating instructions. Emergency personnel should inspect the equipment and become familiar with the colors and labels of the leads. When placing the electrodes on the patient, proper skin preparation and use of proper electrodes are essential for a good signal quality. If necessary and if time permits, prepare the patient's skin for electrode application; clean oily or sweaty skin with an alcohol pad, and shave or clip excess hair at the electrode site. When acquiring a 12-lead ECG from a quiet, supine patient, place the limb electrodes anywhere along the ankles and wrists (figure 11.11a). When it is difficult for the patient to remain motionless because of shivering, muscle tremors, or transport vehicle movement, better results are often obtained if you place limb electrodes on the patient's thorax (figure 11.11b). The limb leads attached to electrodes are as follows:

- Right arm (RA): Usually white
- Left arm (LA): Usually black
- Right leg (RL): Usually green
- Left leg (LL): Usually red

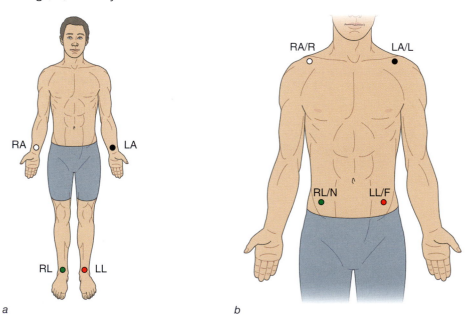

FIGURE 11.11   Twelve-lead ECG limb electrode placement for (a) a motionless patient or (b) a patient who is moving.

When placing the precordial electrodes across the chest, it is imperative to palpate and locate the V1 position (fourth intercostal space), because this space is the reference point for locating the placement of the remaining 5 leads. To locate the V1 position, do the following:

1. Place your finger on top of the jugular notch.

2. Move your finger slowly downward about 1-1/2 inches (3.8 cm) until you feel a slight horizontal ridge or elevation. This ridge is the angle of Louis, where the manubrium joins the body of the sternum.

3. Locate the second intercostal space on the right side of the patient's chest, lateral to and just below the angle of Louis.

4. Move your finger down 2 more intercostal spaces to the fourth intercostal space, which is the V1 position.

Place the remaining leads in the following locations (figure 11.12). When placing electrodes on female patients, always place leads V3 through V6 under the breast rather than on the breast.[53]

- V1: Fourth intercostal space, at the right sternal margin
- V2: Fourth intercostal space, at the left sternal margin
- V3: Fifth rib, between leads V2 and V4
- V4: Fifth intercostal space, on the left midclavicular line
- V5: Left anterior axillary line, at the horizontal level of V4
- V6: Left midaxillary line, at the same horizontal level as V4 and V5

To acquire and transmit the 12-lead ECG, follow the manufacturer instructions specific to the machine. Attach the electrodes to the patient as described previously. Then follow these steps:

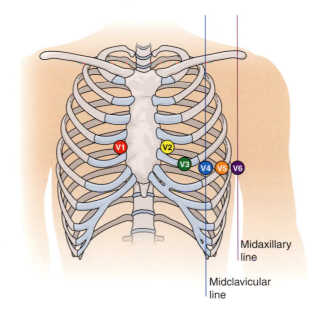

FIGURE 11.12 Locations of leads V1 through V6 in a 12-lead ECG.

- Attach the 12-lead cable wires to the electrodes on the patient.
- Attach the V-lead cable to the 12-lead ECG cable.
- Attach the 12-lead cable to the machine.
- Arrange the 12-lead cable such that it is neat and not dangling or looped. Ensure that the cable is not pulling on individual electrodes.
- To monitor the patient, select the monitor mode.
- To print a 12-lead report, select the recorder mode.

To transmit the 12-lead report to a fax machine, select the transmission mode. Be mindful that transmission of 12-lead ECG data using cellular phones can be less reliable than transmission using landline connections. A strong signal and stationary transmission will improve the transmission's success rate. Follow the directions provided with your cellular phone.[53]

device for rescue breaths, and a fourth retrieves and sets up a defibrillator). Moreover, providers are encouraged to simultaneously perform some steps (e.g., checking for breathing and pulse at the same time) in an effort to reduce the time to first compressions.[3]

In addition, supplemental oxygen (10-15 L/min flow rate) should be administered to patients with breathlessness, signs of heart failure, shock, or an oxygen saturation less than 94% (measure on a pulse oximeter); review chapter 5 for oxygen administration.[52] For a patient who is not breathing, oxygen must be administered with a resuscitation mask with an oxygen inlet or a bag-valve mask (see chapter 10 for emergency ventilation techniques). CPR should continue until ACLS-trained or higher-level HCPs take over or the patient starts to move.[3] Early detection, prompt CPR, rapid activation of EMS, and early defibrillation are vital, because the greatest factor affecting survival after SCA is the time from arrest to defibrillation.[51]

Chain of Survival

Easy access to defibrillators and first-responder AED programs improves survival from SCA by increasing the likelihood that SCA patients will receive CPR and early defibrillation. Emergency cardiac care requires an organized and practiced response by HCPs trained and equipped to recognize SCA, activate the EMS system, provide CPR, and use an AED. The American Heart Association describes these 4 links in a chain of survival to emphasize the time-sensitive interventions for people experiencing SCA:[6,54]

1. Early recognition of the emergency and activation of EMS. (Call 9-1-1.)

2. Early CPR, which can double or triple the victim's chance of survival.

3. Early defibrillation with delivery of a shock within 3 minutes of collapse can produce survival rates as high as 75%.

4. Early ACLS followed by post-resuscitation care delivered by HCPs.

Early Recognition

For any athlete who has collapsed and is unresponsive, SCA should be suspected and an AED should be applied as soon as possible for rhythm analysis. Myoclonic jerking is often present after collapse from SCA and should not be mistaken for a seizure. In addition, occasional or agonal gasping should not be mistaken for normal breathing. Provide cardiopulmonary resuscitation while the AED is being retrieved, and apply the AED as soon as possible. Minimize interruptions in chest compressions by stopping only for rhythm analysis and defibrillation.[51]

Early CPR and Defibrillation

Access to early defibrillation is essential. A goal of less than 3 minutes from the time of collapse (1 minute is ideal) to delivery of the first shock is strongly recommended.[51] Initially, check for a pulse to determine whether CPR is necessary, limiting the time to avoid delay in initiation of chest compressions. Ideally, the pulse check is performed simultaneously with the check for no breathing or agonal gasping to minimize delay in detection of cardiac arrest and initiation of CPR. (Lay rescuers do not check for a pulse.)[3] As quickly as possible after recognition of cardiac arrest, begin chest compressions (C-A-B *not* A-B-C) rather than breaths to minimize time to initiation of the first chest compression. Initially, you should take no more than 10 seconds to check for a pulse; if you do not definitely feel a pulse within that time, start chest compressions. Effective, quality chest compressions are essential for providing blood flow during CPR. For

---

Basic Life Support Sequence

1. Check the scene for safety. If applicable, have the referee stop the game.

2. Check for level of consciousness (LOC) using the AVPU scale (see chapter 4).

3. Activate emergency medical services (EMS) at this time or after checking breathing and pulse.

4. Check for absence of breathing or agonal gasping, and check pulse (ideally simultaneously). Activate the emergency action plan (EAP). If you are the lone HCP, also retrieve the AED and other emergency equipment; if you are not alone, a partner can retrieve it. This step must occur immediately after checking for absence of normal breathing and absent pulse identifies cardiac arrest.

5. Immediately begin CPR, using the AED when available.

6. When the second provider arrives, provide 2-person CPR and use the AED.

this reason, all patients in cardiac arrest should receive chest compressions.[3]

Early, rapid defibrillation is the treatment of choice for VF of short duration, such as for patients of witnessed out-of-hospital cardiac arrest. If the provider witnesses the collapse, the provider should apply the AED and use the defibrillator, if necessary, as soon as it is available.[10] Defibrillation through deployment of electric energy terminates VF and allows the normal cardiac pacemakers to stop firing, thereby stopping the heart, which in turn resumes firing and hopefully produces an effective rhythm if the heart tissue is still viable. AEDs are easy to use, even by untrained people, and they are extremely accurate in recommending a shock only when VF or rapid VT is present.[5] Quality chest compressions are important both before and after defibrillation, because they provide a small but critical amount of blood flow to the heart and brain and increase the likelihood that defibrillation will restore a normal rhythm in time to prevent neurologic damage. Chest compressions create blood flow by increasing intrathoracic pressure and directly compressing the heart. When CPR is initiated, survival rate declines 3% to 4% per minute for every minute defibrillation is delayed.[3] Thus, CPR can greatly improve survival from witnessed SCA for any given time interval to defibrillation. Resuming CPR immediately after shock delivery is also critical given that many victims are in PEA or asystole for several minutes after defibrillation, and CPR is needed to provide perfusion.[5] It is essential to initiate CPR early and deliver chest compressions of sufficient quality.

During states of low blood flow such as CPR, oxygen delivery to the heart and brain is limited by blood flow rather than by arterial oxygen content. Rescue breaths are less important than chest compressions during the first few minutes of resuscitation from witnessed VF cardiac arrest. Further, an AT or HCP performing CPR alone should not interrupt chest compressions for ventilation or advanced airway placement.[12] However, because blood flow is typically the major limiting factor to oxygen delivery during CPR, it is theoretically important to maximize the oxygen content of arterial blood by maxi-

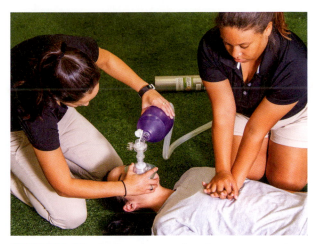

FIGURE 11.13 Performing quality chest compressions with ventilation using a bag-valve mask maximizes oxygen delivery during basic life support.

mizing inspired oxygen concentration. Maximal inspired oxygen can be achieved with high-flow oxygen (15 L/min) into a resuscitation bag-valve mask (figure 11.13) or an advanced airway.[55] The use of oropharyngeal airways (see chapter 10) in patients with cardiac arrest may aid in the delivery of adequate ventilation with a bag-valve mask by preventing the tongue from occluding the airway. However, incorrect insertion of an oropharyngeal airway can displace the tongue and cause airway obstruction. For more information on airway maintenance, see chapter 10.

Early Advanced Cardiac Life Support

HCPs with additional training can provide ACLS, which includes the ability to insert advanced airways, initiate intravenous (IV) access, read and interpret ECGs, and understand emergency pharmacology. Many HCPs have ACLS training, often through local hospitals or college and university health professions programs, including the following:

- Athletic trainers
- Physicians (MD and DO)

Treatable Causes of Cardiac Arrest: The Hs and Ts

Hs	Ts
Hypoxia	Toxins
Hypovolemia	Tamponade (cardiac)
Hydrogen ion (acidosis)	Tension pneumothorax
Hypokalemia or hyperkalemia	Thrombosis, pulmonary
Hypothermia	Thrombosis, coronary

- Pharmacists (PharmD)
- Dentists (DDS)
- Advanced practice professionals, such as physician assistants (PA) and nurse practitioners (NP)
- Respiratory therapists (RT)
- Nurses (RN)
- Paramedics (EMT-P)

The ACLS-trained HCPs quickly search for possible reversible causes of cardiac arrest (see Treatable Causes of Cardiac Arrest: The Hs and Ts).[55] Based on their diagnosis, more specific treatments are provided. These treatments may be medical, such as IV injection of an antidote for drug overdose, or surgical, such as insertion of a chest tube for those with tension pneumothoraxes or hemothoraxes.[12]

Pharmacologic Intervention for Cardiac Emergencies

ATs should be prepared to administer or assist the patient in taking prescribed or over-the-counter medications for treatment of cardiac symptoms (table 11.3). If the patient

TABLE 11.3 Over-the-Counter and Prescribed Medications for Acute Cardiac Symptoms

Medication	Dose and route of administration	Indications and contraindications
Aspirin (acetylsalicylic acid), preferably nonenteric (coated) aspirin	Oral, chewable tablet, 160-325 mg	*Indication:* Hemodynamically stable patients with cardiac symptoms or ACS *Contraindication:* History of aspirin allergy or evidence of recent gastrointestinal bleeding; do not administer aspirin or NSAIDs because of increased risk of the following: • Increased bleeding time from platelet inhibition • Mortality • Reinfarction • Hypertension • Heart failure • Myocardial rupture
Nitroglycerin	Sublingual or aerosol Up to 3 doses at 3- to 5-minute intervals until pain is relieved or low BP limits its use	*Indication:* ACS patients diagnosed by a physician with ischemic discomfort such as angina pectoris *Contraindications:* Do not provide nitrates in patients with the following: • Right ventricular infarction • Hypotension (systolic blood pressure <90 mm Hg or ≥30 mm Hg below baseline) • Extreme bradycardia (<50 bpm), or • Tachycardia in the absence of heart failure (>100 bpm) • Dehydration
Oxygen	Inhaled High-flow supplemental oxygen at 10 to 15 L/min	*Indications:* Patients who are hypoxemic (i.e., oxygen saturation <94%) or have unknown oxygen saturation[3]
Saline or colloids	Intravenous	*Indications:* To increase circulating blood volume[12]
Additional cardiac medications; e.g., adrenaline (epinephrine), amiodarone, atropine, verapamil, bicarbonate, calcium, potassium and magnesium	Injection	*Indications:* ACLS providers based on patient vital signs, ECG, symptoms, or other physiologic parameters

ACLS = advanced cardiac life support; ACS = acute coronary syndrome; ECG = electrocardiogram; NSAIDS = nonsteroidal anti-inflammatory drugs

Based on Kleinman et al. (2015); Neumar et al. (2010); O'Connor et al. (2015); Link et al. (2015).

has not taken aspirin (acetylsalicylic acid) and has no history of aspirin allergy and no evidence of recent gastrointestinal bleeding, ATs should give adult, conscious patients 1 tablet of chewable nonenteric aspirin (160-325 mg) as soon as an AMI is suspected.[3,52] For hemodynamically stable patients with ACS, it is reasonable to consider the early administration of nitroglycerin, although insufficient evidence exists to support or refute the routine administration of nitroglycerin in the prehospital setting in patients with a suspected ACS.[3] Patients diagnosed with ACS that have ischemic discomfort, such as angina pectoris, should receive up to 3 doses of sublingual or aerosol nitroglycerin at 3- to 5-minute intervals until pain is relieved or low BP limits its use (see chapter 5). However, the use of nitrates is contraindicated in patients with right ventricular infarction, hypotension (systolic <90 mm Hg or ≥30 mm Hg below baseline), extreme bradycardia (<50 bpm), or tachycardia in the absence of heart failure (>100 bpm).[52] Prehospital HCPs should administer supplementary oxygen to hypoxemic (oxygen saturation <94%) patients or those with unknown oxygen saturation.[3] The next steps for ACLS providers is insertion of IV lines (see chapter 5) and placement of advanced airway devices (see chapter 10). Commonly used ACLS drugs, such as epinephrine and amiodarone, are also administered.[56] Amiodarone is a first-line antiarrhythmic agent given during cardiac arrest because it has been clinically demonstrated to improve the rate of **return of spontaneous circulation (ROSC)** and hospital admission in adults with refractory VF or pulseless VT.[12] Other arrhythmogenic disorders, such as CPVT, are treated with beta blockers or verapamil, a calcium-channel blockers.[49]

Post-Resuscitation Care

Signs of ROSC associated with significant respiratory effort after cardiac arrest include breathing, coughing, or movement and a palpable pulse or a measurable BP. These signs indicate that CPR may cease while monitoring vital signs and awaiting arrival of transport. Prior to and during transport to the ED, the patient should be placed in a recovery position that is stable, near true lateral, with the head dependent, and with no pressure on the chest to impair breathing.[3]

Emergency Preparedness for Sudden Cardiac Arrest

Comprehensive emergency planning is needed for high school and college athletic programs or any venue for training or competition; it ensures effective and efficient response to cardiac emergencies.[5] Health professionals and organizational administrators must recognize the

current American Heart Association guidelines, which call for the availability and use of AEDs, and that defibrillation is considered a component of basic life support.[57] Once SCA has occurred, preparation is the key to survival. Public access to AEDs and established EAPs greatly improve the likelihood of survival.[51] All EAPs should include medical or HCP oversight, appropriate training of anticipated HCPs in CPR and AED use, coordination with the EMS system, appropriate device maintenance, and an ongoing quality improvement program. The EAP should be specific to each athletic venue and encompass emergency communication, personnel, equipment (and location of equipment), and transportation to appropriate emergency facilities.[5]

Emergency Action Plan Specific to Sudden Cardiac Arrest

Every school or other institution that sponsors athletic activities should have a written and structured EAP (see chapter 3). A cardiac-specific EAP should be tailored to each athletic venue and should include an effective communication system, training of likely first responders in CPR and AED use, acquisition of the necessary emergency equipment, a coordinated and practiced response plan, and access to early defibrillation.[54,58] Access to early defibrillation is essential, and a target goal of less than 3 minutes (1 minute is ideal)[59] from the time of collapse to the first shock is strongly recommended. Prompt recognition of SCA, early activation of EMS, the presence of a trained provider to initiate CPR, and access to early defibrillation are critical in the management of SCA. In any collapsed and unresponsive athlete, SCA should be suspected and an AED applied as soon as possible for rhythm analysis and defibrillation, if needed.[5] All necessary equipment should be placed in a central location that is highly visible and accessible; multiple AEDs may be needed for larger facilities. The cardiac-specific EAP should identify the person or group responsible for documenting personnel training, equipment maintenance, actions taken during the emergency, and evaluation of the emergency response. The EAP should be developed and coordinated in consultation with local EMS personnel, school public safety officials, on-site first responders, and school administrators. The EAP should be coordinated and integrated into the local EMS agency and should be posted at every venue and near appropriate telephones and include the address of the venue and specific directions to guide EMS personnel.[51] Finally, the EAP should be reviewed and practiced at least annually with certified athletic trainers, team and consulting physicians, athletic training students, school and institutional safety personnel, administrators, and coaches.[5]

Post-CPR Recovery Position

1. Raise the patient's arm alongside the ear on your side of the patient *(a)*.
2. Flex the patient's elbow on the opposite arm *(b)*.
3. Grasp the patient's opposite arm with the hand closest to the shoulder and behind the knee with the other hand *(c)*.
4. Carefully roll the patient toward you, placing the patient's hand beneath the face *(d)*.

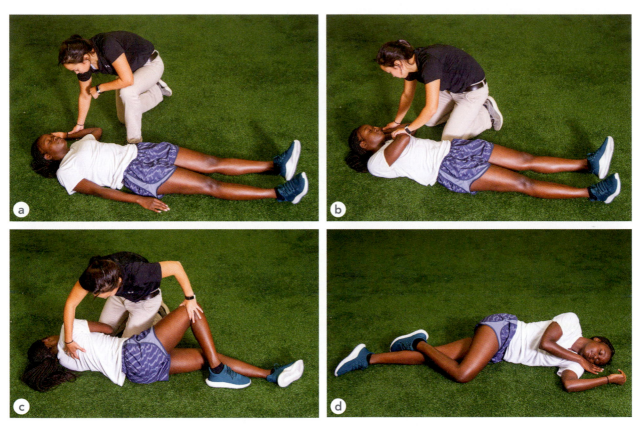

FIGURE 11.14

Personnel for Cardiac Emergencies

The first person responding to a cardiac emergency may vary widely. It may be a coach or a game official, an AT, an EMT, or a physician. Because of the variety in personnel and equipment necessary in responding to a cardiac emergency, an EAP must be developed specifically for cardiac emergencies for each venue. Emergency training requires personnel to be familiar with the use of AED, oxygen, and advanced airways. With a plan in place and rehearsed, these differently trained people will be able to work together as an effective team when responding to cardiac emergencies. The EAP should outline which person is responsible for activating EMS and retrieving

the AED. Coaches and those traveling with athletes should be provided emergency information about the student-athletes, including relevant medical history, medications, personal contact information, and contact information for HCPs.[5] In addition, all personnel associated with practices, competitions, skills instruction, and strength and conditioning activities should have current certification in CPR and training in the use of AEDs and at a minimum.[57]

Equipment for Cardiac Emergencies

All necessary emergency equipment should be at the site or quickly accessible, and personnel must be trained in advance to use it properly (see Emergency Equipment Necessary for Management of Cardiac Emergencies). Resuscitation equipment should be placed in a central location that is highly visible and near a telephone or other means of activating EMS. In the school setting, all school staff should be instructed on the location of emergency equipment.

If a HCP is unfamiliar with the school or where an AED is located, a school administrator should be asked to provide verbal instructions to find and use the AED. All necessary equipment should be on-site, quickly accessible, in good operating condition, and checked on a regular basis. Emergency equipment and medications should be assembled in a code bag (called a *go bag*) and stored in an easily accessible central location at each venue, and personnel must be trained in advance to use it properly. The EMS centers should be notified of the specific type of AED and the exact location of the AED on school grounds.[5] Emergency cardiac care emphasizes use of the bag-valve mask in emergency resuscitation and the use of emergency oxygen and advanced airways in emergency care. HCPs should be appropriately trained to use these devices (refer to chapter 10), and providers should limit use to devices for which they have been trained. Finally, emergency personnel should regularly rehearse the use of equipment, and the emergency equipment that is available should be appropriate for the level of training of the emergency medical professionals and the venue.[57]

Clinical Decision Making

Patients who are unresponsive and not breathing normally are highly likely to be in cardiac arrest. If the patient is unresponsive with abnormal or absent breathing, it is reasonable for the AT or emergency professional to assume that the patient is in cardiac arrest (figure 11.15). It is essential to rapidly detect SCA by appropriately recognizing a range of clinical presentations and descriptions.[3] Differential diagnosis of nontraumatic exercise-related syncope or presyncope includes sudden cardiac arrest, exertional heatstroke, heat exhaustion, hyponatremia, hypoglycemia, exercise-associated collapse, exertional sickling, neurocardiogenic syncope, seizures, and pulmonary embolus. These conditions should be differentiated from cardiac causes of collapse, including cardiac arrhythmias, valvular disorders, coronary artery disease, cardiomyopathies, ion channel disorders (channelopathies), and other cardiac diseases.

Evidence: Cardiovascular Screening

SCD in athletes is a tragic and potentially preventable event. Almost all professional organizations advocate pre-participation cardiac screening, which according to the American Heart Association is "justifiable, necessary, and compelling on the basis of ethical, legal,

Emergency Equipment Necessary for Management of Cardiac Emergencies

- Gloves (nonlatex or nonallergenic)
- AED for early defibrillation (Check batteries annually and before events or competitions)
- Personal protection for rescue breathing (pocket mask or barrier-shield device)
- Bag-valve mask, supplemental oxygen, oral and nasopharyngeal airways, and lubricant
- Advanced airways (e.g., endotracheal tube, Combitube, or laryngeal mask airway)
- Additional supplies, including heavy-duty emergency shears for equipment and clothing removal and exposing the chest, a towel for drying skin on the chest, and a razor for shaving chest hair
- Aluminum chlorhydrate (antiperspirant) (useful for AED leads to stick to sweaty skin)
- Extra AED pads (for damaged or misplaced pads)
- IV start packs, tubing, normal saline solution (1,000-mL bags)
- Emergency cardiac medications, including aspirin and nitroglycerin for use on-site for chest pain without cardiac arrest, or until transport arrives

Note: Large institutions or sport facilities with distant or multiple sites require duplicate equipment. Emergency equipment must be accessible and not be locked in a closet, cabinet, or room, which could delay emergency care. Installing audible alarms that sound when the cabinet door is opened may decrease risk of theft or vandalism.[60]

Using an AED

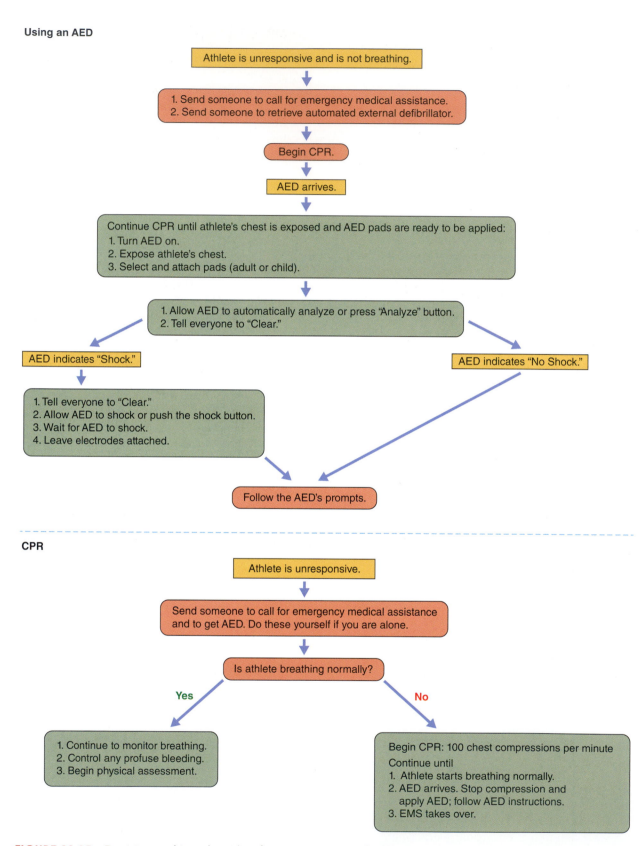

CPR

FIGURE 11.15 Decision-making algorithm for management of SCA.

and medical grounds." Although a controversial topic, pre-participation screening is viewed by many as an important public health initiative.[14(p97)] Much debate occurs worldwide regarding the implementation and extent of pre-participation screening for athletes; the main issue is the balance between lives saved; athletes tested; psychological, ethical, and legal issues; and economic cost. Increased education and awareness about prevention of SCD, including early ECGs and accessibility to AEDs can help prevent sudden cardiac death in athletes as well as nonathletes.[21]

Pre-participation screening may help to reduce the incidence of sudden death, although equal focus should be given to evaluation of the family history to identify victims of sudden death.[23] Using the pre-participation physical examination and cardiac screening, including family and personal history, physical examination, and resting ECG, may identify people at risk and has the potential to decrease the risk of SCD in athletes. The topic is controversial, but a combination of screening including the ECG has a high sensitivity for underlying disease in younger athletes. Unfortunately, specificity and sensitivity of screening without the use of ECG is very low. Detection of asymptomatic conditions should be improved with standardized history forms and attention to episodes of exertional syncope or presyncope, chest pain, a personal or family history of SCA or a family history of exercise intolerance, selective use of ECGs in high-risk athletes (as described earlier), and a stronger knowledge base for HCPs.[23] Cardiovascular screening will never be able to identify all athletes at risk, so adequate preparedness is vital in case of a potentially fatal event at the sporting arena or other facility.[14] Further research is needed to understand whether additional tests such as echocardiograms can improve sensitivity, and whether they can be performed with acceptable cost-effectiveness and acceptable false-positive rate.

Evidence: Factors Affecting Survival After Sudden Cardiac Arrest

The single greatest factor affecting survival after out-of-hospital cardiac arrest is the time interval from arrest to defibrillation. The probability of successful defibrillation for VF-related SCA diminishes rapidly over time, with survival rates declining 7% to 10% per minute for every minute that defibrillation is delayed.[3] Survival after SCA is unlikely once VF has deteriorated to asystole.[5] The presence of AEDs in schools and other institutions provides a means of early defibrillation, not only for young athletes but also for other people on campus who may experience an unexpected cardiac arrest

 RED FLAG

In any athlete who has collapsed in the absence of trauma, suspicion for sudden cardiac arrest should be high until normal airway, breathing, and circulation are confirmed. Agonal respiration or occasional gasping should not be mistaken for normal breathing and should be recognized as a sign of SCA. Similarly, myoclonic jerking or seizurelike activity shortly after collapse should also be treated as SCA until proven otherwise. If no pulse is palpable, the patient should be treated for SCA, and CPR should be initiated immediately.[51]

such as older school employees, spectators, and visitors on campus. At National Collegiate Athletic Association (NCAA) Division I universities, Drezner et al.[61] found that older nonstudents, such as spectators, coaches, and officials, accounted for 77% of SCA cases at collegiate sporting venues. Placement of AEDs at these venues provided a significant survival benefit for older nonstudents, with a 54% overall immediate resuscitation rate. In a case series of 9 collegiate athletes with SCA,[62] all 9 athletes had a witnessed arrest, and most received immediate assessment by an AT skilled in basic life support and CPR. Seven athletes received defibrillation, with an average time from cardiac arrest to defibrillation of 3.1 minutes. Despite a witnessed collapse, timely CPR, and prompt defibrillation in most cases, only 1 of 9 (11%) athletes in this cohort survived—an unexpected finding given the young age, otherwise good health and physical conditioning of the athletes, and early reported defibrillation. Successful resuscitations using AEDs reported in the public media demonstrate the lifesaving potential of access to defibrillation on the athletic field and highlight the need for improved and uniform resuscitation strategies for SCA in athletes.[5]

Summary

Sudden cardiac death (SCD) in athletes aged less than 35 years is most commonly caused by an underlying genetic heart disorder;[4,21,39] however, up to half of all SCDs may be associated with a structurally normal heart at postmortem examination and are referred to as autopsy-negative sudden unexplained deaths. Systematic and intense physical training can lead to changes in the heart; however, these changes are not always detrimental. Much debate occurs worldwide regarding the implementation and extent of pre-participation screening for athletes, with the main issue being the balance between lives saved; athletes tested; psychological, ethical, and legal issues; and the economic cost. Further effort is needed to prevent these largely avoidable cardiac deaths. Providing increased education and awareness about SCD, better-designed athletic equipment (e.g., safety balls, effective chest-wall protectors), training in CPR, and improved accessibility to AEDs can help prevent SCD in athletes as well as nonathletes.[4,21,39]

 Go to the web study guide to complete the case studies for this chapter.

CHAPTER 12

Injuries and Illnesses of the Abdominopelvic Region

After reading this chapter, you will be able to do the following:

- Describe the relevant anatomical components of the abdomen and pelvis.

- Recognize medical emergencies involving the abdomen and pelvis.

- Evaluate and make appropriate referral for emergent conditions of the abdomen and pelvis.

- Ask appropriate history questions relating to emergent conditions of the reproductive system.

Trauma or illness of the abdominopelvic region has many challenges. Many of the organs contained within the abdomen are not firmly fixed to an exact place, and therefore specific location of pain is often difficult. In addition, contents within the peritoneum have diffuse pain sensors and often refer pain to areas away from the injury and even external to the abdominal cavity. The trauma can cause a significant amount of internal bleeding before the patient displays signs of shock, possibly delaying recognition or treatment. It is therefore important to have a high level of suspicion for severe trauma with any blunt-force blow to the abdomen. Injuries and acute conditions of the pelvis present their own challenges; asking thorough history questions in a clear, unambiguous, and anatomically correct manner is paramount. It is unlikely these conditions will be evaluated by inspection and palpation in the athletic setting, and knowing when to refer is important.

Overview of Anatomical Structures in the Abdomen and Pelvis

Unlike organs in the safety of the rib cage in the thorax, structures located within the abdomen and pelvis have little bony protection. In the abdomen and pelvis, protection arises from musculature and organs and tissues that lie in close proximity to one another. This brief review covers key bones and muscles that play a role in protection. Abdominal cavities and quadrants are discussed prior to the key organs that can sustain acute trauma.

Bones

The abdomen and pelvis are somewhat protected by bony structures of the body. The spine safeguards the posterior aspects of the entire abdomen, with the thoracic spine functioning as bony attachments to each of the 12 ribs. The lower ribs serve as bony defense to the liver, spleen, and kidneys; but the majority of the digestive and all of the reproductive anatomy are unprotected by the spine or pelvis.

The bowl-like pelvis serves to provide support to the abdomen and its contents, but it does little in the way of bony protection for the organs within the abdomen and pelvis. The pelvis is made up of 2 separate bones (ilia) that are joined posteriorly by the sacrum (figure 12.1). Anteriorly, the 2 ilia join at the pubic crest. The pelvis provides attachment points for abdominal muscles and for muscles of the hip and thigh.

Muscles

In addition to the musculature of the trunk discussed in chapter 10, the musculature of the abdomen also contributes to protecting the contents of the abdomen and pelvis. Collectively, these muscles support internal organs and assist in respiration and defecation.

Anteriorly, the rectus abdominis is the predominant muscle of the abdomen (figure 12.2). It arises from the pubis in the anterior center of the pelvis and inserts superiorly at the xiphoid of the sternum and costal cartilage of the fifth through seventh ribs. Other relevant anterior muscles are the internal and external oblique muscles and transverse abdominis.

Posteriorly, the deep muscles of the spine—iliocostalis thoracis, spinalis thoracis, and longissimus thoracis—make up the primary protection of the posterior abdomen. These thoracis muscles all attach on the ribs, and the first aspect of each muscle name indicates its function. The iliocostalis thoracis arises from the ilium and travels to the ribs (costalis), the spinalis thoracis, and the longissimus thoracis. The latissimus dorsi provides superficial coverage over these deeper muscles.

Cavities

The abdominal cavity holds all the organs of digestion, as well as many that regulate healthy hemostasis. Within the abdominal cavity is the peritoneum, a thin membrane that lines organs. The peritoneum houses the gallbladder, spleen, tail of the pancreas, and appendix. It also holds the stomach, small intestine, and aspects of the large colon. The mesentery, a tissue that is actually several folds in the peritoneum, helps maintain the contents of the peritoneum in a loose anatomical position within the cavity. Conversely, organs external to the peritoneum such as the liver and kidneys are firmly fixed to their location through strong ligaments to other structures. This difference is important to consider when evaluating a person with an abdominal injury, because structures within the peritoneum move and shift slightly. The mesentery supplies lymph and blood to the contents of the peritoneum.

Fluid generated by the peritoneum provides support to the organs and other contents of the membrane. It prevents friction between contents within the peritoneum and supplies nutrients to them.

External to the peritoneum is the retroperitoneum (behind the peritoneum). This area does not have the benefit of the protective serous material that contents of the peritoneum have. Organs in the retroperitoneum include both kidneys, proximal ureters, the remainder of the pancreas, and the descending colon. Tissues in the retroperitoneum are generally fixed and therefore not able to move much, which is different from the contents within the peritoneum. Another space, the subperitoneum (below the peritoneum), holds the urinary bladder.

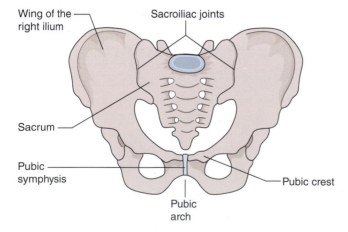
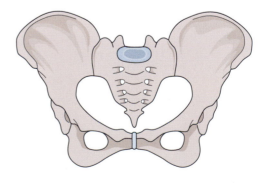

FIGURE 12.1   Anterior aspect of the male and female pelvis.

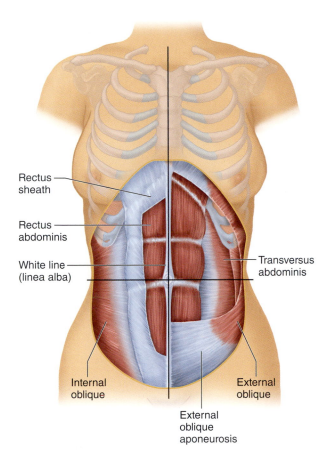

Rectus sheath

Rectus abdominis

White line (linea alba)

Transversus abdominis

Internal oblique

External oblique

External oblique aponeurosis

FIGURE 12.2 Anterior musculature of the abdomen.

Although relatively not understood, neurological sensation is different within the peritoneum in that sensation there is vague, diffuse, and nonspecific. Insult to contents in the peritoneum tends to result in referred pain to another part of the body outside of the thorax. Organs such as the kidneys and liver have direct innervation and thereby have definite pain sensations at the site of damage.

Quadrants

The linea alba (literally "white line") is an anatomical line that lies from the xiphoid to the pubic juncture, and divides the umbilicus in half in the sagittal plane. It is visible on lean, fit patients, but important nonetheless because it divides the abdominal quadrants. A vertical imaginary line through the umbilicus completes the division of the four quadrants of the abdomen (see figure 12.2). These quadrants are named in reference to the patient; for example, the upper-right quadrant (URQ) is on the patient's right side. The upper quadrants begin under the ribs at the diaphragm and end at the invisible transverse line across the umbilicus. The lower quadrants begin at the navel and continue inferiorly through to the bowl of the pelvis. Table 12.1 lists the organs typically found in each quadrant.

Organs

This section is a brief review of the organs in the abdominopelvic region specific to this chapter. It is not intended to be a comprehensive discussion of physiology, but a brief overview of the anatomical placement and function of the organs that are discussed in this chapter (figure 12.3).

Liver

The liver is one of the largest organs in the body, and apart from the brain, it has the most functions. For the gastrointestinal system, the liver metabolizes carbohydrates, proteins, and fats to keep energy levels consistent. One of its primary roles is to store glucose as glycogen and collect fat-soluble vitamins and iron for future use, but it is said that over 500 functions occur within the liver.[1] It resides in the majority of the URQ, under the diaphragm, above the stomach, and to the right of the pancreas.

A capsule surrounds the liver, similar to the pericardium of the heart; it is named Glisson's capsule after the British physician who discovered it. This capsule consists of strong connective tissue that contains the hepatic arteries, veins, and ducts. Glisson's capsule protects the parenchyma (functioning tissue of the organ). The term *parenchyma* is not specific to the liver; it is used to describe the functioning aspect of other organs. Injuries to the liver are described in relation to the amount to damage done to Glisson's capsule (e.g., subcapsular, capsular).

TABLE 12.1 **Abdominal Quadrants and Contents**

Upper-right quadrant (URQ)	Upper-left quadrant (ULQ)	Lower-right quadrant (LRQ)	Lower-left quadrant (LLQ)
Liver	Spleen	Appendix	Distal left ureter
Gallbladder	Stomach	Distal right ureter	Left ovary
Tail of the pancreas	Small intestine*	Right ovary	Left fallopian tube
Small intestine*	Transverse colon*	Right fallopian tube	Small intestine*
Transverse colon*	Descending colon*	Small intestine*	Descending colon*
Ascending colon*		Ascending colon*	

*Aspects of this tissue are in this quadrant but may be in others as well.

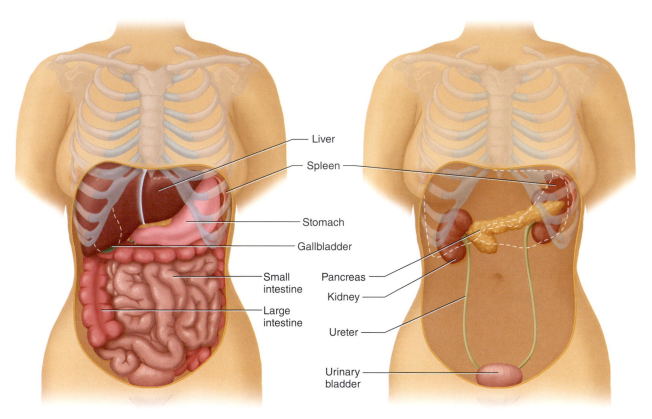

FIGURE 12.3   Structures of the abdominal cavity.

The gallbladder is located under the liver, and they work together to store and process fats in digestion. The liver has aspects of it both within and external to the perineum. Injury to it can present in referred pain to the right shoulder or as an acute, sharp pain over the organ, depending on the area of the liver injured. That being said, the liver also has a remarkable ability to regenerate; a small but healthy portion of a liver will grow and adapt to the size of the host and reassume all usual functions.[2]

Spleen

The spleen resides in the ULQ under the left lower rib cage, where it is usually protected unless it is inflamed, such as it would be in mononucleosis or other blood disorders, or in pregnancy. It is less protected in children, because a child's rib cage is still pliable and does not completely cover the spleen as it does in an adult's rib cage. To palpate a healthy spleen, the practitioner would palpate under the lower borders of the left ribs.

The spleen's main function is filtering blood and providing antibodies, but it serves several other key hemodynamic functions, too. One can live without a spleen; in its absence the marrow of long bones and certain glands will take over the majority of its functions. People who have a **splenectomy** may be more predisposed to infections.

As with the liver, the spleen has a capsule composed of fibroblastic connective tissue and smooth muscle. Protected by the capsule is the parenchyma, termed the same as the liver, which is the functioning tissue of the spleen. This organ is highly vascular; at any time it holds 5% to 6% of cardiac output while filtering 10% to 15% of total blood volume per minute.[3]

Kidneys

The primary role of the fist-sized kidneys is to maintain hemostasis. This paired solid organ is vital to life, but a person will do quite well with only one functioning kidney. Kidneys are located outside of the peritoneal cavity (retroperitoneal), along the lower thoracic spine, and largely under the final ribs. Each kidney is surrounded by a closed retroperitoneal space, which retards extra capsule bleeding by pressure in the space. Muscles of the posterior thorax and adipose tissue protect these organs. The kidneys are attached to the diaphragm and move slightly with breathing. Their function is to maintain fluid balance, remove waste from blood, and regulate both blood pressure and red blood cells in the body. They are highly vascular organs and are supplied by renal arteries, which are direct offshoots of the largest artery in the body, the aorta. The kidneys are also vital in the production of urine, which is why one sign of kidney trauma is **hematuria**. Each kidney has its own ureter that drains urine to the urinary bladder, from where a single urethra expels urine by voluntary muscular contraction to outside the body proper.

Appendix

Formally called the vermiform appendix, the appendix is a tiny pouch with no discernible function. Located in the LRQ at the juncture of the small and large intestines, it is not firmly attached to anything. Its free-floating position is one reason it is challenging to palpate or elicit pain when palpated in a specific spot. The appendix lies within the peritoneum, which means it tends to have referred or diffuse pain as a symptom (**McBurney's point**) instead of pain directly over the organ such as with the liver and kidneys. One can live without an appendix, and it is often removed if inflamed (**appendicitis**).

Female Reproductive System

This section discusses only internal structures that may present with acute, life-threatening conditions to women. The 2 areas discussed are the ovaries and fallopian tubes. The anatomical placement of these tissues is discussed, but their endocrine functions are not reviewed in this text.

Ovary   Most women are born with 2 ovaries, 1 in each lower quadrant (figure 12.4). The ovary is a walnut-sized organ that holds eggs. It is suspended from the uterus and fallopian tube and has a bit of movement; it is not firmly fixed to anything else. The ovary is within the peritoneal cavity, therefore patients with ovarian pain report non-specific locations of discomfort.

At birth, the ovary has all the eggs the woman will ever have. Following a series of endocrine functions, an egg is released approximately each month beginning in puberty (around age 10-12) until menopause (about age 50). When an egg is released, it is not released directly into the associated fallopian tube but rather in close proximity to it.

One can live without ovaries. In addition, a woman can become pregnant without ovaries if an embryo is implanted in her uterus and the embryo is viable.

Fallopian Tube   The fallopian tubes are bilateral projections off uterus. Each one functions as a con-duit to transport the egg from the ovary to the host uterus for implantation and growth into an embryo, then fetus. When an egg is released from the ovary, tiny projections at the terminal end of the fallopian tube, called fimbriae, lure the egg to the tube, and muscular contractions move the egg along the fallopian tube to the uterus. If the egg is not fertilized by sperm, menses occurs; the lining of the uterus that was produced to host the embryo is shed (by way of contractions) through the vagina.

Testicles

Most males are born with 2 testicles that reside external to the body in their individual scrotal sacs (figure 12.5). The testes produce sperm, and the epididymis above each testis serves as a repository for sperm. The scrotum is a bifurcated sac that houses each testis and epididymis as well as the spermatic cords. Spermatic cords allow the individual testis to swing freely within the confines of the scrotum. The cord is a group of vesicles, artery, nerve,

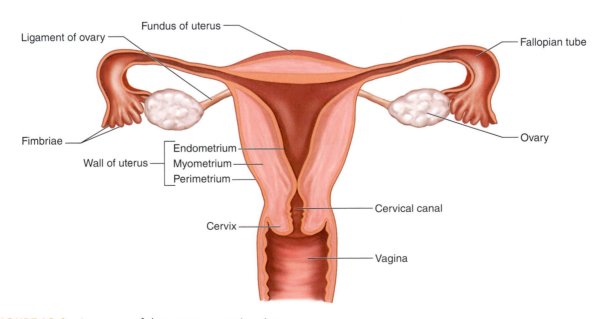

FIGURE 12.4 Anatomy of the uterus, anterior view.

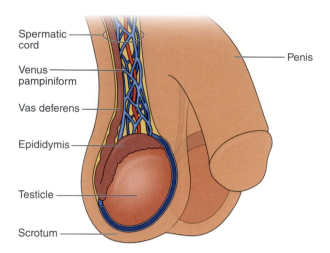

FIGURE 12.5   Anatomy of the testicles.

and duct. Sperm needs to be maintained at a temperature about 2°F to 3°F cooler than the body. Muscles within the scrotum, the dartos and cremaster muscles, contract to raise the scrotum when it is colder outside and relax in the warmer conditions to lower the testes farther from the body. More testicular injuries occur in warmer weather than in colder weather, because they are less protected.

Trauma to Abdominal Organs

Blunt abdominal trauma is a common lead cause of mortality and morbidly in all age groups.[4] Although rare in athletics, abdominal injuries must be quickly recognized as potentially life-threatening and referred to the nearest trauma center as soon as possible. The ability to properly evaluate the abdomen in acute situations is critical, and this brief review is relevant for the conditions that follow. In addition to relevant history questions, the skills of observation, auscultation, palpation, and percussion are necessary for a complete abdominal evaluation. Observation of the region is important and telling. The health care provider (HCP) should inspect for overt trauma, rigidity, bruising, and scrapes. In addition, any distended region should be noted, as well as abdominal symmetry throughout the breathing sequence.

Following observation is auscultation (using a stethoscope to listen for sounds in each of the quadrants of the abdomen). Auscultation occurs in a quiet room; the HCP listens carefully in each area for the quality and quantity of the noise heard. Palpation always follows auscultation in the abdomen, because palpation could elicit sounds not present during auscultation. For both auscultation and palpation, the patient is supine or hook lying (knees bent and feet on the table). Palpation occurs using 2 methods. During the first pass over the abdomen, the HCP uses fingertips, seeking information on size and shape of superficial abdominal organs, the presence of fluid or gas, and areas of pain or tenderness. In the absence of significant pain, the HCP may palpate deeper, usually 1 to 1-1/2 inches (3-4 cm) into the abdomen to determine shape of organs, swelling, masses, fluid, and pain.

Percussion is the final aspect of abdominal evaluation preceding special tests or diagnostic exams. This technique requires 2 fingers tapping over specific regions in the abdomen; the HCP gains insight from the noise elicited from the tapping of the clinician's fingers. This insight occurs in 2 manners; the HCP taps on the abdomen either directly or indirectly by tapping her fingers on the fingers of her opposite hand. HCPs use a specific sequence for percussion, as illustrated in figure 12.6.

Injuries to the Liver and Spleen

Trauma to the liver is a potentially catastrophic event. The mechanism is typically a blunt-force injury, such as a blow from a knee, elbow, shoulder, head, or helmet of an opponent; or physical contact with an unyielding source, such as boarding in ice hockey or indoor soccer, or a fall of a skateboarder on a rail. Because of the close proximity of other organs, it is often associated with other internal damage. Patients may initially complain of the wind being knocked out of them, but they can rapidly deteriorate from internal bleeding and shock.

The spleen is second behind the liver as the most damaged organ from blunt-force trauma.[5] As an organ wholly within the peritoneum, the spleen is not firmly fixed to the abdominal walls, and it has diffuse pain receptors. When injured, the pain is often referred to the upper-left shoulder, in a phenomenon known as Kehr's sign. A ruptured spleen is a life-threatening situation, but diagnosis is sometimes challenging and the spleen has an ability to form a loose hematoma to deter further blood loss. The hematoma is fragile and can tear away, causing hemorrhage. In one documented incident, a

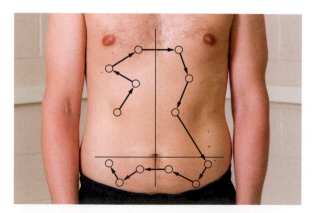

FIGURE 12.6   Sequence for percussion of the abdomen.

football player continued to play after injury, rationalizing his abdominal pain was the result of an earlier spicy meal. His condition was eventually recognized, but by the time he was evaluated and diagnosed using computed tomography (CT) at the hospital, nearly 52% of his total blood volume was contained within his abdomen.[6] Recognition and referral were paramount in his eventual full return to sports.

Incidence and Epidemiology

The main mechanisms of trauma to the liver in sport are direct blow and deceleration injury.[7] Trauma to the liver can have devastating consequences; it is not typically injured alone but in conjunction with other organs.[8] There is a dearth of recent research related to abdominal and pelvic injury rates in the athletic population, but estimates are that up to 10% of abdominal injuries result from sports participation.[9]

One of the biggest problems with diagnosing splenic injuries is the seemingly benign manner in which an injury occurs. The most trivial contact can elicit a significant injury later on. Initial evaluation does not always determine the outcome of the injury, because many times the athlete shakes off the collision as incidental and thinks the only consequence is a momentary loss of breath, or the athlete does not associate any abdominal discomfort with the earlier insult. Typical mechanisms of injury (MOIs) have been a blow to the abdomen; collision with an opponent; fall on a soccer ball or football; mountain biking or motocross accident; and blow to the abdomen from a boogie board, snowboard, surfboard, lacrosse ball or baseball.[3]

In a study of Chinese military hospitals, nearly 8,000 patients were treated for a splenic injury in a 9-year period. In these patients, who were largely men (84%), the average hospital stay was 18 days, and mortality rates were low (0.11% if treated by operation, 0.15% if nonoperative).[10] An interesting aspect of this research was that up to 45% of the total blunt abdominal trauma studied also presented with injury to the spleen.[10]

Risk Factors

Because blunt-force trauma is a main cause of actual trauma to the liver, avoiding situations that could introduce MOI is key. Athletes who have a history of hepatitis or other chronic hepatic conditions should exercise caution and secure physician clearance before engaging in sports involving contact and collision. In sports that require protective padding, such as American football, men's lacrosse, or ice hockey, the chest protector is insufficient to protect the liver, and no commercial padding is available that is unique to provide sufficient safety from harm to the liver.

Certain medical conditions, pregnancy, infectious mononucleosis, and some blood disorders can enlarge the spleen (**splenomegaly**). This enlargement can predispose a person to splenic injury, because the spleen swells beneath the costal margins of the left lower ribs, making it more susceptible to insult. The term *fragile* has been associated with splenomegaly.

Nontraumatic splenic ruptures have been seen in cases of acute mononucleosis. Patients with mononucleosis who have had a ruptured spleen had no relationship with severity of symptoms and the susceptibility of rupture.[11] In a study of 29 patients diagnosed with mononucleosis, all had enlarged spleens (with an average of 50%-60% enlarged), and half of them also had enlargement of the liver (**hepatomegaly**).[11]

Another risk factor for injury to the spleen is its ability to splint itself, which can lead to delayed splenic rupture. Anatomically, a child's spleen has a thicker capsule with a larger proportion of smooth muscle than does the adult spleen. Children have a parenchyma that is more pliable, so when injured, the combination of the thicker capsule and ability of the smooth muscle to contract arterioles allows the pediatric spleen to self-splint, whereas adults have largely lost that ability.[3]

Signs and Symptoms

Regarding injuries to the liver, in addition to the initial sense of loss of breath, patients report sharp URQ pain that may radiate to the right shoulder. Signs may also be subtle at onset, and reevaluation is paramount. Depending on whether the injury to the liver is intraperitoneal or retroperitoneal, pain may be acute, or it may be diffuse and throughout the entire abdomen. Nausea and vomiting are not unusual, but they may not present initially.[7] The HCP may have to link the initial thoracic or abdominal blow to the delayed signs and symptoms, but more so in splenic injuries than in liver trauma. Abdominal guarding may occur, especially if internal bleeding is present, and the patient may go into shock. Patients who present with anxiety, dyspnea, pale and sweaty skin, and confusion should elicit immediate transfer by ambulance to a trauma center; these signs indicate shock.

Initial signs and symptoms of a spleen injury include an athlete reporting a feeling of the air being knocked out of him. Vague abdominal pain or distress may follow, but the athlete may attribute it to something else such as stomach upset from a previous meal.[6] Some athletes try to continue to participate but at a decreasing level. Other findings include pain upon palpation on the lower-left ribs and ULQ, abdominal guarding, swelling, and muscle spasm. Nausea and an urge to defecate have also been reported.[6] The condition can deteriorate to disorientation, confusion, and shock. Signs of shock include thready

History Questions for Evaluating a Blow to the Abdomen

- What happened? (Obtain MOI.)
- Have you been ill recently?
- Have you seen the physician recently?
- Have you recently been diagnosed with a sore throat or mononucleosis?
- Have you been very tired lately?

pulse, pale and sweaty skin, and lowering blood pressure. Typically, blood loss is critical by the time blood pressure is altered. Kehr's sign does not usually present immediately, because it is from blood in the abdomen irritating the phrenic nerve and diaphragm.

Field Assessment Techniques

Patients with intra-abdominal trauma may initially present as an acute, dramatic event, or with a seemingly benign blow to the chest or abdomen accompanied by a temporary loss of breath. On the field, evaluate level of consciousness (LOC) and for shock. Palpate the ribs for pain or crepitus, and palpate the abdomen for pain in each quadrant. Assess for generalized abdominal pain and muscle guarding (abdominal rigidity). Evaluate vital signs, including pulse, respiration, blood pressure, and oxygen saturation levels. The overriding caution is to be clinically suspicious of any blow to the chest or abdomen, and reevaluate often. Given the various muscular attachments that affect the trunk and hip motions, assessing full trunk and hip ranges of motion is also critical.

Resist the urge to allow the patient to dictate return to participation (RTP) without a full evaluation. Although many initially report merely the wind being knocked out of them, it is wise to perform a brief exam to determine the need to continue to monitor the situation. Depending on the findings, assess for full trunk and hip ranges of motion, and determine RTP or conclude that a more thorough evaluation is warranted. Then, remove the patient from the field, assess vital signs, and measure oxygen saturation.

Types and Sequencing

The most widely used grading system for liver trauma is the American Association for the Surgery of Trauma (AAST) grading system. AAST also uses similar scales for spleen and kidney trauma to distinguish levels of damage, from relatively minor to catastrophic. The AAST scale uses these 6 grades to liver trauma (I-VI) that begin with *(I)* a subcapsular hematoma with less than 10% surface area involved, moving to *(II)* a capsular tear less than 1 centimeter, *(III)* a subcapsular hematoma of 10%

to 50% in surface area, all the way to *(VI)* a vascular injury, where the hepatic artery is avulsed.[1,12,13] Injuries in the lower-grade range (I-V) correspond with increasing challenges in liver damage, whereas grade VI is fatal. Grades I and II are categorized as minor liver trauma and collectively represent 80% to 90% of all liver injuries.[7]

The classification used to grade splenic injury is also the AAST splenic injury scale and is similar to the liver injury scale by the same group (AAST). The splenic injury scale is ranked I to V; the first 2 have the same criteria (hematoma, subcapsular, less than 10%, etc.), and V denotes a fractured spleen. Fifty-eight percent of spleen trauma is usually grade I or II.[13]

Diagnostic Accuracy

On the field, only clinical suspicion and abnormal vital signs are available to determine whether the trauma to the liver or spleen is sufficient to warrant transportation to the nearest trauma center. Once there, diagnostic choices vary depending on the responsiveness of the patient. Unconscious patients with a history consistent with intra-abdominal trauma, and who are hemodynamically unstable, may undergo a **diagnostic peritoneal lavage (DPL)**, which is an emergent procedure. If results are positive, surgical exploration of the abdomen via **laparotomy** occurs to determine whether the source of bleeding can be surgically rectified. More common is a diagnostic ultrasound.[14] Studies have demonstrated an 85% sensitivity and 95% specificity of detecting intra-abdominal trauma.[7] Ultrasound is noninvasive, is quick, and does not subject the patient to radiation.

As with intrathoracic diagnoses, CT is the gold standard for intra-abdominal and pelvic injury.[15] The challenges with CT testing are the amount of time it takes, radiation exposure, and cost. It is not the best choice for a patient with acute injury or with failing or unstable vital signs.

The CT is most reliable for diagnosis of a splenic injury. It is most often used with a contrast agent (dye) to discern usual space from blood-filled space. Ultrasound is also successful for detecting blood in the abdominal cavity (hemoperitoneum). As mentioned previously, ultrasound is quick, accurate, and without radiation. As with liver trauma, using DPL is an option for hemodynamically unstable patients in emergent cases.

Clinical Prediction Rules

Because of anatomical differences in the spleen between children and adults, 75% to 93% of children with splenic injuries resulting from blunt trauma may be treated by observation alone, whereas only 35% to 65% of adults with the same MOI are successfully treated by observation.[3]

Immediate Management Techniques

Patients presenting with dyspnea and who are pale, tachycardic, and hypotensive should be managed as critical. If after removal from the playing surface the patient is still not recovering, activate emergency medical services (EMS), and continue to monitor the patient's vital signs. Provide supplemental oxygen (12-15 L/min via a non-rebreather mask) as a precaution, and treat for shock if necessary. Although the initial vital sign readings may not be unusual, repeated assessment findings can indicate underlying trauma.

Once the decision has been made to remove the athlete from participation and vital signs have been obtained, the only outcomes are to continue to monitor or activate EMS for transportation to a trauma center. The deciding factors are the same as with liver trauma, namely, worsening vital signs, any sign of shock, or pain levels not diminishing.

Contraindications

Until it has been definitively determined that the patient is not going to be transported to a trauma center, refrain from providing fluids or food. Should an emergency procedure be required, the presence of contents in the stomach would complicate any operative procedure.

Criteria for Deciding to Transport for Further Medical Examination
The decision to transport must occur before the patient becomes unstable. Hemodynamically unstable patients are in a life-or-death crisis; do not wait until this situation presents itself to call EMS. Be certain transportation is to a level I trauma center, because it is better to travel a bit farther to it than arrive at a hospital that is poorly equipped for immediate surgery.

Patients with a mechanism of blunt force or deceleration injury to the abdomen should be carefully evaluated and watched. Transportation by ambulance to a trauma center is necessary if the patient has deteriorating vital signs, any sign of shock, or pain that is not reducing. Tachycardia coupled with hypotension is alarming and grounds for immediate referral and activation of emergency medical services for passage to the nearest trauma center.

Transportation Techniques   While awaiting transportation, and during the ride, place the patient in a comfortable position. For abdominal trauma, a hook-lying position is advisable because it reduces pressure on the abdomen. Supply supplemental oxygen, and continue to monitor vital signs (pulse, respiration, blood pressure, oxygen saturation). Upon determination that transportation is necessary, place the patient in a **modified Trendelenburg position** with the feet and legs elevated slightly, and provide supplemental oxygen. The modified Trendelenburg position is used to prevent **hypovolemic shock** and facilitate venous return to the heart and brain. Although the research is scanty, it is touted in treatment for shock and for acute abdominal and pelvic organ injury.[7,16]

Injury to the Kidneys

Although it is uncommon, traumatic injury to the kidney occurs in sport and activity. A direct blow to the lower posterior rib cage can injure a kidney, especially in lean people who have less protection from adipose tissue. In sports involving collision, the regulation chest pads offer inadequate protection for preventing injuries to the lower ribs and kidneys, but an added posterior back plate is good posterior protection if worn correctly. This pad is attached superiorly to the bottom of the posterior chest pads, but it is not otherwise attached. It requires a tight fitting jersey to cover the pad and firmly secure it to the body (figure 12.7). If uncovered, the loose flapping back pad can actually cause damage to the kidney if it

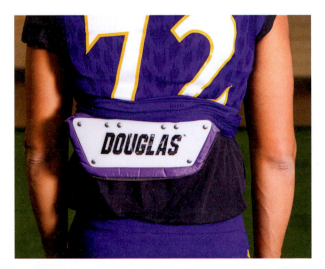

FIGURE 12.7   A football back plate pad can be adequate protection from kidney injury if an athlete wears a jersey over the pad to firmly secure it.

flips perpendicular to the body when the athlete falls. A circular flack vest is also used for protection to the entire lower rib cage and kidneys. However, it is not often worn, because it adds weight and bulk to the athlete.

Incidence and Epidemiology

Overall, renal trauma yields approximately 3% of all trauma admissions to hospitals.[17] A multiyear study of patients with kidney injury reporting to level 1 trauma centers found that of the 320 patients who met the criteria, 18% (59 patients) had sports-related kidney trauma. The main culprits were skiing, snowboarding, and contact sports; but bicycling was also mentioned.[18] Three percent of these patients with sports-related kidney trauma had to undergo a **nephrectomy**.

A study reviewing 240 high school varsity sports over 2 years showed that while adolescents do injure their kidneys during sport, it is far less often than other sport-related injuries. In total 18 kidney and 17 testicular traumas were reported in the over 4-million athlete exposures. American football (12 injuries) and soccer (girls 2, boys 1) contributed the majority of the kidney injuries.[19] None of these injuries required surgical intervention, and all healed without incident.

Risk Factors

Because this section is on kidney trauma and not kidney disease, the only risk factors are contact or collision sports, or falling on an unyielding object (e.g., horseback riding, skateboarding, BMX biking). At one time, having one kidney was a reason to disqualify a person from sports participation, especially those activities where injury to the remaining kidney is possible. In 1994, the American Academy of Pediatrics (AAP) allowed children with a single kidney to participate in contact and collision sports but provided no other guidance regarding participation.[19]

Signs and Symptoms

Given the anatomical attachment of the kidneys to the diaphragm, injury to a kidney will elicit painful breathing; kidneys move slightly with respiration. This injury is excruciating because the kidneys have direct innervation, unlike the intra-abdominal organs such as the spleen or appendix. Yet, similar to intra-abdominal blunt-force trauma, signs and symptoms of kidney injury are dyspnea, tachycardia, and later, hypotension. Hematuria is a delayed sign as well. It has been reported that the degree of hematuria is related to the severity of renal trauma, but renal insult and absence of blood in the urine were also reported.[17] In relatively minor kidney contusions, athletes report hematuria post-practice, but they do not relate a blow to the kidney as significant to disclose unless asked.

Field Assessment Techniques

A kidney injury should be suspected of any athlete fall resulting from a blow to the posterior lower ribs or flank area. Other mechanisms include falling on the posterior flank or hitting an unbending object with the same area. Preliminary complaints may be shortness of breath or dyspnea, but in some cases it resolves quickly. Uncommon, but possible, are nausea, dizziness, and abdominal pain.[21] Upon inspection, an early mark (but not yet ecchymosis) may show where the blow or fall occurred, indicating the area of impact. If the mark is over the anatomical area of the kidney (near the spinal column, under the last ribs), at minimum a kidney contusion is suspected. Palpate the ribs and abdomen, seeking areas of pain, discomfort, or swelling. Depending on the results of the evaluation, either determine RTP readiness or remove the athlete from play and continue to monitor the situation.

Types and Sequencing

As with the liver and spleen, trauma to the kidneys is graded according to the AAST. The scale differs for kidney trauma from the aforementioned organs in that a grade I contusion has the presence of hematuria (microscopic or gross), and a grade I hematoma extends only to the subcapsular area without parenchymal laceration. Grade II lacerations are less than 0.4 inches (1 cm) parenchymal depth, but without urinary extravagation; and grades II through V each have larger tears and advancing detrimental urinary sequelae.

Idiopathic Hematuria

Without related trauma, hematuria has been reported following sporting activity; it is sometimes called sports hematuria. The hematuria may be gross (visible to the naked eye) or microscopic, and it often follows strenuous practices or events, including high-intensity or long-duration practices. Causes have been attributed to dehydration, foot-strike hemolysis, nonsteroidal anti-inflammatory drugs (NSAIDs), hypoxic kidney damage, increased circulation rate, and myoglobinuria release.[20] Treatment is to ensure that no blunt trauma injury occurred, and repeat urine dipstick analysis the next day. Unresolving hematuria, or that accompanied with pain or fever, should be referred to a nephrologist.

Kidney Stones

Kidney stones are a relatively common condition of the urinary system that can manifest acutely. Salts that crystalize within the ureters, urinary bladder, or urethra create the stones, which often form a blockage. Because of the crystallization, acute kidney stones can create pain on either side of the back (either ureter), over the pubis (bladder), or anywhere along the urethra. Sudden acute pain, hematuria, nausea, and vomiting are common signs and symptoms, but abdominal sounds are within the normal limits. This condition is often corrected without treatment, but pain medication may be necessary. A patient presenting with fever should be referred immediately to rule out infection. Once the stone passes, the patient is usually free of symptoms but may have residual hematuria from the stone scraping or stretching the urethra.

Diagnostic Accuracy

For hemodynamically unstable patients, intravenous urography (IVU) is optimal. In this procedure, contrast dye is introduced intravenously, followed by abdominal radiography 10 minutes later. HCPs perform this procedure before conducting any intra-abdominal exploration.[17] The IVU determines the anatomical sufficiency of both kidneys and their respective ureters; but the disadvantages include multiple radiographic images and therefore high doses of radiation.

The best diagnostic imaging for stable patients is the CT scan. It is both sensitive and specific for parenchymal lacerations, infarcts, as well as lesions or bleeding to surrounding organs, including the liver, spleen, and pancreas.[17] Ultrasound is an alternative diagnostic tool, because it is noninvasive and does not use radiation. However, its accuracy is operator dependent.

Clinical Prediction Rules

Research has shown that 40% of patients with sports-related kidney trauma were hemodynamically unstable.[18] This number is significant because of the danger that kidney trauma presents in sports, and one should consider a low level of suspicion for substantial damage with each injury.

Immediate Management Techniques

Patients who are having challenges with pain, dyspnea, or worsening signs and symptoms should have their vital signs monitored. In kidney injury, vital signs are usually within normal ranges, but having these data is important. Patients who deteriorate or do not improve should be referred to a level I trauma center.

Criteria for Deciding to Transport for Further Medical Examination
Deciding to activate EMS for rapid transportation to a level I trauma center is dependent on a clinical suspicion of trauma to the kidney. As mentioned earlier, hematuria is usually not an acute sign, and it is not in itself a reason to call an ambulance. Patients who display any indication of shock should be treated and transported. Treatment for shock includes raising the feet or legs above the heart and keeping the patient warm.

Transportation Techniques
While waiting for the ambulance, keep the patient warm, if in shock. Place the patient in a comfortable position, which may be hook lying. Administer supplemental oxygen (12-15 L/min using a non-rebreather mask).

Appendicitis

Unlike other conditions covered so far in this chapter, appendicitis is a medical condition not brought about by trauma. It is an inflammation of the lining of the vermiform appendix (figure 12.8) that may spread to other areas if left untreated. Without intervention, complications

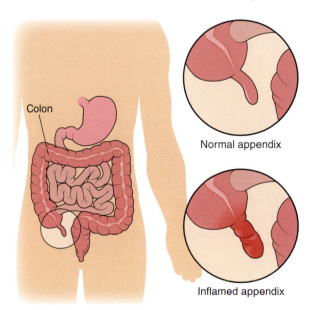

Colon

Normal appendix

Inflamed appendix

FIGURE 12.8 Appendicitis is an inflammation of the appendix in the LRQ.

from appendicitis can be fatal. The only true cure is an appendectomy (surgical removal of the appendix).

Incidence and Epidemiology

With a reported 379,000 cases of appendicitis in the United States annually, it is an emergency but a common one. The incidence of appendicitis has gradually reduced over the years, and it is lower in countries that have a higher dietary intake of fiber.[22]

Risk Factors

Diet is thought to be one factor that is attributed to appendicitis. A high-fiber diet allows food to pass more swiftly through the digestive system, perhaps alleviating the chance that food particles will get trapped in the appendix. Appendicitis is more common in the youth, as the mean age is 6-10 years, and the median age of appendectomy is 22 years.[23]

Signs and Symptoms

The initial presentation of appendicitis is typically anorexia, with nonspecific periumbilical pain. Later, nausea and LRQ pain may occur; although vomiting occurs in half of appendicitis cases.[23] A small number of patients suffer constipation or diarrhea. Patients may have a slightly elevated body temperature. Other findings are rebound tenderness, abdominal rigidity, and guarding. Patients tend to lie supine or on their sides with the hips flexed and knees drawn toward the chest to relieve pain. Symptoms tend to last about 48 hours prior to intervention.

Because of its lack of fixation, a few accessory signs are used to further confirm suspected appendicitis besides the traditional McBurney's point pain (figure 12.9). McBurney's point is found one-third of the distance between the anterior superior iliac spine of the right ilium and the umbilicus. Is it a spot of palpation for an inflamed appendix.

Two signs that will cause LRQ pain are the obturator sign (internal and external rotation of a fixed flexed hip), and the psoas sign (pain with resistive flexion or extension of the right hip).[23]

Two other signs indicating appendicitis, or rather, peritonitis, are Rovsing's sign (LRQ pain when palpating the LLQ) and **Dunphy's sign**. It is also related to peritonitis; it is sharp pain in the LRQ caused by a cough.[23]

Field Assessment Techniques

It is unlikely a person will have an acute bout of appendicitis while participating in recreation or sports. More possible is an athlete who is ill or feels poorly and complains of a gastrointestinal-like illness. Patients who

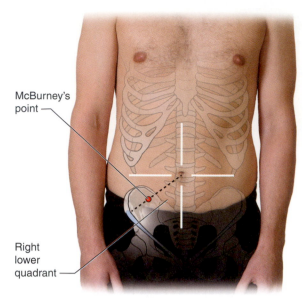

FIGURE 12.9   McBurney's point.

complain of abdominal pain absent any trauma should have a thorough personal history assessment.

Diagnostic Accuracy

Although laboratory studies are usually performed, they generally rule out other conditions. A complete blood count may or may not have elevated white blood cells. A urinalysis will be normal but will also rule out a urinary tract infection (**UTI**).

A CT with contrast (oral or rectal) is the most useful diagnostic tool for patients with unusual appendicitis. A multidetector CT (MDCT) has an unusually high sensitivity and specificity for diagnosing acute appendicitis with values of 98.5% and 98%, respectively.[23] As with the other organ trauma discussed in this chapter, use of CT has its drawbacks, namely, cost and exposure to radiation. Ultrasonography is an option, but is not informative if the appendix is normal, because it is not usually viewed. In addition, given the anatomic variances of appendixes, ultrasound is not the best choice for accuracy in diagnosing appendicitis.

Clinical Prediction Rules

Pain migration is a sentinel symptom of appendicitis. As a distinguishing feature, pain beginning midabdomen and moving to the LRQ has a sensitivity and specificity of 80%, with a positive likelihood of 3.18 for appendicitis.[23]

Immediate Management Techniques

Immediate management of suspected appendicitis is to take any vital signs and assessments that could assist in diagnosis. Vital signs of heart rate, respiration, and blood

History Questions for a Suspected Gastrointestinal Illness

- When did you begin to feel unwell?
- Where exactly is your pain? Has it moved?
- When was the last time you ate, and what did you eat?
- Do you have food allergies or reactions? If so, to what?
- Do you have any chronic gastrointestinal conditions (e.g., gastroesophageal reflux disease, gastritis, Crohn's disease, celiac disease)?
- When was your last normal bowel movement?
- Do you feel nauseated?
- Have you vomited in the last 24 hours? If so, how often? When was the last time?
- Have you had diarrhea in the last 24 hours? If so, how often? When was the last time?
- What have you been eating or drinking since you began to feel poorly?

pressure should be within normal range, as should pulse oximetry. Body temperature may be slightly elevated. A dipstick urine analysis with be within normal limits, but it is helpful in eliminating any urological issues.

Criteria for Deciding to Transport for Further Medical Examination   Patients with vague abdominal pain that has been present for a day and has migrated to the LRQ should be sent to a physician for evaluation. The physician's office should have access to advanced diagnostic studies, including CT or ultrasound, as well as basic laboratory assessments for differential diagnoses. Upon further investigation, the patient may be referred for a surgical consultation.

Acute Abdominopelvic Concerns for Female Athletes

Both ruptured ovarian cysts and ectopic pregnancy are discussed together in this section, because they largely present with similar signs and symptoms and can both be emergent situations. Each typically occurs in women who have reached puberty, but sometimes either can occur absent a primary menses.

Ovarian cysts come in many sizes and with symptoms. A woman can have a minute cyst every month and be unaware of it; or a cyst can continue to grow, become painful, and possibly rupture. Many types of cysts are attributed to the ovary, but the makeup of them is immaterial to this segment. This section discusses only ruptured ovarian cysts.

An ectopic pregnancy occurs when an egg released by the ovary is fertilized and begins to divide and grow in any area other than the uterus. The most common anatomical area is within the fallopian tube as the egg is headed toward the uterus. An ectopic pregnancy can damage the fallopian tube, causing challenges in future conception.

Incidence and Epidemiology

Ovarian cysts tend to occur most from infancy through adolescence when girls are hormonally active, but they are common through the reproductive ages. It is uncommon for ovarian cysts to be cancerous.[24] In fact, 70% to 80% of follicular cysts resolve without intervention.[24] Ectopic pregnancy can occur in any woman with functioning ovaries, from the onset of puberty until menopause.

About 1% to 2% of all pregnancies in the United States are ectopic pregnancies.[25] One study showed that 90% of ectopic pregnancies occur in women who have previously been pregnant. When compared with Caucasian women, women of other races are twice as likely to have ectopic pregnancies.[26]

Risk Factors

Whereas neither ovarian cysts nor ectopic pregnancy can be fully prevented, certain known factors can make one more susceptible to these conditions. One can mitigate the chances by appreciating known risk factors and controlling behaviors that can contribute to these gynecological issues.

Risk factors for ovarian cysts include cigarette smoking, infertility treatment, pregnancy, and tubal ligation.[24] Based on epidemiological studies, women who have been pregnant have a greater risk of ectopic pregnancy than those in their first pregnancy. Other identified risk factors include older maternal age, cigarette smoking and secondhand smoke, use of intrauterine device (IUD), and infertility.[25]

Untreated, a ruptured ovarian cyst or ectopic pregnancy can lead to loss of a fallopian tube or ovary, or even death.

Signs and Symptoms

Signs and symptoms for both these conditions can be similar. A ruptured ovarian cyst may range from relatively pain free, to indicators similar to an ectopic pregnancy. These signs and symptoms include abdominal pain, vaginal bleeding, nausea or vomiting, and abdominal tenderness. Amenorrhea (absence of menstrual cycle) is common with both. Weakness, syncope, and circulatory collapse have occurred with both conditions.[26,27] Referred pain to the shoulder has also been reported.[27]

Separate from the urgent attention a rupture ovarian cyst or ectopic pregnancy presents is mittelschmerz. Mittelschmerz is mid-cycle pain from ovulation when the physiologic release of the egg causes fluid release that results in pain. Because this condition is associated with ovulation, the patient's time of cycle can be an indicator of this benign, self-limiting condition.

Field Assessment Techniques

The female patient who complains of lower-quadrant abdominal pain that is dissimilar from her usual menses pain should have a thorough history performed. Determine whether the patient is mid cycle or not, and whether or not she has had similar symptoms before. Ask whether she is experiencing vaginal bleeding (if not during her menses). If the patient's abdominal pain gets worse, she is not mid cycle, and she appears to be deteriorating, refer to a gynecologist. If she is mid cycle, the pain is episodic (not constant), and she has no vaginal bleeding or signs of syncope, then reevaluate and determine RTP status.

Diagnostic Accuracy

In laboratory testing, a urine test assessing for beta-human chorionic gonadotropic hormone can confirm pregnancy, as will a serum analysis. This test is important for determining whether or not the patient is pregnant. The hormone will be present regardless if the pregnancy is in the uterus, fallopian tube, or elsewhere, and it can indicate an ectopic event continuant with other signs. If the patient is not stable, hematocrit may be determined.

The preferred diagnostic tool for either ovarian cyst or ectopic pregnancy is ultrasonography.[27] This procedure is

effective without radiation, and it is expeditious. It is also less expensive than CT. Many athletic training facilities use diagnostic ultrasound in determining the extent of damage in musculoskeletal as well as other injuries.

Immediate Management Techniques

Immediate management for either of these gynecological issues includes a good and thorough patient history. It is appropriate to question the patient about certain aspects of her prior menstrual history (see Clinical Skills: History Questions Concerning the Reproductive System). When questioning the patient, ask her whether she has a female friend, teammate, or roommate she wishes to be present when you ask the history questions (regardless of the clinician's gender).

Criteria for Deciding to Transport for Further Medical Examination   Patients who are declining, have worsening pain or vital signs, or are clinically unstable should be transferred by ambulance to a level I trauma center. Transportation for these 2 gynecological conditions is only because the patient's condition has deteriorated and the patient is in need of urgent intervention. If the patient is communicative and has normal vital signs, but signs or symptoms suggest an abdominal or gynecological issue, refer her immediately to a gynecologist (to be seen immediately). If the patient is in shock or is declining, activate EMS for transportation to the nearest level I trauma center.

Acute Trauma to Male Genitals

The two testes-threatening acute injuries discussed here are contusion of the testicle and testicular torsion. They are similar in several ways and are discussed together. The MOI for both can be either a direct hit or a glancing blow to the testes. A contusion results from blood accumulating within the testis or between the testis and the scrotum. A torsion injury causes infarct (an area of dead tissue) due to the spermatic cord twisting to a point where nutrients no longer reach the individual testis.

When evaluating a patient with an acute testicular trauma, history and MOI are key, as are the ability to be professional, reassuring, and clear with your terms and instructions.

Incidence and Epidemiology

In a 2-year study published in 2012 of sports-related urological injury, 23,666 injuries were reported via a high school injury surveillance.[19] Regardless of MOI, high school sport-related testicular trauma was reported

🚩 **RED FLAG**

Regardless of the HCP's gender, it is prudent to have a person of the patient's gender present for history questions concerning reproductive organs.

History Questions Concerning the Reproductive System

Women

- When was the first day of your last menstrual cycle (period)?
- Are your periods regular?
- Do you usually have heavy periods?
- Have you had a history of ovarian cysts?

Men

- Did you recently get hit in your testicles or groin?
- Does your testicle feel heavy or swollen?
- Does your testicle feel twisted or higher than usual?

---

highest in American football, with injuries noted in soccer and wrestling.[19] Another study listed lacrosse as the sport with the highest incidence of testicular trauma (48.5% of all testicular trauma), with wrestling (32.8%), baseball (21%), and American football (17.8%) following.[28]

One study showed an 11% tendency for testicular torsion among family members.[29] A relationship also exists between the time of torsion and detorsion, and the salvage of the testis. If detorsion occurs within 6 hours of injury, the salvage rate is 97.2%. If the time frame is between 7 and 12 hours, the salvage rate is 79.3%; at 13 to 24 hours, testicle survival rate is 54%; and the salvage rate after 24 hours is only 18.1%.[30]

Risk Factors

In collision sports, a protective scrotal cup is worn to protect the male genitalia. However, in a study of 731 male high school athletes, only 12.9% wore the cup in these sports.[28] The American Academy of Pediatrics Committee on Sports Medicine has allowed boys with 1 functioning testicle to play sports, albeit a protective cup may be mandated by the physician. Warmer weather is reported to be related to testicular trauma, due in part to the scrotum allowing the testes to be farther from the body proper to remain cooler.

Signs and Symptoms

Usually, athletes sustaining testicular trauma are initially unable to communicate effectively due to pain. They may be nauseated, vomiting, hyperventilating, and pale. Patients with testicular contusions present with a swollen testicle, sometimes to the point where the scrotum appears stretched to capacity. Testicular torsion presents with a higher testicle than typical for the patient, or a transverse lying of the affected testis.[31]

All present with pain for less than 24 hours; but some, typically prepubescent and adolescent patients, may describe thigh or abdominal pain instead of scrotal pain. Young boys complaining of abdominal pain should be questioned about the exact mechanism of injury and location of pain. Cases have occurred with a history of a blunt-force trauma to the testicle, but absence of pain. In this situation either the hematoma or torsion has progressed to a point of infarcted testis.[32]

Field Assessment Technique

On the field, the only assessment of testicular trauma is one of patient history, including whether or not he was hit in the testicles directly (contusion), or it was a glancing blow (contusion or torsion), or neither (torsion).

Send the athlete with a male HCP to a private place for observation. If it is not possible, send the athlete to a private place for self-examination. Clearly tell him to notice, then come back and describe whether he has scrotal swelling, asymmetry, or deformity. Be very clear to ask whether one testicle is higher than the other, and if this is unusual. Ask the athlete if one testis looks sideways, and if either is painful to touch. Any abnormality to either testicle that is observed or reported should be referred immediately to a urologist.

Diagnostic Accuracy

An ultrasound of the scrotum is effective because it can elicit whether the testicle and spermatic cord are anatomically compliant. When performed in conjunction with the ultrasound, a Doppler study confirms whether or not the vascular structures of the testis are intact and whether blood flow is occurring normally within the scrotum.

Reducing Testicular Torsion

Testicular detorsion that occurs within 6 hours of injury has the highest testicle salvage rate.[30,31] Therefore, once torsion is recognized, you have plenty of time to get the patient to a urologist for manual detorsion or, if it fails, surgical detorsion. The following text is intended to describe the procedure for manual detorsion; it is not intended as a tool to apply on the field or in the clinic immediately after torsion.

The patient can be standing or supine. Presented with a testicular torsion, the physician holds the affected testicle with the thumb and forefinger, and rotates the testicle 180° outward in a medial-to-lateral direction.[31] This process may have to be repeated 2 to 3 times, using pain relief as a guide. Following detorsion, the patient will need immediate Doppler studies to confirm that usual blood flow is returning to the affected testis.[30,31,34]

Clinical Prediction Rules

A study of 138 children with testicular pain lasting less than 24 hours, nausea or vomiting, and a testicle positioned superiorly, found that when 2 or more of these findings were present, 100% had testicular torsion with 0% false positives.[33]

Immediate Management Techniques

Following recognition of a testicular torsion or the patient reporting one, immediate referral to a urologist or other qualified HCP is necessary to reduce the torsion. If this procedure is performed outside of a clinic or hospital, the clinician trained in detorsion should have another male (relative, friend, teammate) present when the procedure is being completed.

Criteria for Deciding to Transport for Further Medical Examination   If a patient describes deformity in the testes and sustains an acute onset of pain, he should be referred for further evaluation as soon as possible that day. Unless the patient is going into or is already in shock, or is hemodynamically unstable, transportation is not necessary. However, the patient must be immedi-ately referred to a urologist for a same-day appointment. If transportation is used in the case of testicular torsion, ensure ahead of time that a urologist will be available at the hospital, or transport to a level I trauma center.

Summary

Assessment of the acute abdomen is often challenging; pain is not always focal, and symptoms are not specific. People who present with an identifiable trauma should be carefully evaluated, monitored, and reassessed often, because intra-abdominal bleeding is not always obvious, nor does it happen within a specific time frame. Some athletes are reported to continue to participate in spite of traumatic damage to abdominal organs. When an athlete wants to return to sport without full medical clearance, exercise caution in terms of what you allow the athlete to do.

Assessment of organs in the pelvic region relies largely on the ability of the HCP to ask clear and unambiguous history questions, and providing distinct things for the patient to assess. Ectopic pregnancy, ruptured ovarian cysts, and testicular trauma can all be organ- or life-threatening situations and must be treated as such.

 Go to the web study guide to complete the case studies for this chapter.

CHAPTER 13

Life-Threatening Metabolic Emergencies

Human metabolism requires consistency. Any altering of the physiology, no matter how slight, can affect the whole body. If it is not addressed and corrected, the end result can be catastrophic. Metabolism begins when foods and fluids are ingested. The process of converting calories into energy to keep the body functioning properly occurs in many places, but the pancreas is a key player. Diabetes, **hyperglycemia** (excessive glucose in the blood), and **hypoglycemia** (lower-than-normal amount of glucose in the blood) are the central metabolic emergencies discussed in this chapter.

Overview of the Anatomical Structures in Metabolic Emergencies

This section is reprinted, by permission, from K. Walsh Flanagan and M. Cuppett, *Medical Conditions in the Athlete*, 3rd ed. (Champaign, IL: Human Kinetics, 2017), 345-346.

The disorders discussed here are related to the pancreas, a gland with both exocrine and endocrine functions. The pancreas lies with its ends laterally touching the spleen (figure 13.1) and the duodenum of the small intestine medially.

The pancreas is the primary gland secreting the hormones insulin and glucagon. Insulin stimulates liver, muscle, and fat cells to absorb glucose in the blood and to store it in muscle and liver as glycogen.[1] The pancreas also produces somatostatin from the endocrine glands, called islets of Langerhans. The islets comprise four cell types, but only the 2 primary cell types, alpha and beta, are discussed here. Alpha cells produce glucagon, whereas beta cells secrete insulin.

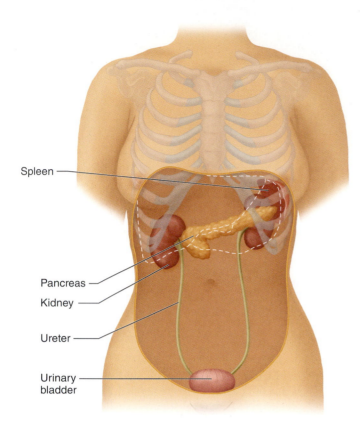

Spleen

Pancreas

Kidney

Ureter

Urinary
bladder

FIGURE 13.1   Location of the pancreas.

When serum glucose (blood sugar) is high, beta cells are stimulated to produce insulin. The secreted insulin then allows muscle, blood, and fat cells to absorb glucose out of the blood, effectively lowering blood sugar to normal ranges. The alpha cells of the islets of Langerhans secrete glucagon, which has the opposite effect of insulin. If blood sugar is low, glucagon is secreted where it has the most effect—the liver. Glucagon stimulates liver cells to break down stored glycogen into glucose and release it into the bloodstream, increasing serum levels of glucose. Glucagon also stimulates muscle to manufacture glucose from stored protein by means of gluconeogenesis. The human body functions best when glucose levels are relatively constant within the bloodstream. Because most body functions rely on glucose in some form, severely fluctuating levels can have profound sequelae.[1]

Diabetes

Parts of this section are reprinted, by permission, from K. Walsh Flanagan and M. Cuppett *Medical Conditions in the Athlete*, 3rd ed. (Champaign, IL: Human Kinetics, 2017), 347-348.

Diabetes mellitus (DM) is a disease in which the body is unable to produce or use insulin effectively. Type 1 diabetes, formerly insulin-dependent diabetes mellitus (IDDM), is characterized by the body's inability to

produce insulin, which is needed for the proper use and storage of carbohydrates. Type 1 DM is caused by auto-immune-mediated destruction of pancreatic beta cells, which are responsible for producing insulin, and there appears to be a hereditary link in people with type 1 DM.[1]

Type 2 DM, formerly non–insulin-dependent diabetes mellitus (NIDDM), makes up the remaining 90% of diabetes cases.[2] This form of DM is related to the body's inability to use insulin effectively because of a combination of resistance to insulin as well as an overall decreased production of insulin, not always, but most often due to obesity. Type 2 DM results more from an insulin resistance syndrome. In addition to numerous environmental and physiological reasons for insulin resistance, the main cause is excess body fat (body mass index—BMI—over 25) linked primarily to a sedentary lifestyle and an excess consumption of calories.[3]

Type 1 diabetes is not preventable. Type 2 diabetes, however, is a condition whose onset and severity can be greatly decreased if not eliminated with adequate exercise and a proper diet.[1] Because this textbook is about acute and emergency care, the focus is on the patient who has type I diabetes. However, the recognition, evaluation, and treatment are the same for both types 1 and 2.

Incidence and Epidemiology

Data from the Centers for Disease Control and Prevention state that over 100 million Americans have diabetes or prediabetes.[4] Diabetes mellitus affects 9.4% of the population, or roughly 30.3 million people, in the United States. An additional 84.1 million Americans have prediabetes, with 9 of 10 people unaware they have the condition. The risk for death among people with diabetes is nearly twice that of people of the same age range without diabetes.[1,4]

Type 1 DM accounts for roughly 10% of the total number of cases, and its onset usually occurs in people less than 20 years of age. The incidence of diabetes is known to increase with age. It is the leading cause of end-stage renal disease in the United States and is a primary cause of blindness and foot and leg amputations in adults. Over 79,000 people with diabetes will die annually due to complications of this disease, which is the seventh leading cause of death in the United States.[5] It is also known to cause neuropathy (nerve damage) in up to 70% of diabetic patients. Individuals with diabetes are twice as likely as persons without diabetes to develop cardiovascular disease.[1,2]

Risk Factors

Certain factors can predispose people to type 2 diabetes. Women can be affected by gestational diabetes, usually occurring in the third trimester of pregnancy and typically resolving in the postpartum period. These individuals are more likely to develop type 2 DM later on in life. Uncontrolled high blood pressure and high cholesterol are also risk factors for type 2 DM, as is being over the age of 45. Certain ethnic populations are at increased risk for diabetes, including Native Americans, African Americans, Asian Americans, and Hispanic Americans.[5] Other causes of type 2 DM are Cushing's syndrome, pancreatic disorders such as pancreatitis, or prolonged medication usage, including glucocorticoids.[1,6] Complications of unmanaged or poorly controlled diabetes include heart disease, ocular challenges including blindness, kidney disease that can lead to renal failure, neuropathies, infections, dental problems, and amputations due to poorly healing distal wounds.[7]

Signs and Symptoms

Whether or not a team includes an athlete with diabetes, all health care providers (HCPs) working with active people should know typical blood glucose values (table 13.1) and what is normal for that specific athlete before, during, and following activity.

The signs and symptoms related to diabetic emergency are varied because of the differing presentations related to serum glucose status, but sometimes they mimic each other. A person with hypoglycemia will present with tachycardia and hyperventilation; whereas one with hyperglycemia will also have hyperventilation and possible cardiac arrhythmia. It is essential to know the patient's medical history, pre-practice blood sugar, and usual readings with activity.

Other salient signs and symptoms depend on whether the patient has too little or too much available serum glucose. The sidebar in the following section, Comparison of Signs and Symptoms for Hypoglycemia and Hyperglycemia, outlines the differences in signs and symptoms between the 2 extremes in blood sugar.

In general, an athlete's performance will begin to deteriorate if his serum glucose is inappropriate for the workload demanded. The athlete may complain of feeling poorly or being weak, or he may even collapse. Prior knowledge of the patient's diabetic status, maintenance history of his blood sugar, and compliance with his medical regimen are all helpful, but current serum glucose must be determined immediately when a patient with diabetes reports any signs or sensations departing from usual ones.

Field Assessment Techniques

It is essential that all athletes with diabetes be identified and meet with HCPs prior to the onset of athletic participation. Having knowledge of who these athletes are, and of their individual management plan, is vital to addressing their unique concerns. The athletic trainer (AT) should know which of her patients has a wearable insulin pump; which patients are on long-acting insulin; and the usual blood glucose readings for those patients before, during, and after practices. Glucometry is an effective and quick assessment that measures blood sugar (serum glucose). It should be used to determine current glucose levels on any athlete known to have diabetes, as well as those with signs or symptoms of hypoglycemia.

Determine the chief complaint and whether it is related to their metabolic condition. If it is, inquire about food and beverage intake (when, how much consumed, what types of foods or beverages). Ask for the time of both last blood sugar reading and last insulin injection (if not wearing a pump); and the amounts of each. Then query signs and symptoms to further assess the situation and take a glucometer reading.

 RED FLAG

Serum blood values vary greatly and can depend on the following:[8,9]

- The individual patient
- Activity type (e.g., aerobic, anaerobic, strenuous)
- Activity timing (after meals or insulin)
- Activity duration
- Environmental conditions (e.g., temperature, altitude, humidity)
- Patient fitness

TABLE 13.1 Typical Blood Glucose Levels

Time at which measurement is taken	Blood serum level (mg/dL)
After fasting for 8 hours	60-80*
2-3 hours after eating	100-140
Random and unplanned	<126

*mg/dL, milligrams of glucose in 100 mL (1 dL) of blood; hypoglycemia is defined as less than 60 mg/dL, and hyperglycemia is defined as greater than 180 mg/dL.

Reprinted by permission from K.W. Flanagan and M. Cuppett, *Medical Conditions in the Athlete*, 3rd ed. (Champaign, IL: Human Kinetics, 2017), 347-352.

Using a Glucometer

1. Wash and sanitize your hands, and put on gloves.
2. Prepare the glucometer with the correct strip for the brand of the device.
3. Load a lancet (needle) in the lancet instrument that is correct for the brand.
4. Use an alcohol pad to clean the desired finger for testing.
5. Place the lancet instrument along the side of a distal finger pad, and press the trigger to release the lancet (a).
6. Allow the blood to collect (Do not squeeze the finger.), and place the testing strip next to the blood to attract the blood droplet to it (b).
7. Read the result from the glucometer.
8. Using alcohol, clean the finger pad again.
9. Remove the used lancet and used testing strip to OSHA-approved receptacles.
10. Remove the gloves, then wash and sanitize your hands.

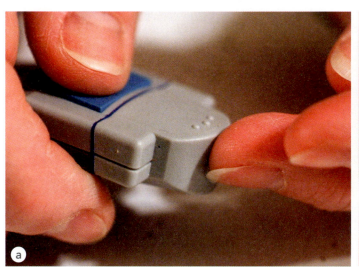
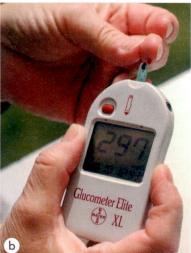

FIGURE 13.2

Diagnostic Accuracy

A common blood test used to diagnose people with diabetes as well as measure effectiveness of overall management and treatment is hemoglobin A1C (also HbA_{1c}). This test is performed in a laboratory and usually requires a sample of a vial of blood, but newer techniques can do the same test using a finger prick. It identifies the concentration of glucose in plasma over time, typically 3 months. Slight differences of opinion exist concerning the recommended A1C values. The International Diabetes Foundation recommends values below 7%; the American Diabetes Association recommends a level of 5.7% or below;[7] and the American College of Endocrinology states an A1C value above 5.5 is indicative of prediabetes.[10] Once diabetes is diagnosed, hemoglobin A1C is also used periodically to monitor plasma glucose levels, to assess effectiveness of therapy strategies.[1]

Immediate Management Techniques

Use a glucometer to assess blood sugar status. Based on the results, determine whether carbohydrate (or glucose) or insulin is necessary. For a patient who has hypoglycemia, administer carbohydrate as prescribed in the following section on hypoglycemia, provided the patient is conscious and able to ingest food. If the patient is unconscious or not responsive, is known to have hypoglycemia, and has a blood glucose level of 70 mg/dL or lower, inject the patient with glucagon and activate emergency medical services (EMS). Armed with the patient's history and blood sugar level, paramedics will be able to administer dextrose intravenously before transportation.

Hyperglycemia is usually an issue of type 1 diabetes. If the pre-exercise blood serum levels are above 250 mg/dL, urinary ketones should be assessed with a dipstick urine test. **Ketonuria** is suggestive of tissue breakdown and unmanaged diabetes. The algorithm for hyperglycemia (figure 13.3) begins with observing the patient's signs and symptoms, beginning with the deep breathing sign called **Kussmaul breathing**. Using these observations,

the HCP will make decisions following the algorithm to recognize and treat hypoglycemia.

If ketonuria is moderate to high, the athlete should avoid exercise, and aggressive measures to lower serum glucose (insulin administration) should begin.[11] Athletes with hyperglycemia but normal ketonuria are allowed to participate as long as serum glucose is assessed every 15 minutes and is demonstrated to be falling.[11]

If you administer insulin, be aware that it should be injected into the **subcutaneous** tissues of the abdomen, upper thigh, or upper arm—and not into the musculature.

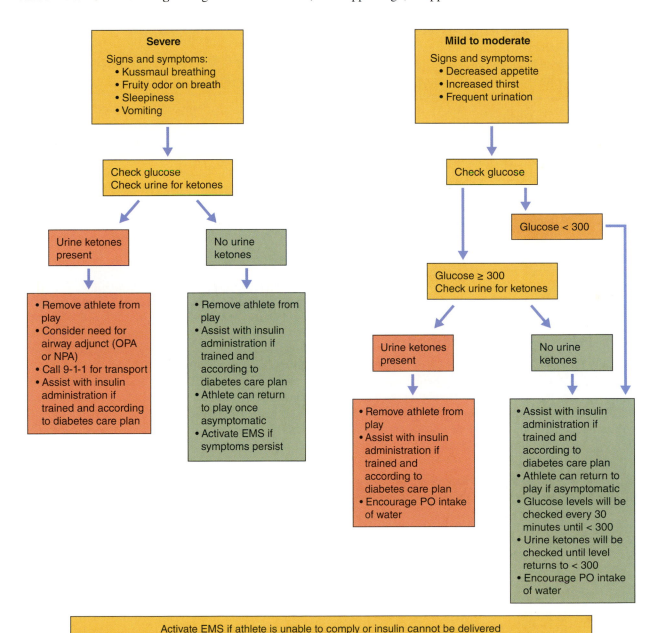

FIGURE 13.3 Algorithm for hyperglycemia.

EMS = emergency medical services; NPA = nasopharyngeal airway; OPA = oropharyngeal airway; PO = orally

Reprinted from Dr. Sharon Rogers Moore.

RED FLAG

Athletes diagnosed with type 1 diabetes should provide extra insulin prescribed for them. The insulin should be kept on hand as the athlete practices, competes, and travels with a team. New, unused needles should be kept in a container with the insulin for quick retrieval.

Contraindications

Extremes in temperature can affect insulin action by reducing its effectiveness. Athletes who have diabetes and are participating in temperatures in the ranges of below 36°F (2.2°C) or above 86°F (30°C) should access their blood sugar levels more frequently.[12] Insulin exposed to extreme conditions should be disposed of if the patient experiences unusual hyperglycemia after using it.[12] Both heat and cold therapies, including hot showers, hot tubs, ice packs, and cold tubs, can affect the delivery of insulin.

Knowing which athletes have diabetes is critical for reasons beyond emergent care. Educating them on the effect of certain therapies can prevent a hypoglycemic or hyperglycemic situation in the future; an athlete may be unaware that the usual dose of insulin can be affected by a simple therapy treatment soon after injection. Thermotherapies may increase insulin absorption rates, whereas cryotherapies may decrease these rates.[12]

Criteria for Deciding to Transport for Further Medical Examination

Typically, a patient with diabetes does not need to be transferred to a hospital unless she is semiconscious or in a coma, does not respond to treatment, or appears to decline. If the blood sugar situation is stable, an evaluation for other underlying conditions must occur. Do not use the patient's medical history as an excuse for any illness or collapse without considering other differential diagnoses that could either contribute or mask another condition.

Transportation Techniques

No unique techniques are necessary for transporting a patient with diabetes to the hospital via ambulance. In the athletic setting, the serum glucose would have been determined and initial treatment already started. However, the patient's medical history (diabetes), recent glucometer readings, as well as treatment provided, should be passed to other HCPs treating the patient.

Hypoglycemia and Hyperglycemia

Anyone can have hypoglycemia regardless of presence or absence of diabetes. Hypoglycemia is the most common adverse effect associated with insulin therapy.[11] Exercise has numerous benefits and is highly recommended for most people with diabetes, but exercise can also trigger hypoglycemia. It takes time, and often trial and error, to establish the correct insulin needs for the demands of the exercise. During this time, the athlete is susceptible to hyperglycemia, hypoglycemia, or both.

Exercise-induced hypoglycemia typically occurs within 6 hours; however, it can be delayed by as much as 48 hours after the completion of activity.[8,9] Nocturnal hypoglycemia is also a concern and a strong reason to have medical staff in overnight housing with athletes. It is helpful at least during the preseason, when all athletes are acclimating to physical and physiological changes in demand as well as their glucose or insulin needs.

Some people with diabetes use a continuous glucose monitor (CGM) that lessens the chance of exercise-induced hypoglycemia.[8,9] The CGM provides consistent serum monitoring and doses when the blood glucose values lower to a pre-established point. However, this

---

Therapies to Be Avoided After Insulin Use

Avoid 1 to 3 hours for rapid-acting insulin; avoid for up to 4 hours for regular insulin.[12]

Thermotherapies to Avoid
- Warm whirlpool
- Sauna
- Shower
- Hot tub
- Bath
- Hydrocollator/hot packs (over injection site)
- Thermal ultrasound (over injection site)

Cryotherapies to Avoid
- Cold whirlpool
- Cold tub
- Ice (over injection site)
- Cold spray (over injection site)

device is not always worn or allowed during competition, and research is not consistent on its effectiveness.[8,9]

Hyperglycemia in an athlete is a serum glucose over 250 mg/dL.[11] It typically results from a lack of insulin, including the athlete who forgot to take a previous dose. It also is triggered by overconsumption, inactivity, illness, stress, or injury.[11] An active athlete who is inactive after injury and who did not scale back the amount of insulin can be at risk for hyperglycemia.

Risk Factors

Hypoglycemia stems from too little available glucose in the bloodstream; if left unrecognized and treated, it can be fatal. In the athletic population, hypoglycemia can be attributed to morning or afternoon workouts without consuming a meal first, causing insufficient caloric intake. Other factors include injecting too much insulin with anticipation of more activity, delayed food intake post-exercise, or alcohol intake postexercise.[11]

Signs and Symptoms

The signs and symptoms of too much or too little available blood sugar are numerous and various. Knowing which signs are associated with which condition is critical. Correctly recognizing the ailment will result in proper treatment, whereas confusing hypoglycemia and hyperglycemia and applying the incorrect remedy can have disastrous consequences.

Field Assessment Techniques

As with the athlete who has diabetes, knowing the medical history of those participating in sport is critical when presented with a fallen athlete. When the glucometer measurement is under 70 mg/dL, the athlete has hypoglycemia. Remove the patient from activity, and provide 15 grams of carbohydrate (figure 13.4).

Examples of suitable carbohydrates include 6 ounces of sweet carbonated beverage, one-half cup of fruit juice, or four glucose tablets.[11] After ingestion, wait 15 minutes, then measure serum glucose again. Waiting the full 15 minutes is critical, because the body needs to absorb and process the carbohydrates enough for it to register on the glucometer; premature measurement can lead to dangerous mistakes. If the measurement is below 80 mg/dL, have the patient consume additional carbohydrates as stated previously, wait another 15 minutes, and measure again. Typically, the patient will respond and serum glucose will rise within 15 to 30 minutes. Injectable glucagon (discussed in the following section) is another resource to use if the patient is noncompliant or unable to ingest calories.

Comparison of Signs and Symptoms for Hypoglycemia and Hyperglycemia

Hypoglycemia (<60 mg/dL)	Hyperglycemia (>180 mg/dL)
• Palpitations	• Weakness
• Tachycardia	• Polyuria
• Anxiety	• Altered vision
• Hyperventilation	• Weight loss
• Blurred vision	• Dehydration
• Shakiness	• Polydipsia
• Weakness	• Hyperventilation
• Diaphoresis	• Hypotension
• Nausea	• Cardiac arrhythmia
• Confusion	• Stupor
• Behavior changes	• Coma
• Hallucinations	
• Hypothermia	
• Seizure	
• Coma	

Reprinted by permission from K.W. Flanagan and M. Cuppett, *Medical Conditions in the Athlete*, 3rd ed. (Champaign, IL: Human Kinetics, 2017), 347-352.

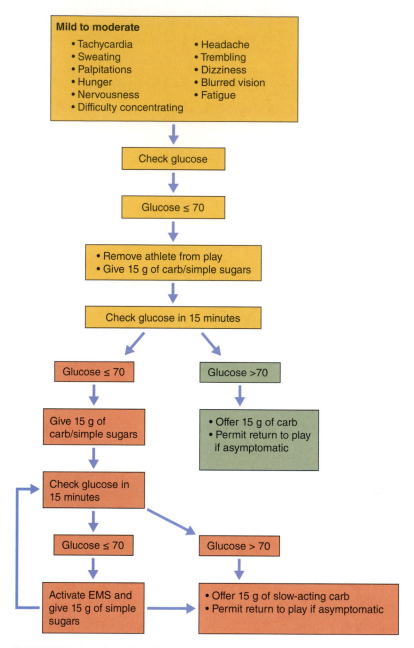

FIGURE 13.4 Algorithm for hypoglycemia.

Reprinted from Dr. Sharon Rogers Moore.

Diagnostic Accuracy

A glucometer is the best, quickest, and most accurate means of assessing blood sugar levels on the field or sidelines. Even if the patient has no diabetic or hypoglycemic history, strongly consider measuring blood sugar in those who exhibit signs or symptoms consistent with hypoglycemia or in the situation of a sudden collapse without mechanism of injury (MOI).

Immediate Management Techniques

Determine blood sugar status via a glucometer. Based on the outcome, deliver treatment; for example, provide a sugary drink, glucose tablets, or glucagon injection for patients with hypoglycemia, and deliver appropriate insulin dosage for hyperglycemia. Calories ingested orally are preferable over glucagon unless the patient is

Administering Glucagon

Glucagon is a hormone that triggers the liver to release glucose into the bloodstream. It can also be used as a treatment for severe hypoglycemia.[13]

- This drug is injected into a patient in the same places insulin is injected (arm or leg muscle) or sometimes in a vein.
- The medicine must be mixed immediately prior to use, and it cannot be prepared ahead of time.
- A glucagon emergency kit has a syringe containing fluid, and a separate bottle.
- Remove the protective needle cover, and insert the needle into the bottle.
- Push the fluid from the syringe into the bottle.
- Remove the syringe from the bottle.
- Gently shake or roll the bottle until the liquid is clear.
- Reinsert the syringe into the bottle, and withdraw the medicine as ordered by a physician.
- Inject glucagon into an arm or leg muscle.

not able to swallow, is semiconscious, or is unconscious. Wait for 15 minutes to see whether the food or beverage consumed has altered serum glucose to a desired level. Exercising with hyperglycemia is not recommended, and activity should cease until serum blood levels are stable and the patient has no signs or symptoms related to diabetic hyperglycemia.[8,9]

Criteria for Deciding to Transport for Further Medical Examination

As with the patient who has diabetes, transportation is not usually necessary. If a blood sugar is obtained and appropriate treatment delivered, wait at least 15 minutes for treatment effect to be noticeable. Both the glucometer reading and symptoms relayed from the patient provide good feedback, but rely on the objective glucometer reading for a true assessment of effectiveness.

Transportation Techniques

A patient with hypoglycemia or hyperglycemia has no unique needs save to provide pharmacological assistance if none was available on-site.

Summary

Metabolic emergencies are those dealing with the ability of the body to produce and metabolize glucose. Athletes with diabetes are in a distinctive category, because they must adjust their insulin and glucose levels to match the ever-changing demands of their physical activity. Knowing who these athletes are, their personal requirements for safe participation, and their diabetes management plan is paramount to quickly identifying and treating episodes of hypoglycemia or hyperglycemia. It is also important to have tools and treatments on hand that can quickly mitigate these conditions, and to know when and how to use them.

 Go to the web study guide to complete the case studies for this chapter.

CHAPTER 14

Exertional Sickling and Rhabdomyolysis

OBJECTIVES

After reading this chapter, you will be able to do the following:

- Describe the clinical definition of exertional rhabdomyolysis and exertional collapse associated with sickle cell trait (ECAST).

- Identify major risk factors for developing exertional rhabdomyolysis and ECAST.

- Assess a patient with signs and symptoms of exertional rhabdomyolysis.

- Describe exertional sickling and ECAST.

- Provide emergency care for a patient with exertional rhabdomyolysis or ECAST.

Two potentially life-threatening conditions related to excessive exercise are exertional rhabdomyolysis (ER) and exertional collapse associated with sickle cell trait (ECAST). Each of these conditions can exist separately, or they can be intertwined. They are important considerations for the athletic trainer (AT) or other health care provider (HCP) who provides medical care to people performing extreme or excessive exercise, particularly at a higher intensity than usual. These pathological conditions are special cases of exertional illness, therefore this chapter discusses their pathophysiology, diagnostic criteria, patient assessment, and emergency management.

Exertional Rhabdomyolysis

Rhabdomyolysis is a potentially life-threatening syndrome characterized by the breakdown of skeletal muscle resulting in the subsequent release of intracellular contents into the circulatory system.[1-7] Rhabdomyolysis is an umbrella term for damage to muscle cells from any cause in which the cell membrane is impaired and the contents leak into bloodstream.[4] This syndrome occurs when muscle injury leads to leakage of muscle cell contents, including electrolytes, myoglobin, potassium, creatine kinase (CK), and other muscle enzymes, into the circulation and extracellular fluid.[3,6-8] Rhabdomyolysis can develop from a variety of causes, such as the following:[1-3,7,9]

- Crush syndrome or traumatic compression of muscles (earthquakes, car accidents, physical torture, abuse)

- Obstruction of blood supply to muscles (ischemia, clots, embolism)

- Electrical shock or lightning
- Prolonged seizures, epilepsy, or cramping
- Extremes in body temperature (hyperthermia, heatstroke)
- Excessive muscle strain or activity
- Extreme, unaccustomed, or novel physical exercise (especially when dehydrated)

ER is characterized by breakdown and necrosis of striated skeletal muscle after engaging in unusually strenuous physical activity.[10] ER can occur in healthy people undertaking vigorous exercise, such as marathon running, military training, or high-intensity resistance training (HIRT).[2,9] ER is increasingly reported in the literature in people performing a novel HIRT exercise program such as CrossFit[2] or Spinning.[6] Other significant causes of ER include excessive muscular activity, such as sporadic strenuous exercise (e.g., preseason football practice or military recruits in boot camp; figure 14.1).[11,12] The more strenuous or prolonged the exercise, the more damage is incurred. Excessive muscular activity results in a state in which ATP production cannot keep up with the demand, subsequently exhausting cellular energy supplies and leading to a disruption of muscle cell membranes. Factors that increase the risk of ER include the following:[13]

- Dehydration and electrolyte disturbances (often resulting from excessive sweating)
- Sickle cell trait (SCT; especially in combination with high altitude or other precipitating factors)
- Extreme heat and humidity
- Exercise-induced asthma
- Fatigue

Strenuous physical exertion can lead to the severe breakdown of skeletal muscle tissue. This breakdown precipitates systemic manifestations of ER that typically include **myoglobinuria**. This syndrome has received considerable attention because of high-profile deaths involving ER in athletes and military personnel. A number of such cases have been attributed to sickle cell trait (SCT), which is described in detail in the next section.[12-17] Large epidemiological studies in warfighters[18] and athletes clearly demonstrate an increased risk for exercise-related sudden death in SCT carriers compared to non-SCT carriers.[19]

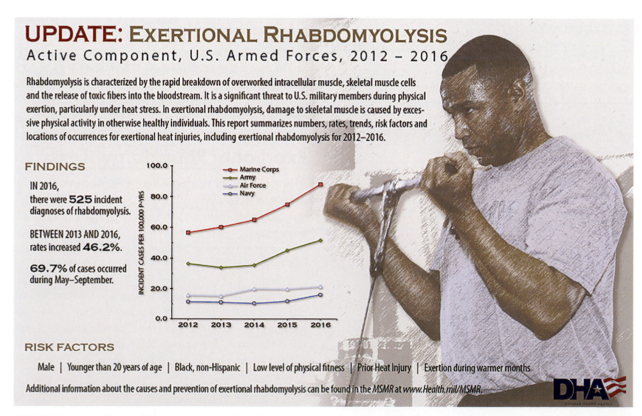

FIGURE 14.1 Infographic on exertional rhabdomyolysis in active-duty U.S. armed forces.

Reprinted from Health.mil. Available: https://health.mil/News/Gallery/Infographics/2017/04/04/Update-Exertional-Rhabdomyolysis-Active-Component-US-Armed-Forces-2012-2016.

Epidemiology of Exertional Rhabdomyolysis

ER is a relatively uncommon condition with an incidence of approximately 29.9 per 100,000 patient years, but it can have very serious consequences of muscle ischemia, cardiac arrhythmia, and death.[10] Risk factors for the development of ER are related to the intensity of the exercise, the conditioning of the participant, hydration, and body temperature, in addition to other potential contributing factors.[6] The National Athletic Trainers' Association (NATA)[20] has identified the following factors that may precipitate ER:

- Performing 2 to 3 minutes of all-out, vigorous, exhaustive, or maximal physical exertion, usually during training and conditioning.
- Sprinting short distances of 800 to 1,600 meters without adequate rest periods.
- Vigorously exercising the first day of preseason or early in the season without adequate acclimatization.
- Sprinting at the end of practice such as gassers or suicide sprints while exhausted or fatigued.

Pathophysiology of Exertional Rhabdomyolysis

Exertional rhabdomyolysis is characterized by the breakdown and necrosis of skeletal muscle after engaging in strenuous or unaccustomed physical activity.[7] Although several mechanisms can lead to skeletal muscle cell damage and death, the common final pathway (figure 14.2) is an increase in intracellular free ionized calcium to a level much higher than normal in the cytoplasm and mitochondria.[7] This increase in intracellular calcium leads to the activation of proteases and production of reactive oxygen species, eventually culminating in the death of the skeletal muscle cells. Necrosis of skeletal muscle cells releases intracellular contents, causing pain, swelling, and potential end-organ damage.[6,7,10]

Exercise-induced muscle damage occurs with strong eccentric component (muscle-lengthening) contractions such as unaccustomed downhill running, plyometrics, and negatives (lowering weights). Secondary factors can exacerbate the damage, such as ischemia from SCT, dehydration, or heat stress.[24] The prominence of muscle stiffness following eccentric exercise, known as delayed-onset muscle soreness (DOMS), is thought to represent local muscle inflammation and sensitization of nociceptors by muscle breakdown products. Exercise-related muscle injury can be considered as a continuum ranging from DOMS to rhabdomyolysis. Symptomatic manifestations may be similar across this spectrum, and cases of ER may be underrecognized or underreported, unfortunately attributing the muscle weakness and myalgia to poor fitness.[2]

Clinical Presentation

ER is a relatively uncommon condition, but if it is not recognized and managed appropriately, it can have

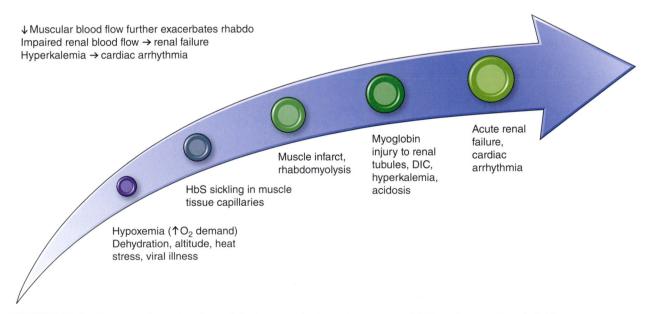

↓ Muscular blood flow further exacerbates rhabdo
Impaired renal blood flow → renal failure
Hyperkalemia → cardiac arrhythmia

Acute renal failure, cardiac arrhythmia

Myoglobin injury to renal tubules, DIC, hyperkalemia, acidosis

Muscle infarct, rhabdomyolysis

HbS sickling in muscle tissue capillaries

Hypoxemia ($\uparrow O_2$ demand) Dehydration, altitude, heat stress, viral illness

FIGURE 14.2 Proposed mechanism of rhabdomyolysis and acute renal failure in exertional sickling.

DIC = disseminated intravascular coagulation; HbS = hemoglobin sickled

Based on Harris et al. (2012); Sherry (1990); George, Delgaudio, and Salhanick (2010).

very serious consequences. ER can be identified with a history of extreme or unaccustomed physical exertion,[25] combined with a clinical examination and followed by laboratory tests. The patient typically presents with pain, tenderness, weakness, and swelling in the affected muscles after engaging in physical activity. Hyperthermia, changes in workout regimen, SCT, certain medications (stimulants and NSAIDs), preexisting illness, or metabolic disorders may predispose an athlete to ER.[10] Even though the final diagnosis of ER is established by laboratory findings, alertness to the syndrome is essential for prompt diagnosis. The 3 primary diagnostic criteria are as follows:[3,20,25-27]

1. Dark, tea-colored urine (myoglobinuria)
   - Appearing 12 to 24 hours after initial muscle damage
2. Myalgia
   - Muscle pain, tenderness, weakness, and edema
3. Elevated serum muscle enzymes
   - Increased CK for 24 to 48 hours then gradual decline

The clinical syndrome of ER comprises acute muscle necrosis with swollen, tender muscles and limb weakness.[3] However, more than half of the patients do not report muscular symptoms. The reddish-brown color of urine is due to myoglobinuria (described later) and constitutes a powerful diagnostic element. Unfortunately, myoglobinuria is observed in approximately half of the cases, and its absence does not exclude the syndrome.[26] Because of the rapid renal clearance of **myoglobin**, it is not a very sensitive indicator.[25] In the clinical examination, muscles may be swollen and sensitive during palpation, while changes in the color of skin are compatible with compression syndrome and muscle necrosis.[7] In severe cases of rhabdomyolysis, general symptoms may include the following:[26,27]

- Malaise or general feeling of illness
- Nausea or vomiting
- Fever
- Electrolyte disturbances
- Tachycardia
- Seizures

Diagnostic Criteria and Tests

Initially, it is important to rule out the 3 most common nontraumatic causes of sudden exertional collapse in healthy people—cardiac conditions, heatstroke, and asthma—followed by exertional sickling collapse.[28] The complete clinical context, including the history and examination findings, should be considered. Dark

 RED FLAG

Clinically, ER presents with severe muscle pain, decreased muscle strength, and myoglobinuria. Patients with these signs and symptoms must be referred for diagnostic testing. Increased myoglobin and CK (because of muscle cell damage or death) are the major laboratory findings which, in combination with the clinical manifestation, lead the clinician to the definitive diagnosis of the syndrome.[7,25-27]

urine without other symptoms may not indicate ER but rather dehydration or other causes of **hematuria**. Acute CK elevation, at least 5 times the upper limit of normal (ULN; > 5,000 U/L), has been suggested, but no absolute cut-off value or clear guidelines are given.[27,29] Criteria that indicate hospitalization is necessary include the following:

- Highly increased CK activity
- Decreased creatinine clearance
- Elevated serum creatinine
- Myoglobinuria
- Metabolic abnormalities
- Signs of compartment syndrome

Creatine Kinase

Patients suspected of having ER should be referred to the emergency department (ED) for full blood laboratory testing, especially CK. An elevated serum CK is the most sensitive and reliable indicator of muscle injury and constitutes the diagnostic hallmark of ER.[3,7,9] In general, CK levels begin to rise approximately 2 to 12 hours after the onset of muscle injury, peak within 24 to 72 hours, and then gradually decline.[7,9] The normal range for CK is 20 to 100 IU/L; however, no universally agreed-upon laboratory definitions exist for ER. Clinically, ER is often diagnosed with elevation of the serum CK to more than 5 times the ULN. Other more recently proposed guidelines suggest a diagnosis of ER should be made only when the serum CK is more than 50 times the ULN.[3,7,9,25,30-33] CK levels more than 10 times the ULN were commonly found in people who were asymptomatic; the implication is that decreased specificity exists when using this cut-off value for ER in athletes or others engaged in vigorous exercise.[25] A 2012 study reported that military recruits undergoing basic training had CK levels greater than 10 times the normal value while remaining asymptomatic.[25]

The serum concentration of CK is used widely as an index of skeletal muscle fiber damage in sport and exercise. Sport training and competition have profound effects on the reference intervals for serum CK, and athletes have higher CK values than nonathletes.[25,34,35] Vigorous or heavy exercise, especially involving eccentric muscle actions (lengthening contractions), often results in perforations in the sarcolemma and damage to sarcomeres leading to increases in circulating CK.[33] The natural history of ER in patients with a serum CK greater than 25,000 U/L is likely benign.[2] In athletes, many cases of exertional rhabdomyolysis are subclinical and may be detected only by an elevated serum CK.[3] Ehlers (2002) found normal CK for American football players during preseason practice to be 5,125 ± 5,518 U/L, or about 30 times normal for men.[35] In fact, CK levels up to 100,000 IU/L are not unusual. In cases where rhabdomyolysis leads to acute renal failure, CK may exceed 15,000 U/L and, on rare occasions, 70,000 U/L; in extreme situations, it can reach even 3,000,000 U/L.[7,30,31]

Myoglobinuria

Exertional rhabdomyolysis leads to leakage of muscle cell contents, including the oxygen binding muscle protein myoglobin.[3,9,32] Myoglobinuria (increased urinary excretion of myoglobin) is the most important consequence of significant muscle breakdown in ER.[3] Myoglobinuria develops once skeletal muscle injury is more than 100 grams.[9,32] Myoglobin elevation occurs before CK elevation, then it is rapidly cleared from the plasma through renal excretion and metabolism. Myoglobin enters the urine when the plasma concentration is more than 1.5 mg/dL and causes the typical reddish-brown discoloration when the urine myoglobin level is more than 100 mg/dL.[3]

Myoglobinuria may be detected either with a urine dipstick (microscopic myoglobinuria) or macroscopically as reddish-brown urine in the case of severe ER.[7] In ER, the level of myoglobin in the serum increases within 1 to 6 hours, reaches its peak in 8 to 12 hours, then returns to normal within 24 hours after the onset of the injury.[9,32] Thus, the detection of myoglobin in the blood or urine is pathognomonic for the diagnosis of rhabdomyolysis, provided that it is made in the initial phases of the syndrome (i.e., within the first 24 hours).[7] Because myoglobin levels may return to normal within 1 to 6 hours after the onset of muscle necrosis, the absence of an elevated serum myoglobin level or of myoglobinuria does not exclude the diagnosis. Myoglobinuria is not present in the majority of ER patients; only 19% of patients with rhabdomyolysis demonstrate myoglobinuria.[9,32,36,37]

When serum myoglobin exceeds 0.3 mg/L, it becomes detectable with a urine dipstick, which is a particularly inexpensive and sensitive test. The main drawback of this technique is that it cannot distinguish whether the actual cause of a positive result is hemoglobin, myoglobin, or hemoglobin-rich red blood cells.[7] A urine dipstick detects heme-rich molecules,[7] but it is not specific to myoglobin in the urine. In ER patients, a urine dipstick screen is not useful to positively detect myoglobinuria, but it may be useful in identifying the absence of myoglobin in the urine, because it has the following:[38]

- Sensitivity (true positive) = 14.3% (95% confidence interval [CI]:
- Specificity (true negative) = 84.9% (95% CI: 71.9-92.8)

In 45% of the cases of rhabdomyolysis, the urine dipstick can be positive for the presence of protein. Proteinuria results from the release of myoglobin and other proteins by the disrupted muscle cells. Macroscopic myoglobinuria (reddish-brown urine) is observed when the concentration of plasma myoglobin exceeds 300 mg/L.[7,9,38]

Complications of Exertional Rhabdomyolysis

ER constitutes a severe medical emergency that requires prompt diagnosis so that its life-threatening complications can be avoided. Although the etiology is multifactorial, all of the potential causes share the same pathophysiological pathway, which involves an increase in intracellular calcium. HCPs should be aware that the pathogenetic mechanisms are strongly linked to the clinical manifestation and laboratory findings of the condition.[7] The major complications of ER include the following:

- Acute renal failure
- Disseminated intravascular coagulation
- Mechanical complications, such as acute compartment syndrome and peripheral nerve injury
- Metabolic derangements, such as hyperkalemia
- Sickling collapse (in patients with SCT) and sudden death

Acute Renal Failure

In ER, acute renal failure (ARF) is a serious complication of ER that may occur 1 to 2 days after initial muscle damage. ARF is rare; only 3% to 7% of ER cases progress to ARF,[24] usually with contributing factors such as dehydration, heat stress, trauma, or underlying disease such as sickle cell trait.[9] Renal tubular obstruction occurs secondary to precipitation of uric acid and myoglobin, which are responsible for a direct toxic effect on the kidneys.[3,9] Decreased renal perfusion is compounded by dehydration, heat stress, or hypotension. In severe cases, **hemodialysis** may be required to remove excess potassium, acid, and phosphate from the blood.[24]

Disseminated Intravascular Coagulation

Disseminated intravascular coagulation occurs in severe rhabdomyolysis and can result in hemorrhagic complications.[9] The systemic effects of this condition are described in chapter 6.

Acute Compartment Syndrome and Peripheral Nerve Injury

The mechanical complications of ER consist of acute compartment syndrome (ACS) and peripheral nerve injury. The associated muscle swelling may exert pressure on peripheral nerves, resulting in neuronal ischemia and causing paresthesia or paralysis. Nerve injury is often proximal, and multiple nerves may be involved in the same extremity. ACS occurs secondary to marked swelling and edema of the involved muscle groups.[9] A compartment pressure test of 30 to 50 mm Hg is an indication for fasciotomy. This complication is rare; 2% of rhabdomyolysis cases progress to ACS. However, ACS may be more common in athletes training beyond their physical ability. For example, in a recent case, 14 high school American football players experienced rhabdomyolysis during summer training after performing an unaccustomed exercise bout. Push-ups and chair dips were performed continuously with almost no rest for intervals of 30 seconds each and then repeated until failure for many athletes. The consequences of this exercise bout resulted in hospitalization of 14 players, 3 of whom required an emergency fasciotomy of their triceps brachii.[39] ACS is further described in chapter 7.

Hyperkalemia

Hyperkalemia constitutes the most life-threatening electrolyte imbalance that results from ER. Because 98% of potassium (K^+) is found in the intracellular space and 60% to 70% of the total cellular mass of the human body consists of skeletal muscle cells, even an acute necrosis of only 100 grams of muscular mass could potentially increase serum measurably. Moreover, hyperkalemia during ER is intensified by the coexistent metabolic acidosis and renal dysfunction, which in combination with hypocalcemia, may cause fatal ventricular arrhythmias.[7]

Patient Assessment

In patients suspected of having ER, the HCP should obtain a detailed history and should be told about any recent intense or unaccustomed exercise. Although the classic symptoms of ER are nonspecific and may not always be present, a high index of suspicion should be present in patients with the classic clinical presentation of muscular aches, weakness, and tea-colored urine. The severity of this condition ranges from mild and not requiring treatment to life-threatening, including complications previously mentioned of acute kidney injury or renal failure, ACS or peripheral nerve injury, disseminated intravascular coagulation, electrolyte derangement, cardiac arrhythmias, and death.[1] Although ER is relatively

rare, the consequences can be fatal; therefore, appropriate emergent treatment should be initiated to limit morbidity and mortality.[10]

Differential Diagnosis

ER evaluation requires a history, physical examination, and serology for definitive diagnosis.[10] Unless a high index of suspicion exists, rhabdomyolysis can be missed, because muscular pain, swelling, and tenderness may not be prominent features and may even be absent. Therefore, the referral to higher-level care for definitive diagnosis of rhabdomyolysis should be made using laboratory tests including serum CK and urine myoglobin. In addition, skeletal muscle biopsy can be used to confirm the diagnosis.[1] Other causes of muscle pain and weakness besides ER should be considered in the appropriate clinical setting. Such causes include acute myopathies, periodic paralysis, polymyositis or dermatomyositis, or Guillain-Barré syndrome. Rhabdomyolysis associated with strenuous exercise or fasting or repeat episodes of rhabdomyolysis suggest an inherited metabolic myopathy.[3,9]

Management of Exertional Rhabdomyolysis

In mild cases, ER may go undiagnosed and could be managed on an outpatient basis with oral hydration and rest. Conservative management with rest and rehydration may be adequate.[2,10] The majority of healthy patients with ER and without comorbidities (e.g., SCT, heat stress, dehydration, trauma) can usually be treated (figure 14.3) with oral or IV rehydration, observed in the ED, and then released. Otherwise, patients should be admitted for IV hydration, diuresis, management of complications, and treatment of the underlying cause. For at least the initial 24 to 48 hours, admission should be in a monitored bed to identify dysrhythmias or renal complications.[3,9] Return to play (RTP) should be determined by assessing risk factors (see Epidemiology of Exertional Rhabdomyolysis) of the patient, including SCT.[10] Correcting modifiable risk factors and managing unmodifiable risk factors are essential for safe RTP. The prognosis and time line for RTP depend on a variety of factors, including severity of the condition and the presence or potential for complications such as ACS, ARF, or hyperkalemia. The patient's physician must be closely consulted and the patient must be closely monitored during the RTP process.

Sickle Cell Trait

SCT is a condition in which a person is heterozygous for the sickle cell mutation in the beta-globin gene (HbAS). Sickle cell trait is most prevalent among persons with African or Mediterranean decent. In the United States, an estimated 7.3% of African-Americans, 0.7% of His-

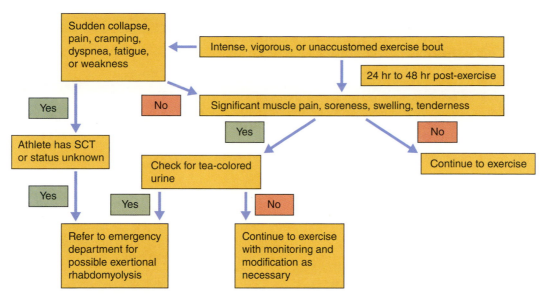

FIGURE 14.3 Decision-making algorithm for ER with and without (or unknown) SCT.

panic people, and 1.6% of U.S. residents overall have SCT.[13] These people are hematologically normal, with no disease and normal **erythrocytes** (red blood cells, or RBCs). A screening test for sickle hemoglobin will be positive, and hemoglobin electrophoresis will reveal that approximately 40% of hemoglobin is HbS. People with SCT experience more ER during vigorous exercise but do not have increased mortality compared to the general population.[13,40]

The U.S. Army has no special recognition or handling of soldiers with SCT before or during physical activity. Instead, the Army uses universal precautions to reduce the risks of dehydration and heat- and exercise-induced illness among all its soldiers. Such measures have been effective in reducing the rates of exercise-related death, regardless of status with respect to sickle cell trait.[13] The NCAA recognizes that precautions can enable student-athletes with SCT to thrive in their sports. These precautions are outlined in the references and in a 2007 NATA consensus statement on sickle cell trait and the athlete.[20] Knowledge of a soldier's or student-athlete's sickle cell status should facilitate prompt and appropriate medical care during a medical emergency.[20,41]

Overview of Clinical Hematology

Hemoglobin (Hb) molecules consist of polypeptide chains with genetically controlled molecular structure. The typical adult Hb molecule (HbA) consists of 2 pairs of protein chains (HbA1 and HbA2). Structural **hemoglobinopathies** involve an abnormal Hb, sickle cell Hb, and designated HbS. The standard description of a patient's Hb composition places the Hb of greatest concentration first (e.g., as in SCT).[44] In oxygenated HbS, much less solubility exists than oxygenated HbA;

it forms a semisolid gel that causes RBCs to deform into a sickle shape at sites of low oxygen. Distorted, inflexible RBCs adhere to the vascular endothelium and plug small arterioles and capillaries, leading to **infarction** and **vaso-occlusion**. Because sickled RBCs are fragile, the mechanical trauma of circulation causes **hemolysis**. Vaso-occlusive crisis (pain crisis) is the most common type caused by ischemia, tissue hypoxia, and infarction—typically of the bones, but also of the spleen, lungs, or kidneys.[44,45]

Several sickle cell syndromes occur as the result of inheritance of HbS from one parent and another hemoglobinopathy from the other parent. **Sickle cell disease (anemia)** is the homozygous inheritance of HbS.[45] Sickle cell disease causes a chronic **hemolytic anemia**. Sickle-shaped RBCs cause vaso-occlusion and are prone to hemolysis, leading to severe pain crises, organ ischemia, and other systemic complications. In the United States, about 0.3% of African Americans have sickle cell anemia (homozygotes); 8% to 13% of African Americans are not anemic (heterozygotes) but have an increased risk of other complications as a result of SCT.[44]

Sickle cell trait is not a disease; it is an inherited red blood cell condition that can affect athletes at all levels. While SCT is not a barrier to playing competitive sports, athletes with SCT have experienced significant physical distress, including collapse and death during intense exercise. The U.S. Armed Forces and the National Collegiate Athletic Association (NCAA)[41] warn that an increased risk exists for medical complications in athletes with SCT during physical exertion, particularly when combined with the following:

- Heat
- Dehydration

NCAA Testing Rule

The NCAA testing rule[42] requires that all student-athletes do the following:

- Be tested for SCT using a Sickledex test or Hb electrophoresis.[43]
- Show proof of a prior test.
- Sign a waiver releasing liability if they decline testing.
- Receive SCT counseling by physicians or certified SCT community counselors who have adequate training.

- Inadequate acclimatization
- Altitude
- Asthma

Epidemiology of Exertional Collapse Associated With Sickle Cell Trait

SCT occurs in 0.8% (1 in 625) Caucasians and 8% (1 in 12) African Americans in the United States (3.1 million people). All newborns in the United States are screened for HbS, but the trait often goes unrecognized. Although SCT is considered benign and asymptomatic, in certain circumstances medical complications can occur. A significantly higher risk of ER was identified among African-American military soldiers with SCT than among those without the trait.[13] A retrospective study of military basic trainees showed that a 40-fold increased risk of sudden death may exist during exertion in males with SCT. In addition, African-American recruits with SCT were 30 times more likely to die during basic training than other African-American recruits. Most deaths were from ER, heatstroke, or acute renal failure.[18] At the time of the investigation, no reports indicated sudden death in female soldiers, nor in soldiers beyond basic training.[46]

SCT-associated sudden death often has components of rhabdomyolysis, heatstroke, disseminated intravascular coagulation, and cardiac arrhythmia. This phenomenon is not limited to soldiers. The relative risk of exertional death for SCT is high. Each year, cases of sudden death are reported in athletes during preseason American football training. According to a large, nationwide study of collegiate football players, African-American football players with SCT are at a 37 times higher risk of exertion-related death compared with their non-SCT counterparts.[28] All deaths in athletes with SCT occurred in African-American Division I football athletes during practice or conditioning.[28] SCT alone is not associated with a higher risk of death than absence of the trait, but SCT is associated with a significantly higher risk of exertional rhabdomyolysis.[13,46]

Studies[13,18,28,25] indicate that the presence of SCT elevates the risks of ER and death while participating in physically demanding activities such as military basic training or preseason football conditioning. According to the National Center for Catastrophic Sports Injury Research and other reports, fatalities that occurred as a result of ER during sports participation had the following common themes:[16,24,47-52]

- Physical exertion
- Intense conditioning drills, often sprinting after 2 to 30 minutes of high-intensity running with limited rest
- Not in game situations, usually plays lasting less than 5 seconds with a rest time of 30 to 45 seconds
- Death most often occurring during conditioning on the first day
- A 66.6 times higher risk of death from SCT complications in college than high school athletes
- Staff being unaware of SCT status of patient deaths
- ER present in 50% of the competitive athlete fatalities associated with SCT

Given the potentially disastrous consequences of SCT and the high frequency of this trait in the population, it is recommended that measures to prevent injury be further instituted. It should be emphasized that ER can occur beyond the traditional periods of military basic training and preseason sports training.[46] An estimate of the number of sickle cell carriers identified and the number of potentially preventable sudden deaths with mandatory SCT screening of NCAA Division I athletes was calculated.[53] Researchers determined that over 2,000 NCAA Division I student-athletes with SCT would be identified under the NCAA SCT screening policy (see NCAA Testing Rule) and that, without intervention, about 7 NCAA Division I student-athletes would die suddenly as a complication of SCT over a 10-year period.[53] Military units and teams that do not ensure gradual acclimatization and year-round physical training should be encouraged to do so. Affected athletes, coaches, and ATs should be educated that maintenance of adequate hydration and avoidance of both high-altitude training sites and of substances that may cause dehydration, such as alcohol, caffeine, antihistamines, and diuretics, can help prevent

SCT-associated collapse and sudden death during exertion. Because sudden death associated with SCT has been shown to occur beyond initial training, it is emphasized that all military units and sports teams should implement these measures.[13,42,46]

Pathophysiology of ECAST

Patients with heterozygous (HbAS) SCT are often asymptomatic; anemia and painful crises are rare.[45] However, people with SCT do have an increased risk of ER and sudden death during sustained, exhausting exercise.[44] Massive sickling, collapse, or sudden death resulting from exposure to high altitudes or extremes of exercise and dehydration have occurred.[45] Intense exercise and heavy exertion cause HbS RBCs to become sickle shaped and accumulate in blood vessels (figure 14.4), causing vaso-occlusion and ischemia. This sickling crisis is exacerbated by heat stress, hypoxia, and dehydration.[28,54]

Patient Assessment of ECAST

In athletes with SCT, it is prudent to assume sickling is occurring, because most athletes that suddenly collapsed

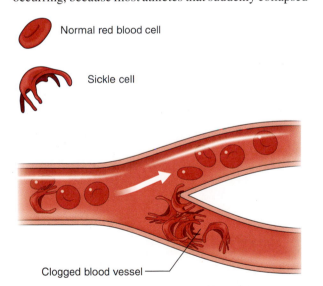

Normal red blood cell

Sickle cell

Clogged blood vessel

FIGURE 14.4 Pathophysiology of sickling collapse.

have died under similar distinctive circumstances. An instantaneous collapse does not occur; rather, a gradual but rapid deterioration occurs with dyspnea, fatigue, weakness, and muscle cramping.[16] Assume athletes with SCT are in sickling crisis when some or all of the following clinical signs are present:[20,54]

- Muscle cramping
- Muscle weakness
- Difficulty breathing or inability to catch breath
- Fatigue
- Pain in the leg(s) or low back

Differential Diagnosis of ECAST

In people with SCT, exertion-induced hypoxia initiates a chain of events that induces sickling, causing vaso-occlusion, potentiating hypoxia and culminating in sudden death. Sickling collapse has a similar presentation to ER (see table 14.1) and heat-related emergencies such as heatstroke (see chapter 15), and it can be mistaken for heat collapse or cardiac collapse. The primary differences with ECAST are the following:[20,47,54,55]

- Core temperature is not elevated.
- It is not necessarily the effects of heat exposure.
- Sudden collapse is precipitated by an exercise-related event with intravascular sickling.
- It often occurs within 30 minutes of on-field windsprints.
- The onset is more precipitous, often with no warning.
- Pain is ischemic rather than because of lactic acidosis.

Management of ECAST

For athletes or soldiers with SCT, intense exertion can cause RBCs to sickle and block blood vessels, especially when present with additional conditions or comorbidities that pose grave risk. For people with severe ER and comorbidities such as SCT (see figure 14.4), intensive

TABLE 14.1   Signs and Symptoms of ECAST Versus Heat Cramps

Heat cramps	ECAST
Often with prodrome of muscle twinges	No prodromal symptoms
Pain that is more excruciating	Pain less than with heat cramps
Hobbling to a halt with muscles that feel locked	Slumping to the ground with weak muscles
Physically writhing and yelling in pain	Lying fairly still, not yelling in pain
Muscles that are visibly contracted and hard	Muscles that look and feel normal
Prolonged recovery with rest, rehydration, electrolyte replacement, and other techniques	Faster recovery when caught early and treated correctly

Based on Eichner (2017); Eichner (2010); Scheinin and Wetli (2009).

care admission may be necessary because an increased risk exists for adverse outcomes of acute kidney injury and death.[2] For an athlete with severe symptoms (CK greater than 5 times the upper limit of normal or dark urine), hospital admission is indicated for IV hydration with normal saline (1-2 L/h) maintaining a urine output of 200 mL/h. Along with IV hydration, monitoring CK levels, kidney function, and electrolyte values must be managed in an inpatient hospital setting where access to monitoring equipment and other services are readily available.[3,10]

Evidence: Factors That Increase Risk of Exertional Rhabdomyolysis

High-intensity resistance training programs such as CrossFit are increasingly popular among personal trainers and physically active people. Clinical outcomes of ER were compared with other causes of rhabdomyolysis in a retrospective cross-sectional study of patients presenting with a serum CK greater than 25,000 U/L (normal range is 20-180 U/L) for 1 year from 2 tertiary referral hospitals in Melbourne, Australia. Records examined identified 12 of 34 cases (35%) that had ER with 10 of 12 (83%) related to HIRT. No acute kidney injury, intensive care admission, or death was found among those with ER. All cases were managed conservatively; 11 were admitted and 9 received IV fluids only. In contrast, patients with rhabdomyolysis from other causes experienced significantly higher rates of intensive care admission (64%, $P = 0.0002$), acute kidney injury (82%, $P = 0.0001$), and death (27%, $P = 0.069$). The researchers concluded that ER resulting from HIRT appears to have a benign course compared with rhabdomyolysis of other etiologies in patients with a serum CK more than 25,000 U/L. Conservative management of ER appears to be adequate, although it requires confirmation in future prospective studies.[2]

Evidence related to the association between SCT and death from ER in soldiers and athletes is limited, but significant publicity has been visible to date. No study has evaluated the relationship between HbAS with exertional rhabdomyolysis and death. However, a database of all digital health encounters for all active-duty Army soldiers in the United States was reviewed to identify 391 cases of exertional rhabdomyolysis in 1.61 million person-months. No statistical difference was observed in the risk of death among soldiers with SCT compared to those without the trait (hazard ratio [HR] 0.99, 95% confidence interval [CI] 0.46-2.13). However, the presence of SCT was associated with an adjusted risk of ER that was 54% higher than that associated with the absence of the trait and a statistically significant increase (HR = 1.54; 95% CI, 1.12-2.12; $P = 0.008$) in the risk of ER among soldiers with SCT compared to those without the trait. The authors of this study concluded that the presence of SCT was not associated with a statistically higher risk of death. However, they identified a statistically significant increased risk of exertional rhabdomyolysis in SCT independent of other risk factors.[13]

Summary

No internationally recognized organization has published validated guidelines for the management of ER.[9] Although SCT is not a barrier to playing competitive sports, athletes with this genetic predisposition have experienced ECAST and death during intense exercise. An increased risk for ER exists in any person who partic-

---

CLINICAL SKILLS

Managing ECAST

- Proactively prepare by developing an emergency action plan (EAP) specific to sickling collapse.
- Treat SCT collapse as a medical emergency; do the following:
  - Check vital signs.
  - Administer high-flow oxygen (10-15 L/min).
  - Cool the athlete, if necessary.
  - Monitor the patient for slow mental responses or vital signs decrease.
- Call 9-1-1, attach an AED, start an IV, and transport the patient to the hospital as quickly as possible.
- Inform the ED to expect explosive rhabdomyolysis and grave metabolic complications.

Based on National Athletic Trainers' Association (2007); Eichner (2010); Scheinin and Wetli (2009).

ipates in extremely intense physical exercise to which he is unaccustomed. In addition, in athletes with SCT, during intense physical exertion the risk of ECAST is especially high, particularly when combined with heat stress, dehydration, or altitude. It is prudent to implement universal precautions to reduce the risks of dehydration and heat- and exercise-induced illness among all physically active people. Such measures are effective in reducing the rates of exercise-related death, regardless of SCT status. Using precautions and having knowledge of a person's sickle cell status facilitate prompt and appropriate medical care during a medical emergency. Athletes with SCT can thrive and participate in all sports. Being aware and using simple precautions may prevent deaths.[20,41]

 Go to the web study guide to complete the case studies for this chapter.

CHAPTER 15

Environmental Emergencies

OBJECTIVES

After reading this chapter, you will be able to do the following:

- Recognize life-threatening environmental emergencies.

- Explain the medical consequences of environmental emergencies (lightning, heatstroke, hypothermia, frostbite, and altitude).

- Justify the use of gold-standard diagnostic tools for heat and cold weather illnesses.

- Differentiate among the various altitude-related emergencies.

- Manage injuries resulting from environmental conditions.

Environmental emergencies fall into 2 categories—those in which a person cannot adapt, and those for which a person can acclimate or prepare. A person cannot adapt to lightning; all one can do is avoid being in situations where it is more likely to be struck. In other environmental conditions (e.g., heat, cold, altitude), a person can acclimate and prepare ahead of time to mitigate the effects of these conditions. This chapter discusses these situations and medical consequences of them, as well as treatment for those affected negatively by environment.

Lightning Emergencies

Lightning is one of the most dangerous environmental conditions. One strike can result in mass casualties (table 15.1). A single bolt can strike a playing field, and the ramification of that strike can radiate out, affecting nearly everyone in the area. This event is called a ground current and is the most common cause of lightning fatality.[1]

A mistake people often make is assuming cloud-to-cloud lighting (lightning in the sky) is not capable of injuring anyone. Any lightning is dangerous; the next bolt can strike the ground and people. The most dangerous aspect of lightning is to ignore it in the distance, or assume one is safe when sheltered from the rain. Thunder is the sound that accompanies lightning. Hearing thunder is an audible clue to move to a solid, fully enclosed, substantial building and wait for the storm to pass. The best place to wait out the storm is within a building where people live and work, and one that has plumbing and electricity.[3]

TABLE 15.1 **Methods and Effects of Lightning Strikes**

Type of lightning strike	Description	Percentage of fatalities*
Side flash	Lightning hits an object, then the victim (tree, pole, umbrella, tent, etc.)	30%-35%
Ground current	Lightning hits the ground, then radiates out to affect everyone in a certain radius of the hit	50%-55%
Direct strike	Lightning strikes a person directly	3%-5%
Upward streamer	When a person is a part of the lightning channel as it makes contact with the earth	10%-15%
Contact injury/conduction	Lightning hits a building and travels through the plumbing, electrical wires, and other channels to reach people (e.g., showering or washing dishes during a storm, swimming in pools, using a device that is plugged into the wall)	3%-5%

*Percentage of lightning-caused fatalities attributed to each type of lightning strike.

Data from Cooper and Holle (2010).

Incidence and Epidemiology

The United States has a geographical preponderance for lighting strikes. The southeast, Colorado, and Arizona lead fatalities annually; and Florida, Texas, and North Carolina are consistently in the top 10. Other notable states with high fatalities because of lightning are Mississippi and Missouri.[4]

In the period between 2006 and 2016 in the United States, 352 people died from lightning strikes, and 64% of the deaths occurred during recreation and leisure activities.[5] Lightning struck and killed more males (277) than females (75); and Friday, Saturday, and Sunday were the days of the week with the highest numbers of fatalities. Of the sporting events during that decade, soccer, golf and running attributed the most deaths to lightning.[5]

In the United States, lightning tends to strike more between April and October; July is the month with the greatest number of lightning strikes and resulting deaths. In addition, most people who are killed by lightning are struck during the late afternoon to early evening.[6]

Medical Consequences of Lightning Strikes

Medical consequences of lightning strikes are immediate, and long-term outcomes are numerous. Acute trauma data report that 50% of people struck by lightning will suffer a ruptured tympanic membrane.[7] Other non–life-threatening effects are fractures and contusions from being thrown by the air explosion resulting from lightning, concussions, and ocular trauma. Other immediate and usually temporary signs and symptoms include tinnitus, blindness, dizziness, confusion, and burns. Burns associated with lightning are largely from the flash of super-heated air

heating objects (e.g., watches, rings, metal piercings, necklaces, zippers, and snaps); these objects retain the heat long enough to burn the patient.[8]

Cardiac arrest is the cause of death in people struck by lightning. When struck, the heart may stop, which in turn retards respiration. Because of the autorhythmicity of cardiac tissue, the heart may attempt to restart; but without respiration, the heart will cease. Survivors often state that their heart "stopped twice," which is true. In most trauma situations, rescuers are trained to treat the living first, but when treating victims of lightning strikes, the opposite is true. Victims of lightning strike who are moving or groaning have an airway and a beating heart, and most likely they will survive. In lightning triage, rescuers treat the apparently dead first, because those people are likely in cardiac arrest.

Nearly every body system can be affected by lightning strikes, but the neurological system takes the biggest toll. The long-term effects include anxiety attacks, sleep disturbances, chronic pain syndromes, peripheral nerve neuropathies, and post-concussion-like syndromes. Other issues include late-onset cataracts, seizures, chronic fatigue, and long-term psychological repercussions. Many people never fully recover or return to their personality or activities from before the strike.[7-10]

Signs and Symptoms

It is usually obvious when someone sustains a lightning strike injury, because a thunderstorm is present. For those who are conscious, assess for fractures and dislocations. Orthopedic injuries occur from falling, objects falling on the patient, or from being thrown by the concussive shockwave of the lightning. Patients may be dazed or confused and may display concussion-like symptoms.

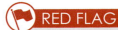

Field Assessment Techniques

Caution is paramount for rescuers who attend to those struck by lightning. Although people who are struck by lightning are safe to touch and assess, the danger is in the environment. It must be certain that the storm has passed and that the health care professional (HCP) and others are in no danger of being struck by another lightning bolt. This can be crudely measured by tracking the last sound of thunder or flash of lightning. When 30 minutes have passed without either the sound of thunder or the sight of a lightning flash, it is safe to resume activities and be outdoors. Until such time, the rescuer is in danger of becoming a victim.[6] People who use lightning detectors should use caution; few independent scientific data exist to support their reliability. Only a few real-time, satellite-driven platforms exist that are validated by research, so use the National Weather Service *"When thunder roars, go indoors!"* slogan to always be mindful of impending dangerous weather.

The emergency examination procedures (discussed in chapter 4) should be followed. Ensure the scene is safe to enter, and that no active storm is in the area. Evaluate the patient for effective airway, breathing, circulation, and disability (ABCD); assess levels of consciousness (using Glasgow Coma Scale; GCS), and determine possible spinal injury. If the patient is unconscious, assume spinal injury and maintain inline stabilization. For conscious patients, assess for level of consciousness and for concussion-like symptoms. If the patient is uncommunicative, assume cervical spine injury and prevent spinal movement. Determine existence of fractures or dislocations, and immobilize them. For minor injuries (e.g., dizziness, confusion, tinnitus, contusions, burns), evaluate briefly to determine whether the patient can be moved to the sideline or indoor facility for more extensive evaluation.

Diagnostic Accuracy

No specific diagnostic tools exist to determine whether a person was struck by lightning, but unique signs show whether a patient is unaware of being struck and the injury was not observed. A victim of an unwitnessed lightning strike may be unconscious or semiconscious. The person may appear to have clothes ripped or torn, leading some people to consider whether the person was attacked. This phenomenon occurs when the heat of lightning flashing over a person rapidly raises to a point where it can cause sweat to heat to steam, which in turn can cause clothing to tear or split.

One sign unique to lightning victims is the Lichtenberg figure. This distinctive marking is only found on victims of lightning strike and resembles a feathering pattern on the skin. Once thought to be a burn, it is a temporary dermal discoloration that may present with a burn or scaling. They appear within 24 hours and typically dissipate within 2 days.[8,11,12]

Immediate Management Techniques

Because no acute unique injures occur from lightning strikes, patients are to be treated for the trauma sustained. Establish airway, breathing and circulation, and apply an automated external defibrillator (AED) if justified. Recognize and stabilize possible cervical spine injuries, fractures, and dislocations. Determine whether the patient is stable and whether transportation to a medical facility is necessary.

Many victims of lightning strikes do not seek further medical attention if their injures are minor and manageable.[7-9] Patients who sustain ocular and tympanic injuries should be referred to the appropriate medical specialist. Contusions and minor burns can be managed without further medical attention.

If mass casualties occur, determine who is unresponsive and evaluate them first. Assess airway, breathing, and circulation, then begin cardiopulmonary resuscitation (CPR) if warranted. In this situation, always assume a cervical spinal injury and maintain cervical inline stabilization. Designate a specific person to retrieve and apply an AED if necessary. Emergency medical services (EMS) should be activated if anyone is unresponsive.

Criteria for Deciding to Transport for Further Medical Examination

Consider transporting victims of lightning strike to a health care facility as one would any other patient. In other words, transport anyone who is unresponsive, semiconscious, or has signs of shock. Patients who are unstable, have open fractures, have dislocations, or show possibility of a cervical spine injury must be stabilized to prevent further damage and sent via ambulance to an appropriate medical facility.

Transportation Techniques

No unique transportation techniques are for patients who have been struck by lightning. If you have made the decision to send a patient to the hospital, move that patient into the ambulance with consideration for the injuries sustained. For example, patients with head injuries should be sent with their heads slightly raised, whereas those in shock should be transported with their legs raised.

Heat-Related Emergencies

Many heat-related illnesses are possible, ranging from muscular twitches to fainting to exertional heatstroke (EHS). EHS is the only true heat-related life-threatening emergency, and it is the only heat illness discussed here. As the name suggests, EHS is brought about by the combination of exertion (working out), temperature (including air and humidity), and other factors. A person can acclimate to the hot weather if given the time and cautiously increasing the activity duration slowly in the hot environment. Heatstroke is preventable in many aspects, including paying close attention to the weather (air temperature, ambient temperature, humidity, wind, sunshine), the heat and humidity trends in the local area, clothing and equipment worn, work-to-rest ratio, and hydration and food intake.[13] Other salient factors include medical conditions, body mass, poor conditioning, medications, prior history of heat illness, and other predispositions that can exacerbate heat illness.[14]

Incidence and Epidemiology

Although the overall risk of EHS is low, its consequences can be fatal. According to the National Center for Catastrophic Sport Injury Research, 148 deaths have occurred since 1955 (56 since 1996) due to EHS in football.[17]

Rates are highest across all levels of football (youth, high school, and collegiate) during the preseason and lower during youth practices and high school games.[18] Athletics are not alone in EHS injury; the U.S. military forces also have significant data. Fort Benning, Georgia and Fort Bragg, North Carolina led a 14-year study period with over 1,400 heat-related illnesses each, and nearly 3,500 incidents were reported from military bases in North and South Carolina combined (table 15.2).[19]

Medical Consequences of Heatstroke

The systemic physiological effects of untreated EHS are many. The rising internal temperature denatures proteins and cellular membranes, causing an inflammatory response.[20] As a reaction, the body relocates an aspect of bacteria usually found in the gastrointestinal system, which can promulgate a sepsis reaction systemically, and therefore begins a coagulation reaction throughout organs.[20] Aside from death, EHS can elicit multi-organ failure, acute respiratory distress syndrome, and coma. Organ failure can become irreversible and the long-term sequelae catastrophic.

Signs and Symptoms

If the weather is hot or humid, be suspicious of EHS for any athlete who presents with any of these signs of symptoms. The 2 cardinal signs of EHS are a rectal

Exertional Hyponatremia

Exertional **hyponatremia** is often associated with heat illness, but it is not caused by heat. Hyponatremia is usually self-imposed overhydration, and it can have dire consequences, including death. Athletes who hyperhydrate in fear of cramping or poor performance cause an imbalance of sodium in their blood. Other causes of hyponatremia are fluid loss from vomiting or diarrhea, certain medications, medical conditions, or chronic conditions.[15,16] Untreated, hyponatremia can lead to extracellular swelling; hepatic, renal, or cardiac failure; pneumonia; and encephalopathies. In severe cases, mortality rate can be as high at 50%.[16]

Signs and symptoms range from headache and malaise to systemic swelling, nausea, lethargy, dyspnea, and delirium. Depending on the body system most affected, the signs and symptoms will correspond with it; for example, chest pain corresponds with cardiac and pulmonary sequelae, and concussion-like or drunken-like actions correspond with cerebral edema. Normal sodium levels in the blood are usually within the range of 135-145 mEq/L, and the severity of symptoms increases with each level decrease of serum sodium (mild is 130-134 mEq/L; moderate, 125-129 mEq/L; and severe, <124 mEq/L).[16] Diagnosis occurs with urine and serum osmolality and urine sodium concentration. Handheld analyzers have made diagnosis quick and efficient, even in the athletic situation.

Depending on the severity of hyponatremia (based on laboratory results), treatment ranges from a wait-and-watch approach to correcting serum sodium with intravenous solution mixtures containing **NaCl**, the concentration and frequency of which are contingent on the dearth of NaCl concentration in the blood.

TABLE 15.2 **Heat Illness in American Military Personnel (2002-2016)**

Military branch	Total heat-related illness cases	EHS cases	Other heat illness injuries
Air Force	205	16	189
Army	1,441	205	1, 236
Marine Corps	734	151	583
Navy	156	29	127
Totals for 2002-2016	**2,536**	**401 (15.8%)**	**2,135 (84.1%)**

Data from Lilley (2017).

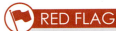 RED FLAG

Signs and symptoms of exertional heatstroke include the following:

- Sudden collapse
- Central nervous system (CNS) dysfunction (acts concussed)
- Rectal temperature over 105°F (40.5°C)
- Hot skin
- Sweaty or dry skin
- Seizure

temperature over 105°F (40.5°C) and central nervous system dysfunction, namely, concussion-like behaviors.[21] Strictly from an observational standpoint, the athlete may be disoriented, confused, or dizzy, and his performance may be deteriorating. EHS patients tend to have **dia-**phoretic and hot skin. The presence or absence of sweat should not be a deterrent to consider EHS, given other feedback. Complaints of muscular cramping, headache, weakness, or dry mouth are worth continued exploration. Nausea, vomiting, or diarrhea can occur prior to collapse.[14,20-23]

Sudden collapse, seizure, altered consciousness, or coma can occur and will likely transpire if not rapidly diagnosed and treated.[21,22] Vital signs can diminish with time, especially if the patient is untreated.

Field Assessment Techniques

A person who has heatstroke presents with concussion-like symptoms, which include confusion, stupor, dizziness, personality changes, and acting combative or complacent. A rapid decision must be made to assess core temperature using a rectal thermometer to diagnose EHS (figure 15.1). Every minute delay to diagnose EHS via rectal thermometry is critical.

CLINICAL SKILLS

Taking a Rectal Temperature

1. Place patient in a side-lying position with the top knee bent.
2. Place a towel over the patient's hips.
3. Wash and sanitize your hands, and don gloves.
4. Lower the patient's pants and underwear to below the gluteal fold.
5. Prepare the thermometer (have correct thermometer; clean instrument with alcohol).
6. Apply the thermometer sleeve and lubricant.
7. Lift the patient's top buttock to visualize the rectum.
8. Insert the thermometer into the rectum 1-1/2 inches (3.5 cm).
9. If using a **thermistor thermometer**, insert the flexible probe 4-6 inches (10-15 cm) past the anal sphincter into the rectum.
10. Wait for a digital reading.
11. Remove the thermometer, dispose of the sleeve, and clean the thermometer with alcohol.
12. If using a thermistor thermometer, the measuring aspect may remain in the patient's rectum until cooling temperature of 102°F (38.8°C) has been reached.

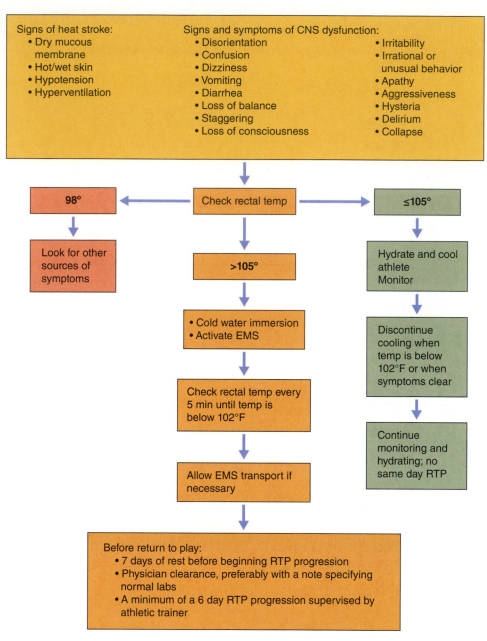

Signs of heat stroke:
• Dry mucous membrane
• Hot/wet skin
• Hypotension
• Hyperventilation

Signs and symptoms of CNS dysfunction:
• Disorientation
• Confusion
• Dizziness
• Vomiting
• Diarrhea
• Loss of balance
• Staggering
• Loss of consciousness
• Irritability
• Irrational or unusual behavior
• Apathy
• Aggressiveness
• Hysteria
• Delirium
• Collapse

Check rectal temp

98°

Look for other sources of symptoms

≤105°

Hydrate and cool athlete
Monitor

>105°

• Cold water immersion
• Activate EMS

Check rectal temp every 5 min until temp is below 102°F

Allow EMS transport if necessary

Discontinue cooling when temp is below 102°F or when symptoms clear

Continue monitoring and hydrating; no same day RTP

Before return to play:
• 7 days of rest before beginning RTP progression
• Physician clearance, preferably with a note specifying normal labs
• A minimum of a 6 day RTP progression supervised by athletic trainer

FIGURE 15.1 Decision tree for EHS.

Diagnostic Accuracy

Rectal thermometer recording of core temperature is the gold standard above all other external deceives (aural, oral, temporal, or axillary measurements) for accurate reading of internal temperature. Only gastrointestinal temperature measured with a swallowed capsule comes close to its accuracy.[24-26]

Rectal thermometers come in 2 varieties (figure 15.2). One is a thermometer, which is rigid, and typically digital. The most common digital thermometers have blue (oral) and red (rectal) attachments. A thermistor thermometer is a flexible device that can remain in an EHS patient for the duration of treatment. It is attached to a small, pager-like device that maintains constant readings. Although expensive, it alleviates the need to remove the athlete from the cold tub to reinsert the digital thermometer and assess core temperature.

A sudden collapse in heat can also be an indicator of exertional sickling and exertional rhabdomyolysis (ER; see chapter 14). Both of these conditions can be fatal if not recognized and treated. The medical staff should know the sickle cell status of each athlete prior to the onset of any activity in order to ensure proper monitoring. Patients diagnosed with sickle cell disease or sickle cell

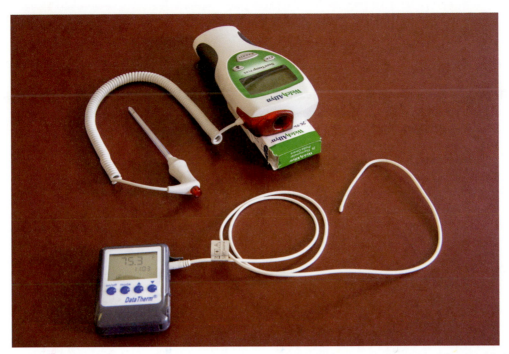

FIGURE 15.2 Both of these digital thermometers measure rectal (core) temperature. The WelchAllyn unit is interchangeable with a blue oral thermometer. The DataTherm unit is designed to have the sensor remain in the anus while cooling measures are administered to the body.

trait must be carefully supervised in activity. As the name suggests, ER involves muscular tissue breakdown, and the chief complaints are related to muscular weakness and muscular pain. Although EHS and exertional sickling and rhabdomyolysis have sudden collapse in common, only EHS patients will have a core (measured via rectal thermometer) temperature of 105°F (40.5°C) or higher.

Immediate Management Techniques

Aggressive, whole-body rapid cooling is critical to mitigate the risk of death due to EHS. Patients are to be immersed (trunk and extremities) into a cold-water tub or pool (figure 15.3).[14,15] Equipment and excess clothing should be removed while the patient is in the cold water, and the patient's head and neck are supported to prevent slipping into the water. This step will allow cooling to begin while the timely process of equipment removal occurs.[14] The water temperature is 35°F to 59°F (1.7°C to 15°C) and has continuous movement, by stirring or some other method, to maintain the cold temperature on the body to increase the cooling effectiveness.

Absent cold-water immersion, data show that the next best options are wet, iced towels and fans. Remove all equipment and most clothing (all but undergarments) from the patient, and place the cold, wet towels on the chest, axilla, and groin. The towels must be wet and switched often to be of any benefit. Do not ring out the

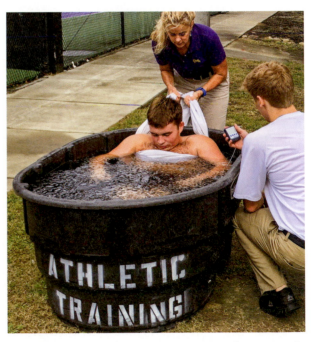

FIGURE 15.3 Cold-water immersion is the most reliable treatment for heatstroke.
Courtesy of Katie Walsh Flanagan

iced towels prior to applying them to the patient. The wet, iced towel and fan combination is not as effective as cold-water immersion. It is imperative to understand that cold-water immersion is the most reliable way of treating EHS, and all other techniques are inferior in rapidly lowering core temperature.[14,22,26]

Most patients experiencing heatstroke are semiconscious, combative, or noncompliant with instructions, and forcing fluids is not recommended. The crisis is not one of dehydration, but one of thermoregulatory collapse. Immediate cold-water immersion is critical to ameliorate the effects of rising core temperature.

If appropriate, following cold-water immersion, an intravenous (IV) treatment may be started. In patients whose mental status deteriorates, or if initially presented with severe symptoms, IV hypertonic saline (3%-5%) is indicated. This delivery of saline rapidly corrects the symptoms of EHS.[14,15,20] Chapter 5 contains more information on IV therapy.

Criteria for Deciding to Transport for Further Medical Examination

Patients with a core temperature of 105°F or greater (≥40.5°C) are cooled until their core temperature lowers to 102°F (38.9°C). After reaching this internal temperature, the patient is then transported via an ambulance to a hospital.

Patients who have a physician on site during the diagnosis and immediate (within 30 minutes from diagnosis) cooling treatment may not be required to be transported to a hospital. If the patient is symptom free 1 hour after cooling, at that time the physician can determine whether or not further medical attention is necessary.[14]

If a physician is not on-site, all patients diagnosed with EHS via rectal temperature should be transported

RED FLAG

It is imperative to rapidly cool all patients with ESH in a cold-water immersion tub *before* transporting for further medical care. The rectal temperature reading should be lowered to 102°F (38.9°C) prior to removing the patient from the cooling process and transporting.

to a hospital after cooling is complete; that is, the core temperature is measured below 102°F (38.9°C).[14]

Cold-Related Emergencies

The 2 primary cold-related emergencies are hypothermia and frostbite. Both have degrees of damage, and both can be limb- or life-threatening. Although these 2 environmental cold conditions are discussed in this section, the focus is on the more severe aspects of each. Typically, environmental cold injuries can be prevented with proper planning, clothing, hydration, and food intake. Exercising in the water, fog, rain, or wind can attribute to a hypothermia injury, as does being more lean. As with other weather-related conditions, having a solid awareness of the current and projected local weather is key, as are the topography, wind conditions, and environmental trends in the region. Wind can contribute considerably to the effects of cold weather, athletes should use caution when exercising outdoors in cooler weather if the wind is a factor (figure 15.4).

Temperature (°F)

Calm	40	35	30	25	20	15	10	5	0	−5	−10	−15	−20	−25	−30	−35	−40	−45
5	36	31	25	19	13	7	1	−5	−11	−16	−22	−28	−34	−40	−46	−52	−57	−63
10	34	27	21	15	9	3	−4	−10	−16	−22	−28	−35	−41	−47	−53	−59	−66	−72
15	32	25	19	13	6	0	−7	−13	−19	−26	−32	−39	−45	−51	−58	−64	−71	−77
20	30	24	17	11	4	−2	−9	−15	−22	−29	−35	−42	−48	−55	−61	−68	−74	−81
25	29	23	16	9	3	−4	−11	−17	−24	−31	−37	−44	−51	−58	−64	−71	−78	−84
30	28	22	15	8	1	−5	−12	−19	−26	−33	−39	−46	−53	−60	−67	−73	−80	−87
35	28	21	14	7	0	−7	−14	−21	−27	−34	−41	−48	−55	−62	−69	−76	−82	−89
40	27	20	13	6	−1	−8	−15	−22	−29	−36	−43	−50	−57	−64	−71	−78	−84	−91
45	26	19	12	5	−2	−9	−16	−23	−30	−37	−44	−51	−58	−65	−72	−79	−86	−93
50	26	19	12	4	−3	−10	−17	−24	−31	−38	−45	−52	−60	−67	−74	−81	−88	−95
55	25	18	11	4	−3	−11	−18	−25	−32	−39	−46	−54	−61	−68	−75	−82	−89	−97
60	25	17	10	3	−4	−11	−19	−26	−33	−40	−48	−55	−62	−69	−76	−84	−91	−98

Wind (mph) — row labels on left side.

Frostbite occurs in: 30 min | 10 min | 5 min

Windchill (°F) = 35.74 + 0.6215T − 35.75(V$^{0.16}$) + 0.4275T(V$^{0.16}$)
T = air temperature (°F)   V = wind speed (mph)

FIGURE 15.4 The effects of wind chill on temperature.

Incidence and Epidemiology

According to the Centers for Disease Control and Prevention (CDC), 13,419 hypothermia-related deaths occurred in the United States between 2003 and 2013. The death rate was higher for males (67%) and the elderly.[27,28] The greatest number of cases of hypothermia reporting to emergency departments was in urban settings, and those cases were attributed to exposure. The prevailing etiologies were alcoholism, drug use, mental illness, and homelessness.[27] The next largest group of people with hypothermia was people engaging in outdoor activities, including hunting, skiing, climbing, boating, and swimming.[27]

Medical Consequences of Cold-Related Emergencies

The effect of environmental cold is a multisystem one, leading to possible loss of a body part or death. The primary physiological response to cold is vasoconstriction. The body shunts blood flow away from extremities to protect the core. As a response, shivering ensues. Shivering intensity is related to the degree of cold and triggers an increased oxygen uptake as well as additional muscular recruitment.[29] A point comes when the system is overwhelmed and cannot sustain shivering, and this is when the more dangerous effects of cold exposure begin.

The most affected organs are the skin, brain, peripheral nervous system, and heart. Cold-induced bronchoconstriction can occur, particularly in people with a history of asthma. Without recognition and treatment, peripheral digits can develop necrosis and require amputation. Skin grafts of dead tissue may be required of the nose, ears, or other exposed body parts. The longer the exposure is, the more serious and ominous the outcome.

Signs and Symptoms

The signs and symptoms of a cold injury depend on the severity and duration of exposure to the cold environment. Tables 15.3 and 15.4 display the range of cold injury and their respective signs and symptoms.

Field Assessment Techniques

Having awareness of the weather and the possibility of a cold injury is the first step to assessing a person who appears injured. Acknowledge that even if the temperature is not unduly cold, those who are lean, ill, dehydrated, or hypoglycemic will react to cold sooner than others. Look for signs of shivering (or not), skin color, and observable vital signs that indicate distress. Evaluate

TABLE 15.3   **Signs and Symptoms of Injuries Elicited by Environmental Cold: Hypothermia**

Sign or symptom	Mild hypothermia	Moderate hypothermia	Severe hypothermia
Core temperature	98.6°F-95°F (37°C-35°C)	94°F-90°F (37°C-35°C)	Below 90°F (below 32°C)
Dermatological	Pale skin	Cyanosis	
Motor control	Impaired fine motor control	Impaired gross motor control	
Central nervous system	Typically conscious Amnesia Lethargy	Impaired mental function Loss of consciousness	Usually comatose
Shivering	Vigorous	Absent	Absent
Blood pressure	Within normal limits	Decreased/difficult to measure	Hypotension
Respiration	Within normal limits	Depressed	Severely depressed Pulmonary edema
Cardiovascular	Within normal limits	Depressed pulse rate; cardiac arrhythmias	Bradycardia Spontaneous ventricular fibrillation Cardiac arrest
Ocular		Dilated pupils	
Other	Polyuria Rhinorrhea	Slurred speech Muscle rigidity	Rigidity

Based on Cappaert et al. (2008).

TABLE 15.4   **Signs and Symptoms of Injuries Elicited by Environmental Cold: Frostbite**

Sign or symptom	Mild or superficial frostbite	Deep frostbite
Skin texture	Dry Waxy Edema	Hard Waxy Vesicles present
Skin color	Erythema White Blue-gray patches	White Black Purple
Skin palpation	Cold, firm skin	Immobile to palpation Poor circulation in area
Patient complaints	Transient burning or tingling	Burning, throbbing, shooting pain
Other		Progressive tissue necrosis Neurapraxia Hemorrhagic blistering (within 36-72 hours)

Based on Cappaert et al. (2008).

mental status. Knowing the signs and symptoms will help determine the next steps. Regardless of the level or type of cold injury, remove the athlete from the field of play to an area free of wind, preferably indoors to warmer temperature. A vehicle (car, team bus) is an excellent choice if space indoors is not readily available.

Diagnostic Accuracy

A rectal thermometer that is specific for cold injuries can read to at least 90°F (32.2°C), and it is the best indicator of a true cold environment emergency. Other signs and symptoms can provide helpful indicators, but the rectal thermometer is the true measure of core temperature.[30]

Immediate Management Techniques

Take the patient out from the cold environment into a place without wind and preferably indoors. Remove

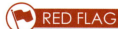 RED FLAG

- Make sure a rectal thermometer that is capable of measuring body temperatures below 90°F (32.2°C) is available.

- If possible, use a thermistor thermometer to determine core temperature. Although expensive, a flexible thermistor thermometer probe is the best choice for environmental emergencies. It has the ability to provide constant monitoring because the recording aspect of the thermometer remains in the patient's rectum during assessment and treatment.

wet or damp clothing, and replace it with warm, dry clothing or blankets, covering the patient from head to toe.[30,31] Measure respiration, pulse, and blood pressure to establish a baseline. Take the rectal temperature with a thermometer suitable for low body temperatures. If a core temperature below normal is registered, rewarm the patient using heat (hydrocollator, heating pad). Apply heat only on the trunk, chest, axilla, and groin in order to prevent **afterdrop**, which can cause arrhythmias and death.[30] If the patient is conscious and is able to consume fluids or food, supply warm beverages and foods containing 6% to 8% carbohydrate. The carbohydrate concentration will facilitate metabolism and heat production.[30,31]

In more severe cases of hypothermia, CPR may be necessary, as may be supplemental oxygen if the respiration is depressed or pulse oxygen is low. If CPR is initiated, send a designated person for the AED, and have others continue the rewarming of the axilla and groin. The trunk should continue to be rewarmed once cardiopulmonary status has been stabilized.

In frostbite, only specific (usually distal) tissues are involved, but that does not negate the fact that a person can still experience hypothermia as well as frostbite. Treat hypothermia first; after you initiate the rewarming, attend to the frostbite. If the frostbite cannot be addressed at the time, wrap damaged tissues in dry towels or cloths to prevent worsening damage. Rewarming can be as simple as applying the damaged tissue to another warm body part or submerging the injured area in warm water that is 98°F to 104°F (37°C-40°C).[30]

Criteria for Deciding to Transport for Further Medical Examination

Deciding to transport a patient who was subjected to a cold-weather emergency and is not improving is an

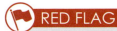

urgent matter. If the patient does not rapidly (within 15 to 20 minutes) recover from rewarming and warm fluids or food (if able), signal an ambulance to transport to a hospital where warming techniques are more advanced and include warm IV fluids. Likewise, a patient who is semiconscious, unconscious, or in need of cardio or pulmonary assistance must be transported via ambulance immediately.

Transportation Techniques

The critical aspect of transporting a cold-weather emergency patient, be it by private vehicle or ambulance, is to not allow any warmed tissues to become reinjured by cold. To that effect, provide warm blankets or clothing to surround the patient, and keep switching the material so that the warmer clothing is closer to the patient's body. One method is for you to warm clothes by wearing them, then remove the warmed clothes and place them closest to the skin on the patient, while donning the cooler clothing to warm it up similarly. In an ambulance, paramedics have materials to keep the patient warm.

If the patient is dyspneic, raise the trunk to assist breathing. Similarly, if the patient is in shock, raise the foot end of the gurney to assist with blood flow to the heart.

Altitude-Related Emergencies

Altitude-related emergencies are a group of medical consequences from high altitude. The 3 most common are acute mountain sickness (AMS), high-altitude cerebral edema (HACE), and high-altitude pulmonary edema (HAPE). AMS is common and treatable; unrecognized, it can progress to HACE or HAPE. HACE is the extreme end stage of AMS.[33]

In general, *high altitude* refers to elevations over 4,800 feet (1,500 m), with moderate altitude listed from 6,400 to 11,200 feet (2,000-3,500 m). United States ski resorts fall into the moderate category, and **hypoxia** and altitude sickness are common at these elevations.[32] Very high

altitude ranges from 11,200 to 18,000 feet (3,500-5,600 m), with extreme altitude listed at over 18,000 feet (5,600 m). In very high altitude, patients can sustain extreme **hypoxemia**, which can occur during sleep or exercise.

One can acclimate to the changing altitude with patience and training, with the exception of extreme altitude. In this situation, people must continue to progressively acclimatize to different altitudes before beginning to ascend again.[32]

Incidence and Epidemiology

AMS has been reported at U.S. ski resorts with incidence ranges from 10% to 40%, but it depends on the rate of ascents and maximum altitude attained.[32] A large study in Colorado concluded that 71% of tourists had at least some symptoms of AMS after ascending to altitudes of 6,900 to 9,700 feet (2,103-2,956 m).[34] Other studies concluded symptoms of AMS are more often associated with the rate of ascension and the altitude itself.[34]

HACE and HAPE are most common at altitudes of 11,200 to 18,000 feet (3,500-5,600 m).[32] HAPE is much more common than is HACE.[34]

Medical Consequences of Altitude-Related Emergencies

The primary culprit for all altitude-related illnesses is hypoxia. The unavailability of the oxygen saturation that a person is used to at lower levels initiates a cascade of physiological changes, beginning with increased respiration. Biofeedback in the body limits hyperventilation, but renal adaptations adjust over the first few days, allowing breathing to return to what is appropriate for the physiological demand. This is why a person is short of breath the first few days at altitude but then adjusts. Initial cerebral response to elevation is an increase in blood flow, which in turn reflects as a headache. Cardiac reactions include tachycardia and hypertension.[32,34] Hemoglobin concentration raises at high altitude, which is one reason that many U.S. athletes train at Colorado Springs, Colorado, where the altitude is 6,035 feet (1,839 m), prior to competitions that take place at lower levels. Increased hemoglobin allows more oxygen to be distributed through the blood. The longer one is at a sustained altitude, the more the adaptation (acclimatization) is to the elevation.

People who experiences symptoms of AMS and can stay at that altitude will do better than those who continue to climb. AMS is usually self-limiting, and symptoms abate in 1 to 3 days.[32] Acetazolamide is a prescription oral diuretic often used to prevent and treat the symptoms of altitude sickness, and it can be taken prior to ascent as well as after symptoms appear.

Those who continue to ascend with symptoms will likely progress to HACE, which can lead to coma within hours to days if unrecognized and treated.[32,34] It is rare for HACE to occur without AMS first, or with concomitant HAPE, but HACE can rapidly progress to coma and death from brain herniation.[33]

Signs and Symptoms

Symptoms of AMS tend to develop within the first hours at high altitude (above 8,000 ft or 2,438 m), but they can take up to 48 hours to appear. Patients complain of a hangover-like feeling, with headache, dizziness, lightheadedness, nausea, vomiting, or anorexia. Reduced urination is common because of fluid retention.[32] Unlike other illnesses, patients do not experience associated fever or muscle aches. The Lake Louise Consensus criteria assist in diagnosing AMS. A headache is mandatory in the criteria, in addition to at least 1 more symptom. The symptoms are in 3 categories—gastrointestinal (anorexia, nausea, vomiting), constitutional (lightheadedness, dizziness, weakness, fatigue), or insomnia.[35] Upon examination a patient with AMS will have little objective presentation beyond complaints. Edema may be observable in places, but all vital signs present within normal limits.

A patient who complains of AMS-like symptoms, but who is also **ataxic** or has concussion-like symptoms, is considered to have HACE and should be treated for HACE until that diagnosis is eliminated.[32] End-stage HACE patients appear to have more severe neurological repercussions, such as a stroke or transient ischemic attack, but it is actually worsening HACE. To be diagnosed with HAPE, one must present with a minimum of 2 signs and 2 symptoms while, or after, gaining elevation (table 15.5).[34]

People with HAPE typically present with signs and symptoms 1 to 3 days after substantial gain in elevation, and they often occur with exercise. A nonproductive cough may occur, which may graduate to a cough with sputum, and later can become tinged with blood. Fatigue is likely the first symptom, which presents challenges when evaluating an athlete who is competing or training.[34] Other noteworthy findings are a fever and engorged cervical veins, and possible lowered oxygen saturation levels measured using a pulse oximeter.

Field Assessment Techniques

If an athlete appears unwell during competition at high altitude, assume residual AMS and evaluate for symptoms. It does not benefit the athlete to continue participation; thus, the athlete should be removed from activity. If the athlete presents with respiratory or concussion-like complaints, evaluate in a place off the activity area.

Determine whether an injury occurred within the past 24 to 48 hours that may illicit high altitude–like symptoms. Regardless if the athlete sustained another previous injury, keep a level of suspicion for altitude-related illnesses.

Take a history of the home altitude of the patient, how rapid the ascension was to the current elevation, duration on the mountain, and onset and duration of the symptoms. Evaluate vital signs of respiration and heart rates, cardiac and pulmonary auscultation, and pulse oximetry. If these numbers all are within normal ranges, consider AMS, but observe for worsening symptoms. With history and physical data, determine the next step, which would be rest, return to lower elevation, seek medical attention for prescription for acetazolamide, or transport to a hospital for further evaluation. Acetazolamide is a diuretic and acts by decreasing edema around the heart and lungs. It addresses glaucoma and congestive heart failure in the same manner. As a pharmacological intervention, it is intended as a short-term response to a bigger problem.

Diagnostic Accuracy

AMS has no definitive diagnostic tools save for a good history. For patients with HACE, magnetic resonance imaging (MRI) will demonstrate neurological changes associated with HACE, and computed tomography (CT) will assist in eliminating stroke, hematomas, or other intracranial defects. Although hypoxia is the initial culprit in these conditions, pulse oximetry is not useful in diagnosing or treating AMS or HACE. However, pulse oximetry is indicated in diagnosing HAPE.[32,34]

For patients suspected of having HAPE, a chest radiograph is useful to confirm HAPE but also can exclude other conditions. As aforementioned, pulse oximetry will be remarkable in patients with HAPE, because the pulmonary edema interferes with regular oxygen exchange.

TABLE 15.5   **Signs and Symptoms of High-Altitude Pulmonary Edema (HAPE)**

Signs	Symptoms
Rales or wheezing in at least 1 lung lobe	Dyspnea at rest
Central cyanosis	Reported cough
Tachypnea	Chest tightness or congestion
Tachycardia	Weakness or decreased exercise tolerance

Based on Kale (2016).

HACE and HAPE are most common at altitudes of 11,200 to 18,000 feet (3,500-5,600 m).[34]

Immediate Management Techniques

If the patient appears to have AMS, remove her from participation in order to rest. The drug acetazolamide may assist in alleviating the symptoms, but signs and symptoms will abate within a few days without treatment. Supplemental low-flow oxygen, 0.5 to 1 L/minute (via nasal cannula) has been effective. The use of hyperbaric chamber therapy is not unheard of, but it is not necessary.

At the first sign of ataxia or altered consciousness, assume HACE and begin descent. Administering supplemental oxygen (2-4 L/min) with a high-flow mask or nasal cannula can help with symptoms, but the key treatment is to descend at least 3,000 feet (914 m).[33] Unlike AMS, the drug acetazolamide will not affect those with HACE. The drug dexamethasone may be effective in conjunction with supplemental oxygen, with the critical treatment goal of getting the patient to lower altitude.[33]

Treatment for patients suspected of HACE is also descent of at least 3,000 feet (914 m). The medications dexamethasone and acetazolamide have been effective in treating symptoms of HACE, but the descent is the critical aspect of treatment.[33]

Patients with suspected AMS and HAPE may benefit from portable hyperbaric chamber treatment. These chambers range from lightweight, coated-fabric bags with manual pumps, to more sustainable containers (e.g., Gamow bag, Certec, PAC). The patient is placed wholly within a chamber, and treated with 2 pounds per square inch (psi) atmosphere, which is equivalent to an approximate drop in elevation of 5,249 feet (1,600 m).[32,37] The treatment lasts 1 hour, then the patient is reevaluated for improvement in symptoms. Patients with HACE should not use the hyperbaric chamber as a replacement for descending to lower altitude.[32]

Criteria for Deciding to Transport for Further Medical Examination

Patients who appear unstable, are in respiratory distress, or have an altered mental status should be transferred via ambulance to a hospital.

Transportation Techniques

When deciding to transport a patient with suspected HAPE or HACE, confirm the patient will be delivered to a level I trauma center or a hospital with capability of handling altitude-related emergencies. If either pulmonary or cerebral edema is suspected, transport with the head and trunk slightly elevated to alleviate unnecessary pressure.

Summary

Environmental medical emergencies are largely preventable. One can avoid lightning danger by not being outdoors during a thunderstorm; and a person can dress, acclimate, and prepare for heat, cold and altitude situations. When an athlete suddenly collapses in these extreme conditions, a high suspicion must be considered for an environmental injury. Having access to the correct tools, such as a rectal thermometer, and knowing when and how to use them is paramount. In addition to the knowledge gained in this chapter, take time to refresh on emergency action plans specific to the environment and the diagnostic tools necessary, and practice both as often as possible.

 Go to the web study guide to complete the case studies for this chapter.

Model Exposure Control Plan

This form may be used, revised, and implemented as needed. Sections in brackets should be replaced with your facility information.

Policy

The [your facility name] is committed to providing a safe and healthful work environment for our entire staff. In pursuit of this goal, the following exposure control plan (ECP) is provided to eliminate or minimize occupational exposure to blood-borne pathogens in accordance with OSHA standard 29 *CFR* 1910.1030, "Occupational Exposure to Bloodborne Pathogens."

The ECP is a key document to assist our organization in implementing and ensuring compliance with the standard, thereby protecting our staff. This ECP includes the following:

- Program administration and contact information
- Determination of exposure
- Implementation of various methods of exposure control
- Postexposure evaluation and follow-up
- Communication of hazards to staff and training
- Recordkeeping
- Procedures for evaluating circumstances surrounding exposure incidents
- Implementation methods for these elements of the standard are discussed in the subsequent pages of this ECP.

Program Administration and Contact Information

- [Name of responsible person or department] is (are) responsible for implementation of the ECP. [Name of responsible person or department] will maintain, review, and update the ECP at least annually, and whenever necessary to include new or modified tasks and procedures.
  - Contact location/phone number/email: [information here]
- Staff who are determined to have occupational exposure to blood or other potentially infectious materials (OPIM) must comply with the procedures and work practices outlined in this ECP.
- [Name of responsible person or department] will provide and maintain all necessary personal protective equipment (PPE), engineering controls (e.g., sharps containers), labels, and red bags as required by the standard. [Name of responsible person or department] will ensure that adequate supplies of the aforementioned equipment are available in the appropriate sizes.
  - Contact location/phone number/email: [information here]
- [Name of responsible person or department] will be responsible for ensuring that all medical actions required by the standard are performed and that appropriate employee health and OSHA records are maintained.
  - Contact location/phone number/email: [information here]s
- [Name of responsible person or department] will be responsible for training, documentation of training, and making the written ECP available to staff and administrators.
  - Contact location/phone number/email: [information here]

Exposure Determination

List of all job classifications at our facility in which all staff have occupational exposure. Included is a list of tasks and procedures, or groups of closely related tasks and procedures, in which occupational exposure may occur for these individuals:

Job title	Department/location	Task/procedure

NOTE: Part-time, temporary, contract, and per diem staff are covered by the blood-borne pathogens standard. The ECP should describe how the standard will be met for these staff.

Methods of Implementation and Control

This facility identifies the need for changes in engineering controls and work practices through [Examples: Review of OSHA records, employee interviews, committee activities, etc.]. We evaluate new procedures and new products regularly by [describe the process, literature reviewed, supplier info, products considered].

- All staff will use universal precautions.
- Engineering controls and work practice controls will be used to prevent or minimize exposure to blood-borne pathogens. The specific engineering controls and work practice controls used are listed here:
  - [For example: non-glass capillary tubes, needleless systems]
- Sharps disposal containers are inspected and maintained or replaced by [Name of responsible person or department] every [list frequency] or whenever necessary to prevent overfilling.
- PPE is provided to our staff at no cost to them.
  - Training in the use of the appropriate PPE for specific tasks or procedures is provided by [Name of responsible person or department].
- The types of PPE available to staff are as follows:
  - [gloves, eye protection, etc.]
  - PPE is located [List location] and may be obtained through [Name of responsible person or department]. (Specify how staff will obtain PPE and who is responsible for ensuring that PPE is available.)

All staff using PPE must observe the following precautions:

- Wash hands immediately or as soon as feasible after removing gloves or other PPE.
- Remove PPE after it becomes contaminated and before leaving the work area.
- Used PPE may be disposed of in [List appropriate containers for storage, laundering, decontamination, or disposal.]
- Wear appropriate gloves when it is reasonably anticipated that there may be hand contact with blood or OPIM, and when handling or touching contaminated items or surfaces; replace gloves if

torn, punctured, or contaminated, or if their ability to function as a barrier is compromised.

- Utility gloves may be decontaminated for reuse if their integrity is not compromised; discard utility gloves if they show signs of cracking, peeling, tearing, puncturing, or deterioration.
- Never wash or decontaminate disposable gloves for reuse.
- Wear appropriate face and eye protection when splashes, sprays, spatters, or droplets of blood or OPIM pose a hazard to the eye, nose, or mouth.
- Remove immediately or as soon as feasible any garment contaminated by blood or OPIM, in such a way as to avoid contact with the outer surface.

The procedure for handling used PPE is as follows: *(May refer to specific procedure by title or number and last date of review; include how and where to decontaminate face shields, eye protection, resuscitation equipment.)*

- Housekeeping
  - Regulated waste is placed in containers that are closable, constructed to contain all contents and prevent leakage, appropriately labeled or color-coded (see the following section "Labels"), and closed prior to removal to prevent spillage or protrusion of contents during handling.
- The procedure for handling sharps disposal containers is as follows: [may refer to specific procedure by title or number and last date of review]
- The procedure for handling other regulated waste is as follows: [may refer to specific procedure by title or number and last date of review]
- Contaminated sharps are discarded immediately or as soon as possible in containers that are closable, puncture resistant, leak proof on sides and bottoms, and appropriately labeled or color coded. Sharps disposal containers are available at [must be easily accessible and as close as feasible to the immediate area where sharps are used].
- Bins and pails (e.g., wash or emesis basins) are cleaned and decontaminated as soon as feasible after visible contamination.
- Broken glassware that may be contaminated is only picked up using mechanical means, such as a brush and dustpan.
- Laundry
  - The following contaminated articles will be laundered by this company: [List of article laundered]

- Laundering will be performed by [Name of responsible person or department) at (time and/or location].
- The following laundering requirements must be met:
  - Handle contaminated laundry as little as possible, with minimal agitation.
  - Place wet contaminated laundry in leak-proof, labeled or color-coded containers before transport. Use [specify either red bags or bags marked with the biohazard symbol] for this purpose.
  - Wear the following PPE when handling or sorting contaminated laundry: [List appropriate PPE].
- Labels
  - The following labeling methods are used in this facility:
  - Equipment to be labeled [label type (size, color)]
  - [specimens, contaminated laundry, etc.] [red bag, biohazard label]
  - [Name of responsible person or department] is responsible for ensuring that warning labels are affixed or red bags are used as required if regulated waste or contaminated equipment is brought into the facility. Staff members are to notify [Name of responsible person or department] if they discover regulated waste containers, refrigerators containing blood or OPIM, contaminated equipment, etc., without proper labels.

Hepatitis B Vaccination

[Name of responsible person or department] will provide training to staff on hepatitis B vaccinations, addressing safety, benefits, efficacy, methods of administration, and availability.

- The hepatitis B vaccination series is available [at no cost after initial employee training and within 10 days of initial assignment] to all staff identified in the exposure determination section of this plan. Vaccination is encouraged unless
  1. documentation exists that the employee has previously received the series,
  2. antibody testing reveals that the employee is immune, or
  3. medical evaluation shows that vaccination is contraindicated.
- However, if an employee declines the vaccination, the employee must sign a declination form.

Staff who decline may request and obtain the vaccination at a later date at no cost. Documentation of refusal of the vaccination is kept at [List location].

Postexposure Evaluation and Follow-Up

Should an exposure incident occur, contact [Name of responsible person] at the following number _____.

[Name of responsible person or department] ensures that the health care professional evaluating an employee after an exposure incident receives the following:

- A description of the employee's job duties relevant to the exposure incident
- Route(s) of exposure
- Circumstances of exposure
- If possible, results of the source individual's blood test
- Relevant employee medical records, including vaccination status
- [Name of responsible person or department] provides the employee with a copy of the evaluating health care professional's written opinion within 15 days after completion of the evaluation.

Employee Training

All staff who have occupational exposure to blood-borne pathogens receive initial and annual training conducted by [Name of responsible person or department]. (Brief description of their qualifications.)

All staff who have occupational exposure to blood-borne pathogens receive training on the epidemiology, symptoms, and transmission of blood-borne pathogen diseases. In addition, the training program covers, at a minimum, the following elements:

- Copy and explanation of the OSHA blood-borne pathogen standard
- An explanation of our ECP and how to obtain a copy
- An explanation of methods to recognize tasks and other activities that may involve exposure to blood and OPIM, including what constitutes an exposure incident
- An explanation of the use and limitations of engineering controls, work practices, and PPE
- An explanation of the types, uses, location, removal, handling, decontamination, and disposal of PPE
- An explanation of the basis for PPE selection

Training records are completed for each employee upon completion of training. These documents will be kept for at least 3 years at [Location of records]. The training records include the following:

- Dates of the training sessions
- Contents or a summary of the training sessions
- Names and qualifications of persons conducting the training

- Names and job titles of all persons attending the training sessions

Employee training records are provided upon request to the employee or the employee's authorized representative within 15 working days. Such requests should be addressed to [Name of responsible person or department].

Adapted from OSHA, *Model Exposure Control Plan*, Appendix D (Washington, DC: OSHA).

APPENDIX B

SCAT-5

The SCAT-5 is used in people aged 13 years and over who are suspected of having sustained a concussion. It contains both an immediate (on-field) and off-field assessment. The SCAT-5 is presented on the following pages; it is also available at http://scat5.cattonline.com/.

SCAT5©

SPORT CONCUSSION ASSESSMENT TOOL — 5TH EDITION

DEVELOPED BY THE CONCUSSION IN SPORT GROUP

FOR USE BY MEDICAL PROFESSIONALS ONLY

supported by

Patient details

Name: _____

DOB: _____

Address: _____

ID number: _____

Examiner: _____

Date of Injury: _____ Time: _____

WHAT IS THE SCAT5?

The SCAT5 is a standardized tool for evaluating concussions designed for use by physicians and licensed healthcare professionals[1]. The SCAT5 cannot be performed correctly in less than 10 minutes.

If you are not a physician or licensed healthcare professional, please use the Concussion Recognition Tool 5 (CRT5). The SCAT5 is to be used for evaluating athletes aged 13 years and older. For children aged 12 years or younger, please use the Child SCAT5.

Preseason SCAT5 baseline testing can be useful for interpreting post-injury test scores, but is not required for that purpose.Detailed instructions for use of the SCAT5 are provided on page 7. Please read through these instructions carefully before testing the athlete. Brief verbal instructions for each test are given in italics. The only equipment required for the tester is a watch or timer.

This tool may be freely copied in its current form for distribution to individuals, teams, groups and organizations. It should not be altered in any way, re-branded or sold for commercial gain. Any revision, translation or reproduction in a digital form requires specific approval by the Concussion in Sport Group.

Recognise and Remove

A head impact by either a direct blow or indirect transmission of force can be associated with a serious and potentially fatal brain injury. If there are significant concerns, including any of the red flags listed in Box 1, then activation of emergency procedures and urgent transport to the nearest hospital should be arranged.

Key points

- Any athlete with suspected concussion should be REMOVED FROM PLAY, medically assessed and monitored for deterioration. No athlete diagnosed with concussion should be returned to play on the day of injury.

- If an athlete is suspected of having a concussion and medical personnel are not immediately available, the athlete should be referred to a medical facility for urgent assessment.

- Athletes with suspected concussion should not drink alcohol, use recreational drugs and should not drive a motor vehicle until cleared to do so by a medical professional.

- Concussion signs and symptoms evolve over time and it is important to consider repeat evaluation in the assessment of concussion.

- The diagnosis of a concussion is a clinical judgment, made by a medical professional. The SCAT5 should NOT be used by itself to make, or exclude, the diagnosis of concussion. An athlete may have a concussion even if their SCAT5 is "normal".

Remember:

- The basic principles of first aid (danger, response, airway, breathing, circulation) should be followed.

- Do not attempt to move the athlete (other than that required for airway management) unless trained to do so.

- Assessment for a spinal cord injury is a critical part of the initial on-field assessment.

- Do not remove a helmet or any other equipment unless trained to do so safely.

© Concussion in Sport Group 2017

Echemendia RJ, *et al. Br J Sports Med* 2017;**51**:851–858. doi:10.1136/bjsports-2017-097506SCAT5   851

1

IMMEDIATE OR ON-FIELD ASSESSMENT

The following elements should be assessed for all athletes who are suspected of having a concussion prior to proceeding to the neurocognitive assessment and ideally should be done on-field after the first first aid / emergency care priorities are completed.

If any of the "Red Flags" or observable signs are noted after a direct or indirect blow to the head, the athlete should be immediately and safely removed from participation and evaluated by a physician or licensed healthcare professional.

Consideration of transportation to a medical facility should be at the discretion of the physician or licensed healthcare professional.

The GCS is important as a standard measure for all patients and can be done serially if necessary in the event of deterioration in conscious state. The Maddocks questions and cervical spine exam are critical steps of the immediate assessment; however, these do not need to be done serially.

STEP 1: RED FLAGS

Name: _____
DOB: _____
Address: _____
ID number: _____
Examiner: _____
Date: _____

RED FLAGS:

- Neck pain or tenderness
- Double vision
- Weakness or tingling/ burning in arms or legs
- Severe or increasing headache
- Seizure or convulsion
- Loss of consciousness
- Deteriorating conscious state
- Vomiting
- Increasingly restless, agitated or combative

STEP 2: OBSERVABLE SIGNS

Witnessed ☐   Observed on Video ☐

Lying motionless on the playing surface	Y	N
Balance / gait difficulties / motor incoordination: stumbling, slow / laboured movements	Y	N
Disorientation or confusion, or an inability to respond appropriately to questions	Y	N
Blank or vacant look	Y	N
Facial injury after head trauma	Y	N

STEP 3: MEMORY ASSESSMENT
MADDOCKS QUESTIONS[2]

"I am going to ask you a few questions, please listen carefully and give your best effort. First, tell me what happened?"

_____

_____

Mark Y for correct answer / N for incorrect

What venue are we at today?	Y	N
Which half is it now?	Y	N
Who scored last in this match?	Y	N
What team did you play last week / game?	Y	N
Did your team win the last game?	Y	N

Note: Appropriate sport-specific questions may be substituted.

STEP 4: EXAMINATION
GLASGOW COMA SCALE (GCS)[3]

Time of assessment			
Date of assessment			
Best eye response (E)			
No eye opening	1	1	1
Eye opening in response to pain	2	2	2
Eye opening to speech	3	3	3
Eyes opening spontaneously	4	4	4
Best verbal response (V)			
No verbal response	1	1	1
Incomprehensible sounds	2	2	2
Inappropriate words	3	3	3
Confused	4	4	4
Oriented	5	5	5
Best motor response (M)			
No motor response	1	1	1
Extension to pain	2	2	2
Abnormal flexion to pain	3	3	3
Flexion / Withdrawal to pain	4	4	4
Localizes to pain	5	5	5
Obeys commands	6	6	6
Glasgow Coma score (E + V + M)			

CERVICAL SPINE ASSESSMENT

Does the athlete report that their neck is pain free at rest?	Y	N
If there is NO neck pain at rest, does the athlete have a full range of ACTIVE pain free movement?	Y	N
Is the limb strength and sensation normal?	Y	N

In a patient who is not lucid or fully conscious, a cervical spine injury should be assumed until proven otherwise.

© Concussion in Sport Group 2017
Echemendia RJ, *et al. Br J Sports Med* 2017;**51**:851–858. doi:10.1136/bjsports-2017-097506SCAT5

852

Sport Concussion Assessment Tool - 5th edition. *Br J Sports Med* 2017; 51:851-858. Reprinted by permission.

385

OFFICE OR OFF-FIELD ASSESSMENT

Please note that the neurocognitive assessment should be done in a distraction-free environment with the athlete in a resting state.

STEP 1: ATHLETE BACKGROUND

Sport / team / school: _____

Date / time of injury: _____

Years of education completed: _____

Age: _____

Gender: M / F / Other

Dominant hand: left / neither / right

How many diagnosed concussions has the
athlete had in the past?: _____

When was the most recent concussion?: _____

How long was the recovery (time to being cleared to play)
from the most recent concussion?: _____ (days)

Has the athlete ever been:

Hospitalized for a head injury?	Yes	No
Diagnosed / treated for headache disorder or migraines?	Yes	No
Diagnosed with a learning disability / dyslexia?	Yes	No
Diagnosed with ADD / ADHD?	Yes	No
Diagnosed with depression, anxiety or other psychiatric disorder?	Yes	No

Current medications? If yes, please list:

_____

_____

_____

_____

_____

_____

Name: _____

DOB: _____

Address: _____

ID number: _____

Examiner: _____

Date: _____

2

STEP 2: SYMPTOM EVALUATION

The athlete should be given the symptom form and asked to read this instruction paragraph out loud then complete the symptom scale. For the baseline assessment, the athlete should rate his/her symptoms based on how he/she typically feels and for the post injury assessment the athlete should rate their symptoms at this point in time.

Please Check: ☐ Baseline ☐ Post-Injury

Please hand the form to the athlete

	none	mild		moderate		severe	
Headache	0	1	2	3	4	5	6
"Pressure in head"	0	1	2	3	4	5	6
Neck Pain	0	1	2	3	4	5	6
Nausea or vomiting	0	1	2	3	4	5	6
Dizziness	0	1	2	3	4	5	6
Blurred vision	0	1	2	3	4	5	6
Balance problems	0	1	2	3	4	5	6
Sensitivity to light	0	1	2	3	4	5	6
Sensitivity to noise	0	1	2	3	4	5	6
Feeling slowed down	0	1	2	3	4	5	6
Feeling like "in a fog"	0	1	2	3	4	5	6
"Don't feel right"	0	1	2	3	4	5	6
Difficulty concentrating	0	1	2	3	4	5	6
Difficulty remembering	0	1	2	3	4	5	6
Fatigue or low energy	0	1	2	3	4	5	6
Confusion	0	1	2	3	4	5	6
Drowsiness	0	1	2	3	4	5	6
More emotional	0	1	2	3	4	5	6
Irritability	0	1	2	3	4	5	6
Sadness	0	1	2	3	4	5	6
Nervous or Anxious	0	1	2	3	4	5	6
Trouble falling asleep (if applicable)	0	1	2	3	4	5	6

Total number of symptoms:	of 22
Symptom severity score:	of 132
Do your symptoms get worse with physical activity?	Y N
Do your symptoms get worse with mental activity?	Y N
If 100% is feeling perfectly normal, what percent of normal do you feel?	

If not 100%, why?

_____

_____

_____

Please hand form back to examiner

© Concussion in Sport Group 2017

Echemendia RJ, *et al. Br J Sports Med* 2017;**51**:851–858. doi:10.1136/bjsports-2017-097506SCAT5

853

3

STEP 3: COGNITIVE SCREENING
Standardised Assessment of Concussion (SAC)[4]

ORIENTATION

	0	1
What month is it?	0	1
What is the date today?	0	1
What is the day of the week?	0	1
What year is it?	0	1
What time is it right now? (within 1 hour)	0	1
Orientation score		of 5

IMMEDIATE MEMORY

The Immediate Memory component can be completed using the traditional 5-word per trial list or optionally using 10-words per trial to minimise any ceiling effect. All 3 trials must be administered irrespective of the number correct on the first trial. Administer at the rate of one word per second.

Please choose EITHER the 5 or 10 word list groups and circle the specific word list chosen for this test.

I am going to test your memory. I will read you a list of words and when I am done, repeat back as many words as you can remember, in any order. For Trials 2 & 3: I am going to repeat the same list again. Repeat back as many words as you can remember in any order, even if you said the word before.

List	Alternate 5 word lists					Score (of 5) Trial 1	Trial 2	Trial 3
A	Finger	Penny	Blanket	Lemon	Insect			
B	Candle	Paper	Sugar	Sandwich	Wagon			
C	Baby	Monkey	Perfume	Sunset	Iron			
D	Elbow	Apple	Carpet	Saddle	Bubble			
E	Jacket	Arrow	Pepper	Cotton	Movie			
F	Dollar	Honey	Mirror	Saddle	Anchor			
	Immediate Memory Score					of 15		
	Time that last trial was completed							

List	Alternate 10 word lists					Score (of 10) Trial 1	Trial 2	Trial 3
G	Finger	Penny	Blanket	Lemon	Insect			
	Candle	Paper	Sugar	Sandwich	Wagon			
H	Baby	Monkey	Perfume	Sunset	Iron			
	Elbow	Apple	Carpet	Saddle	Bubble			
I	Jacket	Arrow	Pepper	Cotton	Movie			
	Dollar	Honey	Mirror	Saddle	Anchor			
	Immediate Memory Score					of 30		
	Time that last trial was completed							

CONCENTRATION

DIGITS BACKWARDS

Please circle the Digit list chosen (A, B, C, D, E, F). Administer at the rate of one digit per second reading DOWN the selected column.

I am going to read a string of numbers and when I am done, you repeat them back to me in reverse order of how I read them to you. For example, if I say 7-1-9, you would say 9-1-7.

Concentration Number Lists (circle one)

List A	List B	List C			
4-9-3	5-2-6	1-4-2	Y	N	0
6-2-9	4-1-5	6-5-8	Y	N	1
3-8-1-4	1-7-9-5	6-8-3-1	Y	N	0
3-2-7-9	4-9-6-8	3-4-8-1	Y	N	1
6-2-9-7-1	4-8-5-2-7	4-9-1-5-3	Y	N	0
1-5-2-8-6	6-1-8-4-3	6-8-2-5-1	Y	N	1
7-1-8-4-6-2	8-3-1-9-6-4	3-7-6-5-1-9	Y	N	0
5-3-9-1-4-8	7-2-4-8-5-6	9-2-6-5-1-4	Y	N	1

List D	List E	List F			
7-8-2	3-8-2	2-7-1	Y	N	0
9-2-6	5-1-8	4-7-9	Y	N	1
4-1-8-3	2-7-9-3	1-6-8-3	Y	N	0
9-7-2-3	2-1-6-9	3-9-2-4	Y	N	1
1-7-9-2-6	4-1-8-6-9	2-4-7-5-8	Y	N	0
4-1-7-5-2	9-4-1-7-5	8-3-9-6-4	Y	N	1
2-6-4-8-1-7	6-9-7-3-8-2	5-8-6-2-4-9	Y	N	0
8-4-1-9-3-5	4-2-7-9-3-8	3-1-7-8-2-6	Y	N	1
		Digits Score:			of 4

MONTHS IN REVERSE ORDER

Now tell me the months of the year in reverse order. Start with the last month and go backward. So you'll say December, November. Go ahead.

Dec - Nov - Oct - Sept - Aug - Jul - Jun - May - Apr - Mar - Feb - Jan	0 1
Months Score	of 1
Concentration Total Score (Digits + Months)	of 5

Echemendia RJ, *et al. Br J Sports Med* 2017;**51**:851–858. doi:10.1136/bjsports-2017-097506SCAT5

854

Sport Concussion Assessment Tool - 5th edition. Br J Sports Med 2017; 51:851-858. Reprinted by permission.

387

4

STEP 4: NEUROLOGICAL SCREEN

See the instruction sheet (page 7) for details of test administration and scoring of the tests.

Can the patient read aloud (e.g. symptom check-list) and follow instructions without difficulty?	Y	N
Does the patient have a full range of pain-free PASSIVE cervical spine movement?	Y	N
Without moving their head or neck, can the patient look side-to-side and up-and-down without double vision?	Y	N
Can the patient perform the finger nose coordination test normally?	Y	N
Can the patient perform tandem gait normally?	Y	N

BALANCE EXAMINATION

Modified Balance Error Scoring System (mBESS) testing[5]

Which foot was tested
(i.e. which is the non-dominant foot)
☐ Left
☐ Right

Testing surface (hard floor, field, etc.) _____

Footwear (shoes, barefoot, braces, tape, etc.) _____

Condition	Errors
Double leg stance	of 10
Single leg stance (non-dominant foot)	of 10
Tandem stance (non-dominant foot at the back)	of 10
Total Errors	of 30

Name:	_____
DOB:	_____
Address:	_____
ID number:	_____
Examiner:	_____
Date:	_____

5

STEP 5: DELAYED RECALL:

The delayed recall should be performed after 5 minutes have elapsed since the end of the Immediate Recall section. Score 1 pt. for each correct response.

Do you remember that list of words I read a few times earlier? Tell me as many words from the list as you can remember in any order.

Time Started _____

Please record each word correctly recalled. Total score equals number of words recalled.

_____
_____
_____

Total number of words recalled accurately: of 5 or of 10

6

STEP 6: DECISION

Domain	Date & time of assessment:		
Symptom number (of 22)			
Symptom severity score (of 132)			
Orientation (of 5)			
Immediate memory	of 15 of 30	of 15 of 30	of 15 of 30
Concentration (of 5)			
Neuro exam	Normal Abnormal	Normal Abnormal	Normal Abnormal
Balance errors (of 30)			
Delayed Recall	of 5 of 10	of 5 of 10	of 5 of 10

Date and time of injury: _____

If the athlete is known to you prior to their injury, are they different from their usual self?
☐ Yes ☐ No ☐ Unsure ☐ Not Applicable
(If different, describe why in the clinical notes section)

Concussion Diagnosed?
☐ Yes ☐ No ☐ Unsure ☐ Not Applicable

If re-testing, has the athlete improved?
☐ Yes ☐ No ☐ Unsure ☐ Not Applicable

I am a physician or licensed healthcare professional and I have personally administered or supervised the administration of this SCAT5.

Signature: _____

Name: _____

Title: _____

Registration number (if applicable): _____

Date: _____

SCORING ON THE SCAT5 SHOULD NOT BE USED AS A STAND-ALONE METHOD TO DIAGNOSE CONCUSSION, MEASURE RECOVERY OR MAKE DECISIONS ABOUT AN ATHLETE'S READINESS TO RETURN TO COMPETITION AFTER CONCUSSION.

© Concussion in Sport Group 2017
Echemendia RJ, *et al. Br J Sports Med* 2017;**51**:851–858. doi:10.1136/bjsports-2017-097506SCAT5

855

CLINICAL NOTES:

_____

_____

_____

_____

Name: _____

DOB: _____

Address: _____

ID number: _____

Examiner: _____

Date: _____

_____

_____

_____

_____

_____

_____

_____

_____

✂ ·

CONCUSSION INJURY ADVICE

(To be given to the person monitoring the concussed athlete)

This patient has received an injury to the head. A careful medical examination has been carried out and no sign of any serious complications has been found. Recovery time is variable across individuals and the patient will need monitoring for a further period by a responsible adult. Your treating physician will provide guidance as to this timeframe.

If you notice any change in behaviour, vomiting, worsening headache, double vision or excessive drowsiness, please telephone your doctor or the nearest hospital emergency department immediately.

Other important points:

Initial rest: Limit physical activity to routine daily activities (avoid exercise, training, sports) and limit activities such as school, work, and screen time to a level that does not worsen symptoms.

1) Avoid alcohol

2) Avoid prescription or non-prescription drugs without medical supervision. Specifically:

a) Avoid sleeping tablets

b) Do not use aspirin, anti-inflammatory medication or stronger pain medications such as narcotics

3) Do not drive until cleared by a healthcare professional.

4) Return to play/sport requires clearance by a healthcare professional.

Clinic phone number: _____

Patient's name: _____

Date / time of injury: _____

Date / time of medical review: _____

Healthcare Provider: _____

© Concussion in Sport Group 2017

Contact details or stamp

Echemendia RJ, *et al. Br J Sports Med* 2017;**51**:851–858. doi:10.1136/bjsports-2017-097506SCAT5

Sport Concussion Assessment Tool - 5th edition. Br J Sports Med 2017; 51:851-858. Reprinted by permission.

INSTRUCTIONS

Words in *Italics* throughout the SCAT5 are the instructions given to the athlete by the clinician

Symptom Scale

The time frame for symptoms should be based on the type of test being administered. At baseline it is advantageous to assess how an athlete "typically" feels whereas during the acute/post-acute stage it is best to ask how the athlete feels at the time of testing.

The symptom scale should be completed by the athlete, not by the examiner. In situations where the symptom scale is being completed after exercise, it should be done in a resting state, generally by approximating his/her resting heart rate.

For total number of symptoms, maximum possible is 22 except immediately post injury, if sleep item is omitted, which then creates a maximum of 21.

For Symptom severity score, add all scores in table, maximum possible is 22 x 6 = 132, except immediately post injury if sleep item is omitted, which then creates a maximum of 21x6=126.

Immediate Memory

The Immediate Memory component can be completed using the traditional 5-word per trial list or, optionally, using 10-words per trial. The literature suggests that the Immediate Memory has a notable ceiling effect when a 5-word list is used. In settings where this ceiling is prominent, the examiner may wish to make the task more difficult by incorporating two 5–word groups for a total of 10 words per trial. In this case, the maximum score per trial is 10 with a total trial maximum of 30.

Choose one of the word lists (either 5 or 10). Then perform 3 trials of immediate memory using this list.

Complete all 3 trials regardless of score on previous trials.

"I am going to test your memory. I will read you a list of words and when I am done, repeat back as many words as you can remember, in any order." The words must be read at a rate of one word per second.

Trials 2 & 3 MUST be completed regardless of score on trial 1 & 2.

Trials 2 & 3:

"I am going to repeat the same list again. Repeat back as many words as you can remember in any order, even if you said the word before."

Score 1 pt. for each correct response. Total score equals sum across all 3 trials. Do NOT inform the athlete that delayed recall will be tested.

Concentration

Digits backward

Choose one column of digits from lists A, B, C, D, E or F and administer those digits as follows:

Say: *"I am going to read a string of numbers and when I am done, you repeat them back to me in reverse order of how I read them to you. For example, if I say 7-1-9, you would say 9-1-7."*

Begin with first 3 digit string.

If correct, circle "Y" for correct and go to next string length. If incorrect, circle "N" for the first string length and read trial 2 in the same string length. One point possible for each string length. Stop after incorrect on both trials (2 N's) in a string length. The digits should be read at the rate of one per second.

Months in reverse order

"Now tell me the months of the year in reverse order. Start with the last month and go backward. So you'll say December, November ... Go ahead"

1 pt. for entire sequence correct

Delayed Recall

The delayed recall should be performed after 5 minutes have elapsed since the end of the Immediate Recall section.

"Do you remember that list of words I read a few times earlier? Tell me as many words from the list as you can remember in any order."

Score 1 pt. for each correct response

Modified Balance Error Scoring System (mBESS)[5] testing

This balance testing is based on a modified version of the Balance Error Scoring System (BESS)[5]. A timing device is required for this testing.

Each of 20-second trial/stance is scored by counting the number of errors. The examiner will begin counting errors only after the athlete has assumed the proper start position. The modified BESS is calculated by adding one error point for each error during the three 20-second tests. The maximum number of errors for any single condition is 10. If the athlete commits multiple errors simultaneously, only

one error is recorded but the athlete should quickly return to the testing position, and counting should resume once the athlete is set. Athletes that are unable to maintain the testing procedure for a minimum of five seconds at the start are assigned the highest possible score, ten, for that testing condition.

OPTION: For further assessment, the same 3 stances can be performed on a surface of medium density foam (e.g., approximately 50cm x 40cm x 6cm).

Balance testing – types of errors

1. Hands lifted off iliac crest
2. Opening eyes
3. Step, stumble, or fall
4. Moving hip into > 30 degrees abduction
5. Lifting forefoot or heel
6. Remaining out of test position > 5 sec

"I am now going to test your balance. Please take your shoes off (if applicable), roll up your pant legs above ankle (if applicable), and remove any ankle taping (if applicable). This test will consist of three twenty second tests with different stances."

(a) Double leg stance:

"The first stance is standing with your feet together with your hands on your hips and with your eyes closed. You should try to maintain stability in that position for 20 seconds. I will be counting the number of times you move out of this position. I will start timing when you are set and have closed your eyes."

(b) Single leg stance:

"If you were to kick a ball, which foot would you use? [This will be the dominant foot] Now stand on your non-dominant foot. The dominant leg should be held in approximately 30 degrees of hip flexion and 45 degrees of knee flexion. Again, you should try to maintain stability for 20 seconds with your hands on your hips and your eyes closed. I will be counting the number of times you move out of this position. If you stumble out of this position, open your eyes and return to the start position and continue balancing. I will start timing when you are set and have closed your eyes."

(c) Tandem stance:

"Now stand heel-to-toe with your non-dominant foot in back. Your weight should be evenly distributed across both feet. Again, you should try to maintain stability for 20 seconds with your hands on your hips and your eyes closed. I will be counting the number of times you move out of this position. If you stumble out of this position, open your eyes and return to the start position and continue balancing. I will start timing when you are set and have closed your eyes."

Tandem Gait

Participants are instructed to stand with their feet together behind a starting line (the test is best done with footwear removed). Then, they walk in a forward direction as quickly and as accurately as possible along a 38mm wide (sports tape), 3 metre line with an alternate foot heel-to-toe gait ensuring that they approximate their heel and toe on each step. Once they cross the end of the 3m line, they turn 180 degrees and return to the starting point using the same gait. Athletes fail the test if they step off the line, have a separation between their heel and toe, or if they touch or grab the examiner or an object.

Finger to Nose

"I am going to test your coordination now. Please sit comfortably on the chair with your eyes open and your arm (either right or left) outstretched (shoulder flexed to 90 degrees and elbow and fingers extended), pointing in front of you. When I give a start signal, I would like you to perform five successive finger to nose repetitions using your index finger to touch the tip of the nose, and then return to the starting position, as quickly and as accurately as possible."

References

1. McCrory et al. Consensus Statement On Concussion In Sport – The 5th International Conference On Concussion In Sport Held In Berlin, October 2016. British Journal of Sports Medicine 2017 (available at www.bjsm.bmj.com)

2. Maddocks, DL; Dicker, GD; Saling, MM. The assessment of orientation following concussion in athletes. Clinical Journal of Sport Medicine 1995; 5: 32-33

3. Jennett, B., Bond, M. Assessment of outcome after severe brain damage: a practical scale. Lancet 1975; i: 480-484

4. McCrea M. Standardized mental status testing of acute concussion. Clinical Journal of Sport Medicine. 2001; 11: 176-181

5. Guskiewicz KM. Assessment of postural stability following sport-related concussion. Current Sports Medicine Reports. 2003; 2: 24-30

© Concussion in Sport Group 2017

Echemendia RJ, *et al. Br J Sports Med* 2017;**51**:851–858. doi:10.1136/bjsports-2017-097506SCAT5

857

CONCUSSION INFORMATION

Any athlete suspected of having a concussion should be removed from play and seek medical evaluation.

Signs to watch for

Problems could arise over the first 24-48 hours. The athlete should not be left alone and must go to a hospital at once if they experience:

- Worsening headache
- Drowsiness or inability to be awakened
- Inability to recognize people or places
- Repeated vomiting
- Unusual behaviour or confusion or irritable
- Seizures (arms and legs jerk uncontrollably)
- Weakness or numbness in arms or legs
- Unsteadiness on their feet.
- Slurred speech

Consult your physician or licensed healthcare professional after a suspected concussion. Remember, it is better to be safe.

Rest & Rehabilitation

After a concussion, the athlete should have physical rest and relative cognitive rest for a few days to allow their symptoms to improve. In most cases, after no more than a few days of rest, the athlete should gradually increase their daily activity level as long as their symptoms do not worsen. Once the athlete is able to complete their usual daily activities without concussion-related symptoms, the second step of the return to play/sport progression can be started. The athlete should not return to play/sport until their concussion-related symptoms have resolved and the athlete has successfully returned to full school/learning activities.

When returning to play/sport, **the athlete should follow a stepwise, medically managed exercise progression, with increasing amounts of exercise.** For example:

Graduated Return to Sport Strategy

Exercise step	Functional exercise at each step	Goal of each step
1. Symptom-limited activity	Daily activities that do not provoke symptoms.	Gradual reintroduction of work/school activities.
2. Light aerobic exercise	Walking or stationary cycling at slow to medium pace. No resistance training.	Increase heart rate.
3. Sport-specific exercise	Running or skating drills. No head impact activities.	Add movement.
4. Non-contact training drills	Harder training drills, e.g., passing drills. May start progressive resistance training.	Exercise, coordination, and increased thinking.
5. Full contact practice	Following medical clearance, participate in normal training activities.	Restore confidence and assess functional skills by coaching staff.
6. Return to play/sport	Normal game play.	

In this example, it would be typical to have 24 hours (or longer) for each step of the progression. If any symptoms worsen while exercising, the athlete should go back to the previous step. Resistance training should be added only in the later stages (Stage 3 or 4 at the earliest).

Written clearance should be provided by a healthcare professional before return to play/sport as directed by local laws and regulations.

Graduated Return to School Strategy

Concussion may affect the ability to learn at school. The athlete may need to miss a few days of school after a concussion. When going back to school, some athletes may need to go back gradually and may need to have some changes made to their schedule so that concussion symptoms do not get worse. If a particular activity makes symptoms worse, then the athlete should stop that activity and rest until symptoms get better. To make sure that the athlete can get back to school without problems, it is important that the healthcare provider, parents, caregivers and teachers talk to each other so that everyone knows what the plan is for the athlete to go back to school.

Note: If mental activity does not cause any symptoms, the athlete may be able to skip step 2 and return to school part-time before doing school activities at home first.

Mental Activity	Activity at each step	Goal of each step
1. Daily activities that do not give the athlete symptoms	Typical activities that the athlete does during the day as long as they do not increase symptoms (e.g. reading, texting, screen time). Start with 5-15 minutes at a time and gradually build up.	Gradual return to typical activities.
2. School activities	Homework, reading or other cognitive activities outside of the classroom.	Increase tolerance to cognitive work.
3. Return to school part-time	Gradual introduction of schoolwork. May need to start with a partial school day or with increased breaks during the day.	Increase academic activities.
4. Return to school full-time	Gradually progress school activities until a full day can be tolerated.	Return to full academic activities and catch up on missed work.

If the athlete continues to have symptoms with mental activity, some other accomodations that can help with return to school may include:

- Starting school later, only going for half days, or going only to certain classes
- More time to finish assignments/tests
- Quiet room to finish assignments/tests
- Not going to noisy areas like the cafeteria, assembly halls, sporting events, music class, shop class, etc.
- Taking lots of breaks during class, homework, tests
- No more than one exam/day
- Shorter assignments
- Repetition/memory cues
- Use of a student helper/tutor
- Reassurance from teachers that the child will be supported while getting better

The athlete should not go back to sports until they are back to school/learning, without symptoms getting significantly worse and no longer needing any changes to their schedule.

© Concussion in Sport Group 2017
Echemendia RJ, et al. Br J Sports Med 2017;**51**:851–858. doi:10.1136/bjsports-2017-097506SCAT5

Sport Concussion Assessment Tool - 5th edition. *Br J Sports Med* 2017; 51:851-858. Reprinted by permission.

391

GLOSSARY

accreditation—Granting of approval by an official review board after specific requirements have been met. The review is based on self-assessment, peer assessment, and judgment. The purpose of accreditation is public accountability.

active infection—A virus or bacterium that is actively replicating and potentially causing symptoms (opposite of a **latent infection**).

activities of daily living (ADLs)—Term used in health care to refer to daily self-care activities (e.g., feeding, bathing, dressing, grooming, work, homemaking, and leisure) as a measure of functional status, particularly in regard to post-injury or disability.

acute coronary syndrome—A spectrum of coronary artery obstruction resulting from atherosclerosis (narrowing of coronary arteries), leading to acute ischemia of cardiac muscle tissue and resulting in stable or unstable angina or acute myocardial infarction.

acute myocardial infarction (AMI or MI)—Also called cardiac arrest or heart attack, it occurs when one of the coronary arteries is blocked, causing ischemia and damage to the myocardium. The most common symptoms are chest pain, pressure, or discomfort that may also be in the shoulder, arm, back, neck, or jaw (referred pain).

advanced cardiac life support (ACLS)—A set of clinical interventions for the urgent treatment of cardiac arrest, stroke, and other life-threatening medical emergencies, as well as the knowledge and skills to deploy those interventions.

advanced-level emergency medical care—Care that has greater potential benefit to the patient, but also greater potential risk to the patient if improperly or inappropriately performed, is more difficult to attain and maintain competency in, and requires significant background knowledge in basic and applied sciences. These include invasive and pharmacological interventions.

afterdrop—A physiological condition of cold injury where rewarming extremities causes dilation of the vessels, sending metabolic byproducts and cold blood from the extremities to the core of the body. The result can be fatal.

against medical advice (AMA)—Also called discharge against medical advice (DAMA), a term used when a patient leaves a health care facility or refuses treatment against the advice of the health care provider. Widespread ethical and legal consensus is that competent patients (or their authorized surrogates) are entitled to decline recommended treatment.

agonal gasping—Abnormal respiration pattern and brainstem reflex that may also be called gasping respiration or agonal breathing. Characterized by gasping and labored breathing that may also have vocalizations and myoclonic activity.

allergen—Substance that triggers an immune response.

allergy—Condition caused by immune system hypersensitivity (atopy) to an allergen in the environment that is generally harmless to most people.

ambulatory care or **outpatient care**—Medical care provided in a setting outside of the hospital, including diagnosis, observation, consultation, treatment, intervention, and rehabilitation services.

anaphylactoid—Adverse reaction that is not IgE mediated and typically not life-threatening.

anaphylaxis—Severe and often fatal systemic allergic reaction in a sensitized individual upon exposure to a specific antigen (as wasp venom or penicillin); characterized by respiratory distress, fainting, itching, and hives.

aneurysm—A bulge or ballooning and weakened area in the wall of an artery; it may occur in the coronary arteries, aorta (as in Marfan syndrome), or brain.

angina pectoris—Chest pain, pressure, or squeezing feeling in the chest as a result of ischemia of the myocardium from obstruction or spasm of the coronary arteries. The patient may also experience discomfort in the neck, jaw, shoulder, back, or arm. Also called angina.

angioedema—Edema of the deep dermis and subcutaneous tissues caused by acute mast cell–mediated reaction from exposure to drug, venom, dietary, pollen, or other allergens.

anisocoria—Unequal size of the pupils. It is a sign of brain trauma. However, this condition affects 20% of the population, and it is generally considered harmless in them.

ankle mortise—Technical name for the ankle joint. It is formed by the distal tibia and fibula and talus.

anomalous coronary arteries—Also called coronary artery anomalies, they are congenital malformations of coronary vessels, often found in combination with other congenital heart defects associated with sudden cardiac death.

antibiotic—Drug that kills or stops the growth of bacteria; examples include penicillin and ciprofloxacin.

antibiotic resistance—Ability of bacteria to resist the effects of an antibiotic. The bacteria are not killed, and their growth is not stopped. Resistant bacteria survive exposure to antibiotics and continue to multiply in the body, potentially causing more harm and spreading to other animals or people.

antigens—Elicit an antibody response activated by B- and T-cell receptors.

antimicrobial—Agent that kills microorganisms or stops their growth.

antiseptic—Substance applied to living tissue or skin to reduce the possibility of infection.

aortic dissection—A tear in the aorta resulting in surging of blood into the thoracic cavity.

apnea—Temporary or permanent cessation of breathing.

appearance of impropriety—A phrase referring to a situation in which an outside person without knowledge of the specific circumstances may question the ethics of the situation. For example, a male AT examining a female patient's chest for a contusion, although within the scope of practice, may appear to be improper touching. It is common practice to avoid even the appearance of impropriety.

appendicitis—An inflammation of the vermiform appendix.

arachnodactyly—Literally "spider fingers," a condition in which, compared to the palm of the hand and arch of the foot, the fingers and toes are abnormally long and slender. Often associated with Marfan syndrome.

arrhythmia—Also called *cardiac dysrhythmia* or *irregular heartbeat*, in which the heartbeat is irregular, too fast, or too slow. *See* **dysrhythmia**.

articulation—The connection or junction between bones that allows varying degrees of movement.

aseptic technique—Preparation of equipment or anatomic site prior to an administration of medication or procedure, in a manner to avoid contamination of the equipment and site in an effort to reduce changes of infection caused by the procedure or medication delivery. Procedure performed under sterile conditions.

aspiration—The accidental sucking in of fluid or particles into the trachea or lungs.

asthenic—Slender build and slight muscular development; ectomorphic.

asystole—Abnormal heart rhythm during cardiac arrest in which no discernible electrical activity appears on the ECG monitor; also called flatline.

ataxic—Pertaining to an uncoordinated or staggering movement, gait, or posture.

athlete's heart—Also called athletic heart syndrome (AHS), athletic bradycardia, or exercise-induced cardiomegaly, athlete's heart is a benign, nonpathologic enlargement of the heart, often with sinus bradycardia.

atlas—First cervical vertebra, named for the Greek Titan in mythology who was said to hold the world on his shoulders; so too does the atlas support the cranium.

atopy (atopic)—Predisposition toward developing certain allergic hypersensitivity reactions.

aura—Warning sign to a migraine or seizure; sometimes described as déjà vu; lightheadedness; or change in taste, smell, hearing, or vision.

auscultation—Using a stethoscope to listen to sounds within the body, such as heart, lungs, other organs, or gastrointestinal sounds.

autoimmune disorder—An immunologically triggered inflammatory response attacks the body's own tissues.

autopsy-negative sudden unexplained death—Sudden cardiac death that is associated with a structurally normal heart at postmortem examination.

avascular necrosis—Death of osseous tissue due to lack of blood supply. It can result from fractures, dislocations, or other medical conditions that obstruct blood flow to an area of bone.

axis—The second cervical vertebra. Identified by the superior projection (dens) by which the atlas articulates and allows for cervical rotation.

bacteremia—Presence of bacteria in the blood, which is usually a sterile environment.

baseline vital signs—Assessment obtained upon initial contact with the patient representing initial level to compare future assessments (serial vitals). Baseline vital signs include pulse, respiration, blood pressure, pain, pulse oximetry, and sometimes temperature.

basophil—Type of white blood cell that is an immune cell with granules of histamine released during allergic reactions and asthma.

beta-lactams—Class of broad-spectrum antibiotics, consisting of all antibiotic agents that contain a beta-lactam ring in their molecular structures, including penicillin derivatives (penams), cephalosporins (cephems), monobactams, and carbapenems.

biohazardous materials—Waste contaminated with potentially infectious agents (e.g., blood, body fluids, and human cell lines), or other materials considered a threat to public health or the environment.

biotelemetry—Automated communications process to remotely monitor measurements such as ECG or vital signs from a remote site transmitted wirelessly to receiving equipment.

blanching—Applying gentle pressure on an area of skin (usually fingernails) causes the skin to turn a lighter shade before resuming its natural color. Abnormal findings indicate a temporary obstruction of blood flow or poor perfusion.

blowout fracture—Deformity of orbital floor, typically resulting from blunt trauma; results in inability to look upward.

bodily fluids—Liquids that originate from inside the body, including blood, urine, saliva, and sputum.

bolus—The administration of a discrete amount of medication or drug within a specific time in order to raise its concentration in the blood to an effective level.

bradyarrhythmia—Abnormal rhythm with a heart rate under 60 beats per minute (bpm) in an adult.

Brugada syndrome—An inherited disorder of cardiac electrophysiology causing an increased risk of syncope and sudden death.

buckling effect—When the vertebral column receives an axial load that is greater than the force it can structurally withstand, the force must be dissipated, causing a disruption within the column at the weakest point.

cachexia (wasting syndrome)—Loss of weight, muscle atrophy, fatigue, weakness, and significant loss of appetite in someone who is not actively trying to lose weight.

Canadian C-Spine Rule—A set of guidelines that clinicians and emergency medical personnel use to determine if a cervical spine injury is present.

carbapenems—Antibiotics used for the treatment of infections known or suspected to be caused by multidrug-resistant (MDR) bacteria, primarily used for people who are hospitalized.

cardiac channelopathies—Congenital or acquired diseases relating to disturbed function of cardiac muscle cell ion channel subunits or the proteins that regulate them.

cardiac output—The amount of blood the heart pumps through the circulatory system in a minute; determined by stroke volume and heart rate.

cardiomyopathy—A disease of the myocardium causing functional impairment in which the left ventricular walls are hypertrophied (thickened) without an obvious cause. A major cause of sudden cardiac death.

catastrophic injury—A severe injury to the spine, spinal cord, brain, severe fractures, and may include other injuries or illnesses causing permanent injury or death.

catheter—Flexible tube inserted through a narrow opening into a body cavity for removing fluid, particularly the bladder.

cauda equina—A bundlelike structure of spinal nerve fibers that extends caudally (inferiorly); often referred to as "tail-like" structure. Hence the name; *cauda equina* is Latin for "horse's tail."

chief complaint—The primary symptom that a patient states as the reason for seeking medical care.

closed-ended questions—Questions answered with a simple "yes" or "no," or with a specific piece of information.

closed fracture—A fracture that does not penetrate the surrounding skin.

coagulation—The process of blood changing from a liquid to a gel, forming a blood clot and resulting in hemostasis.

coagulopathy—Literally "bleeding disorder," an impaired ability of the blood to coagulate (form clots), causing a tendency toward prolonged or excessive bleeding.

collaborative health care—Also known as integrated health care, the concept of bringing together providers, delivery, management, and organization of health care services related to diagnosis, treatment, care, rehabilitation, and health promotion.

collaborative practice—*See* **interprofessional practice**.

collateral circulation—An alternate circulatory pathway through adjacent blood vessels when a major vein or artery is impaired or obstructed.

colonized—When a disease-causing organism is present in or on the body but is not causing illness. A HCP can be colonized and become a carrier and spread infection to other health care workers and patients.

comminution—Many fragments.

Commission on Accreditation of Athletic Training Education (CAATE)—Accrediting agency verifying that academic programs instruct the competencies within the curriculum. Eligibility for the AT certification exam is contingent upon completion of an accredited program.

commotio cordis—Latin for "agitation of the heart," is an often lethal disruption of heart rhythm resulting from a direct blow to the precordial region at a critical time during the cardiac cycle, causing cardiac arrest.

communicable disease—Condition or illness that can be spread from one person or species to another.

community care—Clinic that provides access to high-quality, affordable, and comprehensive primary and preventive medical, dental, and mental health care often to medically underserved and uninsured people.

compartment syndrome—Increased pressure within a fascial compartment (lower leg, upper extremity or abdomen) that obstructs capillary blood flow or tissue perfusion. Acute compartment syndrome is a medical emergency.

conflict of interest—A situation in which a person or organization is involved in multiple interests, financial or otherwise, one of which could possibly corrupt the motivation or decision-making of that individual or organization.

continuous quality improvement—Programs and strategies that help an institution or organization improve efficiency, health care quality, and patient outcomes.

contrecoup injury—Head injury; occurs on the side opposite the site of impact.

conus medullaris—Tapered, distal end of the spinal cord.

cosmesis—Preservation, restoration, or bestowing beauty, such as a surgical correction of a disfiguring defect or cosmetic improvements made by a surgeon following incisions.

coup injury—Head injury; occurs under the site of impact.

covered entity—A provider of health care services and any other person or organization that furnishes, bills, or is paid for health care in the normal course of business. Health care providers (e.g., physicians, hospitals, and clinics) are covered entities if they transmit health information in electronic form in connection with a transaction for which a HIPAA standard has been adopted.

crepitus—Grinding, creaking, or grating sound or sensation produced by friction between bone and cartilage or the fractured parts of a bone. Crepitus is also found in severe cases of tendinitis.

cricoid pressure (also Sellick's maneuver)—A technique used in endotracheal intubation to reduce the risk of regurgitation.

critical—Patient presents with symptoms of a life-threatening illness or injury with a high probability of mortality if immediate intervention is not begun to prevent further airway, respiratory, hemodynamic, and/or neurologic instability.

critical incident—Any event outside the usual experience that is emotionally distressing (e.g., evokes reactions of intense fear, helplessness, or horror) and may involve a perceived threat to one's own safety or the safety of someone else.

crystalloid—A solution that contains water, electrolytes, and in some cases dextrose; may be hypotonic, isotonic, or hypertonic in its makeup with respect to body fluids.

cultural competence—An attitude of respect and awareness for patients from cultures different from the HCP's own.

cyanosis or **cyanotic**—Bluish discoloration of skin, nail beds and mucous membranes caused by decreased local circulation or decreased oxygen saturation of the blood.

debridement—Removing dead, damaged, or infected tissue to improve the healing potential of the remaining viable (healthy) tissue.

decerebrate—Position in which arms are adducted and extended, wrist and fingers flexed, neck extended, with feet often in plantar flexion. This position indicates an injury to the upper brain stem.

decorticate—Position in which arms are flexed with fingers flexed, legs extended, and feet plantar flexed. This position is indicative of severe brain injury.

deep vein thrombosis (DVT)—Clotting of blood in a deep vein of an extremity (usually calf or thigh) or the pelvis, it is the primary cause of pulmonary embolism.

dehiscence—Complication in which a wound ruptures along a surgical incision. Risk factors include age, collagen disorders, diabetes, obesity, poor knotting or grabbing of stitches, and trauma to the wound after surgery.

dens—The most pronounced feature on cervical vertebra 2; allows for lateral rotation of the head. Also called the odontoid process.

dermographism—Literally "skin writing," the most common form of physical urticaria with an exaggerated whealing tendency when the skin is stroked; also called dermatographic urticaria or dermatographism.

diagnostic peritoneal lavage (DPL)—A procedure to determine the presence of blood within the peritoneal cavity. It involves inserting a catheter below the umbilicus and withdrawing fluid to assess for blood.

diaphoresis or **diaphoretic**—Profuse perspiration or covered with sweat.

diaphoretic—Pertaining to sweating.

differential diagnosis—The process of differentiating between 2 or more conditions that present similar clinical signs and symptoms.

dislocation—One bone being forced out of its proper alignment completely.

disposition—General attitude or mood, tendency to act or think in a particular way, or tendency to develop a disease or condition.

disseminated intravascular coagulation (DIC)—Condition in which small blood clots develop throughout the bloodstream, blocking small blood vessels. The increased clotting depletes the platelets and clotting factors needed to control bleeding, causing excessive bleeding.

distracting injury—An injury that initially draws the patients' pain/attention away from another, potentially more serious injury. It is an injury that "distracts" the patient who may not realize that he or she has another injury.

diuresis—Physiologic process of increased urine production in the kidneys as part of homeostatic maintenance of body fluid balance.

dorsal root—Transmits sensory nerve signals forming the afferent portion of the spinal nerve (posterior root ganglion).

drop foot—Condition (transient or permanent) in which the patient cannot perform dorsiflexion. Plantar flexion is intact.

Dunphy's sign—A sign including right-sided abdominal pain, which can be associated with coughing, that can indicate appendicitis.

dysphagia—Difficulty swallowing.

dysphonia—Speech difficulty.

dyspnea—Shortness of breath; difficult or labored breathing.

dysrhythmia—Medical condition causing irregular heart rate. *See also* **arrhythmia**.

ecchymosis—Collection of blood under the skin; bruise.

edema—Fluid retention, may be systemic or localized.

electronic health record (EHR)—A longitudinal electronic record of patient health information generated by one or more encounters in any care delivery setting. EHRs typically contain information such as the patient's demographics, contact information, vital signs, allergies, medical history, current and past medications, immunizations, radiology reports, and laboratory data.

electronic medical record (EMR)—Digital version of the traditional paper-based medical record. The EMR represents a medical record within a single facility, such as a doctor's office or a clinic.

embolism—Lodging of an embolus (especially in an artery) causing occlusion, infarction, and tissue death as a result of blocking the blood supply.

embolus—Blood clot (**thrombus**) or other blockage-causing piece of material, such as a fat globule (fat embolism), bubble of air or other gas (gas embolism), inside a blood vessel.

emergency action plan (EAP)—A written document required by particular OSHA standards [29 CFR 1910.38(a)] with the purpose of facilitating and organizing employer and employee actions during workplace emergencies.

emergency medical services (EMS)—Also known as emergency medical systems, it is a local, regional, state, or national organization of emergency medical personnel, equipment, and supplies designed to function in a coordinated fashion.

emergency physician—A specialist who typically works at an emergency department to care for acutely ill patients and provides advanced cardiac life support, trauma care such as fractures and soft tissue injuries, and management of other life-threatening situations.

emergent—Patient presents with symptoms of an illness or injury that may progress in severity or result in complications with a high probability for morbidity if treatment is not begun quickly.

emesis—Vomiting.

emotional intelligence—Recognizing one's own and other people's emotions and using this information to guide thinking and behavior and adjust emotions based on the situation or setting.

enteral route—Delivery of medications through gastrointestinal system.

envenomation—Process by which venom is injected by the bite (or sting) of a venomous animal.

eosinophilic esophagitis—Also called allergic esophagitis, an allergic inflammatory condition of the esophagus that involves eosinophils, a type of white blood cell. Symptoms are swallowing difficulty, food impaction, vomiting, and heartburn.

epidemiology—Characterization of injury occurrence, identification of risk factors, and the strength of effect of those factors, as well as potentially protective factors related to the development and evaluation of injury prevention strategies and programs.

epinephrine—Medication that is the first-line treatment for anaphylaxis.

epinephrine auto-injector—A self-injectable form of epinephrine.

epistaxis—Unexplained or uncontrolled bleeding from the nose.

erythrocyte (red blood cell)—A biconcave disc without a nucleus containing the red-colored pigment hemoglobin that transports oxygen and carbon dioxide to and from the tissues.

exercise-induced anaphylaxis (EIA)—Rare disorder where anaphylaxis occurs after physical activity resulting in pruritus, hives, flushing, wheezing, and GI involvement, including nausea, abdominal cramping, and diarrhea.

exposure control plan (ECP)—Required by the standard precautions ensuring that procedures are in place to protect health care providers from exposures to blood and other body fluids.

exsanguinating hemorrhage—A medical emergency with extensive blood loss due to internal or external bleeding that is enough to cause death.

exsanguination—Sufficient loss of blood to cause death. Not all blood must be lost to cause death.

extension posturing—Also known as decerebrate posturing; a posture in which the patient arches the back and extends arms straight and parallel to the body as a result of compression on the lower brain stem.

extracardiac—Outside the heart.

Family Educational Rights and Privacy Act (FERPA)—Federal law that protects the privacy of student education records and applies to all public schools.

fasciotomy—A procedure where incisions are made into the fascia; the incisions relieve pressure in the affected compartment.

febrile—Presenting with elevated temperature or signs and symptoms of a fever.

field (on-site) diagnosis—Determination of possible causes of patient condition in the prehospital setting by emergency medical service providers.

field triage—Process of decision making to transport injured patients to the appropriate hospital or trauma center.

flexion posturing—Also known as decorticate posturing, a posture in which the patient arches the back and flexes the arms inward as a result of compression on the upper brain stem.

fluid resuscitation (IV fluid therapy)—Volume depletion resulting from fluid lost from the extracellular space. Acute hemorrhage is the leading cause of acute life-threatening intravascular volume loss requiring aggressive fluid resuscitation to maintain tissue perfusion.

fomite—Any nonliving object or substance capable of carrying infectious organisms and hence transferring them from one person to another.

food-dependent exercise-induced anaphylaxis (FDEIA)—Disorder in which anaphylaxis develops when exercise takes place within a few hours of ingesting a specific food. It is the combination of the food and exercise that precipitates attacks, whereas the food and exercise are each tolerated independently.

FOOSH—Acronym for fall on an outstretched hand. Describes the mechanism of injury.

gastroenteritis—Inflammation of the lining of the stomach and intestines, causing an acute onset of severe vomiting and diarrhea.

general counsel—The main lawyer or chief legal officer for an institution, school district company, or governmental department with a primary responsibility of risk management.

general impression—The initial contact with the patient in which the provider gets an overview of the patient's general appearance and level of distress.

germicide—A substance that kills germs or other microorganisms; an antiseptic.

global positioning system (GPS)—A system of satellites, computers, and receivers that is able to determine the precise positional and velocity data and global time synchronization for air, sea, and land travel.

Good Samaritan law—Legal protection for someone who voluntarily renders aid to an injured person during an emergency. The law grants immunity; if an error is made while rendering emergency medical care, there can be no legal liability for damages in court.

gurney—A wheeled stretcher used for transporting hospital patients.

habitus—Physical characteristics of a person, especially appearance and constitution as related to disease.

hand hygiene—Cleaning hands by using handwashing (washing hands with soap and water), antiseptic hand wash, antiseptic hand rub (alcohol-based hand sanitizer including foam or gel), or surgical hand antisepsis.

hazardous material (HAZMAT)—Any item or chemical that, when being transported or moved, is a risk to public safety or the environment.

health care–associated infection (HAI)—Infection from receiving medical treatment in a health care facility—a major, yet preventable, threat to patient safety.

health care informatics—Also known as clinical informatics, the application of informatics and information technology to deliver health care services and management of health data through the use of computers and computer technology.

health care system—Diverse HCPs who collaborate in order to direct their specialized capabilities toward common goals for the patient.

health informatics—Acquiring, storing, retrieving, and using health care information to foster better collaboration among a patient's various HCPs.

Health Insurance Portability and Accountability Act (HIPAA)—U.S. Federal law that sets the standard for protecting sensitive patient data and protected health information.

hemarthrosis—Blood located within the joint space. Potential indication of soft tissue damage within a joint. Typically observed on X-rays or noted when the joint capsule is drained and blood is extracted with joint fluids.

hematemesis—Vomiting fresh blood.

hematochezia—Bloody stools containing bright red blood may indicate bleeding near the external opening of the colon.

hematuria—Blood in the urine. Gross hematuria is visible blood, whereas microscopic hematuria is only discovered via urine analysis or urine dipstick.

hemiparesis—Muscular weakness on one side of the body, often the result of a stroke.

hemodialysis—Also simply called dialysis, it is a process of purifying blood by extracorporeal removal of waste products such as creatinine and urea and free water from the blood when the kidneys are not functioning properly or are in renal failure.

hemoglobin—The iron-containing protein that carries oxygen from the lungs to the tissues.

hemoglobinopathies—Genetic mutations of the hemoglobin molecule resulting in HbS or other disorders.

hemolysis—Rupture or lysis of RBCs (erythrocytes) and the release of their contents (cytoplasm) into surrounding fluid (e.g., blood plasma).

hemolytic anemia—Hereditary or acquired erythrocyte membrane disorders relating to abnormal erythrocyte membrane, cell metabolism, or hemoglobin structure.

hemoptysis—Coughing or spitting up blood, usually from an injury to the lung or respiratory tract.

hemorrhage (bleeding)—Blood loss, especially when copious. Blood loss inside the body is called *internal hemorrhage* and blood loss outside of the body is called *external hemorrhage*.

hemostasis—Process of cessation of blood loss from a damaged vessel.

hepatomegaly—Enlargement of the liver.

high-concentration oxygen—Supplemental oxygen provided to maintain blood oxygen saturation above 95%. Provide 100% oxygen at a flow rate of 10-12 L/min via nasal cannula, non-rebreather mask, or endotracheal tube.

histamine—Produced by basophils and by mast cells found in nearby connective tissues. Increases permeability of the capillaries to white blood cells and some proteins, to allow them to engage pathogens in infected tissues.

hives—*See* **wheals** or **urticaria**.

Homan's sign—Calf discomfort elicited by ankle dorsiflexion with the knee extended that occasionally occurs with distal leg DVT but is neither sensitive nor specific.

host—Organism that harbors a pathogen, providing nourishment and shelter.

hypercapnia—Arterial concentrations of carbon dioxide more than 50 mm Hg, typically caused by inadequate respiration.

hypercoagulable—Excessive blood clotting, or failure to break down and remove clots. May travel through body limiting or blocking blood flow.

hyperglycemia—Excessive glucose in the blood, typically due to diabetes.

hypernatremia—Excessive serum sodium levels, specifically more than 145 mmol/L.

hyperoxemia—Increased oxygen content of the blood.

hypersensitivity reaction—An immune response that leads to tissue injury.

hypertension—Abnormal elevation in blood pressure and a major risk factor for coronary artery disease, stroke, and heart failure. Classified as prehypertension, stage 1 (mild), stage 2 (moderate), and emergency (severe) hypertension.

hypertensive crisis—Emergency with severe elevations in blood pressure (>180/120 mm Hg) associated with evidence of new or worsening organ damage.

hypertrophic cardiomyopathy (HCM)—Condition in which the left ventricle becomes thickened resulting in the heart being less able to pump blood effectively. Complications include heart failure, an irregular heartbeat, and sudden cardiac death.

hypoglycemia—A condition where patients' blood glucose is ≥70 mg/dL.

hyponatremia—A condition whereby the amount of sodium is diluted in the blood, usually caused by overhydration. It can be life-threatening.

hypoperfusion—Decreased blood flow to an organ or tissue.

hypotension—Low blood pressure (<90 mm Hg systolic and 60 mm Hg diastolic). Often normal in trained athletes at rest.

hypothermia—Potentially dangerous decrease in body temperature.

hypovolemic shock—A life-threatening loss of blood, often internal, where 20% or more of the person's blood volume is external to the circulatory system; also termed hemorrhagic shock.

hypoxemia—Abnormally low oxygen level in arterial blood, which can lead to tissue hypoxia.

hypoxia—A decreased level of oxygenation at the cellular level.

iatrogenic pneumothorax—A pneumothorax caused by a medical procedure, such as thoracentesis or central venous catheter insertion.

icterus—*See* **jaundice.**

immunity—Ability of an organism to resist infection by the action of specific antibodies or sensitized white blood cells.

immunoglobulin E antibodies (IgE)—Antibody proteins produced by the immune system's plasma cells with an essential role in type I hypersensitivity.

incident command system (ICS)—Facilitates a consistent response that allows agencies to work together using common terminology and operating procedures controlling personnel, facilities, equipment, and communications at a single incident scene.

index of suspicion—Initial impression of the likelihood of a disease or condition.

infarction—A local area of necrosis (death) due to lack of oxygen. Obstruction of blood flow, commonly due to embolism, thrombosis, artery blockages, rupture, mechanical compression, or vasoconstriction.

infectious disease—Medical condition caused by the growth and spread of small, harmful organisms within the body.

infiltration—Introduction of a parenteral fluid or medication to tissues outside of a vein, resulting from movement of the needle or cannula from within a vein into the surrounding tissue; signs or symptoms include decreased flow rate, swelling, and discomfort at the site.

Institute of Medicine (IOM)—Now recognized as the Health and Medicine Division of the National Academies, it is a U.S. governmental office that provides unbiased, evidence-based, and authoritative information on issues relating to biomedical science, medicine, and health, and serves as an adviser to the nation to improve health.

intensive care unit (ICU) or **critical care unit**—A hospital unit that has special equipment and specially trained personnel for the care of seriously ill patients who require immediate and continuous attention.

interprofessional practice or **collaborative practice**—When multiple HCPs from different professional backgrounds work together with patients, families, caregivers, and communities to deliver the highest quality of care.

intravenous (IV) catheter—A plastic sheath that is inserted over a needle into a vein for supplying medications or nutrients directly into the bloodstream.

ischemia—Inadequate blood supply to an organ or tissue (especially the myocardium), causing a shortage of oxygen and glucose needed for cellular metabolism.

jaundice—Also known as icterus; a yellowish or greenish pigmentation of the skin and sclera of the eyes due to high bilirubin levels. Commonly associated with itchiness, pale feces, or dark urine.

Kehr's sign—Referred pain at the left shoulder from trauma to the spleen.

Kendrick Extrication Device (K.E.D)—Specialized device used for extricating spine-injured patients from places where the traditional long spine board may not fit (e.g., bouldering, gymnastic foam pits, front seats of cars).

ketonuria—Ketones in the urine, suggesting the body is breaking down more readily available sources for fuel rather than glucose. Also called ketoaciduria.

Korotkoff sounds—Blood flow sounds that are heard while taking BP with a sphygmomanometer and stethoscope over the brachial artery in the antecubital fossa. These sounds appear and disappear as the blood pressure cuff is inflated and deflated. Named after Dr. Nikolai Korotkoff, a Russian physician who discovered them in 1905.

Kussmaul breathing—Abnormal deep, fast, and sighing respiration indicating possible diabetic ketoacidosis.

lactated Ringer's (LR) solution—Mixture of sodium chloride, sodium lactate, potassium chloride, and calcium chloride in water. It is used for replacing fluids and electrolytes in those who have low blood volume or low blood pressure.

laparotomy—A surgical incision into the abdomen to access the contents of the cavity; used for exploration, diagnosis, or surgical purposes.

latent infection—A hidden or dormant infection that is asymptomatic but capable of manifesting symptoms under particular circumstances or if activated (*see* **active infection**).

lipohemarthrosis—Radiographic findings of fat infiltration and fluid into the joint capsule. Fat molecules are hydrophobic and therefore separate from the fluid creating 2 layers, observable on radiographic imaging.

log-roll—SMR technique in which the patient is rolled on his side and the long spine board is placed behind him. It has been shown to cause the most motion of all techniques, but it requires the lowest number of people.

long QT syndrome—Also called torsades de pointes, a genetic channelopathy in which a rapid, irregular QRS complex exists on the ECG baseline that may degenerate into ventricular fibrillation.

lucid interval—Temporary improvement in patient with a TBI, after which the patient rapidly deteriorates.

lymphadenopathy (adenopathy, lymphadenitis)—Disease of the lymph nodes, in which they are abnormal in size, number, or consistency. Lymphadenopathy of an inflammatory type (the most common type) is lymphadenitis, producing swollen or enlarged lymph nodes.

malocclusion—Imperfect positioning of teeth when jaws are closed.

Marfan syndrome—A genetic disorder of connective tissue; the most serious complication involves the heart and aorta with an increased risk of mitral valve prolapse and aortic aneurysm.

mass care (or casualty) incident (MCI)—Incident in which emergency medical services resources, such as personnel and equipment, are overwhelmed by the number and severity of casualties.

McBurney's point—Pain one-third of the way between the umbilicus and anterior superior iliac spine of the ilium, indicating possible appendicitis.

mechanism of injury (MOI)—Manner in which a physical injury or tissue damage occurred.

medical oversight—Supervision usually provided by a medical director, typically a physician in emergency medicine or pediatric emergency medicine who is responsible for actions of the emergency care team.

medical specialty—A field of practice focused on specific knowledge and skills required for the prevention, diagnosis, and management of a particular condition.

melena—Black, foul-smelling, tarry stool that contains digested blood.

menorrhagia—Excessive or prolonged menstrual blood flow.

methicillin—An antibiotic that is a beta-lactam and semi-synthetic derivative of penicillin, formerly used in the treatment of bacterial infections caused by *Staphylococcus* bacteria, which have become resistant to commonly used penicillin-related antibiotics (e.g., methicillin-resistant *S. aureus*, or MRSA).

microbess—Relating to a microorganism (e.g., bacterium) causing disease.

modified Trendelenburg position—Position in which a person is supine with the feet elevated 15°-30° above the heart as a means of reducing intra-abdominal pressure and facilitating venous return to the heart. It is used as a treatment for shock.

multidrug-resistant organisms (MDROs)—Microorganism with resistance to multiple antibiotics that pose a serious threat for hospitalized patients.

multiperson lift and slide—Formerly called the 6+ person lift or the lift and slide, this technique has demonstrated the least amount of motion in the severely injured spine, but it requires the greatest number of personnel.

multiple organ failure (MOF)—Severe, life-threatening condition that develops subsequent to an acute injury or illness and characterized by a hypometabolic, immunodepressed state with clinical and biochemical evidence of decreased functioning of the body's organ systems.

myocardial infarction—A heart attack; literally, it means the death of the heart muscle.

myoclonic jerking—Uncontrollable jumps, jolts, twitches, jerks, or other seizurelike activities caused by sudden muscle contractions (positive myoclonus) or brief lapses of contraction (negative myoclonus).

myoglobin—Oxygen-binding protein in muscle tissue that is only found in the bloodstream after muscle injury. It is an abnormal finding, and it can be diagnostically relevant when found in blood or urine (*see* **myoglobinuria**).

myoglobinuria—Presence of myoglobin in the urine, usually associated with rhabdomyolysis or muscle destruction.

NaCl—The chemical abbreviations for sodium (Na) and chloride (Cl); together they form salt.

nature of illness (NOI)—Expression of an illness or disease and its meaning(s) to the patient and significant others.

nebulized—Turned into fine mist.

needlestick injury—*See* **percutaneous exposure incident**.

nephrectomy—Surgical removal of a kidney.

NEXUS criteria—An algorithm used by emergency medical personnel and clinicians to determine if cervical spine radiographs are warranted.

non-rebreather mask—A soft mask that conforms to the tissues of the face; when connected to an oxygen supply, it delivers 60-100% inspired supplemental oxygen.

normal saline (NS)—*See* **saline**.

nosocomial—Of or pertaining to a hospital, especially infections acquired in the hospital setting.

notice of privacy practices—Pamphlet or brochure that focuses on privacy issues and concerns, prompting people to have discussions with their health care providers and exercise their rights.

obtundation—State or condition characterized by a reduced level of consciousness with diminished responsiveness to stimuli.

occult—Hidden or concealed.

occupational exposure—Reasonably anticipated skin, eye, mucous membrane, or parenteral contact with blood or other potentially infectious materials (OPIM) that may result from the performance of the employee's duties.

oliguria—Diminished urine output in relation to fluid intake.

open-ended question—A question phrased as a statement requiring a thoughtful and detailed response rather than a one-word response.

open fracture—Often called a compound fracture, a fracture that results in a wound to the skin, exposing the underlying soft tissue or osseous tissue to the external environment.

oral immunotherapy (OIT)—Regular administration of small amounts of allergen (food) by mouth; also called oral desensitization.

orchiectomy—Surgical removal of a testicle.

OSHA—Occupational Safety and Health Administration; a U.S. agency that regulates health and safety in the workplace.

osmotic demyelination syndrome—Previously termed central pontine myelinolysis, neurological damage in the brain stem, often the result of overly aggressive correction of hyponatremia.

other potentially infectious materials (OPIM)—Any body fluid that is visibly contaminated with blood and all body fluids in situations where it is difficult or impossible to differentiate between body fluids.

outpatient care—*See* **ambulatory care**.

Paget-Schroetter syndrome (effort thrombosis)—Medical condition involving upper-extremity deep vein thrombosis (DVT) in which blood clots form in the deep veins of the arms, usually in the axillary or subclavian veins.

palliation—To make something less painful or harmful.

parenteral route—Delivery of medications outside the gastrointestinal system, usually through injection or insertion of an indwelling catheter.

patent airway—Open pathway for gas exchange between a patient's lungs and the atmosphere.

pathogen—An agent that causes infection or disease, especially a microorganism, such as a bacterium, virus, or fungus.

patient care report (PCR)—Document of all patient care and pertinent patient information that serves as a method for data collection.

patient-centered care or **participatory care**—Process in which both the patient and HCP contribute to the medical decision-making process. HCPs explain treatments and alternatives to patients to provide the necessary resources for patients to choose the treatment option that best aligns with their unique cultural and personal beliefs.

patient presentation—Organized account of the patient's history and physical examination.

pectus excavatum—Also known as sunken chest or funnel chest, a congenital deformity of the chest in which the sternum and ribs are concave (caved in) on the anterior thorax.

percutaneous—Access via a needle puncture (or other approved puncture device) that does not include surgical access using a scalpel.

percutaneous exposure incident—Also called **needlestick injury**, the penetration of skin by a needle or other sharp object, which was in contact with blood, tissue, or other body fluid before the exposure.

percutaneous technique—Delivery of medication through the skin.

perfusion—Circulation of blood within an organ or tissue with adequate amounts of oxygen and nutrients to meet the cells' needs.

petechiae—Small intradermal or mucosal hemorrhages.

pneumatic antishock garment (PASG)—A medical compression garment used to treat severe blood loss to improve survival for people with trauma; they are controversial and may worsen outcomes. Also known as medical antishock trousers (MAST).

positive feedback—Process in which small disturbances become larger, causing further change in the same direction.

positive-pressure ventilation—Ventilation provided using a tight-fitting mask that covers the nose or both the nose and mouth.

post-concussive syndrome—Complex disorder characterized by continuation of concussion symptoms for weeks and even months after the initial injury.

post-phlebitic syndrome—Medical condition that may occur as a long-term complication of deep vein thrombosis (DVT).

post-traumatic stress disorder (PTSD)—A mental disorder that can develop after a person is exposed to a traumatic event, such warfare, violent personal assault such as rape, or other life-threatening events. Symptoms may include disturbing thoughts, feelings, or dreams related to the events, mental or physical distress to trauma-related cues, attempts to avoid trauma-related cues, and an increase in the fight-or-flight response.

practice act—A statute defining scope of practice defined by each state's licensure laws. In athletic training, the entire practice act, including accompanying rules, constitutes the law governing athletic training practice within a state.

prehospital care report—*See* **patient care report.**

premonitory symptoms—Also called prodrome, an early symptoms indicating the onset of a disease or illness

primacy of the patient—Advocating for the patient's best interests and well-being and protecting the patient from undue harm.

primary care—The day-to-day health care by a HCP that is usually the first contact for patients within a health care system.

Privacy Rule—*See also* **Health Insurance Portability and Accountability Act (HIPAA)**. National standard for protection of individuals' medical records and other personal health information and applies to health plans, health care facilities, and health care providers that conduct health care transactions electronically.

protected health information (PHI)—Any information about health status, provision of health care, or payment for health care that can be linked to a specific person.

protocol—A set of instructions describing the process to follow. Also, a medical guideline for investigating a particular set of findings in a patient or method to control a certain disease.

pruritus—Severe skin itching.

psychological first aid (PFA)—A technique used by mental health and disaster response workers to help people of all ages in the immediate aftermath of a catastrophic incident, campus violence, natural disaster, or terrorism.

ptosis—Droopy upper eyelid.

pulmonary embolism—Sudden blockage of a major artery in the lung by a blood clot.

pulse points—Areas of the body where the heart rate can be palpated by compressing an artery against a bone. The most common pulse points are the radial and carotid pulse; however distal sensation is often palpated at the posterior tibial artery or brachial artery.

pulseless electric activity (PEA)—Also known as electromechanical dissociation, PEA is a form of cardiac arrest in which an abnormal heart rhythm and electrical activity are observed on ECG, but the heart is unable to generate a pulse and supply blood to the body.

purpura—Larger areas of mucosal or skin hemorrhage.

pyrogenic reaction—Sudden onset of fever, chills, backache, headache, nausea, and vomiting as a result of being exposed to foreign proteins, such as those found in bacteria or fungi.

recumbence—Lying in the supine position or on the back.

regulation—A rule or a statute that prescribes the management, governance, or operating parameters for a given group. It tends to be a function of administrative agencies to which a legislative body has delegated authority to promulgate rules or regulations. Most regulations are intended to protect the public health, safety, and welfare.

reprocessing—Sterilization, disinfection, or cleaning of a reusable medical device.

respiratory arrest—An absence of breathing; apnea.

respiratory distress—Difficulty breathing resulting in increased effort to maintain adequate ventilation and oxygenation.

respiratory failure—Inability to maintain adequate ventilation and oxygenation.

return of spontaneous circulation (ROSC)—Resumption of sustained perfusing cardiac activity associated with significant respiratory effort after cardiac arrest, often after CPR and AED have been administered. Signs include breathing, coughing, or movement and a palpable pulse or a measurable BP.

return to participation or **return to play (RTP)**—A decision to allow a patient to resume physical activity. Responsibility for this decision lies with the medical director or team physician and is often implemented by an athletic trainer.

Reye's syndrome—Emergency illness, primarily affecting children and teenagers, that targets the body's organs. Most severe effects are to the liver and brain, presenting with rapid severe neurological impairments or symptoms. While the cause is unknown, the condition is often associated with aspirin use during fever, therefore aspirin is not recommended for treatment of fever in patients under 19 years of age.

rhabdomyolysis—Condition with rapid breakdown of damaged skeletal muscle.

rhinorrhea—Condition in in which the nasal cavity fills mucus fluid and is a common symptom of allergies (hay fever) or certain diseases such as the common cold; also known as runny nose.

risk management—Identification, assessment, and application of resources to minimize, monitor, and control the probability and impact of unfortunate events.

SAC—Space available for the spinal cord. The cerebrospinal fluid space around the spinal cord.

saline—Also normal saline (NS) or sodium chloride injection, a sterile, nonpyrogenic solution for fluid and electrolyte replenishment in single-dose containers for intravenous administration.

scoop stretcher—Rigid device used to pick up injured patient off ground and place on secondary SMR device.

scope of practice—Defined parameters of various duties or services that may be provided by a person with specific credentials. Whether regulated by rule, statute, or court decision, it represents the limits of services a person may legally perform.

second impact syndrome—Condition in which a second concussion occurs prior to a first concussion completely resolving, causing rapid and severe decompensation of the patient.

seesaw breathing—Breathing pattern with complete (or partial) airway obstruction during which the patient's diaphragm descends, causing the abdomen to lift and the chest to sink. When the diaphragm relaxes, the process is reversed.

Segond sign—Avulsion fracture of the lateral tibial condyle and may indicate injury to the anterior cruciate ligament.

self-awareness—Being aware of one's self through examination of one's emotional reactions; and understanding how one's attitudes, perceptions, past and present experiences, and relationships create a lens through which one sees the world and the people in it.

sensitization—Induction of an allergic response.

sepsis—Potentially life-threatening complication of an infection in which chemicals released into the bloodstream to fight the infection trigger inflammatory responses throughout the body.

serial vitals—Periodic monitoring of vital signs, most commonly to include blood pressure, heart rate, respiratory rate, and pulse oximetry.

sharps—Medical devices with sharp points or edges that can puncture or cut skin (e.g., needles, scalpels).

shock—Also called *circulatory shock*, it is a life-threatening medical condition in which low blood perfusion to tissues results in cellular injury and inadequate tissue function. Signs of shock include hypotension, tachycardia, weak pulse, and signs of poor end-organ perfusion (e.g., confusion, loss of consciousness).

shunting—Redirecting blood, usually by constriction of smooth muscle in arterioles.

sickle cell disease (anemia)—A hemoglobinopathy that causes a chronic hemolytic anemia. The disease occurs almost exclusively in black people and is caused by homozygous inheritance of HbS. Sickle-shaped RBCs cause vaso-occlusion and are prone to hemolysis, leading to severe pain crises, organ ischemia, and other systemic complications. Prognosis is poor; however, with treatment, the life span of homozygous patients is more than 50 years. Common causes of death are acute chest syndrome, intercurrent infections, pulmonary emboli, infarction of a vital organ, and renal failure.

sign—Objective evidence of disease that can be detected by someone other than the individual affected by the disease.

sinus bradycardia—A normal sinus rhythm in which the heart rate is low—less than 60 bpm. Highly conditioned athletes often have sinus bradycardia as a result of training in which the heart contraction is more efficient and produces a greater cardiac output with each heartbeat.

sinus rhythm—Also called normal sinus rhythm (NSR), it is the normal cardiac rhythm in which myocardial depolarization begins at the sinus node. Characterized by the presence of correctly oriented P waves on the ECG resulting in the normal heart rate (60-100 bpm in adults).

situational awareness—Ability to identify, process, and comprehend critical elements of information about what is happening in an emergency situation.

somnolence—A strong desire for sleep or sleeping for unusually long periods.

spinal motion restriction (SMR)—The cumulative processes of securing a patient with a suspected spine injury to a rigid immobilization device. Formally referred to as *spinal immobilization*.

splenectomy—Surgical removal of the spleen.

splenomegaly—Enlargement of the spleen.

standard precautions—Minimum infection prevention practices that apply to all patient care, regardless of suspected or confirmed infection status of the patient, in any setting where health care is delivered.

sterilization—Process that eliminates, removes, kills, or deactivates all forms of life and other microbial agents (bacteria, viruses) present in a specified region, such as a surface, a volume of fluid, or medication.

straddle lift and slide—A SMR technique typically used on smaller patients because the rescuers straddle/stand over the patient to lift her. The technique is very similar to the multiperson lift and slide.

subcutaneous—Tissue in the fatty layer that is below the skin and above the muscle.

subcutaneous emphysema—Air under the skin of the chest wall; caused by chest trauma.

subluxation—Occurs when one bone is forced out of its proper alignment completely, but it reduces on its own.

sudden arrhythmic death syndrome (SADS)—Also called sudden adult death syndrome or sudden unexpected death syndrome (SUDS), it is sudden unexpected death of adolescents and adults sometimes associated with channelopathies including long QT syndrome, Brugada syndrome, and catecholaminergic polymorphic ventricular tachycardia.

suture—A stitch.

symptom—Subjective evidence of disease that is experienced by the individual affected by the disease.

syncope—Also called *fainting* or *passing out*, a temporary loss of consciousness and muscle posture, characterized by a fast onset, short duration, and spontaneous recovery. Often as a result of hypotension and temporary insufficient blood flow to the brain.

syndesmotic joint—Joint that has a strong and tight articulation via strong fibrous tissue only allowing for minimal movement between the articulations.

systemic inflammatory response syndrome (SIRS)—Serious, potentially life-threatening condition related to sepsis where there is pathophysiological systemic inflammation, organ dysfunction, and organ failure.

systems thinking—A business management discipline that concerns an understanding of a system by examining the linkages and interactions between the components that comprise the entirety of that defined system.

tachyarrhythmia—Rapid irregular heartbeat.

tachycardia—Rapid heart rate, usually defined as more than 100 beats per minute in adults.

tachypnea—Abnormally rapid breathing rate, more than 20 breaths/min in adults.

talar dome—Superior surface of the talus that articulates with the distal end of the tibia (tibial plafond).

team-based health care—Provision of health services to individuals, families, and their communities by at least two health providers who work collaboratively with patients and their caregivers to accomplish shared goals and achieve coordinated, high-quality care.

telangiectasias—Small dilated blood vessels near the surface of the skin or mucous membranes, measuring between 0.5 and 1 mm in diameter; spider veins.

tetraplegia—Quadriplegia; paralysis of all 4 extremities.

therapeutic behaviors—Interpersonal communication skills that are consciously applied by the HCP in both verbal and nonverbal ways.

thermistor thermometer—A thermometer with a flexible measuring unit that remains in a patient until desired core temperature is reached.

thrombi—Many blood clots, or a group of clots; the plural of thrombus.

thrombocytopenia—Low blood platelet count.

thrombosis—Formation of a blood clot that obstructs the flow of blood through a blood vessel.

thrombus (clot)—Final product of blood coagulation in hemostasis. A healthy response to injury to prevent bleeding (as opposed to a harmful **thrombosis**).

thunderclap—Sudden severe headache, often described as "the worst headache."

tibial plafond—Distal articular portion of the tibia.

transmission—Passing a pathogen-causing communicable disease from an infected host to an individual to cause infection.

traumatic event—An incident that causes physical, emotional, spiritual, or psychological harm. The person experiencing the distressing event may feel threatened, anxious, or frightened and will need support and time to recover and regain emotional and mental stability.

triage—The process of determining the priority of patients' treatments based on the severity of their condition.

Triple Aim—A framework developed by the Institute for Healthcare Improvement that describes an approach to optimizing health system performance.

tripod position—In a patient experiencing respiratory distress (or when an athlete is winded or out of breath), the person sits or stands leaning forward supporting the upper body with hands on the knees or another surface.

turgor—Elasticity of the skin or its ability to change shape and return to normal.

type I hypersensitivity reaction—Also known as immediate hypersensitivity, an allergic reaction provoked by reexposure to a specific allergen.

unsecured PHI—An impermissible use or disclosure under the Privacy Rule that compromises the security or privacy of the protected health information.

urticaria—A skin rash triggered by a reaction to food, medicine, or other irritants. Symptoms include itchy, raised, red, or skin-colored welts on the skin's surface; also known as **hives**.

UTI—Urinary tract infection. An infection along the urinary tract that includes the ureters, urethra, and urinary bladder.

vaccine—A substance used to stimulate the production of antibodies and provide immunity against one or several diseases. Usually an agent resembling a disease-causing microorganism or a weakened or dead form of a microbe.

Valsalva maneuver—Attempting to exhale with the nostrils and mouth, or the glottis closed, increasing intrathoracic pressure, as when bracing to lift a heavy object or blowing up a balloon.

vancomycin—Antimicrobial drug often used to treat infections caused by enterococci.

vasoconstriction—Narrowing of the blood vessels resulting from contraction of the muscular wall and increasing blood pressure.

vaso-occlusion (vaso-occlusive crisis)—Occurs when the microcirculation is obstructed by sickled RBCs, resulting in an infarction, ischemic tissue injury, and pain.

venipuncture—A procedure in which a needle is inserted into the lumen of a vein.

venous thromboembolism (VTE)—A blood clot that starts in a vein. *See also* **deep vein thrombosis** and **pulmonary embolism**.

ventral root—Transmits motor nerve signals forming the efferent portion of the spinal nerve (anterior root ganglion).

ventricular fibrillation (V-fib, VF)—An arrhythmia in which uncoordinated myocardial contraction in ventricles causes quivering rather than properly contracting. This uncoordinated contraction of the ventricles causes significantly reduced cardiac output and cardiac arrest.

ventricular tachycardia (V-tach, VT)—A potentially life-threatening arrhythmia in which improper cardiac electrical activity causes tachycardia starting in the ventricles. May lead to ventricular fibrillation, asystole, and sudden death.

vertebral foramen—The space or canal through which the spinal cord passes.

violation—Deliberate deviation from an operating procedure, standard, or rule.

vital signs—Most commonly includes blood pressure, heart rate, respiratory rate, and pulse oximetry.

Volkmann's contracture—A flexion contracture, more commonly observed in the upper extremity, is the result of prolonged vascular obstruction. Hallmark sign is a clawlike deformity of the wrist, hand, and fingers. Passive extension of fingers is restricted.

wheals—Dermal edema or fluid collected in the layer of skin below the surface, temporarily raising the skin, typically reddened, and usually accompanied by itching; also called **hives**.

willful neglect—Conscious, intentional failure or reckless indifference to the obligation to comply with the administrative simplification provision violated.

within normal limits (WNL)—No abnormal results occurred during testing.

Wolff-Parkinson-White syndrome (WPW)—A disorder of the cardiac electrical system caused by an abnormal accessory electrical conduction pathway between the atria and the ventricles.

REFERENCES

CAATE STANDARDS

1. BOC Standards of Professional Practice. Board of Certification website. www.bocatc.org/system/document_versions/versions/69/original/boc-standards-of-professional-practice-2018- 20171113.pdf?1510606441. Published October 2017. Accessed February 1, 2018.

CHAPTER 1

1. Gawande A. Cowboys and Pit Crews. *The New Yorker.* 2011; https://www.newyorker.com/news/news-desk/cowboys-and-pit-crews. Accessed September 28, 2018.

2. Mitchell P, Wynia M, Golden R, et al. *Core Principles and Values of Effective Team-Based Health Care.* Washington, DC: Institute of Medicine. 2012.

3. Gilbert JH, Yan J, Hoffman SJ. A WHO report: Framework for action on interprofessional education and collaborative practice. *J Allied Health.* 2010;39 Suppl 1:196-197.

4. Agency for Healthcare Research and Quality. TeamSTEPPS 2.0 Curriculum Guide. 2010. https://www.ahrq.gov/teamstepps/index.html.

5. Bodenheimer T. Building teams in primary care: Lessons learned. 2007. www.chcf.org/~/media/MEDIA%20LIBRARY%20Files/PDF/PDF%20B/PDF%20BuildingTeamsInPrimaryCareLessons.pdf. Accessed March 23, 2017.

6. Interprofessional Education Collaborative. Core competencies for interprofessional collaborative practice: 2016 update. 2016. https://nebula.wsimg.com/2f68a39520b03336b41038c370497473?AccessKeyId=DC06780E69ED19E2B3A5&disposition=0&alloworigin=1. Accessed September 12, 2018.

7. Alastair B. Crossing the Quality Chasm: A New Health System for the 21st Century. Washington, DC: Institute of Medicine; 2001.

8. The Modern Nurse. The importance of interprofessional collaboration in healthcare. 2016. https://www.discovernursing.com/nursing-notes/importance-interprofessional-collaboration-healthcare#.WNUmFVUrJhG. Accessed March 24, 2017.

9. Board of Certification. Standards of professional practice. 2017. http://www.bocatc.org/athletic-trainers. Accessed September 12, 2018.

10. Courson R, Goldenberg M, Adams KG, et al. Inter-association consensus statement on best practices for sports medicine management for secondary schools and colleges. *J Athl Train.* 2014;49(1):128-137.

11. Scheid D. Room for change. *NATA News.* 2011; March:10-13.

12. Laursen RM. A patient-centered model for delivery of athletic training services. *Athl Ther Today.* 2010;15(3):1-3.

13. Herring SA, Kibler WB, Putukian M. Team physician consensus statement: 2013 update. *Med Sci Sports Exerc.* 2013;45(8):1618-1622.

14. National Highway Traffic Safety Administration. Emergency medical responder scope of practice. 2004. https://www.nremt.org/rwd/public/document/emr. Accessed March 29, 2017.

15. American College of Emergency Physicians. Definition of emergency medicine. 2017. https://www.acep.org/patient-care/policy-statements/definition-of-emergency-medicine/#sm.0001dplf3yu97ewkxls26j8lpbwfv. Accessed April 1, 2017.

16. Kellermann A. The future of emergency care in the United States. *Med Gen Med.* 2006;8(3):36-36.

17. Kellermann AL. Defining the future of emergency care. *Ann Emerg Med.* 2006;48(2):135-137.

18. World Health Organization. Patient safety curriculum guide. Multi-professional patient safety curriculum guide. 2012. www.who.int/patientsafety/education/curriculum/Curriculum_Tools/en. Accessed March 30, 2017.

19. Kaldy J. Safe patient transitions: Getting patients safely from one health care setting to the next requires diligent communications among providers. *Provider.* 2008; 34:22-35.

20. Institute for Healthcare Improvement. SBAR technique for communication: A situational briefing model. www.ihi.org/resources/Pages/Tools/SBARTechniqueforCommunicationASituationalBriefingModel.aspx. Accessed March 4, 2017.

21. Boyle DK, Kochinda C. Enhancing collaborative communication of nurse and physician leadership in two intensive care units. *J Nurs Adm.* 2004;34(2):60-70.

22. WHO. Patient safety curriculum guide—Multi-professional. 2011. http://www.who.int/patientsafety/education/mp_curriculum_guide/en/. Accessed September 12, 2018.

23. NATA. Code of Ethics. 2016. www.nata.org/membership/about-membership/member-resources/code-of-ethics. Accessed July 12, 2017.

24. Commission on Accreditation of Athletic Training Education. CAATE athletic training education competencies, 6th ed. 2018. https://caate.net/wp-content/uploads/2014/06/5th-Edition-Competencies.pdf. Accessed April 29, 2015.

25. College of Nurses of Ontario. Therapeutic nurse-client relationship practice standards. 2006. www.cno.org/globalassets/docs/prac/41033_therapeutic.pdf. Accessed September 12, 2018.

26. Nurses Association of New Brunswick. Standards for the therapeutic nurse-client relationship. 2015. www.nanb.nb.ca/media/resource/NANB-StandardsOfPractice-RegisteredNurses-2012-E.pdf. Accessed March 22, 2017.

27. Pollack A, Beck R. *Advanced Emergency Care and Transportation of the Sick and Injured.* Sudbury, MA: Jones and Bartlett; 2012.

28. Stickley T. From SOLER to SURETY for effective non-verbal communication. *Nurse Educ Pract.* 2011;11(6):395-398.

29. Mayer JD, Roberts RD, Barsade SG. Human abilities: Emotional intelligence. *Annu Rev Psychol.* 2008;59:507-536.

30. Patak L, Wilson-Stronks A, Costello J, et al. Improving patient-provider communication: A call to action. *J Nurs Adm.* 2009;39(9):372-376.

CHAPTER 2

1. Courson R, Goldenberg M, Adams KG, et al. Inter-association consensus statement on best practices for sports medicine management for secondary schools and colleges. *J Athl Train.* 2014;49(1):128-137.

2. International Organization for Standardization. Risk management—Principles and guidelines. 2009. https://www.iso.org/obp/ui/#iso:std:iso:31000:ed-1:v1:en. Accessed July 31, 2017.

3. Board of Certification Inc. BOC facility principles. 2013. http://www.bocatc.org/. Accessed April 10, 2016.

4. Centers for Disease Control and Prevention. Recommended vaccines for healthcare workers. 2017. https://www.cdc.gov/vaccines/adults/rec-vac/hcw.html. Accessed April 25, 2017.

5. Collaborators on Mortality and Causes of Death. Global, regional, and national age-sex specific all-cause and cause-specific mortality for 240 causes of death, 1990-2013: A systematic analysis for the Global Burden of Disease Study 2013. *Lancet Infect Dis.* 2014;385(9963):117-171.

6. Centers for Disease Control and Prevention. Antimicrobial resistance. 2017. https://www.cdc.gov/drugresistance/about.html. Accessed April 26, 2017.

7. Centers for Disease Control and Prevention. Tuberculosis (TB). 2016. https://www.cdc.gov/tb/topic/basics/default.htm. Accessed April 26, 2018.

8. National Health and Medical Research Council. Clinical educators guide for the prevention and control of infection in healthcare. 2010. https://www.nhmrc.gov.au/_files_nhmrc/publications/attachments/cd33_icg_clinical_ed_guide_web.pdf. Accessed April 25, 2017.

9. Siegel J, Rhinehart, E, Jackson M, Chiarello L. Guideline for isolation precautions: Preventing transmission of infectious agents in healthcare settings. 2007. http://www.cdc.gov/ncidod/dhqp/pdf/isolation2007.pdf. Accessed April 11, 2017.

10. Siegel J, Rhinehart E, Jackson M, Chiarello L. Management of multidrug-resistant organisms in healthcare settings. 2006. https://www.cdc.gov/hicpac/pdf/mdro/mdroguideline2006.pdf. Accessed April 26, 2017.

11. Centers for Disease Control and Prevention. Guide to infection prevention for outpatient settings: minimum expectations for safe care. 2016. http://www.cdc.gov/HAI/prevent/prevent_pubs.html. Accessed April 25, 2017.

12. Occupational Safety and Health Administration. Quick Reference guide to the bloodborne pathogens standard. 2010. https://www.osha.gov/SLTC/bloodbornepathogens/bloodborne_quickref.html Accessed April 11, 2017.

13. Centers for Disease Control and Prevention. Diseases and organisms in healthcare settings. 2014. https://www.cdc.gov/hai/organisms/organisms.html. Accessed July 17, 2017.

14. OSHA. Employee exposure to bloodborne pathogens. 2007. https://www.osha.gov/SLTC/etools/hospital/hazards/univprec/univ.html. Accessed April 17, 2017.

15. Occupational Safety and Health Administration. Healthcare wide hazards MDRO—Multidrug-resistant organisms. 2002. https://www.osha.gov/SLTC/etools/hospital/hazards/mro/mro.html. Accessed April 26, 2017.

16. National Institute for Occupational Safety and Health. Preventing exposures to bloodborne pathogens among paramedics. 2010. https://www.cdc.gov/niosh/docs/wp-solutions/2010-139/pdfs/2010-139.pdf. Accessed April 11, 2017.

17. Mathur P. Hand hygiene: Back to the basics of infection control. *Indian J Med Res.* 2011;134(5):611-620.

18. Boyce JM, D P. CDC guideline for hand hygiene in healthcare settings. *MMWR Morb Mort Wkly Rep.* 2002;51(RR-16):1-48.

19. Centers for Disease Control and Prevention. Safe injection practices to prevent transmission of infections to patients. 2007. https://www.cdc.gov/injectionsafety/ip07_standardprecaution.html. Accessed April 26, 2017.

20. Centers for Disease Control and Prevention. Workbook for designing, implementing, and evaluating a sharps injury prevention program. 2008. https://www.cdc.gov/sharpssafety/pdf/sharpsworkbook_2008.pdf. Accessed April 26, 2017.

21. National Institute for Occupational Safety and Health. Preventing needlestick injuries in health care settings. 1999. https://www.cdc.gov/niosh/docs/2000-108/pdfs/2000-108.pdf. Accessed April 26, 2017.

22. Rutala W, Weber D. Guideline for disinfection and sterilization in healthcare facilities. 2008. https://www.cdc.gov/hicpac/Disinfection_Sterilization/acknowledg.html. Accessed April 27, 2017.

23. US Food and Drug Administration. Reprocessing of single use devices. 2005. https://www.fda.gov/iceci/compliance-manuals/compliancepolicyguidancemanual/ucm073887.htm. Accessed July 31, 2017.

24. US Food and Drug Administration. Reprocessing of reusable medical devices. 2017. https://www.fda.gov/MedicalDevices/ProductsandMedicalProcedures/ReprocessingofReusableMedicalDevices/ucm20081513.htm. Accessed July 31, 2017.

25. McDonnell G, Russell D. Antiseptics and disinfectants: Activity, action, and resistance. *Clin Microbiol Rev.* 1999;12(1):147-179.

26. World Health Organization. Methods of Sterilization. *The International Pharmacopoeia.* 6th ed. 2016. http://apps.who.int/phint/pdf/b/Jb.7.5.9.pdf.

27. US Environmental Protection Agency. Selected EPA-registered disinfectants. 2016. https://www.epa.gov/pesticide-registration/selected-epa-registered-disinfectants. Accessed August 2, 2017.

28. Beam JW, Buckley B, Holcomb WR, Ciocca M. National Athletic Trainers' Association position statement: Management of acute skin trauma. *J Athl Train.* 2016;51(12):1053-1070.

29. Centers for Disease Control and Prevention. Guide to infection prevention for outpatient settings. 2015. http://www.cdc.gov/hai/pdfs/guidelines/Ambulatory-Care+-Checklist_508_11_2015.pdf. Accessed October 23, 2016.

30. Occupational Safety and Health Administration. Bloodborne pathogens standards. 2001. https://www.osha.gov/pls/oshaweb/owadisp.show_document?p_table=STANDARDS&p_id=10051. Accessed April, 11, 2017.

31. Van der Molen HF, Zwinderman KA, Sluiter JK, Frings-Dresen MH. Interventions to prevent needle stick injuries among health care workers. *Work (Reading, Mass).* 2012;41 Suppl 1:1969-1971.

32. Pollack A, Beck R. *Advanced Emergency Care and Transportation of the Sick and Injured.* Sudbury, MA: Jones and Bartlett; 2012.

33. American Academy of Pediatrics. Consent for emergency medical services for children and adolescents. *Pediatrics.* 2003;(3):703.

34. NATA. Best practice guidelines for athletic training documentation. 2017. https://www.nata.org/sites/default/files/best-practice-guidelines-for-athletic-training-documentation.pdf. Accessed May 1, 2018.

35. Moore GP MP, Fider C, Moore MJ. What emergency physicians should know about informed consent. *Acad Emerg Med.* 2014;21(8):922-927.

36. McGrane K, Moore GP, Cookman L. Special report: Good Samaritan Law and the emergency physician: Where are you covered? *ED Legal Letter* [serial online]. 2009. Available from: InfoTrac Health Reference Center Academic, Ipswich, MA. Accessed September 12, 2018.

37. Howie WO, Howie BA, McMullen PC. To assist or not assist: Good Samaritan considerations for nurse practitioners. *J Nurse Pract.* 2012;8(9):688.

38. Gulam H DJ. A brief primer on Good Samaritan law for health care professionals. *Aust Health Rev.* 2007(3):478.

39. US Department of Health and Human Services. HIPAA for professionals. 1996. https://www.hhs.gov/hipaa/for-professionals/security/laws-regulations/index.html. Accessed July 13, 2017.

40. US Department of Health and Human Services. Standards for privacy of individually identifiable health information. 2015. https://www.hhs.gov/hipaa/for-professionals/privacy/guidance/introduction/index.html. Accessed September 12, 2018.

41. US Department of Health and Human Services. Model notices of privacy practices. 2014. https://www.hhs.gov/hipaa/for-professionals/privacy/guidance/model-notices-privacy-practices/index.html. Accessed May 1, 2018.

42. US Department of Health and Human Services. HHS strengthens HIPAA enforcement. 2009. https://wayback.archive-it.org/3926/20131018161347/http://www.hhs.gov/news/press/2009pres/10/20091030a.html. Accessed May 1, 2018.

43. US Department of Health and Human Services. Breach notification rule. 2013. https://www.hhs.gov/hipaa/for-professionals/breach-notification/index.html. Accessed May 1, 2018.

44. HIPAA Survival Guide. HITECH Act Summary. 2017. http://www.hipaasurvivalguide.com/hitech-act-text.php. Accessed September 12, 2018.

45. US Department of Health and Human Services and US Department of Education. Joint guidance on the application of the Family Educational Rights and Privacy Act (FERPA) and the Health Insurance Portability and Accountability Act of 1996 (HIPAA) to student health records. 2008. https://www2.ed.gov/policy/gen/guid/fpco/doc/ferpa-hipaa-guidance.pdf. Accessed July 13, 2017.

46. Commission on Accreditation of Athletic Training Education. CAATE Athletic Training Education Competencies, 6th ed. 2018; https://caate.net/wp-content/uploads/2014/06/5th-Edition-Competencies.pdf. Accessed April 29, 2015.

47. Nurses Service Organization. Defensive documentation. 2017. www.nso.com/risk-education/individuals/articles/Defensive-Documentation. Accessed August 2, 2017.

48. EMTResource.com. SOAPM is used for EMS documentation. 2014. http://www.emtresource.com/resources/documentation/soapm/#more-198. Accessed August 2, 2017.

49. EMTResource.com. ICHART is used for EMS documentation. 2014. www.emtresource.com/resources/documentation/ichart. Accessed August 2, 2017.

50. Alfandre DJ. "I'm going home": Discharges against medical advice. *Mayo Clin Proc.* 2009;84.(3):255-260.

51. Alfandre D. From "I'm not staying!" to "I'm not leaving!": Ethics, communication, and empathy in complicated medical discharges. *Mt Sinai J Med.* 2008;75(5):466-471.

52. The Sullivan Group. Emergency medicine risk and safety toolbox. 2017. https://www.thesullivangroup.com/risk_resources/ToolBox/AMA_form.pdf. Accessed August 2, 2017.

53. The Sullivan Group. Do's & don'ts of AMA: Patients who leave against medical advice. 2018. http://blog.thesullivangroup.com/ama-patients-who-leave-against-medical-advice. Accessed May 2, 2018.

54. Levy F, Mareiniss DP, Iacovelli C. The importance of a proper against-medical-advice (AMA) discharge. *J Emerg Med.* 2012;43(3):516-520.

55. Child Welfare Information Gateway. Mandatory reporters of child abuse and neglect. 2016. Washington, DC: U.S. Department of Health and Human Services, Children's Bureau.

CHAPTER 3

1. Centers for Disease Control and Prevention. Child safety and injury prevention. 2016. https://www.cdc.gov/

safechild/sports_injuries/index.html. Accessed February 7, 2017.

2. Tirabassi J, Brou L, Khodaee M, Lefort R, Fields SK, Comstock RD. Epidemiology of high school sports-related injuries resulting in medical disqualification: 2005-2006 through 2013-2014 academic years. *Am J Sports Med.* 2016;(11):2925.

3. Hurtubise JM, Beech C, Macpherson A. Comparing severe injuries by sex and sport in collegiate-level athletes: A descriptive epidemiologic study. *Int J Athl Ther Train.* 2015;20(4):44-50.

4. Casa DJ, Drezner JA. Moving forward faster: the quest to apply evidence-based emergency practice guidelines in high school sports. *J Athl Train.* 2015;50(4):341-342.

5. Boden BP, Breit I, Beachler JA, Williams A, Mueller FO. Fatalities in high school and college football players. *Am J Sports Med.* 2013;41(5):1108-1116.

6. Casa DJ, Almquist J, Anderson SA, et al. The inter-association task force for preventing sudden death in secondary school athletics programs: best-practices recommendations. *J Athl Train.* 2013;48(4):546-553.

7. Kerr ZY, Marshall SW, Dompier TP, Corlette J, Klossner DA, Gilchrist J. College sports-related injuries - United States, 2009-10 through 2013-14 academic years. *MMWR Morb Mortal Wkly Rep.* 2015;64(48):1330-1336.

8. Olympia RP, Brady J. Emergency preparedness in high school-based athletics: A review of the literature and recommendations for sport health professionals. *Phys Sportsmed.* 2013;41(2):15-25.

9. Courson R, Navitskis L, Patel H. Emergency-action planning. *Athl Ther Today.* 2005;10(2):7-76 12p.

10. Occupational Safety and Health Administration (OSHA). Develop and implement an emergency action plan (EAP). 2016. https://www.osha.gov/SLTC/etools/evacuation/implementation.html. Accessed February 7, 2017.

11. Drezner JA, Courson RW, Roberts WO, Mosesso VN, Link MS, Maron BJ. Inter-association Task Force recommendations on emergency preparedness and management of sudden cardiac arrest in high school and college athletic programs: a consensus statement. *J Athl Train.* 2007;42(1):143-158.

12. Drezner JA. Preparing for sudden cardiac arrest--the essential role of automated external defibrillators in athletic medicine: a critical review. *Br J Sports Med.* 2009;43(9):702-707.

13. Hazinski MF, Markenson D, Neish S, et al. Response to cardiac arrest and selected life-threatening medical emergencies - The Medical Emergency Response Plan for Schools - A statement for healthcare providers, policymakers, school administrators, and community leaders. *Circulation.* 2004;109(2):278.

14. Grantham J, Hill N, Siegle J. Boston strong: Heroes among us. *NATA News.* July2013:11-18.

15. Courson R. Preventing sudden death on the athletic field: The emergency action plan. *Curr Sports Med Rep.* 2007;6(2):93-100.

16. Andersen J, Courson RW, Kleiner DM, McLoda TA. National Athletic Trainers' Association position statement: Emergency planning in athletics. *J Athl Train.* 2002;37(1):99-104.

17. Drezner J, Pluim B, Engebretsen L. Prevention of sudden cardiac death in athletes: New data and modern perspectives confront challenges in the 21st century. *Br J Sports Med.* 2009;43(9):625-626.

18. Courson R, Goldenberg M, Adams KG, et al. Inter-association consensus statement on best practices for sports medicine management for secondary schools and colleges. *J Athl Train.* 2014;49(1):128-137.

19. Pollack A, Beck R. *Advanced Emergency Care and Transportation of the Sick and Injured.* Sudbury, MA: Jones and Bartlett; 2012.

20. Fire and Emergency Medical Services (FEMS). FEMS performance charts. 2015. https://fems.dc.gov/page/performance-charts-1-4. Accessed July 5, 2017.

21. American College of Surgeons. Resources for optimal care of the injured patient. 2014. https://www.facs.org/quality-programs/trauma/vrc/resources. Accessed July 5, 2017.

22. Olympia RP, Dixon T, Brady J, Avner JR. Emergency planning in school-based athletics: A national survey of athletic trainers. *Pediatr Emerg Care.* 2007;23(10):703-708.

23. Toresdahl BG, Harmon KG, Drezner JA. High school automated external defibrillator programs as markers of emergency preparedness for sudden cardiac arrest. *J Athl Train.* 2013;48(2):242-247.

24. Pryor RR, Casa DJ, Vandermark LW, et al. Athletic training services in public secondary schools: A benchmark study. *J Athl Train.* 2015;50(2):156-162.

25. Mazerolle SM, Raso S, Pagnotta KD, Stearns R, Casa DJ. Athletic directors' barriers to hiring athletic trainers in high schools. *J Athl Train.* 2015;50(10):1059-1068.

26. NATA. Official statement on athletic health care provider "time outs" before athletic events. 2012. https://www.nata.org/sites/default/files/timeout.pdf. Accessed May 2, 2018.

27. World Health Organization. Patient safety curriculum guide. Multi-professional patient safety curriculum guide. 2012. http://www.who.int/patientsafety/education/curriculum/Curriculum_Tools/en/. Accessed March 30, 2017.

28. Crisis Prevention Institute. Critical incident reporting: The importance of documentation. 2016. http://www.crisisprevention.com/CPI/media/Media/PDF/CriticalIncidentReportingTool2011.pdf. Accessed March 2, 2017.

29. Kellermann A. The future of emergency care in the United States. *Med Gen Med.* 2006;8(3):36.

30. Duckworth R. Mass casualty incident management: Part 11. *EMSWorld.com.* 2012. http://www.emsworld.com/article/10778968/mci-management. Accessed February 7, 2017.

31. Federal Emergency Management Agency (FEMA). Operational templates and guidance for EMS mass incident deployment. 2012. https://www.usfa.fema.gov/operations/ops_ems.html. Accessed August 1, 2016.

32. Hoch D. Preparing an emergency plan: creating a comprehensive emergency plan assures athletic directors that everyone on their staffs is prepared to properly respond. *Coach and Athletic Director.* 2015;l85:10-11.

33. Neal TL. Catastrophic-incident guideline: Building a plan you hope is never used. *Athl Ther Today.* 2005;10(3):18-21.

34. Neal TL, Diamond AB, Goldman S, et al. Inter-association recommendations for developing a plan to recognize and refer student-athletes with psychological concerns at the collegiate level: an executive summary of a consensus statement. *J Athl Train.* 2013;48(5):716-720.

35. Mental Health Coordinating Council. Psychological Injury Management Guide (PIMG). 2016. http://pimg.mhcc.org.au/. Accessed March 2, 2017.

36. Brymer M, Jacobs A, Layne C, et al. Psychological First Aid: Field Operations Guide. 2nd ed. 2006. http://www.nctsn.org/sites/default/files/pfa/english/1-psyfirstaid_final_complete_manual.pdf. Accessed January 25, 2017.

37. American Psychiatric Association (APA). *Diagnostic and Statistical Manual of Mental Disorders.* 5th ed. Arlington, VA: American Psychiatric Publishing; 2013.

38. NATA. ATs care peer-to-peer support program. 2016. https://www.nata.org/membership/about-membership/member-resources/ats-care. Accessed July 5, 2017.

CHAPTER 4

1. New York Department of Health. Patient assessment definitions. Bureau of Emergency Medical Services and Trauma Systems. 2015. https://www.health.ny.gov/professionals/ems/pdf/srgpadefinitions.pdf. Accessed September 24, 2017.

2. Parker M, Magnusson C. Assessment of trauma patients. *Intl J Orthop Trauma Nurs.* 2016;21:21-30.

3. American College of Surgeons, ed. *ATLS: Advanced Trauma Life Support Manual.* Chicago: American College of Surgeons; 2012.

4. Thompson C, Kilroy D, Tesfayohannes B. Trauma: Clinical assessment of the patient with major injuries. *Surgery.* 2003;21:193-196.

5. Mistovich J, Karren K. *Pre-Hospital Emergency Care.* Boston, MA: Pearson; 2014.

6. Limmer D, Mistovich L, Krost W. Scene size-up. 2007. www.emsworld.com/article/10321423/beyond-the-basics-scene-size-up. Accessed July 31, 2016, 2016.

7. Pollack A, Beck R. *Advanced Emergency Care and Transportation of the Sick and Injured.* Sudbury, MA: Jones and Bartlett; 2012.

8. Henry MC, Stapleton ER. *EMT Prehospital Care.* 2nd ed. Burlington, MA: Jones and Bartlett; 2012.

9. Limmer D, Mistovich L, Krost W. Scene safety: Beyond the basics. 2006. www.emsworld.com/article/10322834/beyond-the-basics-scene-safety. Accessed September 13, 2018.

10. Centers for Disease Control and Prevention. Guidelines for field triage of injured patients. 2011. www.cdc.gov/mmwr/pdf/rr/rr6101.pdf. Accessed October 23, 2016.

11. Ratcliff TK, Lincoln EW. Disaster Medicine. In: Stone CK, Humphries RL, eds. *Current Diagnosis & Treatment: Emergency Medicine.* 8th ed. New York, NY: McGraw-Hill Education, Inc.; 2017.

12. Jordan J. Approach to the trauma patient. Merck Manual Professional Version. 2016. https://www.merckmanuals.com/professional/injuries-poisoning/approach-to-the-trauma-patient/approach-to-the-trauma-patient. Accessed September 24, 2017.

13. Kelly CA, Upex A, Bateman DN. Comparison of consciousness level assessment in the poisoned patient using the Alert/Verbal/Painful/Unresponsive Scale and the Glasgow Coma Scale. *Ann Emerg Med.* 2004;44(2):108-113.

14. Madsen J. Overview of incidents involving mass casualty weapons. *Merck Manual Professional Version.* 2017. https://www.merckmanuals.com/professional/injuries-poisoning/mass-casualty-weapons/overview-of-incidents-involving-mass-casualty-weapons#v8982614. Accessed September 24, 2017.

15. Delaney JS, Drummond R. Mass casualties and triage at a sporting event. *Br J Sports Med.* 2002;36(2):85-88; discussion 88.

16. Blackwell T. Prehospital care of the adult trauma patient. *UpToDate.* 2017. https://www.uptodate.com/contents/prehospital-care-of-the-adult-trauma-patient?search=Prehospital%20Care%20of%20the%20Adult%20Trauma%20Patient&source=search_result&selectedTitle=1~150&usage_type=default&display_rank=1. Accessed September 13, 2018.

17. Thim T, Krarup NH, Grove EL, Rohde CV, Lofgren B. Initial assessment and treatment with the Airway, Breathing, Circulation, Disability, Exposure (ABCDE) approach. *Int J Gen Med.* 2012;5:117-121.

18. Singletary EM, Charlton NP, Epstein JL, et al. Part 15: First Aid: 2015 American Heart Association and American Red Cross guidelines update for first aid. *Circulation.* 2015;132:S574-S589.

19. Markenson D, Ferguson JD, Chameides L, et al. Part 17: First aid: 2010 American Heart Association and American Red Cross guidelines for first aid. *Circulation.* 2010;122(S3):S934-946.

20. Tindall SC. Level of Consciousness. In Walker HK, Hall WD, Hurst JW e, eds. *Clinical Methods: The History, Physical, and Laboratory Examinations.* 3rd ed. Boston, MA: Butterworths; 1990.

21. Kleinman ME, Brennan EE, Goldberger ZD, et al. Part 5: Adult basic life support and cardiopulmonary resuscitation quality: 2015 American Heart Association guidelines update for cardiopulmonary resuscitation and emergency cardiovascular care. *Circulation.* 2015;132(18 Suppl 2):S414-435.

22. Link MS, Berkow LC, Kudenchuk PJ, et al. Part 7: Adult advanced cardiovascular life support: 2015 American Heart Association guidelines update for cardiopulmonary resuscitation and emergency cardiovascular care. *Circulation.* 2015;132(18 Suppl 2):S444-464.

23. Mistovich J, Limmer D, Werman H. Trauma assessment for the EMT. *EMS World.* 2011. www.emsworld.com/article/10318988/trauma-assessment-for-the-HCP.

24. Bickley L, Szilagyi P. *Bates' Guide to Physical Examination and History Taking.* 11th ed. Philadelphia, PA: Lippincott Williams & Wilkins; 2013.

25. Venes D. *Taber's Cyclopedic Medical Dictionary.* FA Davis; 2013.

26. Rhoades RA, Bell DR. *Medical Physiology: Principles for Clinical Medicine.* 4th ed. Baltimore, MD: Lippincott Williams & Wilkins; 2013.

27. Marx JA, Rosen P. *Rosen's Emergency Medicine: Concepts and Clinical Practice.* Philadelphia, PA: Elsevier Saunders; 2017.

28. Pickering TG, Hall JE, Appel LJ, et al. Recommendations for blood pressure measurement in humans and experimental animals: Part 1: Blood pressure measurement in humans. *Hypertension.* 2005;45(1):142-161.

29. Whelton PK, Carey RM, Aronow WS, et al. Clinical practice guideline: 2017 ACC/AHA/AAPA/ABC/ACPM/AGS/APhA/ASH/ASPC/NMA/PCNA Guideline for the prevention, detection, evaluation, and management of high blood pressure in adults. A report of the American College of Cardiology/American Heart Association Task Force on Clinical Practice Guidelines. *J Am Coll Cardiol.* 2018;71:e127-e248.

30. Sahu D, Bhaskaran M. Palpatory method of measuring diastolic blood pressure. *J Anaesthesiol Clin Pharmacol.* 2010;26(4):528-530.

31. Eberhardt S. Improve handoff communication with SBAR. *Nursing.* 2014;44(11):17-20.

32. Institute for Healthcare Improvement. SBAR technique for communication: A situational briefing model. www.ihi.org/resources/Pages/Tools/SBARTechniqueforCommunicationASituationalBriefingModel.aspx. Accessed March 4, 2017.

33. Narayan MC. Using SBAR communications in efforts to prevent patient rehospitalizations. *Home Healthc Nurse.* 2013;31(9):504-515; quiz 515-507.

34. Pope BB, Rodzen L, Spross G. Raising the SBAR: How better communication improves patient outcomes. *Nursing.* 2008;38(3):41-43.

35. Powell SK. SBAR-It's not just another communication tool. *Prof Case Manag.* 2007;12(4):195-196.

36. Paffrath T, Lefering R, Flohe S. How to define severely injured patients? An Injury Severity Score (ISS) based approach alone is not sufficient. *Injury.* 2014;45 Suppl 3:S64-69.

37. Deng Q, Tang B, Xue C, et al. Comparison of the ability to predict mortality between the Injury Severity Score and the New Injury Severity Score: A meta-analysis. *Int J Environ Res Public Health.* 2016;13(8):825.

38. Venegas-Borsellino C. Triage and Transport in the Field for the Critically Ill Patient. In Oropello JM, Pastores SM, Kvetan V, eds. *Critical Care.* New York, NY: McGraw-Hill Education; 2017.

39. Baker SP, O'Neill B, Haddon W, Jr., Long WB. The injury severity score: a method for describing patients with multiple injuries and evaluating emergency care. *J Traum.* 1974;14(3):187-196.

40. Osler T, Baker SP, Long W. A modification of the injury severity score that both improves accuracy and simplifies scoring. *J Trauma.* 1997;43(6):922-925; discussion 925-926.

41. Staudenmayer K, Wang NE, Weiser TG, et al. The triage of injured patients: Mechanism of injury, regardless of injury severity, determines hospital destination. *Am Surg.* 2016;82(4):356-361.

CHAPTER 5

1. Board of Certification, Inc. State regulation search. www.bocatc.org. Accessed September 25, 2018.

2. Kahanov L, Roberts J, Wughalter EM. Adherence to drug-dispensation and drug-administration laws and guidelines in collegiate athletic training rooms: A 5-year review. *J Athl Train.* 2010;45(3):299-305.

3. Kahanov L, Furst D, Johnson S, Roberts J. Adherence to drug-dispensation and drug-administration laws and guidelines in collegiate athletic training rooms. *J Athl Train.* 2003;38(3):252-258.

4. CAATE. CAATE 2020 standards for accreditation of professional athletic training programs. https://caate.net/pp-standards/. Accessed April 10, 2018.

5. Casa DJ, Almquist J, Anderson SA, et al. The inter-association task force for preventing sudden death in secondary school athletics programs: Best-practices recommendations. *J Athl Train* 2013;48(4):546-53 doi0.4085/1062-6050-48.4.12. Accessed April 15, 2018.

6. Anderson S, Eichner, ER. Consensus statement: Sickle cell trait and the athlete. *National Athletic Trainers' Association News.* June 2007. www.nata.org/sites/default/files/sicklecelltraitandtheathlete.pdf. Accessed April 9, 2018.

7. Armstrong LE, Casa DJ, et al. American College of Sports Medicine position stand. Exertional heat illness during training and competition. *Med Sci Sports Exerc.* 2007;39(3):556-72. doi0.1249/MSS.0b013e31802fa199. Accessed April 15, 2018.

8. Magnus BC, Miller, MG. *Pharmacology Application in Athletic Training.* Philadelphia, PA: F.A. Davis; 2005.

9. Casa DJ, Guskiewicz KM, Anderson SA, et al. National Athletic Trainers' Association position statement: Preventing sudden death in sports. *J Athl Train.* 2012;47(1):96-118.

10. Drezner JA, Courson RW, Roberts WO, et al. Inter Association Task Force recommendations on emergency preparedness and management of sudden cardiac arrest in high school and college athletic programs: A consensus statement. *Prehosp Emerg Care.* 2007;11(3):253-271. doi0.1080/10903120701204839. Accessed April 15, 2018.

11. Alexander MB, Belle R. *Advance EMT: A Clinical-Reasoning Approach.* Pearson Education; 2012.

12. Hughes RG, Blegen MA. Medication Administration Safety. In Hughes RG, ed. *Patient Safety and Quality: An Evidence-Based Handbook for Nurses.* Rockville, MD: Agency for Healthcare Research and Quality (US); 2008.

13. Adams D, Elliot TS. Skin antiseptics used prior to intra-vascular catheter insertion. *Br J Nurs.* 2007;16(5):278-

280. doi0.12968/bjon.2007.16.5.22997. Accessed April 19, 2018.

14. Veauthier B, Sievers K, Hornecker J. Acute coronary syndrome: Emergency department evaluation and management. *FP Essent*. 2015;437:17-22.

15. Veauthier B, Sievers K, Hornecker J. Acute coronary syndrome: Out-of-hospital evaluation and management. *FP Essent*. 2015;437:11-16.

16. Greenland P, Alpert JS, Beller GA, et al. 2010 ACCF/AHA guideline for assessment of cardiovascular risk in asymptomatic adults: a report of the American College of Cardiology Foundation/American Heart Association Task Force on Practice Guidelines. *J Am Coll Cardiol*. 2010;56(25):e50-103. doi0.1016/j.jacc.2010.09.001. Accessed April 19, 2018.

17. Schrank KS. Cardiac arrest management. Adapting AHA Guidelines 2010 to your EMS protocols. *EMS World*. 2011;40(5):I16-I17.

18. Centers for Disease Control and Prevention. National Center for Health Statistics: Asthma Data for the U.S. www.cdc.gov/nchs/fastats/asthma.htm. Accessed April 15, 2018.

19. Miller MG, Weiler JM, Baker R, Collins J, D'Alonzo G. National Athletic Trainers' Association position statement: Management of asthma in athletes. *J Athl Train*. 2005;40(3):224-245.

20. Johnson DB, Bounds CG. Albuterol. www.statpearls.com/as/pulmonary/17330/. Accessed April 19, 2018.

21. Carhart E, Salzman JG. Prehospital oxygen administration for chest pain patients decreases significantly following implementation of the 2010 AHA guidelines. *Prehosp Emerg Care*. 2014;18(4):471-475. doi0.3109/10903127.2014.912705. Accessed April 19, 2018.

22. Cohen MB, Saunders SS, Wise SK, Nassif S, Platt MP. Pitfalls in the use of epinephrine for anaphylaxis: Patient and provider opportunities for improvement. *Int Forum Allergy Rhinol*. 2017;7(3):276-286. doi0.1002/alr.21884. Accessed April 19, 2018.

23. Chooniedass R, Temple B, Becker A. Epinephrine use for anaphylaxis: Too seldom, too late: Current practices and guidelines in health care. *Ann Allergy Asthma Immunol*. 2017;119(2):108-110. doi0.1016/j.anai.2017.06.004. Accessed April 19, 2018.

24. Kahn PA, Wagner NE, Gabbay RA. Underutilization of glucagon in the prehospital setting. *Ann Intern Med*. 2018;168(8):603-604. doi0.7326/M17-2222. Accessed April 19, 2018.

25. Howell MA, Guly HR. A comparison of glucagon and glucose in prehospital hypoglycaemia. *J Accid Emerg Med*. 1997;14(1):30-32.

26. Adams J. Surgeon General's advisory on naloxone and opioid overdose. 2018. www.surgeongeneral.gov/priorities/opioid-overdose-prevention/naloxone-advisory.html, Accessed April 21, 2018.

27. Seymour CW, Cooke CR, Hebert PL, Rea TD. Intravenous access during out-of-hospital emergency care of noninjured patients: A population-based outcome study. *Ann Emerg Med*. 2012;59(4):296-303. doi0.1016/j.annemergmed.2011.07.021. Accessed April 15, 2018.

28. McDermott BP, Anderson SA, Armstrong LE, et al. National Athletic Trainers' Association position statement: Fluid replacement for the physically active. *J Athl Train*. 2017;52(9):877-895. doi0.4085/1062-6050-52.9.02. Accessed April 15, 2018.

29. Velasquez BJ. IV utilization or access by licensed athletic trainer in clinical setting. *Sport Exerc Med Open J*. 2018;4(1). https://openventio.org/iv-utilization-or-access-by-licensed-athletic-trainer-in-the-clinical-setting/. Accessed September 25, 2018.

30. Fuchs, EJ. Athletic Trainer's Utilization and Clinical Establishment of IV Access and Fluid Administration to Improve Patient Care. 2018. Kentucky Athletic Trainers Society February Regional Meeting. February 25, 2018; Richmond, KY.

31. Casa DJ, Armstrong LE, Kenny GP, O'Connor FG, Huggins RA. Exertional heat stroke: New concepts regarding cause and care. *Curr Sports Med Rep*. 2012;11(3):115-123. doi0.1249/JSR.0b013e31825615cc. Accessed April 15, 2018.

32. Casa DJ, Anderson SA, Baker L, et al. The inter-association task force for preventing sudden death in collegiate conditioning sessions: Best practices recommendations. *J Athl Train*. 2012;47(4):477-480. doi0.4085/1062-6050-47.4.08. Accessed April 15, 2018.

33. Lavery I. Intravenous therapy: Preparation and administration of IV medicines. *Br J Nurs*. 2011;20(4):S28, S30-34. doi0.12968/bjon.2011.20.4.S28. Accessed April 19, 2018.

34. Tuma S, Sepkowitz KA. Efficacy of safety-engineered device implementation in the prevention of percutaneous injuries: a review of published studies. *Clin Infect Dis*. 2006;42(8):1159-1170 doi0.1086/501456. Accessed April 19, 2018.

35. Azar-Cavanagh M, Burdt P, Green-McKenzie J. Effect of the introduction of an engineered sharps injury prevention device on the percutaneous injury rate in healthcare workers. *Infect Control Hosp Epidemiol*. 2007;28(2):165-170. doi0.1086/511699. Accessed April 19, 2018.

36. Jeffery RM, Dickinson L, Ng ND, DeGeorge LM, Nable JV. Naloxone administration for suspected opioid overdose: An expanded scope of practice by a basic life support collegiate-based emergency medical services agency. *J Am Coll Health*. 2017;65(3):212-216. doi0.1080/07448481.2016.1277730. Accessed April 19, 2018.

37. Gulec N, Lahey J, Suozzi JC, Sholl M, MacLean CD, Wolfson DL. Basic and advanced EMS providers are equally effective in naloxone administration for opioid overdose in northern New England. *Prehosp Emerg Care*. 2018;22(2):163-169. doi0.1080/10903127.2017.1371262. Accessed April 19, 2018.

38. Friedman MS, Manini AF. Validation of criteria to guide prehospital naloxone administration for drug-related altered mental status. *J Med Toxicol*. 2016;12(3):270-275. doi0.1007/s13181-016-0549-5. Accessed April 19, 2018.

39. Fellows SE, Coppola AJ, Gandhi MA. Comparing methods of naloxone administration: A narrative review. *J Opioid*

Manag. 2017;13(4):253-260. doi0.5055/jom.2017.0393. Accessed April 19, 2018.

40. Rando J, Broering D, Olson JE, Marco C, Evans SB. Intranasal naloxone administration by police first responders is associated with decreased opioid overdose deaths. *Am J Emerg Med.* 2015;33(9):1201-1204. doi0.1016/j. ajem.2015.05.022. Accessed April 19, 2018.

41. Casa DJ, DeMartini JK, Bergeron MF, et al. National Athletic Trainers' Association position statement: Exertional heat illnesses. *J Athl Train.* 2015;50(9):986-1000. doi0.4085/1062-6050-50.9.07. Accessed April 15, 2018.

42. Jimenez CC, Corcoran MH, Crawley JT, et al. National athletic trainers' association position statement: Management of the athlete with type 1 diabetes mellitus. *J Athl Train.* 2007;42(4):536-545.

43. Ford, J. Nonmedical prescription drug use among college students: A comparison between athletes and nonathletes. *J Am Coll Health.* 2008;57(2):211-219.

44. Knopf, A. Participation in sports reduces teen risk of nonmedical use of prescription opioids and heroin. *CABL.* 2016;32(9):4. doi0.1002/cbl.30152. Accessed September 5, 2018.

45. Kentucky Board of Medical Licensure. KRS 311.903: Prohibited services by licensed athletic trainers, responsibilities and duties of licensed athletic trainers, prohibited billing. kbml.ky.gov/ah/Pages/Athletic-Trainer.aspx. Accessed September 20, 2018.

CHAPTER 6

1. Pollack A, Beck R. *Advanced Emergency Care and Transportation of the Sick and Injured.* Sudbury, MA: Jones and Bartlett; 2012.

2. Rhoades RA, Bell DR. *Medical Physiology: Principles for Clinical Medicine.* 4th ed. Baltimore, MD: Lippincott Williams & Wilkins; 2013.

3. de Moya MA. Shock and Fluid Resuscitation. *Merck Manual Professional Version.* 2013. www.merckmanuals. com/professional/critical-care-medicine/shock-and-fluid-resuscitation/shock. Accessed June 2, 2017.

4. van Oostendorp S, Tan EC, Geeraedts LM. Prehospital control of life-threatening truncal and junctional haemorrhage is the ultimate challenge in optimizing trauma care; a review of treatment options and their applicability in the civilian trauma setting. *Scand J Trauma Resusc Emerg Med.* 2016;24(1):110-110.

5. American College of Surgeons, ed. *ATLS: Advanced Trauma Life Support Manual.* Chicago: American College of Surgeons; 2012.

6. Geeraedts JLMG, Kaasjager HAH, van Vugt AB, Frölke JPM. Review: Exsanguination in trauma: A review of diagnostics and treatment options. *Injury.* 2009;40:11-20.

7. Balk EM, Ellis AG, Di M, Adam GP, Trikalinos TA. Venous thromboembolism prophylaxis in major orthopedic surgery: Systematic review update. *Agency for Healthcare Research and Quality (US).* 2017. https://www.ncbi.nlm. nih.gov/books/NBK476632/. Accessed September 15, 2018.

8. American Heart Association. What is venous thromboembolism (VTE)? 2017. www.heart.org/ HEARTORG/Conditions/VascularHealth/Venous Thromboembolism/What-is-Venous-Thromboembolism-VTE_UCM_479052_Article.jsp#.WvH1c4gvyUk. Accessed May 8, 2018.

9. Douketis JD. Deep venous thrombosis (DVT). *Merck Manual Professional Version.* 2018. www.merckmanuals.com/ professional/cardiovascular-disorders/peripheral-venous-disorders/deep-venous-thrombosis-dvt. Accessed May 5, 2018.

10. Mall NA, Van Thiel GS, Heard WM, Paletta GA, Bush-Joseph C, Bach BR. Paget-Schroetter Syndrome: A review of effort thrombosis of the upper extremity from a sports medicine perspective. *Sports Health.* 2013;5(4):353-356.

11. Melby SJ, Vedantham S, Narra VR, et al. Clinical research study: Comprehensive surgical management of the competitive athlete with effort thrombosis of the subclavian vein (Paget-Schroetter syndrome). *J Vasc Surg.* 2008;47:809-820.e803.

12. Alla VM, Natarajan N, Kaushik M, Warrier R, Nair CK. Paget-Schroetter Syndrome: Review of pathogenesis and treatment of effort thrombosis. *West J Emerg Med.* 2010;11(4):358-362.

13. Douketis J. Deep venous thrombosis (DVT). *Merck Manual Professional Version.* www.merckmanuals.com/ professional/cardiovascular-disorders/peripheral-venous-disorders/deep-venous-thrombosis-dvt. Accessed November 27, 2017.

14. Kearon C, Bauer K. Clinical presentation and diagnosis of the nonpregnant adult with suspected deep vein thrombosis of the lower extremity. *Wolters Kluwer UpToDate.* 2017. www.uptodate.com/contents/clinical-presentation-and-diagnosis-of-the-nonpregnant-adult-with-suspected-deep-vein-thrombosis-of-the-lower-extremity?source=search_result&search=deep%20vein%20 thrombosis%20adult&selectedTitle=2~150. Accessed November 27, 2017.

15. Tubbs RJ, Savitt DL, Suner S. Extremity Conditions. In Tintinalli JE, Stapczynski JS, Ma OJ, Yealy DM, Meckler GD, Cline DM, eds. *Tintinalli's Emergency Medicine: A Comprehensive Study Guide.* New York, NY: McGraw-Hill; 2016.

16. Maier RV. Approach to the Patient with Shock. In Kasper D, Fauci A, Hauser S, Longo D, Jameson JL, Loscalzo J, eds. *Harrison's Principles of Internal Medicine.* 19th ed. New York, NY: McGraw-Hill; 2015.

17. Gutierrez G, Reines HD, Wolf-Gutierrez ME. Clinical review: Hemorrhagic shock. *Crit Care.* 2004;8:373-381.

18. Rice V. Shock, a clinical syndrome: An update. An overview of shock: part 1. *Crit Care Nurse.* 1991;11(4):20-27.

19. Bulger EM, Snyder D, Schoelles K, et al. An evidence-based prehospital guideline for external hemorrhage control: American College of Surgeons Committee on Trauma. *Prehosp Emerg Care.* 2014;18(2):163-173.

20. Rossaint R, Bouillon B, Cerny V, et al. Management of bleeding following major trauma: An updated European guideline. *Critical Care.* 2010;14(2):R52-R52.

21. Colwell C. Initial management of moderate to severe hemorrhage in the adult trauma patient. *Wolters Kluwer UptoDate.* 2017. www-uptodate-com.libproxy.chapman. edu/contents/initial-management-of-moderate-to-severe-hemorrhage-in-the-adult-trauma-patient?source=search_result&search=shock&selectedTitle=9~150. Accessed November 16, 2017.

22. Mistovich J, Karren K. *Pre-Hospital Emergency Care.* Boston, MA: Pearson; 2014.

23. Moake JL. Overview of Hemostasis. *Merck Manual Professional Version.* 2016. www.merckmanuals.com/professional/hematology-and-oncology/hemostasis/overview-of-hemostasis. Accessed June 2, 2017.

24. Trinkman H, Beam D, Hagemann T. Coagulation Disorders. In DiPiro J, Talbert R, Yee G, Matzke G, Wells B, Posey M, eds. *Pharmacotherapy: A Pathophysiologic Approach.* 10th ed. Columbus, OH: McGraw-Hill; 2017.

25. Harper D, Young A, McNaught C-E. The physiology of wound healing. *Surgery (0263-9319).* 2014;32(9):445.

26. Nelson J, Hemphill R. Clotting Disorders. In Tintinalli JE, Stapczynski JS, Ma OJ, Yealy DM, Meckler GD, Cline DM, eds. *Tintinalli's Emergency Medicine: A Comprehensive Study Guide.* New York, NY: McGraw-Hill; 2016.

27. Bates SM, Jaeschke R, Stevens SM, et al. Diagnosis of DVT: Antithrombotic therapy and prevention of thrombosis. 9th ed. American College of Chest Physicians evidence-based clinical practice guidelines. *Chest.* 2012;141(2 Suppl):e351S-e418S.

28. MedlinePlus.com. Blood thinners. 2017. https://medlineplus.gov/bloodthinners.html. Accessed September 15, 2018.

29. Fookes C. Drugs.com. Nonsteroidal anti-inflammatory agents. 2017. www.drugs.com/drug-class/nonsteroidal-anti-inflammatory-agents.html. Accessed September 15, 2018.

30. Leung L. Clinical features, diagnosis, and treatment of disseminated intravascular coagulation in adults. *Wolters Kluwer UpToDate.* 2017. www.uptodate.com/contents/clinical-features-diagnosis-and-treatment-of-disseminated-intravascular-coagulation-in-adults?source=search_result&search=disseminated%20intravascular%20coagulation&selectedTitle=1~150. Accessed November 27, 2017.

31. Moake JL. Overview of coagulation disorders. *Merck Manual Professional Version.* 2016. http://www.merckmanuals.com/professional/hematology-and-oncology/coagulation-disorders/overview-of-coagulation-disorders. Accessed November 27, 2017.

32. Moake JL. Excessive bleeding. *Merck Manual Professional Version.* 2016. http://www.merckmanuals.com/professional/hematology-and-oncology/hemostasis/excessive-bleeding. Accessed November 27, 2017.

33. Henry MC, Stapleton ER. *EMT Prehospital Care.* 2nd ed. Burlington, MA: Jones and Bartlett; 2012.

34. Duncan NS, Moran C. Initial resuscitation of the trauma victim. *Orthop Trauma.* 2010;24(1):1-8.

35. Cannon JW, Rasmussen TE. Severe extremity injury in the adult patient. *Wolters Kluwer UpToDate.* 2017. www.uptodate.com/contents/severe-extremity-injury-in-the-adult-patient?source=search_result&search=peripheral%20vascular%20injury&selectedTitle=1~150. Accessed November 6, 2017.

36. Walsh Flanagan K, Cuppett M. *Medical Conditions in the Athlete.* 3rd ed. Champaign, IL: Human Kinetics; 2017.

37. Singer AJ. Lacerations. *Merck Manual Professional Version.* 2017. www.merckmanuals.com/professional/injuries-poisoning/lacerations-and-abrasions/lacerations#v1110165. Accessed May 13, 2018.

38. Forsch RT. Essentials of skin laceration repair. *Am Fam Phys.* 2008;78(8):945-951.

39. Mankowitz SL. Laceration management. *J Emerg Med.* 2017(3):369.

40. Brancato J. Minor wound preparation and irrigation. *UpToDate.* 2018. www.uptodate.com/contents/minor-wound-preparation-and-irrigation?topicRef=6320&source=see_link#H1. Accessed May 13, 2018.

41. Singer A, Hollander J. Wound Closure In: Tintinalli JE, Stapczynski JS, Ma OJ, Yealy DM, Meckler GD, Cline DM, eds. *Tintinalli's Emergency Medicine: A Comprehensive Study Guide.* New York, NY: McGraw-Hill; 2016.

42. Lipsett S. Closure of minor skin wounds with staples. *UpToDate.* 2017. www.uptodate.com/contents/closure-of-minor-skin-wounds-with-staples. Accessed May 13, 2018.

43. Honsik KA, Romeo MW, Hawley CJ, Romeo SJ, Romeo JP. Sideline skin and wound care for acute injuries. *Curr Sports Med Rep.* 2007;6(3):147-154.

44. Rosen P. *Atlas of Emergency Procedures.* St. Louis, MO: Mosby; 2001.

45. Marx JA, Rosen P. *Rosen's Emergency Medicine: Concepts and Clinical Practice.* Philadelphia, PA: Elsevier Saunders; 2017.

46. Tisherman SA, Schmicker RH, Brasel KJ, et al. Detailed description of all deaths in both the shock and traumatic brain injury hypertonic saline trials of the Resuscitation Outcomes Consortium. *Ann Surg.* 2015;261(3):586-590.

47. Bonta MJ. Approaching shock in the trauma patient. *Emerg Med Rep.* 2009; Available from: InfoTrac Health Reference Center Academic, Ipswich, MA. Accessed September 15, 2018.

48. Wilson M, Davis DP, Coimbra R. Diagnosis and monitoring of hemorrhagic shock during the initial resuscitation of multiple trauma patients: A review. *J Emerg Med.* 2003;24(4):413-422.

49. Foex BA. Systemic responses to trauma. *Br Med Bull.* 1999;54(4):726.

50. Gaieski DF, Mikkelsen ME. Definition, classification, etiology, and pathophysiology of shock in adults. *Wolters Kluwer UpToDate.* 2017. www.uptodate.com/contents/definition-classification-etiology-and-pathophysiology-of-shock-in-adults?source=search_result&search=neurogenic%20shock&selectedTitle=1~22. Accessed November 28, 2017.

51. Nicks BA, Gaillard J. Approach to shock. In Tintinalli JE, Stapczynski JS, Ma OJ, Yealy DM, Meckler GD, Cline

DM, eds. *Tintinalli's Emergency Medicine: A Comprehensive Study Guide.* Columbus, OH: McGraw-Hill; 2016.

52. Singer M, Deutschman CS, Seymour C, et al. The third international consensus definitions for sepsis and septic shock (sepsis-3). *JAMA.* 2016;315(8):801-810.

53. Gaieski DF, Mikkelsen ME. Evaluation of and initial approach to the adult patient with undifferentiated hypotension and shock. *Wolters Kluwer UpToDate.* 2017. www.uptodate.com/contents/evaluation-of-and-initial-approach-to-the-adult-patient-with-undifferentiated-hypotension-and-shock?source=see_link. Accessed November 28, 2017.

54. Britt LD, Weireter JLJ, Riblet JL, Asensio JA, Maull K. Priorities in the management of profound shock. *Surg Clin North Am.* 1996;76:645-660.

55. Singletary EM, Charlton NP, Epstein JL, et al. Part 15: First Aid: 2015 American Heart Association and American Red Cross Guidelines Update for First Aid. *Circulation.* 2015;132:S574-S589.

56. Simons FER, Ardusso LRF, Bil MB, et al. International consensus on (ICON) anaphylaxis. *World Allergy Organ J.* 2014.

57. Kemp SF, Lockey RF. Anaphylaxis: A review of causes and mechanisms. *J Allergy Clin Immunol.* 2002;110:341-348.

58. Khan BQ, Kemp SF. Pathophysiology of anaphylaxis. *Curr Opin Allergy Clin Immunol.* 2011;11(4):319-325.

59. Castells M. Diagnosis and management of anaphylaxis in precision medicine. *J Allergy Clin Immunol.* 2017(2):321.

60. Sicherer SH, Leung DYM. Advances in allergic skin disease, anaphylaxis, and hypersensitivity reactions to foods, drugs, and insects in 2014. *J Allergy Clin Immunol.* 2015;135(2):357.

61. Boyce JA, Austen FK. Allergies, Anaphylaxis, and Systemic Mastocytosis. In Kasper D, Fauci A, Hauser S, Longo D, Jameson JL, Loscalzo J, eds. *Harrison's Principles of Internal Medicine.* 19th ed. New York, NY: McGraw-Hill 2015.

62. Rowe BH, Gaeta TJ. Anaphylaxis, Allergies, and Angioedema. In Tintinalli JE, Stapczynski JS, Ma OJ, Yealy DM, Meckler GD, Cline DM, eds. *Tintinalli's Emergency Medicine: A Comprehensive Study Guide.* New York, NY: McGraw-Hill; 2016.

63. National Institute of Allergy and Infectious Diseases. Anaphylaxis. 2010; https://web.archive.org/web/20150504041904/http://www.niaid.nih.gov/topics/anaphylaxis/Pages/default.aspx. Accessed November 29, 2017.

64. Tran PT, Muelleman RL. Allergy, Hypersensitivity, Angioedema, and Anaphylaxis. In Marx JA, Rosen P, eds. *Rosen's Emergency Medicine: Concepts and Clinical Practice.* Philadelphia, PA: Elsevier Saunders; 2017.

65. Delves PJ. Overview of allergic and atopic disorders. *Merck Manual Professional Version.* 2016. http://www.merckmanuals.com/professional/immunology-allergic-disorders/allergic,-autoimmune,-and-other-hypersensitivity-

disorders/overview-of-allergic-and-atopic-disorders. Accessed June 2, 2017.

66. Delves PJ. Anaphylaxis. *Merck Manual Professional Version.* 2016. www.merckmanuals.com/professional/immunology-allergic-disorders/allergic,-autoimmune,-and-other-hypersensitivity-disorders/anaphylaxis. Accessed November 28, 2017.

67. Warren JS, Strayer DS. Immunopathology. In David S. Strayer, Rubin E, Saffitz JE, Schiller AL, eds. *Rubin's Pathology: Clinicopathologic Foundations of Medicine.* 7th ed. Philadelphia, PA: Wolters Kluwer; 2015.

68. Reber LL, Galli SJ, Hernandez JD. The pathophysiology of anaphylaxis. *J Allergy Clin Immunol.* 2017;140(2):335-348.

69. Simons FER, Ardusso LRF, Bilò MB, et al. World Allergy Organization guidelines for the assessment and management of anaphylaxis. *World Allergy Organ J.* 2011;4(2):13-37.

70. Simons FER, Ebisawa M, Sanchez-Borges M, et al. 2015 update of the evidence base: World Allergy Organization anaphylaxis guidelines. *World Allergy Organ J.* 2015.

71. Sampson HA, Muñoz-Furlong A, Campbell RL, et al. Second Symposium on the Definition and Management of Anaphylaxis: Summary Report—Second National Institute of Allergy and Infectious Disease/Food Allergy and Anaphylaxis Network Symposium. *Ann Emerg Med.* 2006;47(4):373.

72. Campbell RL, Hagan JB, Manivannan V, et al. Food, drug, insect sting allergy, and anaphylaxis: Evaluation of National Institute of Allergy and Infectious Diseases/Food Allergy and Anaphylaxis Network criteria for the diagnosis of anaphylaxis in emergency department patients. *J Allergy Clin Immunol.* 2012;129:748-752.

73. Brown SGA. Food allergy, dermatologic diseases, and anaphylaxis: Clinical features and severity grading of anaphylaxis. *J Allergy Clin Immunol.* 2004;114:371-376.

74. Pumphrey RSH. Lessons for management of anaphylaxis from a study of fatal reactions. *Clin Exp Allergy.* 2000;30(8):1144.

75. Lieberman P, Nicklas RA, Oppenheimer J, et al. The diagnosis and management of anaphylaxis practice parameter: 2010 Update. *J Allergy Clin Immunol.* 2010;126(3):477.

76. Boyce JA, Assa'ad A, Burks AW, et al. Guidelines for the Diagnosis and Management of Food Allergy in the United States: Summary of the NIAID-Sponsored Expert Panel Report. *J Pediatr Nurs.* 2011;26(3):e2.

77. Keet C. Recognition and management of food-induced anaphylaxis. *Pediatr Clin North Am.* 2011;58(2):377-388, x.

78. Dutau G, Micheau P, Juchet A, Rancé F, Brémont F. Exercise and food-induced anaphylaxis. *Pediatr Pulmonol.* 2001;32(S23):48.

79. Bernstein JA, Lang DM, Khan DA, et al. Reviews and feature article: The diagnosis and management of acute and chronic urticaria: 2014 update. *J Allergy Clini Immunol.* 2014;133:1270-1277.e1266.

80. Feldweg AM. Review and feature article: food-dependent, exercise-induced anaphylaxis: Diagnosis and management

in the outpatient setting. *J Allergy Clin Immunol Pract.* 2017;5:283-288.

81. Eller E. Managing exercise food induced anaphylaxis. *Clin Transl Allergy.* 2011;1(Suppl 1):S49.

82. Gummin DD, Mowry JB, Spyker DA, Brooks DE, Fraser MO, Banner W. 2016 Annual Report of the American Association of Poison Control Centers' National Poison Data System (NPDS): 34th Annual Report. *Clin Toxicol.* 2017.

83. Barish RA, Arnold T. Insect stings. *Merck Manual Professional Version.* 2016. http://www.merckmanuals.com/professional/injuries-poisoning/bites-and-stings/insect-stings. Accessed December 2, 2017.

84. Schneir A, Clark RF. Bites and Stings. In Tintinalli JE, Stapczynski JS, Ma OJ, Yealy DM, Meckler GD, Cline DM, eds. *Tintinalli's Emergency Medicine: A Comprehensive Study Guide.* New York, NY: McGraw-Hill; 2016.

85. Page EH. Urticaria (Hives; Wheals). *Merck Manual Professional Version.* 2016. www.merckmanuals.com/professional/dermatologic-disorders/approach-to-the-dermatologic-patient/urticaria. Accessed December 2, 2017.

86. Delves PJ. Angioedema. Merck Manual Professional Version. 2016. https://www.merckmanuals.com/professional/immunology-allergic-disorders/allergic,-autoimmune,-and-other-hypersensitivity-disorders/angioedema. Accessed October 1, 2018.

87. Manivannan V, Decker WW, Stead LG, Li JTC, Campbell RL. Visual representation of National Institute of Allergy and Infectious Disease and Food Allergy and Anaphylaxis Network criteria for anaphylaxis. *Int J Emerg Med.* 2009;2(1):3-5.

88. Campbell RL, Li JTC, Nicklas RA, Sadosty AT. Practice parameter: Emergency department diagnosis and treatment of anaphylaxis: a practice parameter. *Ann Allergy Asthma Immunol.* 2014;113:599-608.

89. Campbell RL. Anaphylaxis: Emergency treatment. In *Merck Manual: Professional Version.* 2017. www.uptodate.com/contents/anaphylaxis-emergency-treatment?source=see_link#H3338251726. Accessed December 4, 2017.

90. World Health Organization. WHO model lists of essential medicines. 2017. www.who.int/medicines/publications/essentialmedicines/en. Accessed December 4, 2017, 2017.

91. Mylan, Inc. About EpiPen. 2017. www.epipen.com/en/hcp/for-health-care-partners/for-school-nurses. Accessed December 4, 2017.

92. Huggins RA, Scarneo SE, Casa DJ, et al. The Inter-Association Task Force document on emergency health and safety: Best-practice recommendations for youth sports leagues. *J Athl Train.* 2017;52(4):384-400.

93. Wauters RH, Banks TA, Lomasney EM. Food-dependent exercise-induced anaphylaxis. *BMJ Case Rep.* 2018;2018:1.

94. Manabe T, Oku N, Aihara Y. Food-dependent exercise-induced anaphylaxis in Japanese elementary school children. *Pediatr Int.* 2018;60(4):329-333.95.

95. Kucera KL, Thomas LC, Cantu RC. National Center for Catastrophic Sport Injury Research (NCCSIR) All Sport Report 1982/83-2015/16. 2017. https://nccsir.unc.edu/files/2013/10/NCCSIR-34th-Annual-All-Sport-Report-1982_2016_FINAL.pdf. Accessed May 9, 2018.

CHAPTER 7

1. Marieb EN. *Human Anatomy.* 8th ed. San Francisco, CA: Pearson Education; 2017.

2. Braun SR, Walker HK, Hall WD, Hurst JW. *Clinical Methods, the History, Physical, and Laboratory Examinations.* Stoneham, MA: Butterworth; 1990.

3. Prentice W. *Principles of Athletic Training: A Competency-Based Approach.* New York, NY: McGraw-Hill Higher Education; 2016.

4. Peskun CJ, Levy BA, Fanelli GC, et al. Diagnosis and management of knee dislocations. *Phys Sportsmed.* 2010;38(4):101-111.

5. Parrett BM, Matros E, Pribaz JJ, Orgill DP. Lower extremity trauma: trends in the management of soft-tissue reconstruction of open tibia-fibula fractures. *Plast Reconstr Surg.* 2006;117(4):1315-1322; discussion 1323-1324.

6. Menkes JS. Initial evaluation and management of orthopedic injuries. In Tintinalli JE, Stapczynski JS, Ma OJ, Yealy DM, Meckler GD, Cline DM, eds. *Tintinalli's Emergency Medicine: A Comprehensive Study Guide.* 8th ed. New York, NY: McGraw-Hill Inc.; 2000:1739-1753.

7. Sandrey MA. Effects of acute and chronic pathomechanics on the normal histology and biomechanics of tendons: A review. *J Sport Rehabil.* 2000;9(4):339-352.

8. Bailón-Plaza A, Van Der Meulen MC. Beneficial effects of moderate, early loading and adverse effects of delayed or excessive loading on bone healing. *J Biomech.* 2003;36(8):1069-1077.

9. Morell DJ, Thyagarajan DS. Sternoclavicular joint dislocation and its management: A review of the literature. *World J Orthop.* 2016;7(4):244.

10. Mirza AH, Alam K, Ali A. Posterior sternoclavicular dislocation in a rugby player as a cause of silent vascular compromise: A case report. *Br J Sports Med.* 2005;39(5):e28-e28.

11. Starkey C, Brown SD. *Examination of Orthopedic & Athletic Injuries.* Philadelphia, PA: FA Davis; 2015.

12. Groh GI. Sternoclavicular Joint Injuries. In *Clavicle Injuries.* Cham, Switzerland: Springer; 2018:145-163.

13. Marker LB, Klareskov B. Posterior sternoclavicular dislocation: an American football injury. *Br J Sports Med.* 1996;30(1):71-72.

14. Salgado R, Ghysen D. Post-traumatic posterior sternoclavicular dislocation: Case report and review of the literature. *Emerg Radiol.* 2002;9(6):323-325.

15. Gurney-Dunlop T, Eid AS, Old J, Dubberley J, MacDonald P. First-time anterior shoulder dislocation natural history and epidemiology: Immobilization versus early surgical repair. *Ann Jt.* 2017;2(11).

16. Atef A, El-Tantawy A, Gad H, Hefeda M. Prevalence of associated injuries after anterior shoulder dislocation: A prospective study. *Int Orthop.* 2016;40(3):519-524.

17. Cunningham NJ. Techniques for reduction of antero-inferior shoulder dislocation. *Emerg Med Australas.* 2005;17(5-6):463-471.

18. Kowalsky MS, Levine WN. Traumatic posterior glenohumeral dislocation: Classification, pathoanatomy, diagnosis, and treatment. *Orthop Clin North Am.* 2008;39(4):519-533.

19. McBride T, Kalogrianitis S. Dislocations of the shoulder joint. *Trauma.* 2012;14(1):47-56.

20. Robinson CM, Aderinto J. Posterior shoulder dislocations and fracture-dislocations. *JBJS.* 2005;87(3):639-650.

21. Goudie EB, Murray IR, Robinson CM. Instability of the shoulder following seizures. *J Bone Jt Surg Br.* 2012;94(6):721-728.

22. Mclaughlin HL. Posterior dislocation of the shoulder. *JBJS.* 1952;34(3):584-590.

23. Zacchilli MA, Owens BD. Epidemiology of shoulder dislocations presenting to emergency departments in the United States. *JBJS.* 2010;92(3):542-549.

24. Donohue MA, Brelin AM, LeClere LE. Management of first-time shoulder dislocation in the contact athlete. *Oper Tech Sports Med.* 2016;24(4):236-241.

25. Khiami F, Gérometta A, Loriaut P. Management of recent first-time anterior shoulder dislocations. *Orthop Traumatol Surg Res.* 2015;101(1):S51-S57.

26. Ufberg JW, Vilke GM, Chan TC, Harrigan RA. Anterior shoulder dislocations: Beyond traction-countertraction. *J Emerg Med.* 2004;27(3):301-306.

27. Robinson CM, Kelly M, Wakefield AE. Redislocation of the shoulder during the first six weeks after a primary anterior dislocation: risk factors and results of treatment. *JBJS.* 2002;84(9):1552-1559.

28. Wheelock M, Clark TA, Giuffre JL. Nerve transfers for treatment of isolated axillary nerve injuries. *Plast Surg.* 2015;23(2):77-80.

29. Karnes JM, Bravin DA, Hubbard DF. Axillary artery compression as a complication of a shoulder dislocation. *J Shoulder Elbow Surg.* 2016;25(3):e61-e64.

30. Rouleau DM, Hebert-Davies J, Robinson CM. Acute traumatic posterior shoulder dislocation. *J Am Acad Orthop Surg.* 2014;22(3):145-152.

31. Sheps DM, Hildebrand KA, Boorman RS. Simple dislocations of the elbow: Evaluation and treatment. *Hand Clin.* 2004;20(4):389-404.

32. Mehlhoff TL, Noble PC, Bennett JB, Tullos HS. Simple dislocation of the elbow in the adult. Results after closed treatment. *JBJS.* 1988;70(2):244-249.

33. Cohen MS, Hill Hastings II. Acute elbow dislocation: Evaluation and management. *J Am Acad Orthop Surg.* 1998;6(1):15-23.

34. Platz A, Heinzelmann M, Ertel W, Trentz O. Posterior elbow dislocation with associated vascular injury after blunt trauma. *J Trauma Acute Care Surg.* 1999;46(5):948-950.

35. Wadström J, Kinast C, Pfeiffer KM. Anatomical variations of the trochlear notch in elbow dislocations. *Z Für Unfallchirurgie Versicherungsmedizin Berufskrankh Off Organ Schweiz Ges Für Unfallmedizin Berufskrankh Rev Traumatol Assicurologie Mal Prof Organe Off Société Suisse Médecine Accid Mal Prof.* 1988;81(1):68.

36. Josefsson PO, Nilsson BE. Incidence of elbow dislocation. *Acta Orthop Scand.* 1986;57(6):537-538.

37. Armstrong A. Simple elbow dislocation. *Hand Clin.* 2015;31(4):521-531.

38. Stoneback JW, Owens BD, Sykes J, Athwal GS, Pointer L, Wolf JM. Incidence of elbow dislocations in the United States population. *JBJS.* 2012;94(3):240-245.

39. Goodman AD, Lemme N, DeFroda SF, Gil JA, Owens BD. Elbow dislocation and subluxation injuries in the National Collegiate Athletic Association, 2009-2010 through 2013-2014. *Orthop J Sports Med.* 2018;6(1). doi: 2325967117750105. Accessed February 2, 2018.

40. Miyazaki AN, Fregoneze M, Santos PD, Sella G do V, Checchia CS, Checchia SL. Brachial artery injury due to closed posterior elbow dislocation: case report. *Rev Bras Ortop.* 2016;51(2):239-243.

41. Borchers JR, Best TM. Common finger fractures and dislocations. *Am Fam Physician.* 2012;85(08):805-810.

42. Ramponi D, Cerepani MJ. Finger proximal interphalangeal joint dislocation. *Adv Emerg Nurs J.* 2015;37(4):252-257.

43. Golan E, Kang KK, Culbertson M, Choueka J. The epidemiology of finger dislocations presenting for emergency care within the United States. *Hand.* 2016;11(2):192-196.

44. Abraham MK, Scott S. The emergent evaluation and treatment of hand and wrist injuries. *Emerg Med Clin.* 2010;28(4):789-809.

45. Mall NA, Carlisle JC, Matava MJ, Powell JW, Goldfarb CA. Upper extremity injuries in the National Football League: part I: Hand and digital injuries. *Am J Sports Med.* 2008;36(10):1938-1944.

46. Fairbairn KJ, Mulligan ME, Murphey MD, Resnik CS. Gas bubbles in the hip joint on CT: An indication of recent dislocation. *AJR Am J Roentgenol.* 1995;164(4):931-934.

47. Court-Brown CM, Heckman JD, McQueen MM, Ricci WM, Tornetta P, McKee MD, eds. *Rockwood and Green's Fractures in Adults.* 8th ed. Philadelphia, PA: Wolters Kluwer Health; 2015.

48. Epstein HC. *Traumatic dislocation of the hip.* Williams & Wilkins. Baltimore, MD; 1980.

49. Pape H-C, Rice J, Wolfram K, Gänsslen A, Pohlemann T, Krettek C. Hip dislocation in patients with multiple injuries: A follow-up investigation. *Clin Orthop Relat Res.* 2000;377:99-105.

50. Anderson K, Strickland SM, Warren R. Hip and groin injuries in athletes. *Am J Sports Med.* 2001;29(4):521-533.

51. Scudese VA. Traumatic anterior hip redislocation. A case report. *Clin Orthop.* 1972;88:60-63.

52. Wetters NG, Murray TG, Moric M, Sporer SM, Paprosky WG, Valle CJD. Risk factors for dislocation after revision total hip arthroplasty. *Clin Orthop Relat Res.* 2013;471(2):410-416.

53. Hak DJ, Goulet JA. Severity of injuries associated with traumatic hip dislocation as a result of motor vehicle collisions. *J Trauma.* 1999;47(1):60-63.

54. Sanders S, Tejwani N, Egol KA. Traumatic hip dislocation--A review. *Bull NYU Hosp Jt Dis*. 2010;68(2):91-96.

55. Suraci AJ. Distribution and severity of injuries associated with hip dislocations secondary to motor vehicle accidents. *J Trauma*. 1986;26(5):458-460.

56. Clegg TE, Roberts CS, Greene JW, Prather BA. Hip dislocations—Epidemiology, treatment, and outcomes. *Injury*. 2010;41(4):329-334.

57. Tornetta 3rd P., Mostafavi HR. Hip dislocation: Current treatment regimens. *J Am Acad Orthop Surg*. 1997;5(1):27-36.

58. Howells NR, Brunton LR, Robinson J, Porteus AJ, Eldridge JD, Murray JR. Acute knee dislocation: An evidence based approach to the management of the multiligament injured knee. *Injury*. 2011;42(11):1198-1204.

59. King JJ, Cerynik DL, Blair JA, Harding SP, Tom JA. Surgical outcomes after traumatic open knee dislocation. *Knee Surg Sports Traumatol Arthrosc*. 2009;17(9):1027-1032.

60. Medina O, Arom GA, Yeranosian MG, Petrigliano FA, McAllister DR. Vascular and nerve injury after knee dislocation: A systematic review. *Clin Orthop Relat Res*. 2014;472(9):2621-2629.

61. Sillanpää PJ, Kannus P, Niemi ST, Rolf C, Felländer-Tsai L, Mattila VM. Incidence of knee dislocation and concomitant vascular injury requiring surgery: a nationwide study. *J Trauma Acute Care Surg*. 2014;76(3):715-719.

62. McDonough EB, Wojtys EM. Multiligamentous injuries of the knee and associated vascular injuries. *Am J Sports Med*. 2009;37(1):156-159.

63. Natsuhara KM, Yeranosian MG, Cohen JR, Wang JC, McAllister DR, Petrigliano FA. What is the frequency of vascular injury after knee dislocation? *Clin Orthop Relat Res*. 2014;472(9):2615-2620.

64. Schenck RC. Classification of Knee Dislocations. In *The Multiple Ligament Injured Knee*. Cham, Switzerland: Springer; 2004:37-49.

65. Wang C, Yang J, Wang S, et al. Three-dimensional motions of distal syndesmosis during walking. *J Orthop Surg*. 2015;10:166.

66. Lievers WB, Adamic PF. Incidence and severity of foot and ankle injuries in men's collegiate American football. *Orthop J Sports Med*. 2015;3(5). doi: 2325967115581593. Accessed January 30, 2018.

67. Wight L, Owen D, Goldbloom D, Knupp M. Pure ankle dislocation: A systematic review of the literature and estimation of incidence. *Injury*. 2017;48(10):2027-2034.

68. Skelley NW, McCormick JJ, Smith MV. In-game management of common joint dislocations. *Sports Health*. 2014;6(3):246-255.

69. McLaughlin JA, Light R, Lustrin I. Axillary artery injury as a complication of proximal humerus fractures. *J Shoulder Elbow Surg*. 1998;7(3):292-294.

70. Murray IR, Amin AK, White TO, Robinson CM. Proximal humeral fractures. *Bone Jt J*. 2011;93(1):1-11.

71. Modi CS, Nnene CO, Godsiff SP, Esler CNA. Axillary artery injury secondary to displaced proximal humeral fractures: A report of two cases. *J Orthop Surg*. 2008;16(2):243-246.

72. Jovanovich EN, Howard JF. Brachial plexus injury in a 6-year-old boy with 100% displaced proximal humeral metaphyseal fracture: A case report. *PM&R*. 2017;9(12):1294-1298.

73. Branch T, Partin C, Chamberland P, Emeterio E, Sabetelle M. Spontaneous fractures of the humerus during pitching: a series of 12 cases. *Am J Sports Med*. 1992;20(4):468-470.

74. Chu SP, Kelsey JL, Keegan TH, et al. Risk factors for proximal humerus fracture. *Am J Epidemiol*. 2004;160(4):360-367.

75. Griffin MR, Ray WA, Fought RL, Melton III LJ. Black-white differences in fracture rates. *Am J Epidemiol*. 1992;136(11):1378-1385.

76. Goulding A. Risk Factors for Fractures in Normally Active Children and Adolescents. In *Optimizing Bone Mass and Strength*. Vol 51. Basel, Switzerland: Karger; 2007:102-120.

77. Stenning M, Drew S, Birch R. Low-energy arterial injury at the shoulder with progressive or delayed nerve palsy. *Bone Jt J*. 2005;87(8):1102-1106.

78. Charles S, Ner I. Displaced proximal humeral fractures: Part II. Treatment of three-part and four-part displacement. *JBJS*. 1970;52(6):1090-1103.

79. Gellman H, Botte MJ. *Fractures of the Distal Radius*. American Academy of Orthopaedic Surgeons Series. Rosemont, IL: American Academy of Orthopaedic Surgeons; 1998.

80. Hanel DP, Jones MD, Trumble TE. Wrist fractures. *Orthop Clin*. 2002;33(1):35-57.

81. Shah NS, Buzas D, Zinberg EM. Epidemiologic dynamics contributing to pediatric wrist fractures in the United States. *Hand*. 2015;10(2):266-271.

82. Kozin SH, Wood MB. Early soft-tissue complications after fractures of the distal part of the radius. *J Bone Jt Surg Am*. 1993;75:144-153.

83. Holden CP, Holman J, Herman MJ. Pediatric pelvic fractures. *J Am Acad Orthop Surg*. 2007;15(3):172-177.

84. Giannoudis PV, Grotz MR, Tzioupis C, et al. Prevalence of pelvic fractures, associated injuries, and mortality: the United Kingdom perspective. *J Trauma Acute Care Surg*. 2007;63(4):875-883.

85. Moreno C, Moore EE, Rosenberger A, Cleveland HC. Hemorrhage associated with major pelvic fracture: A multispecialty challenge. *J Trauma*. 1986;26(11):987-994.

86. Wiens C, Zoga A. Imaging of Rodeo and Equestrian Injuries. In *Imaging in Sports-Specific Musculoskeletal Injuries*. Cham, Switzerland: Springer; 2016:697-720.

87. Brandes S, Borrelli J. Pelvic fracture and associated urologic injuries. *World J Surg*. 2001;25(12):1578-1587.

88. McCabe MP, Savoie III FH. Simple elbow dislocations: Evaluation, management, and outcomes. *Phys Sportsmed*. 2012;40(1):62-71.

89. Demetriades D, Karaiskakis M, Toutouzas K, Alo K, Velmahos G, Chan L. Pelvic fractures: epidemiology and

predictors of associated abdominal injuries and outcomes1. *J Am Coll Surg.* 2002;195(1):1-10.

90. Amorosa LF, Kloen P, Helfet DL. High-energy pediatric pelvic and acetabular fractures. *Orthop Clin.* 2014;45(4):483-500.

91. Shaath MK, Koury KL, Gibson PD, Adams MR, Sirkin MS, Reilly MC. Associated injuries in skeletally immature children with pelvic fractures. *J Emerg Med.* 2016;51(3):246-251.

92. Scott I, Porter K, Laird C, Greaves I, Bloch M. The pre-hospital management of pelvic fractures: Initial consensus statement. *J Paramed Pract.* 2014;6:248-252.

93. Meta M, Lu Y, Keyak JH, Lang T. Young-elderly differences in bone density, geometry, and strength indices depend on proximal femur sub-region: A cross sectional study in Caucasian-American women. *Bone.* 2006;39(1):152-158.

94. Egol K, Koval K, Zuckerman J. *Handbook of Fractures.* 5th ed. Philadelphia, PA: Wolters Kluwer Health; 2015.

95. Sikka R, Fetzer G, Hunkele T, Sugarman E, Boyd J. Femur fractures in professional athletes: A case series. *J Athl Train.* 2015;50(4):442-448.

96. Kay MC, Register-Mihalik JK, Gray AD, Djoko A, Dompier TP, Kerr ZY. The epidemiology of severe injuries sustained by National Collegiate Athletic Association Student-Athletes, 2009-2010 through 2014-2015. *J Athl Train.* 2017;52(2):117-128.

97. Johnson AW, Weiss CB, Wheeler DL. Stress fractures of the femoral shaft in athletes—More common than expected: A new clinical test. *Am J Sports Med.* 1994;22(2):248-256.

98. Pennock AT, Ellis HB, Willimon SC, et al. Intra-articular physeal fractures of the distal femur: A frequently missed diagnosis in adolescent athletes. *Orthop J Sports Med.* 2017;5(10).

99. Pietu G, Lebaron M, Flecher X, Hulet C, Vandenbussche E. Epidemiology of distal femur fractures in France in 2011-12. *Orthop Traumatol Surg Res.* 2014;100(5):545-548.

100. Hant FN, Bolster MB. Drugs that may harm bone: Mitigating the risk. *Cleve Clin J Med.* 2016;83(4):281-288.

101. Albuquerque RP e, Hara R, Prado J, Schiavo L, Giordano V, do Amaral NP. Epidemiological study on tibial plateau fractures at a level I trauma center. *Acta Ortop Bras.* 2013;21(2):109-115.

102. Prentice W. *Arnheim's Principles of Athletic Training: A Competency-Based Approach.* 13th ed. New York, NY: McGraw-Hill; 2009.

103. Mauser N, Gissel H, Henderson C, Hao J, Hak D, Mauffrey C. Acute lower-leg compartment syndrome. *Orthopedics.* 2013;36:619-624.

104. Köstler W, Strohm PC, Südkamp NP. Acute compartment syndrome of the limb. *Injury.* 2004;35(12):1221-1227.

105. Stenroos A, Pakarinen H, Jalkanen J, Mälkiä T, Handolin L. Tibial fractures in Alpine skiing and snowboarding in Finland: A retrospective study on fracture types and injury mechanisms in 363 patients. *Scand J Surgery* 2016;105(3):191-196.

106. Shibuya N, Davis ML, Jupiter DC. Epidemiology of foot and ankle fractures in the United States: An analysis of the National Trauma Data Bank (2007 to 2011). *J Foot Ankle Surg.* 2014;53(5):606-608.

107. Robertson GAJ, Wood AM, Aitken SA, Brown CC. Epidemiology, management, and outcome of sport-related ankle fractures in a standard UK population. *Foot Ankle Int.* 2014;35(11):1143-1152.

108. Su AW, Larson AN. Pediatric ankle fractures: Concepts and treatment principles. *Foot Ankle Clin.* 2015;20(4):705-719.

109. Hansen JT. *Netter's Anatomy Flash Cards.* 3rd ed. Philadelphia, PA: Elsevier; 2010.

110. Bachmann LM, Haberzeth S, Steurer J, Riet G ter. The accuracy of the Ottawa knee rule to rule out knee fractures: A systematic review. *Ann Intern Med.* 2004;140(2):121-124.

111. Cheung TC, Tank Y, Breederveld RS, Tuinebreijer WE, de Lange-de Klerk ESM, Derksen RJ. Diagnostic accuracy and reproducibility of the Ottawa Knee Rule vs the Pittsburgh Decision Rule. *Am J Emerg Med.* 2013;31(4):641-645.

112. Seaberg DC, Yealy DM, Lukens T, Auble T, Mathias S. Multicenter comparison of two clinical decision rules for the use of radiography in acute, high-risk knee injuries. *Ann Emerg Med.* 1998;32(1):8-13.

113. Richman PB, McCuskey CF, Nashed A, et al. Performance of two clinical decision rules for knee radiography. *J Emerg Med.* 1997;15(4):459-463.

114. Bauer SJ, Hollander JE, Fuchs SH, Thode HC. A clinical decision rule in the evaluation of acute knee injuries. *J Emerg Med.* 1995;13(5):611-615.

115. Pires R, Pereira A, Abreu-E-Silva G, et al. Ottawa ankle rules and subjective surgeon perception to evaluate radiograph necessity following foot and ankle sprain. *Ann Med Health Sci Res.* 2014;4(3):432-435.

116. Bachmann LM, Kolb E, Koller MT, Steurer J, Riet G ter. Accuracy of Ottawa ankle rules to exclude fractures of the ankle and mid-foot: Systematic review. *BMJ.* 2003;326(7386):417.

117. Gould SJ, Cardone DA, Munyak J, Underwood PJ, Gould SA. Sideline coverage: When to get radiographs? A review of clinical decision tools. *Sports Health.* 2014;6(3):274-278.

118. Toney CM, Games KE, Winkelmann ZK, Eberman LE. Using tuning-fork tests in diagnosing fractures. *J Athl Train.* 2016;51(6):498-499.

119. Markhardt BK, Gross JM, Monu J. Schatzker Classification of tibial plateau fractures: Use of CT and MR imaging improves assessment. *RadioGraphics.* 2009;29(2):585-597.

120. Runcie H, Greene M. Femoral traction splints in mountain rescue prehospital care: To use or not to use? That is the question. *Wilderness Environ Med.* 2015;26(3):305-311.

121. Lack WD, Karunakar MA, Angerame MR, et al. Type III open tibia fractures: Immediate antibiotic prophylaxis minimizes infection. *J Orthop Trauma.* 2015;29(1):1-6.

122. Murdock M, Murdoch MM. Compartment syndrome: A review of the literature. *Clin Podiatr Med Surg.* 2012;29(2):301-310.

123. Bamba R, Malhotra G, Bueno Jr RA, Thayer WP, Shack RB. Ring avulsion injuries: A systematic review. *HAND.* 2018;13(1):15-22.

124. Kupfer DM, Eaton C, Swanson S, McCarter MK, Lee GW. Ring avulsion injuries: A biomechanical study. *J Hand Surg.* 1999;24(6):1249-1253.

125. Molski M. Replantation of fingers and hands after avulsion and crush injuries. *J Plast Reconstr Aesthet Surg.* 2007;60(7):748-754.

126. DavasAksan A, Durusoy R, Bal E, Kayalar M, Ada S, Tanık FA. Risk factors for occupational hand injuries: Relationship between agency and finger. *Am J Ind Med.* 2012;55(5):465-473.

127. Sorock GS, Lombardi DA, Peng DK, et al. Glove use and the relative risk of acute hand injury: A case-crossover study. *J Occup Environ Hyg.* 2004;1(3):182-190.

128. Urbaniak JR, Evans JP, Bright DS. Microvascular management of ring avulsion injuries. *J Hand Surg.* 1981;6(1):25-30.

129. Kerr ZY, Marshall SW, Dompier TP, Corlette J, Klossner DA, Gilchrist J. College sports-related injuries - United States, 2009-10 through 2013-14 academic years. *MMWR Morb Mortal Wkly Rep.* 2015;64(48):1330-1336.

CHAPTER 8

1. Paluska SA, Lansford CD. Laryngeal trauma in sport. *Curr Sports Med Rep.* 2008;7(1):16-21. doi:10.1097/01.csmr.0000308673.53182.72. Accessed June 7, 2018.

2. Morris S-A, Jones WH, Proctor MR, Day AL. Emergent treatment of athletes with brain injury. *Neurosurgery.* 2014;75 Suppl 4:S96-S105. doi:10.1227/NEU.0000000000000465. Accessed June 7, 2018.

3. Kleiven S. Why most traumatic brain injuries are not caused by linear acceleration but skull fractures are. *Front Bioeng Biotechnol.* 2013;1:15. doi:10.3389/fbioe.2013.00015. Accessed June 7, 2018.

4. Blennow K, Brody DL, Kochanek PM, et al. Traumatic brain injuries. *Nat Rev Dis Primers.* 2016;2:16084. doi:10.1038/nrdp.2016.84. Accessed June 7, 2018.

5. Giza CC, Prins ML, Hovda DA. It's not all fun and games: Sports, concussions, and neuroscience. *Neuron.* 2017;94(6):1051-1055. doi:10.1016/j.neuron.2017.05.003. Accessed June 7, 2018.

6. Bethel J. Emergency care of children and adults with head injury. *Nurs Stand.* 2012;26(43):49-56. doi:10.7748/ns2012.06.26.43.49.c9176. Accessed June 7, 2018.

7. Saatman KE, Duhaime A-C, Bullock R, et al. Classification of traumatic brain injury for targeted therapies. *J Neurotrauma.* 2008;25(7):719-738.

8. Centers for Disease Control and Prevention. *Report to Congress on Mild Traumatic Brain Injury in the United States: Steps to Prevent a Serious Public Health Problem.* Atlanta, GA: CreateSpace; 2014.

9. Sarmiento K, Hoffman R, Dmitrovsky Z, Lee R. A 10-year review of the Centers for Disease Control and Prevention's Heads Up initiatives: Bringing concussion awareness to the forefront. *J Safety Res.* 2014;50:143-147.

10. Licona N, Chung J, Poole J, Laurenson N, Harris O. Prospective tracking and analysis of TBI in veterans and military personnel at Palo Alto DVBIC. *Arch Phys Med Rehabil.* 2015;96(10):e110.

11. Hollander JE, Richman PB, Werblud M, Miller T, Huggler J, Singer AJ. Irrigation in facial and scalp lacerations: Does it alter outcome? *Ann Emerg Med.* 1998;31(1):73-77.

12. Hollander JE, Singer AJ. Laceration management. *Ann Emerg Med.* 1999;34(3):356-367.

13. Pressley JC, Kendig TD, Frencher SK, Barlow B, Quitel L, Waqar F. Epidemiology of bone fracture across the age span in blacks and whites. *J Trauma.* 2011;71(5 Suppl 2):S541-S548.

14. Nelson EL, Melton LJ 3rd, Annegers JF, Laws ER, Offord KP. Incidence of skull fractures in Olmsted County, Minnesota. *Neurosurgery.* 1984;15(3):318-324.

15. Aubry M, Cantu R, Dvorak J, et al. Summary and agreement statement of the First International Conference on Concussion in Sport, Vienna 2001. *Phys Sportsmed.* 2002;30(2):57-63. doi:10.3810/psm.2002.02.176. Accessed June 7, 2018.

16. Pfister T, Pfister K, Hagel B, Ghali WA, Ronksley PE. The incidence of concussion in youth sports: A systematic review and meta-analysis. *Br J Sports Med.* 2016;50(5):292-297.

17. Coronado VG, Haileyesus T, Cheng TA, et al. Trends in sports- and recreation-related traumatic brain injuries treated in US emergency departments: The National Electronic Injury Surveillance System-All Injury Program (NEISS-AIP) 2001-2012. *J Head Trauma Rehabil.* 2015;30(3):185-197. doi:10.1097/HTR.0000000000000156. Accessed June 7, 2018.

18. Harmon KG, Drezner J, Gammons M, et al. American Medical Society for Sports Medicine position statement. *Clin J Sport Med.* 2013;23(1):1-18.

19. Custer A, Sufrinko A, Elbin RJ, Covassin T, Collins M, Kontos A. High baseline postconcussion symptom scores and concussion outcomes in athletes. *J Athl Train.* 2016;51(2):136-141.

20. Broglio SP, Cantu RC, Gioia GA, et al. National Athletic Trainers' Association Position Statement: Management of sport concussion. *J Athl Train.* 2014;49(2):245-265. doi:10.4085/1062-6050-49.1.07. Accessed June 7, 2018.

21. Guskiewicz KM, Valovich McLeod TC. Pediatric sports-related concussion. *PM R.* 2011;3(4):353-364; quiz 364.

22. Marshall SW, Guskiewicz KM, Shankar V, McCrea M, Cantu RC. Epidemiology of sports-related concussion in seven US high school and collegiate sports. *Injury Epidemiology.* 2015;2(1). doi:10.1186/s40621-015-0045-4. Accessed June 7, 2018.

23. McCrory P, Meeuwisse W, Dvořák J, et al. Consensus statement on concussion in sport-the 5th International Conference on Concussion in Sport held in Berlin, October

2016. *Br J Sports Med.* 2017;51(11):838-847. doi:10.1136/bjsports-2017-097699. Accessed June 7, 2018.

24. Pellman EJ, Viano DC. Concussion in professional football. *Neurosurg Focus.* 2006;21(4):1-10.

25. McCrory P. Does second impact syndrome exist? *Clin J Sport Med.* 2001;11(3):144-149.

26. Bey T, Ostick B. Second impact syndrome. *West J Emerg Med.* 2009;10(1):6-10.

27. Mori T, Katayama Y, Kawamata T. Acute hemispheric swelling associated with thin subdural hematomas: Pathophysiology of repetitive head injury in sports. *Acta Neurochir Suppl.* 2006;96:40-43.

28. McCrory P, Meeuwisse WH, Dvořák J, et al. 5th International Conference on Concussion in Sport (Berlin). *Br J Sports Med.* 2017;51(11):837. doi:10.1136/bjsports-2017-097878. Accessed June 7, 2018.

29. Putukian M. Clinical evaluation of the concussed athlete: A view from the sideline. *J Athl Train.* 2017;52(3):236-244. doi:10.4085/1062-6050-52.1.08. Accessed June 7, 2018.

30. Patricios J, Fuller GW, Ellenbogen R, et al. What are the critical elements of sideline screening that can be used to establish the diagnosis of concussion? A systematic review. *Br J Sports Med.* 2017;51(11):888-894.

31. Echemendia RJ, Meeuwisse W, McCrory P, et al. The Sport Concussion Assessment Tool 5th Edition (SCAT5): Background and rationale. *Br J Sports Med.* 2017;51(11):848-850.

32. Davis GA, Purcell L, Schneider KJ, et al. The Child Sport Concussion Assessment Tool 5th Edition (Child SCAT5): Background and rationale. *Br J Sports Med.* 2017;51(11):859-861.

33. McCrea M. Standardized mental status testing on the sideline after sport-related concussion. *J Athl Train.* 2001;36(3):274-279.

34. McCrory P, Meeuwisse WH, Dvořák J, et al. 5th International Conference on Concussion in Sport (Berlin). *Br J Sports Med.* 2017;51(11):837.

35. Rabinowitz AR, Merritt VC, Arnett PA. The return-to-play incentive and the effect of motivation on neuropsychological test-performance: Implications for baseline concussion testing. *Dev Neuropsychol.* 2015;40(1):29-33.

36. Mrazik M, Naidu D, Lebrun C, Game A, Matthews-White J. Does an individual's fitness level affect baseline concussion symptoms? *J Athl Train.* 2013;48(5):654-658.

37. Weber ML, Dean J-HL, Hoffman NL, et al. Influences of mental Illness, current psychological state, and concussion history on baseline concussion assessment performance. *Am J Sports Med. 2018;*46(7):1742-1751.

38. Mannix R, Iverson GL, Maxwell B, Atkins JE, Zafonte R, Berkner PD. Multiple prior concussions are associated with symptoms in high school athletes. *Ann Clin Transl Neur.* 2014;1(6):433-438.

39. Gagnon I, Grilli L, Friedman D, Iverson GL. A pilot study of active rehabilitation for adolescents who are slow to recover from sport-related concussion. *Scand J Med Sci Sports.* 2016;26(3):299-306. doi:10.1111/sms.12441. Accessed June 7, 2018.

40. Zemek R, Barrowman N, Freedman SB, et al. Clinical risk score for persistent postconcussion symptoms among children with acute concussion in the ED. *JAMA.* 2016;315(10):1014-1025. doi:10.1001/jama.2016.1203. Accessed June 7, 2018.

41. Silverberg ND, Iverson GL. Is rest after concussion "the best medicine?": Recommendations for activity resumption following concussion in athletes, civilians, and military service members. *J Head Trauma Rehabil.* 2013;28(4):250-259. doi:10.1097/HTR.0b013e31825ad658. Accessed June 7, 2018.

42. Chrisman SPD, Rivara FP. Physical activity or rest after concussion in youth: Questions about timing and potential benefit. *JAMA.* 2016;316(23):2491-2492. doi:10.1001/jama.2016.17562. Accessed June 7, 2018.

43. Baugh CM, Robbins CA, Stern RA, McKee AC. Current understanding of chronic traumatic encephalopathy. *Curr Treat Options Neurol.* 2014;16(9). doi:10.1007/s11940-014-0306-5. Accessed June 7, 2018.

44. Young LA, Rule GT, Bocchieri RT, Burns JM. Biophysical mechanisms of traumatic brain injuries. *Semin Neurol.* 2015;35(1):5-11. doi:10.1055/s-0035-1544242. Accessed June 7, 2018.

45. K2. Tagge CA, Fisher AM, Minaeva OV, et al. Concussion, microvascular injury, and early tauopathy in young athletes after impact head injury and an impact concussion mouse model. *Brain.* 2018;141(2):422-458.

46. Polderman KH, Tjong Tjin Joe R, Peerdeman SM, Vandertop WP, Girbes ARJ. Effects of therapeutic hypothermia on intracranial pressure and outcome in patients with severe head injury. *Intensive Care Med.* 2002;28(11):1563-1573. doi:10.1007/s00134-002-1511-3. Accessed June 7, 2018.

47. Dunn LT. Raised intracranial pressure. *J Neurol Neurosurg Psychiatry.* 2002;73(suppl 1):i23-i27.

48. Kurland D, Hong C, Aarabi B, Gerzanich V, Marc Simard J. Hemorrhagic progression of a contusion after traumatic brain injury: A review. *J Neurotrauma.* 2012;29(1):19-31. doi:10.1089/neu.2011.2122. Accessed June 7, 2018.

49. Deen HG, Gordon Deen H. Head trauma. *Neurol Clin Neurosci.* 2007:1386-1396.

50. Cripps A, Livingston SC. Differentiating concussion from intracranial pathology in athletes. *J Sport Rehabil.* 2017;26(1):101-108. doi:10.1123/jsr.2015-0043. Accessed June 7, 2018.

51. Dunning J. A meta-analysis of variables that predict significant intracranial injury in minor head trauma. *Arch Dis Child.* 2004;89(7):653-659. doi:10.1136/adc.2003.027722. Accessed June 7, 2018.

52. Ganz JC. The lucid interval associated with epidural bleeding: evolving understanding. *J Neurosurg.* 2013;118(4):739-745.

53. Bir SC, Maiti TK, Ambekar S, Nanda A. Incidence, hospital costs and in-hospital mortality rates of epidural hematoma in the United States. *Clin Neurol Neurosurg.* 2015;138:99-103.

54. Chen H, Guo Y, Chen S-W, et al. Progressive epidural hematoma in patients with head trauma: Incidence, outcome, and risk factors. *Emerg Med Int.* 2012;2012:134905.

55. Stiell IG, Wells GA. The Canadian CT Head Rule. *Lancet*. 2001;358(9286):1014.

56. Mueller FO. Catastrophic head injuries in high school and collegiate sports. *J Athl Train*. 2001;36(3):312-315.

57. Headache Classification Committee of the International Headache Society (IHS). The International Classification of Headache Disorders, 3rd ed. (beta version). *Cephalalgia*. 2013;33(9):629-808. doi:10.1177/0333102413485658. Accessed June 7, 2018.

58. Mitsikostas DD, Ashina M, Craven A, et al. European Headache Federation consensus on technical investigation for primary headache disorders. *J Headache Pain*. 2015;17:5. doi:10.1186/s10194-016-0596-y. Accessed June 7, 2018.

59. Rasmussen BK, Jensen R, Schroll M, Olesen J. Epidemiology of headache in a general population—A prevalence study. *J Clin Epidemiol*. 1991;44(11):1147-1157.

60. Lipton RB, Stewart WF, Diamond S, Diamond ML, Reed M. Prevalence and burden of migraine in the United States: Data from the American Migraine Study II. *Headache*. 2001;41(7):646-657.

61. Lipton RB, Bigal ME, Diamond M, et al. Migraine prevalence, disease burden, and the need for preventive therapy. *Neurology*. 2007;68(5):343-349. doi:10.1212/01.wnl.0000252808.97649.21. Accessed June 7, 2018.

62. Rasmussen BK, Jensen R, Schroll M, Olesen J. Epidemiology of headache in a general population—A prevalence study. *J Clin Epidemiol*. 1991;44(11):1147-1157. doi:10.1016/0895-4356(91)90147-2. Accessed June 7, 2018.

63. Pryse-Phillips W, Findlay H, Tugwell P, Edmeads J, Murray TJ, Nelson RF. A Canadian population survey on the clinical, epidemiologic and societal impact of migraine and tension-type headache. *Can J Neurol Sci*. 1992;19(3):333-339.

64. Schwartz BS. Epidemiology of tension-type headache. *JAMA*. 1998;279(5):381. doi:10.1001/jama.279.5.381. Accessed June 7, 2018.

65. Cohen A. Trigeminal autonomic cephalalgias—A diagnostic and therapeutic overview. *Adv Clin Neurosci Rehabil*. 2014;14(4):12-15.

66. Koppen H, van Veldhoven PLJ. Migraineurs with exercise-triggered attacks have a distinct migraine. *J Headache Pain*. 2013;14:99. doi:10.1186/1129-2377-14-99. Accessed June 7, 2018.

67. Begasse de Dhaem O, Barr WB, Balcer LJ, Galetta SL, Minen MT. Post-traumatic headache: the use of the sport concussion assessment tool (SCAT-3) as a predictor of post-concussion recovery. *J Headache Pain*. 2017;18(1):60. doi:10.1186/s10194-017-0767-5. Accessed June 7, 2018.

68. Hagen K, Wisløff U, Ellingsen Ø, Stovner LJ, Linde M. Headache and peak oxygen uptake: The HUNT3 study. *Cephalalgia*. 2016;36(5):437-444. doi:10.1177/0333102415597528. Accessed June 7, 2018.

69. Cheshire WP, Ott MC. Headache in Divers. *Headache*. 2001;41(3):235-247. doi:10.1046/j.1526-4610.2001.111006235.x. Accessed June 7, 2018.

70. Dodick DW. Diagnosing headache: Clinical clues and clinical rules. *Adv Stud Med*. 2003;3(2):87-92.

71. Ahmed F. Headache disorders: Differentiating and managing the common subtypes. *Br J Pain*. 2012;6(3):124-132. doi:10.1177/2049463712459691. Accessed June 7, 2018.

72. Hu XH, Henry Hu X, Markson LE, Lipton RB, Stewart WF, Berger ML. Burden of migraine in the United States. *Arch Intern Med*. 1999;159(8):813. doi:10.1001/archinte.159.8.813. Accessed June 7, 2018.

73. Diamond S, Bigal ME, Silberstein S, Loder E, Reed M, Lipton RB. Patterns of diagnosis and acute and preventive treatment for migraine in the United States: Results from the American Migraine Prevalence and Prevention Study. *Headache*. 2006;0(0):061117080657014 - ??? doi:10.1111/j.1526-4610.2006.00631.x. Accessed June 7, 2018.

74. Ahmadi A, Schwebel DC, Rezaei M. The efficacy of wet-cupping in the treatment of tension and migraine headache. *Am J Chin Med*. 2008;36(1):37-44. doi:10.1142/S0192415X08005564. Accessed June 7, 2018.

75. Symptom watch: 8 headache red flags and what they mean. United Health Care. www.uhclatino.com/content/lat-muh-clati/oxford/en/mantenerse-saludable/consejos-de-salud-al-instante/consejos-de-salud/observacion-de-sintomas--senales-de-advertencia-de-ocho-tipos-de.html. Accessed January 30, 2018.

76. O'Donnell MJ, Xavier D, Liu L, et al. Risk factors for ischaemic and intracerebral haemorrhagic stroke in 22 countries (the INTERSTROKE study): A case-control study. *Lancet*. 2010;376(9735):112-123. doi:10.1016/S0140-6736(10)60834-3. Accessed June 7, 2018.

77. Praveenya N, Mandava P, Kiranmai T, Mounika P, Reddy U, Anuroop V. Stroke associated risk factors and their incidence in patients admitted to tertiary care hospital. *WJPPS*. 2016;5(10):667-676. doi:10.20959/wjpps201610-7746. Accessed June 7, 2018.

78. Lubis SA, Novitri N. Comparison of post-stroke functional recovery between ischemic and hemorrhagic stroke patients: A prospective cohort study. *AMJ*. 2017;4(2):267-270. doi:10.15850/amj.v4n2.1069. Accessed June 7, 2018.

79. Kroll ME, Green J, Beral V, et al. Adiposity and ischemic and hemorrhagic stroke: Prospective study in women and meta-analysis. *Neurology*. 2016;87(14):1473-1481. doi:10.1212/WNL.0000000000003171. Accessed June 7, 2018.

80. Nordahl H, Osler M, Frederiksen BL, et al. Combined effects of socioeconomic position, smoking, and hypertension on risk of ischemic and hemorrhagic stroke. *Stroke*. 2014;45(9):2582-2587. doi:10.1161/STROKEAHA.114.005252. Accessed June 7, 2018.

81. Rose DZ, Guerrero WR, Mokin MV, et al. Hemorrhagic stroke following use of the synthetic marijuana "spice." *Neurology*. 2015;85(13):1177-1179. doi:10.1212/WNL.0000000000001973. Accessed June 7, 2018.

82. Harris BF, Winn C, Ableman TB. Hemorrhagic stroke in a young healthy male following use of pre-workout supplement Animal Rage XL. *Mil Med*. 2017;182(9):e2030-e2033. doi:10.7205/milmed-d-17-00013. Accessed June 7, 2018.

83. Cohen PA, Zeijlon R, Nardin R, Keizers PHJ, Venhuis B. Hemorrhagic stroke probably caused by exercise combined with a sports supplement containing β-Methylphenyl-ethylamine (BMPEA): A case report. *Ann Intern Med.* May 2015. doi:10.7326/L15-0106. Accessed June 7, 2018.

84. Young C, Oladipo O, Frasier S, Putko R, Chronister S, Marovich M. Hemorrhagic stroke in young healthy male following use of sports supplement Jack3d. *Mil Med.* 2012;177(12):1450-1454. doi:10.7205/milmed-d-11-00342. Accessed June 7, 2018.

85. Liferidge A, Brice J, Overby B, Evenson K. Ability of laypersons to use the Cincinnati Prehospital Stroke Scale. *Prehosp Emerg Care.* 2004;8(4):384-387. doi:10.1016/j.prehos.2004.05.004. Accessed June 7, 2018.

86. Kothari R, Pancioli A, Liu T, Brott T, Broderick J. Cincinnati Prehospital Stroke Scale: Reproducibility and validity. *Ann Emerg Med.* 1999;33(4):373-378. doi:10.1016/S0196-0644(99)70299-4. Accessed June 7, 2018.

87. Powers WJ, Rabinstein AA, Ackerson T, et al. 2018 Guidelines for the early management of patients with acute ischemic stroke: A guideline for healthcare professionals from the American Heart Association/American Stroke Association. *Stroke.* January 2018. doi:10.1161/STR.0000000000000158. Accessed June 7, 2018.

88. The Joint Commission. Facts about stroke certification. www.jointcommission.org/facts_about_joint_commission_stroke_certification. Accessed June 4, 2018.

89. Collard SS, Ellis-Hill C. How do you exercise with epilepsy? Insights into the barriers and adaptations to successfully exercise with epilepsy. *Epilepsy Behav.* 2017;70(Pt A):66-71. doi:10.1016/j.yebeh.2017.03.004. Accessed June 7, 2018.

90. Huff JS, Morris DL, Kothari RU, Gibbs MA, Emergency Medicine Seizure Study Group. Emergency department management of patients with seizures: A multicenter study. *Acad Emerg Med.* 2001;8(6):622-628.

91. Slattery DE, Pollack CV. Seizures as a cause of altered mental status. *Emerg Med Clin North Am.* 2010;28(3):517-534. doi:10.1016/j.emc.2010.03.011. Accessed June 7, 2018.

92. Capovilla G, Kaufman KR, Perucca E, Moshé SL, Arida RM. Epilepsy, seizures, physical exercise, and sports: A report from the ILAE Task Force on Sports and Epilepsy. *Epilepsia.* 2016;57(1):6-12. doi:10.1111/epi.13261. Accessed June 7, 2018.

93. Fisher RS, Cross JH, French JA, et al. Operational classification of seizure types by the International League Against Epilepsy: Position Paper of the ILAE Commission for Classification and Terminology. *Epilepsia.* 2017;58(4):522-530.

94. Epilepsy Foundation. Types of seizures. www.epilepsy.com/learn/types-seizures. Accessed June 4, 2018.

95. Krauss G, Theodore WH. Treatment strategies in the postictal state. *Epilepsy Behav.* 2010;19(2):188-190. doi:10.1016/j.yebeh.2010.06.030. Accessed June 7, 2018.

96. Fisher RS, Engel JJ Jr. Definition of the postictal state: When does it start and end? *Epilepsy Behav.* 2010;19(2):100-104. doi:10.1016/j.yebeh.2010.06.038. Accessed June 7, 2018.

97. Epilepsy Foundation. Getting emergency help. www.epilepsy.com/learn/seizure-first-aid-and-safety/getting-emergency-help. Accessed June 4, 2018.

98. Epilepsy Foundation. Diazepam. www.epilepsy.com/medications/diazepam/advanced. Accessed June 4, 2018.

99. Robinson TW. Valium in the treatment of epilepsy. *Calif Med.* 1970;112(3):63-64.

100. Peeters E. Treatment of epileptic seizures as medical emergencies: A prospective analysis of a decision tree for nonmedically trained staff. *Seizure.* 2000;9(7):473-479. doi:10.1053/seiz.2000.0420. Accessed June 7, 2018.

101. Park E, Abraham MK. Altered mental status and endocrine diseases. *Emerg Med Clin North Am.* 2014;32(2):367-378. doi:10.1016/j.emc.2013.12.007. Accessed June 7, 2018.

102. Hardern RD, Quinn ND. Emergency management of diabetic ketoacidosis in adults. *Emerg Med J.* 2003;20(3):210-213.

103. American Heart Association. Hypertensive crisis: When you should call 9-1-1 for high blood pressure. www.heart.org/HEARTORG/Conditions/HighBloodPressure/GettheFactsAboutHighBloodPressure/Hypertensive-Crisis-When-You-Should-Call-9-1-1-for-High-Blood-Pressure_UCM_301782_Article.jsp#.WnDlmFPwYWo.

104. American Diabetes Association. Hypoglycemia (low blood glucose). www.diabetes.org/living-with-diabetes/treatment-and-care/blood-glucose-control/hypoglycemia-low-blood.html. Accessed June 5, 2018.

105. MayoClinic. Signs and symptoms. Hypothermia. www.mayoclinic.org/diseases-conditions/hypothermia/symptoms-causes/syc-20352682.

106. Nwazue VC, Raj SR. Confounders of vasovagal syncope: Orthostatic hypotension. *Cardiol Clin.* 2013;31(1):89-100.

107. American Heart Association. Syncope (fainting). www.heart.org/HEARTORG/Conditions/Arrhythmia/SymptomsDiagnosisMonitoringofArrhythmia/Syncope-Fainting_UCM_430006_Article.jsp#.WnC0JVPwYWo.

108. Lanier JB, Mote MB, Clay EC. Evaluation and management of orthostatic hypotension. *Am Fam Physician.* 2011;84(5):527-536.

109. Panayiotopoulos CP. Syncopal attacks imitating epileptic seizures. In Panayiotopoulos CP, ed. *Imitators of Epileptic Seizures.* London, UK: Springer London; 2012:9-15.

110. Arlt W, Society for Endocrinology Clinical Committee. Society for Endocrinology Endocrine Emergency Guidance: Emergency management of acute adrenal insufficiency (adrenal crisis) in adult patients. *Endocr Connect.* 2016;5(5):G1-G3.

111. Bornstein SR, Allolio B, Arlt W, et al. Diagnosis and treatment of primary adrenal insufficiency: An Endocrine Society Clinical Practice Guideline. *J Clin Endocrinol Metab.* 2016;101(2):364-389.

112. Aronow WS. Treatment of hypertensive emergencies. *Ann Transl Med.* 2017;5(Suppl 1):S5.

113. American Diabetes Association. Hypoglycemia. www.diabetes.org/living-with-diabetes/treatment-and-care/

blood-glucose-control/hypoglycemia-low-blood.html. Accessed June 5, 2018.

114. McCullough L, Aurora S. Diagnosis and treatment of hypothermia. *Am Fam Physician*. 2004;70(12):2325-2332.

115. Lezama MV, Oluigbo NE, Ouellette JR. Myxedema coma and thyroid storm: Diagnosis and management. http://turner-white.com/pdf/brm_IM_V14P2.pdf. Accessed June 5, 2018.

116. Black AM, Eliason PH, Patton DA, Emery CA. Epidemiology of facial injuries in sport. *Clin Sports Med*. 2017;36(2):237-255. doi:10.1016/j.csm.2016.11.001. Accessed June 7, 2018.

117. Salomone JP. The face of trauma. *JEMS*. 2011;36(4):50-56. doi:10.1016/s0197-2510(11)70089-4. Accessed June 7, 2018.

118. Pollard KA, Xiang H, Smith GA. Pediatric eye injuries treated in US emergency departments, 1990-2009. *Clin Pediatr*. 2012;51(4):374-381. doi:10.1177/0009922811427583. Accessed June 7, 2018.

119. Read SP, Young RC, Flynn HW Jr. Outcomes in bullous retinal detachment. *Am J Ophthalmol Case Rep*. 2017;6:18-20. doi:10.1016/j.ajoc.2016.12.008. Accessed June 7, 2018.

120. Ong HS, Barsam A, Morris OC, Siriwardena D, Verma S. A survey of ocular sports trauma and the role of eye protection. *Cont Lens Anterior Eye*. 2012;35(6):285-287. doi:10.1016/j.clae.2012.07.007. Accessed June 7, 2018.

121. Haring RS, Sheffield ID, Canner JK, Schneider EB. Epidemiology of sports-related eye injuries in the United States. *JAMA Ophthalmol*. 2016;134(12):1382-1390. doi:10.1001/jamaophthalmol.2016.4253. Accessed June 7, 2018.

122. Mishra A, Verma AK. Sports related ocular injuries. *Armed Forces Med J India*. 2012;68(3):260-266. doi:10.1016/j.mjafi.2011.12.004. Accessed June 7, 2018.

123. Wipperman JL, Dorsch JN. Evaluation and management of corneal abrasions. *Am Fam Physician*. 2013;87(2):114-120. www.ncbi.nlm.nih.gov/pubmed/23317075.

124. Rosner M, Treister G, Belkin M. Epidemiology of retinal detachment in childhood and adolescence. *J Pediatr Opthalmol Strabismus*. 1987;Jan-Feb;24(1):42-44.

125. Risk factors for idiopathic rhegmatogenous retinal detachment. The Eye Disease Case-Control Study Group. *Am J Epidemiol*. 1993;137(7):749-757.

126. Khan-Farooqi HR, Chiranand P, Edelstein SL. Epidemiology and outcome of traumatic hyphema: A retrospective case series. *Inv Opthalmol Vis Sci*. 2010;April(51)1314.

127. Carniol ET, Bresler A, Shaigany K, et al. Traumatic tympanic membrane perforations diagnosed in emergency departments. *JAMA Otolaryngol Head Neck Surg*. December 2017. doi:10.1001/jamaoto.2017.2550. Accessed June 7, 2018.

128. Xydakis MS, Bebarta VS, Harrison CD, Conner JC, Grant GA, Robbins AS. Tympanic-membrane perforation as a marker of concussive brain injury in Iraq. *N Engl J Med*. 2007;357(8):830-831. doi:10.1056/NEJMc076071. Accessed June 7, 2018.

129. Patterson R. The Le Fort fractures: Rene Le Fort and his work in anatomical pathology. *Can J Surg*. 1991;34(2):183-184.

130. Reehal P. Facial injury in sport. *Curr Sports Med Rep*. 2010;9(1):27-34. doi:10.1249/jsr.0b013e3181cd2c04. Accessed June 7, 2018.

131. Pieramici DJ. Sports-Related Eye Injuries. *JAMA*. 2017;318(24):2483-2484. doi:10.1001/jama.2017.17560. Accessed June 7, 2018.

132. Batista AM, Ferreira F de O, Marques LS, Ramos-Jorge ML, Ferreira MC. Risk factors associated with facial fractures. *Braz Oral Res*. 2012;26(2):119-125.

133. Sharma H, Chowdhury S, Navaneetham A, Upadhyay S, Alam S. Costochondral graft as interpositional material for TMJ ankylosis in children: A clinical study. *J Maxillofac Oral Surg*. 2015;14(3):565-572.

134. Young EJ, Macias CR, Stephens L. Common dental injury management in athletes. *Sports Health*. 2015;7(3):250-255. doi:10.1177/1941738113486077. Accessed June 7, 2018.

135. Gould TE, Piland SG, Caswell SV, et al. National Athletic Trainers' Association Position Statement: Preventing and managing sport-related dental and oral injuries. *J Athl Train*. 2016;51(10):821-839. doi:10.4085/1062-6050-51.8.01. Accessed June 7, 2018.

136. Jalisi S, Zoccoli M. Management of laryngeal fractures--a 10-year experience. *J Voice*. 2011;25(4):473-479.

137. Mendelsohn AH, Sidell DR, Berke GS, John MS. Optimal timing of surgical intervention following adult laryngeal trauma. *Laryngoscope*. 2011;121(10):2122-2127.

138. Academy for Sports Dentistry Emergency Treatment Card. Academy for Sports Dentistry. www.academyforsportsdentistry.org/treatment-cards. Accessed January 29, 2017.

139. Atkins BZ, Abbate S, Fisher SR, Vaslef SN. Current management of laryngotracheal trauma: Case report and literature review. *J Trauma*. 2004;56(1):185-190. doi:10.1097/01.TA.0000082650.62207.92. Accessed June 7, 2018.

140. Bin Zahid A, Hubbard ME, Dammavalam VM, et al. Assessment of acute head injury in an emergency department population using sport concussion assessment tool - 3rd ed. *Appl Neuropsychol Adult*. 2018;25(2):110-119. doi:10.1080/23279095.2016.1248765. Accessed June 7, 2018.

141. Buckley TA, Munkasy BA, Clouse BP. Sensitivity and specificity of the Modified Balance Error Scoring System in concussed collegiate student athletes. *Clin J Sports Med*. 2018;28(2):174-176. doi: 10.1097/JSM.0000000000000426. Accessed June 7, 2018.

142. Resch J, Driscoll A, McCaffrey N, et al. ImPact test-retest reliability: Reliably unreliable? *J Athl Trn*. 2013;48(4):506-511. doi: 10.4085/1062-6050-48.3.09. Accessed June 7, 2018.

CHAPTER 9

1. National Spinal Cord Injury Statistical Center. *Facts and Figures at a Glance*. Birmingham, AL: University of Alabama at Birmingham; 2017.

2. National Spinal Cord Injury Statistical Center. *Facts and Figures at a Glance*. Birmingham, AL: University of Alabama at Birmingham; 2014.

3. National Collegiate Athletic Association. Student-Athletes. www.ncaa.org/student-athletes. Accessed August 24, 2017.

4. National Federation of State High School Associations. 2016-17 High School Athletics Participation Survey. National Federation of State High School Associations. www.nfhs.org/articles/high-school-sports-participation-increases-for-28th-straight-year-nears-8-million-mark/. Published September 6, 2017. Accessed December 29, 2017.

5. Marieb EN. *Human Anatomy, Global Edition*. 8th ed. San Francisco, CA: Pearson Education; 2017.

6. Broome DR, Hayman LA, Herrick RC, Braverman RM, Glass RB, Fahr LM. Postnatal maturation of the sacrum and coccyx: MR imaging, helical CT, and conventional radiography. *AJR*. 1998;170(4):1061-1066. doi:10.2214/ajr.170.4.9530059. Accessed October 23, 2017.

7. Marieb EN, Hoehn K. *Human Anatomy & Physiology*. 7th ed. San Francisco, CA: Pearson Education; 2007.

8. Swartz EE, Boden BP, Courson RW, et al. National Athletic Trainers' Association position statement: Acute management of the cervical spine–injured athlete. *J Athl Train*. 2009;44(3):306.

9. Blackmore ME, Goswami T, Chancey C. Cervical spinal injuries and risk assessment. 2012. http://cdn.intechopen.com/pdfs/38127/InTech-Cervical_spinal_injuries_and_risk_assessment.pdf. Accessed April 30, 2013.

10. Torg JS, Vegso JJ, O'Neill MJ, Sennett B. The epidemiologic, pathologic, biomechanical, and cinematographic analysis of football-induced cervical spine trauma. *Am J Sports Med*. 1990;18(1):50-57. doi:10.1177/036354659001800109. Accessed September 17, 2012.

11. Hadley M. Guidelines of the American Association of Neurologic Surgeons and the Congress of Neurologic Surgeons: Cervical spine immobilization before admission to hospital. *Neurosurgery*. 2002;50:S7-17.

12. Boden BP, Levin D. Cervical Spine. In *Musculoskeletal and Sports Medicine for the Primary Care Physician*. 4th ed. Boca Raton, FL: Taylor & Francis Group; 2016:423-238.

13. Penning L. Kinematics of cervical spine injury. *Eur Spine J*. 1995;4(2):126-132.

14. Amevo B, Aprill C, Bogduk N. Abnormal instantaneous axes of rotation in patients with neck pain. *Spine*. 1992;17(7):748-756.

15. Meron A, McMullen C, Laker SR, Currie D, Comstock RD. Epidemiology of cervical spine injuries in high school athletes over a ten-year period. *PM&R*. 2018;10(4):365-372. doi:10.1016/j.pmrj.2017.09.003. Accessed April 17, 2018.

16. Nagel DA, Koogle TA, Piziali RL, Perkash I. Stability of the upper lumbar spine following progressive disruptions and the application of individual internal and external fixation devices. *J Bone Joint Surg Am*. 1981;63(1):62-70.

17. Panjabi MM, Hausfeld JN, White AA. A biomechanical study of the ligamentous stability of the thoracic spine in man. *Acta Orthopaedica*. 1981;52(3):315-326.

18. DuBose DN. Changes in space available for the cord when comparing a stable spine to an unstable spine during range of motion testing. 2015. http://search.proquest.com/openview/ca5234692f1efd799554c2030bbd604c/1?pq-origsite=gscholar&cbl=18750&diss=y. Accessed May 24, 2017.

19. Chung SS, Lee CS, Kim SH, Chung MW, Ahn JM. Effect of low back posture on the morphology of the spinal canal. *Skeletal Radiol*. 2000;29(4):217-223.

20. Ching RP, Watson NA, Carter JW, Tencer AF. The effect of post-injury spinal position on canal occlusion in a cervical spine burst fracture model. *Spine*. 1997;22(15):1710.

21. Inufusa A, An HS, Lim TH, Hasegawa T, Haughton VM, Nowicki BH. Anatomic changes of the spinal canal and intervertebral foramen associated with flexion-extension movement. *Spine*. 1996;21(21):2412-2420.

22. Osterholm J, Wilkins R. The Catecholamine Hypothesis of Spinal Cord Injury. In *The Pathophysiology of Spinal Cord Trauma*. Springfield, IL: Thomas; 1978:41-45.

23. Torg JS, Pavlov H, Genuario SE, et al. Neurapraxia of the cervical spinal cord with transient quadriplegia. *J Bone Joint Surg Am*. 1986;68(9):1354.

24. Madhugiri VS, Ambekar S, Roopesh Kumar VR, Sasidharan GM, Nanda A. Spinal aneurysms: Clinicoradiological features and management paradigms. *J Neurosurg Spine*. 2013;19(1):34-48. doi:10.3171/2013.3.SPINE121026. Accessed April 17, 2018.

25. Vuong SM, Jeong WJ, Morales H, Abruzzo TA. Vascular diseases of the spinal cord: Infarction, hemorrhage, and venous congestive myelopathy. *Semin Ultrasound CT MR*. 2016;37(5):466-481. doi:10.1053/j.sult.2016.05.008. Accessed April 17, 2018.

26. NASEMSO Medical Director's Council. National Model: EMS Clinical Guidelines. October 2014. www.nasemso.org/Projects/ModelEMSClinicalGuidelines/documents/National-Model-EMS-Clinical-Guidelines-23Oct2014.pdf. Accessed January 14, 2015.

27. White IV CC, Domeier RM, Millin MG. EMS spinal precautions and the use of the long backboard—resource document to the position statement of the National Association of EMS Physicians and the American College of Surgeons Committee on Trauma. *Prehosp Emerg Care*. 2014;18(2):306-314. doi:10.3109/10903127.2014.884197. Accessed May 4, 2015.

28. Stiell IG, Wells GA, Vandemheen KL, et al. The Canadian C-Spine Rule for radiography in alert and stable trauma patients. *JAMA*. 2001;286(15):1841-1848.

29. Vaillancourt C, Stiell IG, Beaudoin T, et al. The out-of-hospital validation of the Canadian C-Spine Rule by paramedics. *Ann Emerg Med*. 2009;54(5):663-671.e1. doi:10.1016/j.annemergmed.2009.03.008. Accessed October 26, 2017.

30. Hoffman JR, Wolfson AB, Todd K, Mower WR. Selective cervical spine radiography in blunt trauma: methodology of the National Emergency X-Radiography Utilization Study (NEXUS). *Ann Emerg Med*. 1998;32(4):461-469.

31. Purvis TA, Carlin B, Driscoll P. The definite risks and questionable benefits of liberal pre-hospital spinal immobilisation. *Am J Emerg Med*. 2017;35(6):860-866. doi:10.1016/j.ajem.2017.01.045. Accessed October 26, 2017.

32. Abram S, Bulstrode C. Routine spinal immobilization in trauma patients: What are the advantages and disadvantages? *Surgeon*. 2010;8(4):218-222. doi:10.1016/j.surge.2010.01.002. Accessed October 26, 2017.

33. Kornhall DK, Jørgensen JJ, Brommeland T, et al. The Norwegian guidelines for the prehospital management of adult trauma patients with potential spinal injury. *Scand J Trauma Resusc Emerg Med*. 2017;25:2. doi:10.1186/s13049-016-0345-x. Accessed October 17, 2017.

34. Davies G, Deakin C, Wilson A. The effect of a rigid collar on intracranial pressure. *Injury*. 1996;27(9):647-649. doi:10.1016/S0020-1383(96)00115-5. Accessed February 6, 2015.

35. Sheerin F, de Frein R. The occipital and sacral pressures experienced by healthy volunteers under spinal immobilization: a trial of three surfaces. *J Emerg Nurs*. 2007;33(5):447-450. doi:10.1016/j.jen.2006.11.004. Accessed May 10, 2015.

36. Aprahamian C, Thompson BM, Finger WA, Darinz JC. Experimental cervical spine injury model: Evaluation of airway management and splinting techniques. *Ann Emerg Med*. 1984;13(8):584-587.

37. Goutcher CM, Lochhead V. Reduction in mouth opening with semi-rigid cervical collars. *Br J Anaesth*. 2005;95(3):344-348.

38. Prasarn ML, Horodyski M, Scott NE, Konopka G, Conrad B, Rechtine GR. Motion generated in the unstable upper cervical spine during head tilt–chin lift and jaw thrust maneuvers. *Spine J*. 2014;14(4):609-614. doi:10.1016/j.spinee.2013.06.080. Accessed May 4, 2015.

39. Becker DE, Rosenberg MB, Phero JC. Essentials of airway management, oxygenation, and ventilation: part 1: basic equipment and devices. *Anesth Prog*. 2014;61(2):78-83. doi:10.2344/0003-3006-61.2.78. Accessed September 28, 2018.

40. Wendling AL, Tighe PJ, Conrad BP, Baslanti TO, Horodyski M, Rechtine GR. Comparison of four airway devices on cervical spine alignment in cadaver models of global ligamentous instability at C1-2. *Anesth Analg*. 2013;117(1):126-132. doi:10.1213/ANE.0b013e318279b37a. Accessed September 28, 2018.

41. Prasarn M, Conrad BP, Rubery P, et al. Comparison of four airway devices on cervical spine alignment in a cadaver model with global ligamentous instability at C5-6. *Spine*. 2011. doi: 10.1097/BRS.0b013e31822419fe. Accessed September 28, 2018.

42. Burkey S, Jeanmonod R, Fedor P, Stromski C, Waninger KN. Evaluation of standard endotracheal intubation, assisted laryngoscopy (Airtraq), and laryngeal mask airway in the management of the helmeted athlete airway: A Manikin study. *Clin J Sport Med*. 2011;21(4):301-306. doi:10.1097/JSM.0b013e31821d314c. Accessed September 28, 2018.

43. Delaney JS, Al-Kashmiri A, Baylis P-J, Troutman T, Aljufaili M, Correa JA. The assessment of airway maneuvers and interventions in university Canadian football, ice hockey, and soccer players. *J Athl Train*. 2011;46(2):117-125. doi:10.4085/1062-6050-46.2.117. Accessed September 28, 2018.

44. Crosby ET. Airway management in adults after cervical spine trauma. *Anesthesiology*. 2006;104(6):1293-1318.

45. Hastings RH, Wood PR. Head extension and laryngeal view during laryngoscopy with cervical spine stabilization maneuvers. *Anesthesiology*. 1994;80(4):825-831.

46. Crosby ET. Considerations for airway management for cervical spine surgery in adults. *Anesthesiol Clin*. 2007;25(3):511-533.

47. Brimacombe J, Keller C, Künzel KH, Gaber O, Boehler M, Pühringer F. Cervical spine motion during airway management: A cinefluoroscopic study of the posteriorly destabilized third cervical vertebrae in human cadavers. *Anesth Analg*. 2000;91(5):1274-1278.

48. Gerling MC, Davis DP, Hamilton RS, et al. Effects of cervical spine immobilization technique and laryngoscope blade selection on an unstable cervical spine in a cadaver model of intubation. *Ann Emerg Med*. 2000;36(4):293-300.

49. Mihalik JP, Lynall RC, Fraser MA, et al. Football equipment removal improves chest compression and ventilation efficacy. *Prehosp Emerg Care*. 2016;20(5)578-585. doi: 10.3109/10903127.2016.1149649. Accessed September 27, 2018.

50. McCabe JB, Nolan DJ. Comparison of the effectiveness of different cervical immobilization collars. *Ann Emerg Med*. 1986;15(1):50-53. doi:10.1016/S0196-0644(86)80487-5. Accessed October 24, 2017.

51. De Lorenzo RA. A review of spinal immobilization techniques. *J Emerg Med*. 1996;14(5):603-613.

52. Boissy P, Shrier I, Brière S, et al. Effectiveness of cervical spine stabilization techniques. *Clin J Sport Med*. 2011;21(2):80-88.

53. Kleiner DM, Almquist J, Bailes J, et al. Prehospital care of the spine injured athlete: A document from the Inter-Association Task Force for Appropriate Care of the Spine Injured Athlete. *J Athl Train*. 2001;36(1):4-29.

54. Lennarson PJ, Smith D, Todd MM, et al. Segmental cervical spine motion during orotracheal intubation of the intact and injured spine with and without external stabilization. *J Neurosurg Spine*. 2000;92(2):201-206.

55. Bivins HG, Ford S, Bezmalinovic Z, Price HM, Williams JL. The effect of axial traction during orotracheal intubation of the trauma victim with an unstable cervical spine. *Ann Emerg Med*. 1988;17(1):25-29.

56. Tierney RT, Maldjian C, Mattacola CG, Straub SJ, Sitler MR. Cervical spine stenosis measures in normal subjects. *J Athl Train*. 2002;37(2):190.

57. Gabbott DA, Baskett PJ. Management of the airway and ventilation during resuscitation. *Br J Anaesth.* 1997;79(2):159-171.

58. Richter D, Latta LL, Milne EL, et al. The stabilizing effects of different orthoses in the intact and unstable upper cervical spine: a cadaver study. *J Trauma.* 2001;50(5):848-854.

59. Horodyski M, DiPaola CP, Conrad BP, Rechtine GR. Cervical collars are insufficient for immobilizing an unstable cervical spine injury. *J Emerg Med.* 2011;41(5):513-519.

60. Ben-Galim P, Dreiangel N, Mattox KL, et al. Extrication collars can result in abnormal separation between vertebrae in the presence of a dissociative injury: *J Trauma.* 2010;69(2):447-450. doi:10.1097/TA.0b013e3181be785a. Accessed September 27, 2018

61. Lador R, Ben-Galim P, Hipp JA. Motion within the unstable cervical spine during patient maneuvering: The neck pivot-shift phenomenon. *J Trauma Acute Care Surg.* 2011;70(1):247.

62. Aoi Y, Inagawa G, Hashimoto K, et al. Airway scope laryngoscopy under manual inline stabilization and cervical collar immobilization: A crossover in vivo cinefluoroscopic study. *J Trauma Acute Care Surg.* 2011;71(1):32-36. doi:10.1097/TA.0b013e3181e75873. Accessed October 27, 2017.

63. Salomone JP, Pons PT, eds. *Prehospital Trauma Life Support.* 7th ed. St. Louis, MO: Mosby Jems Elsevier; 2011.

64. Del Rossi G, Horodyski MH, Conrad BP, Di Paola CP, Di Paola MJ, Rechtine GR. The 6-plus–person lift transfer technique compared with other methods of spine boarding. *J Athl Train.* 2008;43(1):6.

65. DuBose DN, Zdziarski LA, Scott N, et al. Horizontal slide creates less cervical motion when centering an injured patient on a spine board. *Journal Emerg Med.* 2015. www.sciencedirect.com/science/article/pii/S0736467915010227. Accessed November 20, 2015.

66. Conrad BP, Marchese DL, Rechtine GR, Prasarn M, Del Rossi G, Horodyski MH. Motion in the unstable cervical spine when transferring a patient positioned prone to a spine board. *J Athl Train.* 2013;48(6):797-803. doi:10.4085/1062-6050-48.5.07. Accessed May 11, 2015.

67. Ferno K.E.D. - Kendrick Extrication Device. Emergency Medical Products. www.buyemp.com/product/ferno-ked-kendrick-extrication-device. Accessed August 21, 2017.

68. Howell JM, Burrow R, Dumontier C, Hillyard A. A practical radiographic comparison of short board technique and Kendrick Extrication Device. *Ann Emerg Med.* 1989;18(9):943-946.

69. Winterberger E, Jacomet H, Zafren K, Ruffinen GZ, Jelk B. The use of extrication devices in crevasse accidents: Official statement of the International Commission for Mountain Emergency Medicine and the Terrestrial Rescue Commission of the International Commission for Alpine Rescue intended for physicians, paramedics, and mountain rescuers. *Wilderness Environ Med.* 2008;19(2):108-110. doi:10.1580/07-WEME-CO-1012.1. Accessed October 27, 2014.

70. Casa DJ, Stearns RL. *Preventing Sudden Death in Sport & Physical Activity.* Burlington, MA: Jones & Bartlett; 2016.

71. Del Rossi G, Rechtine GR, Conrad BP, Horodyski M. Are scoop stretchers suitable for use on spine-injured patients? *Am J Emerg Med.* 2010;28(7):751-756.

72. Prasarn ML, Hyldmo PK, Zdziarski LA, et al. Comparison of the vacuum mattress versus the spine board alone for immobilization of the cervical spine injured patient: A biomechanical cadaveric study. *Spine.* June 2017. doi:10.1097/BRS.0000000000002260. Accessed August 22, 2017.

73. Luscombe MD, Williams JL. Comparison of a long spinal board and vacuum mattress for spinal immobilisation. *Emerg Med J.* 2003;20(5):476-478. doi:10.1136/emj.20.5.476. Accessed August 22, 2017.

74. Mok JM, Jackson KL, Fang R, Freedman BA. Effect of vacuum spine board immobilization on incidence of pressure ulcers during evacuation of military casualties from theater. *Spine J.* 2013;13(12):1801-1808. doi:10.1016/j.spinee.2013.05.028. Accessed August 22, 2017.

75. Hamilton RS, Pons PT. The efficacy and comfort of full-body vacuum splints for cervical-spine immobilization. *J Emerg Med.* 1996;14(5):553-559. doi:10.1016/S0736-4679(96)00170-9. Accessed August 22, 2017.

76. EP+R Spider-Strap. www.epandr.com/products/immobilization/straps/spiderStrap.php. Accessed August 22, 2017.

77. EP+R Strap Pak Speed Clips. www.epandr.com/products/immobilization/straps/speedClips.php. Accessed August 22, 2017.

78. Mazolewski P, Manix TH. The effectiveness of strapping techniques in spinal immobilization. *Ann Emerg Med.* 1994;23(6):1290-1295.

79. Prentice W. *Arnheim's Principles of Athletic Training: A Competency-Based Approach.* 13th ed. New York, NY: McGraw-Hill; 2009.

80. Kyle, J. Friday Night Medical Time Out. The Kyle Group. www.kyle-group.com/friday-night-medical-time-out/. Accessed August 22, 2017.

81. Conrad BP, Rossi GD, Horodyski MB, Prasarn ML, Alemi Y, Rechtine GR. Eliminating log rolling as a spine trauma order. *Surg Neurol Int.* 2012;3(Suppl 3):S188-S197. doi:10.4103/2152-7806.98584. Accessed November 11, 2014.

82. Conrad BP, Horodyski M, Wright J, Ruetz P, Rechtine GR. Log-rolling technique producing unacceptable motion during body position changes in patients with traumatic spinal cord injury. *J Neurosurg Spine.* 2007;6(6):540-543.

83. Conrad BP, Marchese DL, Rechtine GR, Horodyski M. Motion in the unstable thoracolumbar spine when spine boarding a prone patient. *J Spinal Cord Med.* 2012;35(1):53-57. doi:10.1179/2045772311Y.0000000045. Accessed May 4, 2015.

84. Del Rossi G, Bodkin D, Dhanani A, Courson RW, Konin JG. Protective athletic equipment slows initiation of CPR in simulated cardiac arrest. *Resuscitation.* 2011;82(7):908-912. doi:10.1016/j.resuscitation.2011.02.022. Accessed September 21, 2015.

85. Waninger KN, Goodbred A, Vanic K, et al. Adequate performance of cardiopulmonary resuscitation techniques during simulated cardiac arrest over and under protective equipment in football: *Clin J Sport Med.* 2014;24(4):280-283. doi:10.1097/JSM.0000000000000022. Accessed September 21, 2015.

86. Swartz EE, Norkus SA, Cappaert T, Decoster LC. Football equipment design affects face mask removal efficiency. *Am J Sport Med.* 2005;33(8):1210-1219.

87. Sherbondy PS, Hertel JN, Sebastianelli WJ. The effect of protective equipment on cervical spine alignment in collegiate lacrosse players. *Am J Sport Med.* 2006;34(10):1675-1679.

88. Palumbo MA, Hulstyn MJ, Fadale PD, O'Brien T, Shall L. The effect of protective football equipment on alignment of the injured cervical spine radiographic analysis in a cadaveric model. *Am J Sport Med.* 1996;24(4):446-453.

89. Gastel JA, Palumbo MA, Hulstyn MJ, Fadale PD, Lucas P. Emergency removal of football equipment: A cadaveric cervical spine injury model. *Ann Emerg Med.* 1998;32(4):411-417.

90. Swartz EE, Mihalik JP, Beltz NM, Day MA, Decoster LC. Face mask removal is safer than helmet removal for emergent airway access in American football. *Spine J.* 2014;14(6):996-1004. doi:10.1016/j.spinee.2013.10.032. Accessed October 13, 2014.

91. Ray R, Luchies C, Frens MA, Hughes W, Sturmfels R. Cervical spine motion in football players during 3 airway-exposure techniques. *J Athl Train.* 2002;37(2):172.

92. Jenkins HL, Valovich TC, Arnold BL, Gansneder BM. Removal tools are faster and produce less force and torque on the helmet than cutting tools during face-mask retraction. *J Athl Train.* 2002;37(3):246.

93. Swartz EE, Decoster LC, Norkus SA, Cappaert TA. The influence of various factors on high school football helmet face mask removal: A retrospective, cross-sectional analysis. *J Athl Train.* 2007;42(1):11.

94. Swartz EE, Mihalik JP, Decoster LC, Al-Darraji S, Bric J. Emergent access to the airway and chest in American football players. *J Athl Train.* 2015;50(7):681-687. doi:10.4085/1062-6050-50.4.04. Accessed September 22, 2015.

95. DuBose D, Connoly S, Hatzel B, et al. Motion Created in an unstable cervical spine during the removal of a football helmet: Comparison of techniques. *Athl Train Sports Health Care.* 2015;7(6).

96. Bradney DA, Bowman TG. Lacrosse helmet facemask removal. *J Athl Train.* 2013;48(1):47-56.

97. LaPrade RF, Schnetzler KA, Broxterman RJ, Wentorf F, Wendland E, Gilbert TJ. Cervical spine alignment in the immobilized ice hockey player: A computed tomographic analysis of the effects of helmet removal. *Am J Sport Med.* 2000;28(6):800-803.

98. Waninger KN, Richards JG, Pan WT, Shay AR, Shindle MK. An evaluation of head movement in backboard-immobilized helmeted football, lacrosse, and ice hockey players. *Clin J Sport Med.* 2001;11(2):82-86.

99. Courson R. University of Georgia sports medicine emergency and care best practices. Sports Medicine at UGA. www.georgiadogs.com/ot/sports-medicine/sports-med-conf.html. Accessed September 22, 2015.

100. Dahl MC, Ananthakrishnan D, Nicandri G, Chapman JR, Ching RP. Helmet and shoulder pad removal in football players with unstable cervical spine injuries. *J Appl Biomech.* 2009;25(2):119-32.

101. Horodyski M, DiPaola CP, DiPaola MJ, Conrad BP, Del Rossi G, Rechtine GR. Comparison of the flat torso versus the elevated torso shoulder pad removal techniques in a cadaveric cervical spine instability model. *Spine.* 2009;34(7):687-691.

102. Decoster LC, Shirley CP, Swartz EE. Football face-mask removal with a cordless screwdriver on helmets used for at least one season of play. *J Athl Train.* 2005;40(3):169.

103. Copeland AJ, Decoster LC, Swartz EE, Gattie ER, Gale SD. Combined tool approach is 100% successful for emergency football face mask removal. *Clin J Sport Med.* 2007;17(6):452-457.

104. Gale SD, Decoster LC, Swartz EE. The combined tool approach for face mask removal during on-field conditions. *J Athl Train.* 2008;43(1):14.

CHAPTER 10

1. Melendez S. Rib fracture. 2017. https://emedicine.medscape.com/article/825981-overview. Accessed November 28, 2017.

2. Bansidhar BJ, Lagares-Garcia JA, Miller SL. Clinical rib fractures: Are follow-up chest X-rays a waste of resources? *Am Surg.* 2002;68(5):449-453.

3. Davis S, Affatato A. Blunt chest trauma: Utility of radiological evaluation and effect on treatment patterns. *Am J Emerg Surg.* 2006;24(4):482-486.

4. Rodriguez RM, Anglin D, Langdorf MI, et al. NEXUS chest: Validation of a decision instrument for selective chest imaging in blunt trauma. *JAMA.* 2013;148(10):940-946.

5. Glass E, Thompson J, Cole P, Gause T, Altman G. Treatment of sternoclavicular joint dislocations: A systematic review of 251 dislocations in 24 case studies. *J Trauma.* 2011;70(5):1294-1298.

6. Rudzinski J. Sternoclavicular joint injury. 2017. https://emedicine.medscape.com/article/828642-overview. Accessed November 28, 2017.

7. Morell DJ, Thyagarajan DS. Sternoclavicular joint dislocation and its management: A review of the literature. *World J Orthop.* 2016;7(4):244-250.

8. LaMori JC, Shoheiber O, Mody SH, Bookhart BK. Inpatient resource use and cost burden of deep vein thrombosis and pulmonary embolism in the Unites States. *Clin Ther.* 2015;37(1):62-70.

9. Belohlavek J, Dytrych V, Linhart A. Pulmonary embolism, part 1: Epidemiology, risk factors, and risk stratification, pathophysiology, clinical presentation, diagnosis and nonthrombotic pulmonary embolism. *Exp Clin Cardiol.* 2013;18(2):129-138.

10. Centers for Disease Control and Prevention (CDC). Venous thromboembolism. www.cdc.gov/ncbddd/dvt/data.html. Accessed November 28, 2017.

11. PIOPED Investigators. Value of the ventilation/perfusion scan in acute pulmonary embolism. Results of the prospective investigation of pulmonary embolism diagnosis (PIOPED). *JAMA*. 1990;263(20):2753-2759.

12. Beckman MG, Hooper WC, Critchley SE, Ortel TL. Venous thromboembolism: a public health concern. *Am J Prev Med*. 2010;38(4):S495-501.

13. Dalen JE, Waterbrook AL. Why are nearly all CT pulmonary angiograms for suspected pulmonary embolism negative? *Am J Med*. 2017;130(3):247-248.

14. Saleh J, El-Othmani MM, Saleh KJ. Deep vein thrombosis and pulmonary embolism considerations in orthopedic surgery. *Orthop Clin North Am*. 2017;48(2):127-135.

15. Ouellette E. Pulmonary embolism. 2017. emedicine.medscape.com/article/300901-overview. Accessed November 29, 2017.

16. Boka K. Pulmonary embolism clinical scoring systems. https://emedicine.medscape.com/article/1918940-overview. Accessed November 28, 2017.

17. Daley B. Pneumothorax. 2016; 2017. https://emedicine.medscape.com/article/424547-overview. Accessed November 28, 2017.

18. Mancini M. Hemothorax. 2017. https://emedicine.medscape.com/article/2047916-overview. Accessed November 28, 2017.

19. Peclet MH, Newman KD, Eichelberger MR, Gotschall, CS, Garcia VF, Bowman, LM. Thoracic trauma in children: An indicator of increased mortality. *J Pediatr Surg*. 1990;25(9):961-966.

20. Ebrahimi A, Yousefifart M, Mohammad Kazemi H, et al. Diagnostic accuracy of chest ultrasonography versus chest radiography for identification of pneumothorax: A systematic review and meta-analysis. *J Resp Dis, Thor Surg, Inten Care and TB*. 2014;13(4).

21. Soldati G, Testa A, Sher S, Pignataro G, La Sala M, Silveri NG . Occult traumatic pneumothorax: Diagnostic accuracy of lung ultrasonography in the emergency department. *Chest*. 2008;133(1):204-211.

22. Emond M, Guimont C, Chauney JM, et al. Clinical prediction rule for delayed hemothorax after minor thoracic injury: a multicenter derivation and validation study. *CMAJ*. 2017;5(2):E444-E453.

23. Miller K. Oxygen administration: What is the best choice. 2017. www.rtmagazine.com/2015/10/oxygen-administration-best-choice. Accessed November 28, 2017.

24. EMS Safety. Emergency oxygen administration. 2012. www.emssafetyservices.com/wp-content/uploads/2014/05/In-Depth_O2_A_06-12-12.pdf. Accessed November 28, 2017.

25. American Red Cross. Administering emergency oxygen. 2011. www.redcross.org/images/MEDIA_CustomProductCatalog/m3240082_AdministeringEmergencyOxygenFactandSkill.pdf. Accessed November 29, 2017.

26. Murphy MF, Avegno JL. Extraglottic Devices: Supraglottic Type. In Brown CA, Salles JC, Mick NW, eds. *The Walls Manual of Emergency Airway Management*. 5th ed. Philadelphia, PA: Wolters Kluwer; 2018.

27. Feld F. Airway Management. In Gorse K, Blanc R. Feld F. Radelet M, eds. *Emergency Care in Athletic Training*. Philadelphia, PA: FA Davis; 2010.

28. Laurin EG, Simon LV, Braude DA, Murphy MF. Extraglottic Devices: Retroglottic Type. In Brown CA, Salles JC, Mick NW, eds. *The Walls Manual of Emergency Airway Management*. 5th ed. Philadelphia, PA: Wolters Kluwer; 2018.

29. Morris MJ. Asthma. 2017. https://emedicine.medscape.com/article/296301-overview. Accessed May 14, 2018.

30. Garry JA Exercised-induced asthma. 2017. https://emedicine.medscape.com/article/1938228-overview. Accessed May 14, 2018.

31. See KC, Phua J, Lim TK. Trigger factors in asthma and chronic obstructive pulmonary disease: A single-centre cross-sectional survey. *Singapore Med J*. 2016;266(12):1929-1936.

32. Casa DJ, Guskiewics, KM, Anderson SA, et al. National Athletic Trainers' Association Position Statement: Preventing sudden death in sport. *J Athl Train*. 2012:47(1):96-118.

CHAPTER 11

1. Asif IM, Yim ES, Hoffman JM, Froelicher V. Update: Causes and symptoms of sudden cardiac death in young athletes. *Phys Sportsmed*. 2015;43(1):44-53.

2. Neumar RW, Shuster M, Callaway CW, et al. Part 1: Executive summary: 2015 American Heart Association guidelines update for cardiopulmonary resuscitation and emergency cardiovascular care. *Circulation*. 2015;132(18 Suppl 2):S315-367.

3. Kleinman ME, Brennan EE, Goldberger ZD, et al. Part 5: Adult basic life support and cardiopulmonary resuscitation quality: 2015 American Heart Association guidelines update for cardiopulmonary resuscitation and emergency cardiovascular care. *Circulation*. 2015;132(18 Suppl 2):S414-435.

4. Maron BJ, Doerer JJ, Haas TS, Tierney DM, Mueller FO. Sudden deaths in young competitive athletes: Analysis of 1866 deaths in the United States, 1980-2006. *Circulation*. 2009;119(8):1085-1092.

5. Drezner JA. Inter-Association task force recommendations on emergency preparedness and management of sudden cardiac arrest in high school and college athletic programs: A consensus statement. *J Athl Train*. 2007;42(1):143-159.

6. Henry MC, Stapleton ER. *EMT Prehospital Care*. 2nd ed. Burlington, MA: Jones and Bartlett; 2012.

7. Chugh SS, Reinier K, Teodorescu C, et al. Epidemiology of sudden cardiac death: Clinical and research implications. *Prog Cardiovasc Dis*. 2008;51(3):213-228.

8. Marx JA, Rosen P. *Rosen's Emergency Medicine: Concepts and Clinical Practice*. Philadelphia, PA: Elsevier Saunders; 2017.

9. Black HR, Sica D, Ferdinand K, White WB. AHA/ACC scientific statement: Eligibility and disqualification recommendations for competitive athletes with cardiovascular abnormalities: Task force 6: Hypertension. A scientific statement from the American Heart Association and the American College of Cardiology. *J Am Coll Cardiol.* 2015;66:2393-2397.

10. Berg RA, Hemphill R, Abella BS, et al. Part 5: Adult basic life support: 2010 American Heart Association guidelines for cardiopulmonary resuscitation and emergency cardiovascular care. *Circulation.* 2010;122(18 Suppl 3):S685-705.

11. Zipes DP, Link MS, Ackerman MJ, et al. Eligibility and disqualification recommendations for competitive athletes with cardiovascular abnormalities: Task force 9: Arrhythmias and conduction defects: A scientific statement from the American Heart Association and American College of Cardiology. *Circulation.* 2015;132(22):e315-325.

12. Neumar RW, Otto CW, Link MS, et al. Part 8: Adult advanced cardiovascular life support: 2010 American Heart Association guidelines for cardiopulmonary resuscitation and emergency cardiovascular care. *Circulation.* 2010;122(18 Suppl 3):S729-S767.

13. Boden BP, Breit I, Beachler JA, Williams A, Mueller FO. Fatalities in high school and college football players. *Am J Sports Med.* 2013;41(5):1108-1116.

14. Schmied C, Borjesson M. Sudden cardiac death in athletes. *J Intern Med.* 2014;275(2):93-103.

15. Harmon KG, Asif IM, Klossner D, Drezner JA. Incidence of sudden cardiac death in National Collegiate Athletic Association athletes. *Circulation.* 2011;123(15):1594-1600.

16. Eckart RE, Scoville SL, Campbell CL, et al. Sudden death in young adults: A 25-year review of autopsies in military recruits. *Ann Int Med.* 2004;141(11):829-834.

17. Eckart RE, Shry EA, Burke AP, et al. Sudden death in young adults: An autopsy-based series of a population undergoing active surveillance. *J Am Coll Cardiol.* 2011;58(12):1254-1261.

18. Harmon KG, Drezner JA, Maleszewski JJ, et al. Pathogeneses of sudden cardiac death in National Collegiate Athletic Association athletes. *Circ Arrhythm Electrophysiol.* 2014;7(2):198-204.

19. Harmon KG, Drezner JA, Wilson MG, Sharma S. Incidence of sudden cardiac death in athletes: A state-of-the-art review. *Heart.* 2014;100(16):1227-1234.

20. Asif IM, Rao AL, Drezner JA. Sudden cardiac death in young athletes: What is the role of screening? *Curr Opin Cardiol.* 2013;28(1):55-62.

21. Semsarian C, Sweeting J, Ackerman MJ. Sudden cardiac death in athletes. *Br J Sports Med.* 2015;49(15):1017-1023.

22. Chandra N, Bastiaenen R, Papadakis M, Sharma S. Sudden cardiac death in young athletes: Practical challenges and diagnostic dilemmas. *J Am Coll Cardiol.* 2013;61(10):1027-1040.

23. Patel V, Elliott P. Sudden death in athletes. *Clin Med (Lond).* 2012;12(3):253-256.

24. Pollack A, Beck R. *Advanced Emergency Care and Transportation of the Sick and Injured.* Sudbury, MA: Jones and Bartlett; 2012.

25. Maron BJ, Udelson JE, Bonow RO, et al. Eligibility and disqualification recommendations for competitive athletes with cardiovascular abnormalities: Task force 3: Hypertrophic cardiomyopathy, arrhythmogenic right ventricular cardiomyopathy and other cardiomyopathies, and myocarditis: A scientific statement from the American Heart Association and American College of Cardiology. *Circulation.* 2015;132(22):e273-e280 278p.

26. Terrell T, Pitt J, Asif I. Sudden cardiac death in athletes. *Int J Athl Ther Train.* 2015;20(3):38-45.

27. Winkel BG, Holst AG, Theilade J, et al. Nationwide study of sudden cardiac death in persons aged 1-35 years. *Eur Heart J.* 2011;32(8):983-990.

28. Blauwet LA, Cooper LT. Myocarditis. *Prog Cardiovasc Dis.* 2010;52(4):274-288.

29. Stout M. The Marfan syndrome: Implications for athletes and their echocardiographic assessment. *Echocardiography.* 2009;26(9):1075-1081.

30. Judge DP, Dietz HC. Marfan's syndrome. *Lancet.* 2005;366(9501):1965-1976.

31. Liang D. Marfan history in athletes from family history section. *Curr Sports Med Rep.* 2015;14(4):341-342.

32. Braverman AC, Harris KM, Kovacs RJ, Maron BJ. Eligibility and disqualification recommendations for competitive athletes with cardiovascular abnormalities: Task force 7: Aortic diseases, including Marfan syndrome. *J Am Coll Cardiol.* 2015;66(21):2398-2405 2398p.

33. Yetman AT, Bornemeier RA, McCrindle BW. Long-term outcome in patients with Marfan syndrome: Is aortic dissection the only cause of sudden death? *J Am Coll Cardiol.* 2003;41(2):329-332.

34. Chatard JC, Mujika I, Goiriena JJ, Carre F. Screening young athletes for prevention of sudden cardiac death: Practical recommendations for sports physicians. *Scand J Med Sci Sports.* 2016;26(4):362-374.

35. Glorioso J, Jr., Reeves M. Marfan syndrome: Screening for sudden death in athletes. *Curr Sports Med Rep.* 2002;1(2):67-74.

36. The Marfan Foundation. What is Marfan syndrome? 2014. www.marfan.org/about/marfan. Accessed March 26, 2016.

37. Mitchell BL. Ventricular tachycardia (VT). Merck Manual Professional Version. 2015. www.merckmanuals.com/professional/cardiovascular-disorders/arrhythmias-and-conduction-disorders/ventricular-tachycardia. Accessed September 25, 2017.

38. Mitchell BL. Ventricular fibrillation (VF). Merck Manual Professional Version. 2015. www.merckmanuals.com/professional/cardiovascular-disorders/arrhythmias-and-conduction-disorders/ventricular-fibrillation.

39. Palacio LE, Link MS. Commotio cordis. *Sports Health.* 2009;1(2):174-179.

40. Link MS, Maron BJ, VanderBrink BA, et al. Impact directly over the cardiac silhouette is necessary to produce ventricular fibrillation in an experimental model of commotio cordis. *J Am Coll Cardiol.* 2001;37(2):649-654.

41. Maron BJ, Estes NA, 3rd. Commotio cordis. *N Engl J Med.* 2010;362(10):917-927.

42. Maron BJ, Gohman TE, Kyle SB, Estes NA, 3rd, Link MS. Clinical profile and spectrum of commotio cordis. *J Am Med Assoc.* 2002;287(9):1142-1146.

43. Doerer JJ, Haas TS, Estes NA, 3rd, Link MS, Maron BJ. Evaluation of chest barriers for protection against sudden death due to commotio cordis. *Am J Cardiol.* 2007;99(6):857-859.

44. Ackerman MJ, Zipes DP, Kovacs RJ, Maron BJ. Eligibility and disqualification recommendations for competitive athletes with cardiovascular abnormalities: Task force 10: The cardiac channelopathies: A scientific statement from the American Heart Association and American College of Cardiology. *Circulation.* 2015;132(22):e326-329.

45. Corrado D, Basso C, Rizzoli G, Schiavon M, Thiene G. Does sports activity enhance the risk of sudden death in adolescents and young adults? *J Am Coll Cardiol.* 2003;42(11):1959-1963 1955p.

46. Morita H, Wu J, Zipes DP. The QT syndromes: Long and short. *The Lancet.* 2008(9640):750.

47. Goldenberg I, Moss AJ. Long QT Syndrome. *J Am Coll Cardiol.* 2008;51(24):2291-2300.

48. Chung EH. Brugada ECG patterns in athletes. *J Electrocardiol.* 2015;48(4):539-543.

49. Sumitomo N, Harada K, Nagashima M, et al. Catecholaminergic polymorphic ventricular tachycardia: electrocardiographic characteristics and optimal therapeutic strategies to prevent sudden death. *Heart.* 2003;89(1):66-70.

50. Pflaumer A, Davis AM. Guidelines for the diagnosis and management of catecholaminergic polymorphic ventricular tachycardia. *Heart Lung Circ.* 2012;21(2):96-100.

51. Casa DJ, Guskiewicz KM, Anderson SA, et al. National Athletic Trainers' Association position statement: Preventing sudden death in sports. *J Athl Train.* 2012;47(1):96-118.

52. O'Connor RE, Al Ali AS, Brady WJ, et al. Part 9: Acute coronary syndromes: 2015 American Heart Association guidelines update for cardiopulmonary resuscitation and emergency cardiovascular care. *Circulation.* 2015;132(18 Suppl 2):S483-500.

53. ZOLL Medical Corporation. Non-interpretive 12-lead ECG monitoring. 2002; www.zoll.com/medical-products/product-manuals. Accessed April 16, 2018.

54. Drezner JA, Courson RW, Roberts WO, et al. Inter-association task force recommendations on emergency preparedness and management of sudden cardiac arrest in high school and college athletic programs: A consensus statement. *J Athl Train.* 2007;42(1):143-158.

55. Link MS, Berkow LC, Kudenchuk PJ, et al. Part 7: Adult advanced cardiovascular life support: 2015 American Heart Association guidelines update for cardiopulmonary resuscitation and emergency cardiovascular care. *Circulation.* 2015;132(18 Suppl 2):S444-464.

56. Vanden Hoek TL, Morrison LJ, Shuster M, et al. Part 12: Cardiac arrest in special situations: 2010 American Heart Association guidelines for cardiopulmonary resuscitation and emergency cardiovascular care. *Circulation.* 2010;122(18 Suppl 3):S829-861.

57. Andersen JC, Courson RW, Kleiner DM, McLoda TA. National Athletic Trainers' Association position statement: Emergency planning in athletics. *J Athl Train.* 2002(1):99.

58. Casa DJ, Anderson SA, Baker L, et al. The inter-association task force for preventing sudden death in collegiate conditioning sessions: best practices recommendations. *J Athl Train.* 2012;47(4):477-480.

59. Casa DJ, Almquist J, Anderson SA, et al. The inter-association task force for preventing sudden death in secondary school athletics programs: best-practices recommendations. *J Athl Train.* 2013;48(4):546-553.

60. Andersen J, Courson RW, Kleiner DM, McLoda TA. National Athletic Trainers' Association position statement: Emergency planning in athletics. *J Athl Train.* 2002;37(1):99-104.

61. Drezner JA, Rao AL, Heistand J, Bloomingdale MK, Harmon KG. Effectiveness of emergency response planning for sudden cardiac arrest in United States high schools with automated external defibrillators. *Circulation.* 2009;120(6):518-525.

62. Drezner JA, Rogers KJ. Sudden cardiac arrest in intercollegiate athletes: Detailed analysis and outcomes of resuscitation in nine cases. *Heart Rhythm.* 2006;3(7):755-759.

CHAPTER 12

1. Parks RW, Chrysos E, Diamond T. Management of liver trauma. *Br J Surg.* 1999;86(9):1121-1135. bjs1210 [pii].

2. Michalopulos G. Liver regeneration. *J. Cell Physiol.* 2007;213(2):286-300. https://www.ncbi.nlm.nih.gov/pmc/articles/PMC2701258. Accessed December 21, 2017.

3. Gannon E, Howard T. Splenic injuries in athletes: A review. *Curr Sports Med Rep.* 2010;9(2):111-114.

4. Legome E. Blunt abdominal trauma. 2017. https://emedicine.medscape.com/article/1980980. Accessed December 20, 2017.

5. Martin J, Shah J, Robinson CM, Dariushnia S. Evaluation and management of blunt solid organ trauma. *Tech Vasc Interv Radiol.* 2017;20(4):230-236.

6. Ralston DJ, Scherm MJ. Splenic artery avulsion in a high school football player: A case report. *J Athl Train.* 2004;39(2):201-205. www.ncbi.nlm.nih.gov/pubmed/15173873. Accessed December 20, 2017.

7. Rifat SF, Gilvydis RP. Blunt abdominal trauma in sports. *Curr Sports Med Rep.* 2003;2(2):93-97. www.ncbi.nlm.nih.gov/pubmed/12831665. Accessed December 20, 2017.

8. Khan A. Liver trauma imaging. 2017. https://emedicine.medscape.com/article/370508-overview. Accessed December 20, 2017.

9. Juyia R, Kerr H. Return to play after liver and spleen trauma. *Sport Health.* 2014;6(3):239-245.

10. Chen Y, Qui J, Yang A, Yuan D, Zhou J. Epidemiology and management of splenic injury: An analysis of a Chinese military registry. *Exp Ther Med.* 2017;13(5):2102-2108.

11. Foreman B, Mackler L. Can we prevent splenic rupture for patients with infectious mononucleosis? *J. Fam Pract.* 2005;54(6):536-557.

12. Moore EE, Cogbill TH, Jurkovich GJ, et al. Organ injury scaling: Spleen and liver. (1994 revision) *J Trauma* 1995;38(3):323-324. www.ncbi.nlm.nih.gov/pubmed/7897707. Accessed December 21, 2017.

13. Tinkoff G, Esposito TJ, Reed J, et al. American Association for the Surgery of Trauma Organ Injury Scale I: Spleen, liver, and kidney, validation based on the National Trauma Data Bank. *J. Trauma.* 2008;207(5):646-655. www.ncbi.nlm.nih.gov/pubmed/18954775. Accessed December 21, 2017.

14. Jagminas L. Diagnostic peritoneal lavage. 2017. https://emedicine.medscape.com/article/82888-overview#a2. Accessed December 21, 2017.

15. Juyia RF, Kerr HA. Return to play after liver and spleen trauma. *Sports Health.* 2014;6(3):239-245. doi:10.1177/1941738114528468. Accessed December 21, 2017.

16. Yoneda G, Katagiri S, Yamamoto M. Reverse Trendelenburg position is a safe technique for lowering central venous pressure without decreasing blood pressure than clamping of the inferior vena cava below the liver. *J Hepatobilliary Pancreat Sci.* 2015;Jun 22(6):463-466. www.ncbi.nlm.nih.gov/pubmed/25763776. Accessed December 21, 2017.

17. Lusaya D. Renal trauma. 2017. https://emedicine.medscape.com/article/440811-overview. Accessed December 21, 2017.

18. Patel DP, Redshaw JD, Breyer BN, et al. High-grade renal injuries are often isolated in sports-related trauma. *Injury.* 2015;46(7):1245-1249. www.ncbi.nlm.nih.gov/pubmed/25769197. Accessed December 22, 2017.

19. Grinsell MM, Butz K, Gurka MJ, Gurka KK, Norwood V. Sport-related kidney injury among high school athletes. *Pediatrics.* 2012;130(1):e40-5. www.ncbi.nlm.nih.gov/pubmed/22711726. Accessed December 22, 2017.

20. Jones GR, Newhouse I. Sport-related hematuria: a review. *Clin J Sport Med.* 1997;7(2):119-125.

21. Holmes FC, Hunt JJ, Sevier TL. Renal injury in sport. *Curr Sports Med Rep.* 2003;2(2):103-109. www.ncbi.nlm.nih.gov/pubmed/12831667. Accessed December 22, 2017.

22. Ferris M, Quan S, Kaplan BS, et al. The global incidence of appendicitis: A systematic review of population-based studies. *Ann Surg.* 2017;266(2):237-241. www.ncbi.nlm.nih.gov/pubmed/28288060. Accessed December 22, 2017.

23. Criag S. Appendicitis. 2017. https://emedicine.medscape.com/article/773895-overview#a6. Accessed December 22, 2017.

24. Grabosch S. Ovarian cysts. 2017. https://emedicine.medscape.com/article/255865-overview. Accessed December 22, 2017.

25. Moini A, Hosseini R, Jahangiri N, Shiva M, Akhoond MR. Risk factors for ectopic pregnancy: A case-control study. *J Res Med Sci.* 2014;19(9):844-849. www.ncbi.nlm.nih.gov/pubmed/25535498. Accessed December 22, 2017.

26. Sepillian V. Ectopic pregnancy. 2017. https://emedicine.medscape.com/article/2041923-overview.

27. Webb C. Ovarian cyst rupture. 2017. https://emedicine.medscape.com/article/253620-clinical.

28. Bieniek J, Sumfest J. Sports-related testicular injuries and the use of protective equipment among young male athletes. *Urology.* 2014;84(6):1485-1489.

29. Cubillos J, Palmer JS, Friedman SC, Freyle J, Lowe FC, Palmer LS. Familial testicular torsion. *J Urol.* 2011;185(6):2469-2472. www.ncbi.nlm.nih.gov/pubmed/21555017. Accessed September 28, 2018.

30. Mellick LB, Sinex JE, Gibson RW, Mears K. A systematic review of testicle survival time after a torsion event. *Pediatr Emerg Care.* 2017. doi:10.1097/PEC.0000000000001287. Accessed September 28, 2018.

31. Rupp T. Testicular torsion in emergency medicine. 2017. https://emedicine.medscape.com/article/778086-overview.

32. Terlecki A. Testicular trauma. 2017. https://emedicine.medscape.com/article/441362-overview.

33. Boettcher M, Bergholz R, Krebs T, Wenke K, Aronson D. Clinical predictors of testicular torsion in children. *Urology.* 2012;70(3):670-674.

34. Bowmann JS, Moore JC. Bedside ultrasound of a painful testicle before and after manual detorsion by an emergency physician. *Acad Emerg Med.* 2009;16(4):336.

CHAPTER 13

1. Flanagan KW, Cuppett M. *Medical Conditions in the Athlete.* 3rd ed. Champaign, IL: Human Kinetics; 2017:347-352.

2. Ferri FF. *Ferri's Clinical Advisor.* 19th ed. Philadelphia, PA: Elsevier; 2016:2064.

3. Khardori R. Type 2 diabetes mellitus. https://emedicine.medscape.com/article/117853-overview. Published December 12, 2017. Updated 2017. Accessed January 1, 2018.

4. Centers for Disease Control and Prevention (CDC). More than 100 million Americans have diabetes and prediabetes. www.cdc.gov/media/releases/2017/p0718-diabetes-report.html. Accessed January 2, 2018.

5. Centers for Disease Control and Prevention (CDC). FastStats—Leading causes of death. www.cdc.gov/nchs/fastats/leading-causes-of-death.htm. Accessed January 2, 2018.

6. Porter RS, Kaplan JL, eds. *The Merck Manual.* 19th ed. Whitehouse Station, JN: Merck Sharpe & Dohme Corp; 2011.

7. American Diabetes Association. Diagnosing diabetes and learning about prediabetes. www.diabetes.org/diabetes-basics/diagnosis. Accessed January 2, 2018.

8. Alexandria V. American Diabetes Association Issues new recommendations on physical activity and exercise for people with diabetes. http://www.diabetes.org/news-room/press-releases/2016/ada-issues-new-recommenda-tions-on-physical-activity-and-exercise.html. Accessed January 1, 2018.

9. Colberg SR, Sigal RJ, Yardley JE, et al. Physical activity/exercise and diabetes: a position statement of the American Diabetes Association. *Diabetes Care*. 2016;39(11):2065-2079.

10. Einhorn D. American Association of Clinical Endocrinologists/American College of Endocrinology statement on the use of hemoglobin A1c for the diagnosis of diabetes. *Endocr Pract*. 2010;16(2):155.

11. Macknight JM, Mistry DJ, Pastors JG, Holmes V, Rynders CA. The daily management of athletes with diabetes. *Clin Sports Med*. 2009;28(3):479-495. doi: 10.1016/j.csm.2009.02.005. Accessed December 30, 2017.

12. Jimenez CC, Corcoran MH, Crawley JT, et al. National Athletic Trainers' Association position statement: Management of the athlete with type 1 diabetes mellitus. *J Athl Train*. 2007;42(4):536-545.

13. WedMD. Diabetes: How to give glucagon. www.webmd.com/diabetes/tc/diabetes-how-to-give-glucagon-top-ic-overview#1. Accessed January 2, 2018.

CHAPTER 14

1. Khan FY. Rhabdomyolysis: A review of the literature. *Neth J Med*. 2009;67(9):272-283.

2. Huynh A, Leong K, Jones N, et al. Outcomes of exertional rhabdomyolysis following high-intensity resistance training. *Intern Med J*. 2016;46(5):602-608.

3. Warren JD, Blumbergs PC, Thompson PD. Rhabdomyolysis: A review. *Muscle Nerve*. 2002;25(3):332.

4. Knochel JP. Rhabdomyolysis and myoglobinuria. *Annu Rev Med*. 1982;33(1):435.

5. Bosch X, Poch E, Grau JM. Rhabdomyolysis and acute kidney injury. *N Eng J Med*. 2009(1):62.

6. Brogan M, Ledesma R, Coffino A, Chander P. Freebie rhabdomyolysis: A public health concern. Spin class-induced rhabdomyolysis. *Am J Med*. 2017;130(4):484-487.

7. Giannoglou GD, Chatzizisis YS, Misirli G. The syndrome of rhabdomyolysis: Pathophysiology and diagnosis. *Eur J Intern Med*. 2007;18(2):90-100.

8. Bosch X, Poch E, Grau JM. Rhabdomyolysis and acute kidney injury. *N Engl J Med*. 2009;361(1):62-72.

9. Counselman FL, Lo BM. Rhabdomyolysis. In Tintinalli JE, Stapczynski JS, Ma OJ, Yealy DM, Meckler GD, Cline DM, eds. *Tintinalli's Emergency Medicine: A Comprehensive Study Guide*. New York, NY: McGraw-Hill; 2016.

10. Tietze DC, Borchers J. Exertional rhabdomyolysis in the athlete: A clinical review. *Sports Health*. 2014;6(4):336-339.

11. Smoot MK, Cavanaugh JE, Amendola A, West DR, Herwaldt LA. Creatine kinase levels during preseason camp in National Collegiate Athletic Association Division I football athletes. *Clin J Sports Med*. 2014;24(5):438-440.

12. Gilliam S. Sickle cell trait, rhabdomyolysis, and mortality among US Army Soldiers. *J Emerg Med*. 2016(5).

13. Nelson DA, Deuster PA, Carter R, III, Hill OT, Wolcott VL, Kurina LM. Sickle cell trait, rhabdomyolysis, and mortality among U.S. Army soldiers. *New Eng J Med*. 2016;375:435-442.

14. Tripette J, Hardy-Dessources MD, Romana M, et al. Exercise-related complications in sickle cell trait. *Clin Hemorheol Microcirc*. 2013;55(1):29-37.

15. Shelmadine BD, Baltensperger A, Wilson RL, Bowden RG. Rhabdomyolysis and acute renal failure in a sickle cell trait athlete: A case study. *Clin J Sports Med*. 2013;23(3):235-237.

16. Harris KM, Haas TS, Eichner ER, Maron BJ. Sickle cell trait associated with sudden death in competitive athletes. *Am J Cardiol*. 2012;110(8):1185-1188.

17. Kark JA, Ward FT. Exercise and hemoglobin S. *Semin Hematol*. 1994;31(3):181-225.

18. Kark JA, Posey DM, Schumacher HR, Ruehle CJ. Sickle-cell trait as a risk factor for sudden death in physical training. *N Engl J Med*. 1987;317(13):781-787.

19. Connes P, Harmon KG, Bergeron MF. Pathophysiology of exertional death associated with sickle cell trait: Can we make a parallel with vaso-occlusion mechanisms in sickle cell disease? *Br J Sports Med*. 2013;47(4):190.

20. National Athletic Trainers' Association. NATA Statement on Sickle Cell Trait and the Athlete. www.nata.org/consensus-statements. Accessed June 19, 2014.

21. Center AFHS. Update: Exertional rhabdomyolysis, active component, U.S. Armed Forces, 2009-2013. In. *MSMR*. Vol 21. 2014/04/02 ed: Armed Forces Health Surveillance Center 2014:14-17.

22. Sherry P. Sickle cell trait and rhabdomyolysis: Case report and review of the literature. *Mil Med*. 1990;155(2):59-61.

23. George M, Delgaudio A, Salhanick SD. Exertional rhabdomyolysis--when should we start worrying? Case reports and literature review. *Pediatr Emerg Care*. 2010 26(11):864-866.

24. Sayers SP, Clarkson PM. Exercise-induced rhabdomyolysis. *Curr Sports Med Rep*. 2002;1(2):59.

25. Kenney K, Landau ME, Gonzalez RS, et al. Serum creatine kinase after exercise: Drawing the line between physiological response and exertional rhabdomyolysis. *Muscle Nerve*. 2012;45(3):356-362.

26. Criddle L. Rhabdomyolysis. Pathophysiology, recognition, and management. *Crit Care Nurse*. 2003;23(6):14-22.

27. Atias D, Druyan A, Heled Y. Recurrent exertional rhabdomyolysis: Coincidence, syndrome, or acquired myopathy? *Curr Sports Med Rep*. 2013;12(6):365-369.

28. Harmon KG, Drezner JA, Klossner D, Asif IM. Sickle cell trait associated with a RR of death of 37 times in National Collegiate Athletic Association football athletes: A database with 2 million athlete-years as the denominator. *Br J Sports Med*. 2012;46(5):325-330.

29. Sanchez CE, Jordan KM. Exertional Sickness. *Am J Med*. 2010;123(1):27-30.

30. Burke J, Seda G, Allen D, Knee TS. A case of severe exercise-induced rhabdomyolysis associated with a weight-loss dietary supplement. *Mil Med.* 2007;172(6):656-658.

31. Casares P, Marull J. Over a million creatine kinase due to a heavy work-out: A case report. *Cases J.* 2008;1(1):173.

32. Melli G, Chaudhry V, Cornblath DR. Rhabdomyolysis: An evaluation of 475 hospitalized patients. *Med.* 2005;84(6):377-385.

33. Koch AJ, Pereira R, Machado M. The creatine kinase response to resistance exercise. *J Musculoskelet Neuronal Interact.* 2014;14(1):68-77.

34. Mougios V. Reference intervals for serum creatine kinase in athletes. *Br J Sports Med.* 2007;41(10):674-678.

35. Ehlers GG, Ball TE, Liston L. Creatine kinase levels are elevated during 2-a-day practices in collegiate football players. *J Athl Train.* 2002;37(2):151-156.

36. Braseth NR, Allison EJ, Jr., Gough JE. Exertional rhabdomyolysis in a body builder abusing anabolic androgenic steroids. *Eur J Emerg Med.* 2001;8(2):155-157.

37. Greenberg J, Arneson L. Exertional rhabdomyolysis with myoglobinuria in a large group of military trainees. *Neurology.* 1967;17(3):216-222.

38. Young SE, Miller MA, Docherty M. Urine dipstick testing to rule out rhabdomyolysis in patients with suspected heat injury. *Am J Emerg Med.* 2009;27(7):875-877.

39. Russell M. Combination of intense drill, heat, dehydration, may have sent McMinnville players to hospital. *The Oregonian/OregonLive* Aug 22, 2010.

40. Damon LE, Andreadis C. Blood disorders. In Papadakis MA, McPhee SJ, Rabow MW, eds. *Current Medical Diagnosis and Treatment.* 57th ed. New York, NY: McGraw-Hill; 2018.

41. National Collegiate Athletic Association. NCAA Sports Medicine Handbook. http://www.ncaapublications.com/productdownloads/MD15.pdf . Accessed September 25, 2018.

42. National Collegiate Athletic Association. 2017-2018 NCAA Division I Manual. 2017. www.ncaapublications.com. Accessed Dec 19, 2017.

43. Adams P. Sickle cell trait can take a sudden deadly turn: exercise can transform round red blood cells into dangerous sickle cells. *Am Nurse Today.* 2007 2(11):19-20.

44. Braunstein EM. Hemoglobin S-C Disease. (Sickle Cell Disease). Merck Manual Professional Version. https://www.merckmanuals.com/professional/hematology-and-oncology/anemias-caused-by-hemolysis/hemoglobin-s-c-disease. Accessed September 25, 2018.

45. Benz EJ. Disorders of Hemoglobin In: Kasper D, Fauci A, Hauser S, Longo D, Jameson JL, Loscalzo J, eds. *Harrison's Principles of Internal Medicine.* 19th ed. New York, NY: McGraw-Hill; 2015.

46. Kerle KK, Nishimura KD. Exertional collapse and sudden death associated with sickle cell trait. *Mil Med.* 1996;161(12):766-767.

47. Boden BP, Breit I, Beachler JA, Williams A, Mueller FO. Fatalities in high school and college football players. *Am J Sports Med.* 2013;41(5):1108-1116.

48. Maron BJ, Doerer JJ, Haas TS, Tierney DM, Mueller FO. Sudden deaths in young competitive athletes: Analysis of 1866 deaths in the United States, 1980-2006. *Circulation.* 2009;119(8):1085-1092.

49. Scoville SL, Gardner JW, Magill AJ, Potter RN, Kark JA. Non-traumatic deaths during US Armed Forces basic training, 1977-2001. *Am J Prev Med.* 2004;26(3):205-212.

50. Eichner ER. Sickle cell trait. *J Sport Rehab.* 2007;16(3):197-203.

51. Eckart RE, Scoville SL, Campbell CL, et al. Sudden death in young adults: A 25-year review of autopsies in military recruits. *Ann Int Med.* 2004;141(11):829-834.

52. Eckart RE, Shry EA, Burke AP, et al. Sudden death in young adults: An autopsy-based series of a population undergoing active surveillance. *J Am Coll Cardiol.* 2011;58(12):1254-1261.

53. Tarini BA, Brooks MA, Bundy DG. A policy impact analysis of the mandatory NCAA sickle cell trait screening program. *Health Serv Res.* 2012;47(1 Pt 2):446-461.

54. Eichner ER. Sickle cell trait in sports. *Curr Sports Med Rep.* 2010;9(6):347-351.

55. Scheinin L, Wetli CV. Sudden death and sickle cell trait: Medicolegal considerations and implications. *Am J Forensic Med Pathol.* 2009;30(2):204-208.

CHAPTER 15

1. National Weather Service. Lightning science: Five ways lightning strikes people. Common cause of lightning death. https://www.weather.gov/safety/lightning-struck. Accessed December 27, 2017.

2. Cooper MA, Holle R. Mechanisms of Lightning injury should affect lightning safety messages. *International Lightning Detection Conference Proceeding.* 2010.

3. Walsh KM. Lightning and severe thunderstorms in event management. *Curr Sports Med Rep.* 2012;11(3):131-134. 10.1249/JSR.0b013e3182563e95 [doi].

4. National Weather Service. NWS lightning fatalities. http://www.lightningsafety.noaa.gov/fatalities.shtml. Accessed December 20, 2017.

5. Jensenius J. A detailed analysis of lightning deaths in the United States from 2006 through 2016. http://www.lightningsafety.noaa.gov/fatalities/analysis03-17.pdf. Accessed December 27, 2017.

6. Walsh KM, Cooper MA, Holle R, et al. National Athletic Trainers' Association position statement: Lightning safety for athletics and recreation. *J Athl Train.* 2013;48(2):258-270. doi:10.4085/1062-6050-48.2.25.

7. Cooper MA. Lightning injuries. *Emerg Med Clin North Am.* 1983;1(3):639-641.

8. Cooper MA. Emergent care of lightning and electrical injuries. *Semin Neurol.* 1995;15(3):268-278. doi:10.1055/s-2008-1041032.

9. Cooper MA. Lightning injuries: Prognostic signs for death. *Ann Emerg Med.* 1980;9(3):134-138. S0196-0644(80)80268-X [pii].

10. Cooper MA, Marshburn S. Lightning strike and electric shock survivors, international. *Neuro Rehabilitation.* 2005;20(1):43-47.

11. Cherington M, McDonough G, Olson S, Russon R, Yarnell PR. Lichtenberg figures and lightning: Case reports and review of the literature. *Cutis.* 2007;80(2):141-143.

12. Dutta B. Lichtenberg figure and lightning. *Indian J Dermatol.* 2016;61(1):109-111. 10.4103/0019-5154.174062 [doi].

13. National Athletic Trainers' Association. Inter-Association Task Force on Exertional Heat Illnesses Consensus Statement. https://www.nata.org/sites/default/files/inter-association-task-force-exertional-heat-illness.pdf. Accessed December 31, 2017.

14. Casa DJ, DeMartini JK, Bergeron MF, et al. National Athletic Trainers' Association Position Statement: Exertional heat illnesses. *J Athl Train.* 2015;50(9):986-1000. 10.4085/1062-6050-50.9.07 [doi].

15. Casa DJ, Guskiewicz KM, Anderson SA, et al. National athletic trainers' association position statement: preventing sudden death in sports. *J Athl Train.* 2012;47(1):96-118.

16. Simon EE. Hyponatremia. https://emedicine.medscape.com/article/242166-overview. Accessed December 29, 2017.

17. Kucera KL, Cantu RC. National Center for Catastrophic Sport Injury Research. http://nccsir.unc.edu/reports. Accessed December 29, 2017.

18. Yeargin SW, Kerr ZY, Casa DJ, et al. Epidemiology of exertional heat illnesses in youth, high school, and college football. *Med Sci Sports Exerc.* 2016;48(8):1523-1529. doi:10.1249/MSS.0000000000000934.

19. Lilley K. Heat Illness remains 'significant threat' to troops, despite warnings and guidelines. *Military Times.* 2017;July(19):1.

20. Helman AS. Heat stroke. https://emedicine.medscape.com/article/166320-overview. Accessed December 29, 2017.

21. University of Connecticut Kory Stringer Institute. Heat stroke recognition. https://ksi.uconn.edu/emergency-conditions/heat-illnesses/exertional-heat-stroke/heat-stroke-recognition. Accessed December 29, 2017.

22. Pryor RR, Roth RN, Suyama J, Hostler D. Exertional heat illness: emerging concepts and advances in prehospital care. *Prehosp Disaster Med.* 2015;30(3):297-305. doi:10.1017/S1049023X15004628.

23. Sylvester JE, Belval LN, Casa DJ, O'Connor FG. Exertional heat stroke and American football: What the team physician needs to know. *Am J Orthop (Belle Mead NJ).* 2016;45(6):340-348.

24. Ganio MS, Brown CM, Casa DJ, et al. Validity and reliability of devices that assess body temperature during indoor exercise in the heat. *J Athl Train.* 2009;44(2):124-135. doi:10.4085/1062-6050-44.2.124.

25. Casa DJ, Becker SM, Ganio MS, et al. Validity of devices that assess body temperature during outdoor exercise in the heat. *J Athl Train.* 2007;42(3):333-342.

26. Huggins RA, Scarneo SE, Casa DJ, et al. The Inter-Association Task Force document on emergency health and safety: Best-practice recommendations for youth sports leagues. *J Athl Train.* 2017;52(4):384-400. doi:10.4085/1062-6050-52.2.02.

27. Li J. Hypothermia. https://emedicine.medscape.com/article/770542-overview. Accessed December 30, 2017.

28. Meiman J, Anderson H, Tomasallo C, Centers for Disease Control and Prevention (CDC). Hypothermia-related deaths—Wisconsin, 2014, and United States, 2003-2013. *MMWR Morb Mortal Wkly Rep.* 2015;64(6):141-143.

29. Castellani JW. Prevention of cold injuries during exercise. www.medscape.com/viewarticle/717044_3. Accessed December 30, 2017.

30. Cappaert TA, Stone JA, Castellani JW, et al. National Athletic Trainers' Association position statement: Environmental cold injuries. *J Athl Train.* 2008;43(6):640-658. doi:10.4085/1062-6050-43.6.640.

31. Keller CS. Guidelines for competition in the cold. www.nfhs.org/articles/guidelines-for-competition-in-the-cold/. Accessed December 30, 2017.

32. Harris NS. Altitude illness - Cerebral syndromes. https://emedicine.medscape.com/article/768478-overview. Accessed December 30, 2017.

33. Jensen JD, Vincent AL. Altitude illness, cerebral syndromes, high altitude cerebral edema (HACE).). In *StatPearls.* Treasure Island, FL: StatPearls Publishing LLC; 2017.

34. Kale RM. Altitude-related disorders. https://emedicine.medscape.com/article/303571-overview. Accessed December 30, 2017.

35. The Lake Louise Consensus on the Definition and Quantification of Altitude Illness, p 272-274. In Sutton JR, Coates G, Houston CS, eds. *Hypoxia and Mountain Medicine.* Burlington, VT: Queen City Printers; 1992.

36. Jensen JD, Vincent AL. Altitude illness, pulmonary syndromes, high altitude pulmonary edema (HAPE). In *StatPearls.* Treasure Island, FL: StatPearls Publishing LLC; 2017.

37. Roach RC, Lawley JS, Hackett PH. High-altitude physiology. In Auerbach PS, Cushing TA, Harris NS, eds. *Auerbach's Wilderness Medicine.* 7th ed. Philadelphia, PA: Elsevier; 2017.

INDEX

Note: The italicized *f* and *t* following page numbers refer to figures and tables, respectively.

A

AAP (American Academy of Pediatrics) 336, 341
AAST (American Association for the Surgery of Trauma) 334, 336
Abbreviated Injury Scale (AIS) 102
abbreviations, medical 48, 49*t*
ABCDE assessment approach 83-84, 84*f*, 172, 210, 254
abdominopelvic region 327-342
   bones of 328, 328*f*
   cavities of 328-329
   injuries to 332-342
   musculature of 328, 329*f*
   organs of 329-332, 330-332*f*
   overview 327
   quadrants of 329, 329*t*
abuse, mandated reporting of 45-46
acetazolamide 375-377
acetylsalicylic acid. *See* aspirin
ACLS (advanced cardiac life support) 306, 319-320
ACSM (American College of Sports Medicine) 106, 122
action plans. *See* emergency action plans (EAPs)
active infections 29
acute compartment syndrome (ACS) 215, 358
acute coronary syndromes (ACS) 110, 309-310
acute exertional compartment syndrome 215
acute mountain sickness (AMS) 375-377
acute myocardial infarction (AMI) 309-310, 316
acute renal failure (ARF) 357
adhesive strips 149-150, 149*f*
adolescents. *See* children and adolescents
adrenaline. *See* epinephrine
advanced cardiac life support (ACLS) 306, 319-320
advanced EMTs (AEMTs) 10-13
advanced-level emergency medical care 10
advanced trauma life support (ATLS)
   hemorrhage and 139-140, 153
   hip dislocation and 194
   knee dislocation and 197
   pelvic fracture and 204
   physical examination and 83
   rib fracture and 292
AEDs. *See* automated external defibrillators
AEMTs (advanced EMTs) 10-13

afterdrop 374
against medical advice (AMA) 48, 50-52, 51*f*
Agency for Healthcare Research and Quality 4
agonal gasping 315, 318, 325
AIDS. *See* HIV/AIDS
airborne transmission 30
airway management
   assessment procedures 87
   blind airways 290-291, 290*f*
   nasopharyngeal 288-289, 289*f*, 289*t*
   oropharyngeal 288-290, 289*f*, 289*t*
   overview 115
   rib fractures and 292
   spinal injuries and 256-257, 256*f*
AIS (Abbreviated Injury Scale) 102
albuterol inhalers 111-113, 113*f*, 113*t*
alcohol-based hand sanitizers 34-35
allergens 160, 300
allergic drug reactions 160, 170-171
allergies 60, 62, 160, 163, 165-166
altered mental status 236, 236-237*t*
altitude-related emergencies 375-377
   diagnostic accuracy for 376-377
   field assessment techniques 376
   immediate management techniques 377
   incidence and epidemiology 375
   medical consequences of 375-376
   signs and symptoms of 376, 376*t*
   transport of patients for 377
AMA (against medical advice) 48, 50-52, 51*f*
ambulatory care 3, 5, 28, 39
amenorrhea 340
American Academy of Pediatrics (AAP) 336, 341
American Association for the Surgery of Trauma (AAST) 334, 336
American Association of Poison Control Centers 167
American College of Sports Medicine (ACSM) 106, 122
American Heart Association 110, 115, 233, 318, 321, 323
American Stroke Association 233
AMI (acute myocardial infarction) 309-310, 316
amiodarone 321
ampules, drawing medication from 117, 118, 118*f*
AMS (acute mountain sickness) 375-377
anaphylactoid 160, 163
anaphylaxis 160-177

angioedema and 170, 170*f*
assessment of patients with 171-172, 171*f*
biphasic 120, 173
classification of 160-161, 161*t*
defined 160, 161
differential diagnosis and 164-171
drug-induced 160, 170-171
education and communication of 174
emergency action plans for 174-177, 176*f*
emergency care for 172-175, 172*f*
etiology of 162-163
exercise-induced 166-167, 174, 175
food-dependent exercise-induced 167, 175, 177
food-induced 62, 160, 163, 165-166
from insect bites and stings 167-169, 168*t*
latex allergy and 62, 166
management of 62, 111, 117
pathophysiology of 160-171
pharmacological intervention for 173-174
risk factors for 161-162
signs and symptoms 163-165
transport of patients for 120, 169
urticaria and 160, 164, 169-170, 169*f*
aneurysms 311
angina pectoris 309, 321
angioedema 170, 170*f*
angle shears for face mask removal 270, 270*f*
ankle anatomy 197, 198*f*
ankle dislocation 197-200
   field assessment techniques 199, 199*t*
   immediate management techniques 199-200
   incidence and epidemiology 197-198
   risk factors for 198
   signs and symptoms of 198-199, 198*f*
ankle fractures 208-210, 212, 212*f*
ankle mortise 197
annulus fibrosus 251, 251*f*
anomalous coronary arteries 311
antibacterials 40
antibiotic resistance 33-34, 33*t*
antibiotics 28, 33-34, 33*t*, 40
anticoagulants 141, 142, 143*t*, 227, 297
anticonvulsants 207
antihistamines 111, 166, 167, 169-171, 174
antimicrobials 28, 33-34, 33*t*, 40
antiseptics 34, 35, 40-41
antivirals 28, 40

aortic dissection 311-312
aortic valve 304, 305*f*
apnea 286
appearance of impropriety 22
appendectomy 338
appendicitis 337-339
    clinical prediction rules for 338
    defined 331, 337, 337*f*
    diagnostic accuracy for 338
    field assessment techniques 338
    immediate management techniques
        338-339
    incidence and epidemiology 338
    risk factors for 336
    signs and symptoms of 338, 338*f*
    transport of patients for 339
appendix, structure and function of 331
arachnodactyly 312
arachnoid mater 219
ARF (acute renal failure) 357
arrhythmias 306, 311-315
arrhythmogenic disorders 312-315
arrhythmogenic right ventricular cardio-
        myopathy or dysplasia (ARVD)
        311
arteries of upper and lower extremities
        180-183, 181*f*, 183*f*
arteriosclerosis 309
articulations 179
aseptic technique 38, 110, 127
aspiration 289
aspirin
    anaphylaxis from 171
    anticoagulant effects of 141, 142,
        143*t*
    asthma and 300
    for cardiac emergencies 320*t*, 321
    characteristics of 110*t*
    for headaches 231
    oral administration of 110
asthenic 157
asthma 299-302
    defined 299
    diagnostic accuracy for 300, 302*f*
    exercised-induced 299-300
    field assessment techniques 300, 301*f*
    food allergy and 166
    immediate management techniques
        300-302
    incidence and epidemiology 299-300
    medication administration for 111-
        112, 115-116, 300
    risk factors for 300
    signs and symptoms of 165, 300
    transport of patients for 301-302
asystole 307, 308, 313
ataxia 376, 377
athlete's heart 310
athletic trainers (ATs). *See also* emer-
        gency examinations; medication
        administration
    barriers to hiring of 65
    on Boston Marathon medical team 56
    in collaborative practice 5-6
    core values of 19

medical oversight of 105-106
    practice settings for 7-8
    professional behaviors of 19
    role of 7, 27, 54, 57
    rules and regulations for 7
    scope of practice 105-106
    student practitioners 15
atlas 248, 248*f*, 250
ATLS. *See* advanced trauma life support
atopic disorders 160, 162
atrioventricular (AV) valves 304, 305
ATs. *See* athletic trainers
ATs Care program 74
aura 229-230
auscultation 96-98, 286, 298, 305,
        332
autoimmune disorders 160
automated external defibrillators (AEDs)
    accessibility of 74, 314, 325
    emergency action plans and 55, 59,
        62, 65
    first responder training on use of 9,
        13, 57
    maintenance of 62
    pulmonary embolism and 297
    response time requirements 60, 65
    situations delaying use of 315
    for sudden cardiac arrest 257, 318-
        319, 321-323, 325
autopsy-negative sudden unexplained
        deaths 312
avascular necrosis 206
AV (atrioventricular) valves 304, 305
AVPU scale 83, 86
axial loading 252-253, 252*f*
axillary artery 180, 181*f*, 189, 201
axillary nerve 180, 180*f*
axis 250

B
back plate pads 335-336, 335*f*
bacteremia 31*t*
bag-valve masks 115*t*, 256, 288, 288*f*
balance error scoring system (BESS)
        224*t*, 230
baseline vital signs 91, 94, 122
basic life support (BLS) 306, 315, 318
basilar fractures 221
basophils 160, 161, 169
beta-lactams 33*t*
biohazardous material 41, 41*f*
biotelemetry 315
biphasic anaphylaxis 120, 173
blanching 95
blind airways 115, 290-291, 290*f*
blood
    components of 136, 136*f*
    in eye 240, 240*f*
    glucose levels in 343-345, 345*t*
    oxygen saturation of 97, 99, 99*f*
blood loss. *See* hemorrhage
blood pressure (BP) 96-99, 97*t*, 123,
        304, 305
blowout fractures 241, 241*f*, 242
BLS (basic life support) 306, 315, 318
blunt trauma 145, 238

Board of Certification (BOC) 18, 22-24,
        28, 34, 105
body language 21
bolus 123
Boston Marathon medical team 56
boundaries, professional 22-23
BP. *See* blood pressure
brachial artery 180, 181, 181*f*
bradyarrhythmias 156
bradycardia 306, 308
brain anatomy and physiology 218-
        219, 218*f*
brain stem 218, 218*f*
break tabs 106, 106*f*
breathing. *See* respiratory assessment
bronchial sounds 286
bronchovesicular sounds 286
Brugada syndrome 313
buckling effect 252-253
burnout 18
burns 238, 366

C
CAATE. *See* Commission on Accredi-
        tation of Athletic Training Edu-
        cation
cachexia 170
CAD (coronary artery disease) 308, 309
call-out exchange 70
Canadian C-Spine Rule 254-256, 255*f*
Canadian CT Head Rule 228
capillary refill time (CRT) 95, 96*f*
carbapenems 31*t*, 33*t*
cardiac arrest. *See* sudden cardiac arrest
        (SCA)
cardiac channelopathies 314
cardiac output 138, 139*f*, 304
cardiogenic shock 154, 156, 156*t*, 304
cardiomyopathies 309
cardiopulmonary resuscitation (CPR)
    for anaphylaxis 172
    certification in 8, 322
    Good Samaritan laws and 45
    for hypothermia 374
    post-resuscitation care 321, 322,
        322*f*
    for pulseless patients 87, 88, 158,
        313-314
    for sudden cardiac arrest 257, 315,
        318-319, 325
cardiovascular screening 323, 325
cardiovascular system 303-307. *See also*
        blood; heart; perfusion
    assessment of circulation 87-88
    electrical conduction system of heart
        306-307, 306-307*f*
    function of 303-304
    heart chambers, valves, and vessels
        304-305, 305*f*
    pulmonary and systemic circulations
        304, 304*f*, 306
    responses to blood loss 138
CARE (Concussion Assessment &
        Response: Sport Version) 224
catastrophic events 71-74, 81, 303
catastrophic injuries 54-55, 72-74, 153

catecholaminergic polymorphic ventricular tachycardia (CPVT) 315, 321
catheters 31*t*, 38, 123-124, 123*f*, 127-129
cauda equina 251
CC (costoclavicular) ligament 282, 283*f*, 293
Centers for Disease Control and Prevention (CDC)
 on asthma 111
 on contaminated medical device handling 39
 on diabetes 344
 Guidelines for Field Triage of Injured Patients 81
 hand hygiene guidelines from 35
 HEADS UP Concussion in Youth Sports Initiative 225
 on hypothermia-related deaths 373
 protective practices developed by 31
 on pulmonary embolism 295
 on standard precautions 80
 vaccine recommendations from 29, 29*t*
central nervous system (CNS) 251
cerebellum 218, 218*f*
cerebrovascular accident (CVA). *See* stroke
cerebrum 218, 218*f*
cervical collars 259, 266
cervical spine injuries 85-86, 257-259, 258*f*
cervical vertebra 248-249*f*, 248-251
CGMs (continuous glucose monitors) 348-349
check-back strategy 70
checking routines 16
checklists, use of 17
chemical burns 238
chief complaint 89-91, 90-91*t*
children and adolescents. *See also* parents and guardians
 abuse or neglect of 45-46
 anaphylaxis triggers in 163
 ankle fractures in 208
 appendicitis among 338
 asthma in 111, 299
 bone flexibility in 292
 Colles' fracture among 203
 concussion among 221
 confidentiality and 47
 consent obtained from 44
 IV access in 124
 pelvic fractures in 204
 professional boundaries with 22
 skull fractures among 221
 spleen structure in 330, 333
cholinergic urticaria 169-170
chronic compartment syndrome 215
chronic traumatic encephalopathy (CTE) 225-226
Cincinnati Prehospital Stroke Scale 232-233, 233*t*
circulatory system. *See* cardiovascular system

circumflex artery 180
CK (creatine kinase) 356-357
clavicles 282, 282*f*
closed-ended questions 21-22
closed fractures 184
clot development 141, 141*f*
cluster headaches 229, 229*f*, 231
CNS (central nervous system) 251
coagulation 140
coagulopathy 136, 141
coccyx 248-250, 248*f*
Code of Ethics (NATA) 18, 24
Code of Professional Responsibility (BOC) 18, 22-24
cold-related emergencies 372-375
 diagnostic accuracy for 374
 field assessment techniques 373-374
 immediate management techniques 374-375
 incidence and epidemiology 373
 medical consequences of 373
 signs and symptoms of 373, 373-374*t*
 transport of patients for 374-375
 wind chill and 372, 372*f*
cold-stimulus headaches 230
cold urticaria 169*f*, 170
cold-water immersion 371-372, 371*f*
collaborative health care 4
collaborative practice 4-6. *See also* team-based health care
collateral circulation 182
Colles' fracture 202-203, 203*f*
colonized persons 30, 34
Combitube airway 291, 291*f*
comminution 184
Commission on Accreditation of Athletic Training Education (CAATE)
 on ankle dislocation 199
 on finger dislocation 193
 on medication administration 106, 116-117, 129
 on shoulder dislocation 190
commotio cordis 87, 313-314, 314*f*
communicable diseases 28, 34. *See also specific diseases*
communication
 closed- and open-ended questions in 21-22, 90
 cultural competence and 20, 24
 during emergencies 68-71
 importance of 4
 interpersonal 20-22
 interprofessional 5, 6, 18, 69
 nonverbal 21, 21*t*
 oral reports 69
 as professional attribute 19
 in transfer of care 70, 100-101, 101*t*
community care settings 16
compartment syndrome
 categories of 215
 elbow dislocation and 192
 exertional rhabdomyolysis and 358
 immediate management of 215
 lower-extremities and 207, 209, 214, 214*f*

signs and symptoms of 215
compensated shock 154
competence 19, 47. *See also* cultural competence
computed tomography (CT)
 for appendicitis 338
 for head injuries 221, 226, 228
 for kidney injuries 337
 for liver and spleen injuries 334
 for lower-extremity fractures 209
 for pneumothorax and hemothorax 298
 for pulmonary embolism 296
 for rib fracture 292
 for sternoclavicular joint injury 295
concussion 221-225
 diagnostic accuracy for 224, 224*t*
 field assessment techniques 222-224, 223*t*
 immediate management techniques 224-225
 incidence and epidemiology 221-222
 risk factors for 222
 signs and symptoms of 222
 transport of patients for 225
 types and sequencing 222-224
Concussion Assessment & Response: Sport Version (CARE) 224
confidentiality issues 23, 46-47, 69
conflicts of interest 7, 24
consciousness. *See* level of consciousness (LOC)
consent from patients 20, 43-45
contaminated equipment or surfaces 39-41*t*, 39-42
continuous glucose monitors (CGMs) 348-349
continuous quality improvement 48
contrecoup injury 220
conus medullaris 251
core competencies of team-based health care 5
corneal abrasion 238-239, 239*f*
coronary artery anomalies 311
coronary artery disease (CAD) 308, 309
coronary circulation 304, 306
costoclavicular (CC) ligament 282, 283*f*, 293
cough etiquette 42-43
counseling services 73-74
coup injury 220
covered entities 46
CPR. *See* cardiopulmonary resuscitation
CPVT (catecholaminergic polymorphic ventricular tachycardia) 315, 321
cranial nerve function 222, 223*t*
creatine kinase (CK) 356-357
crepitus 88, 188, 292, 294, 334
crisis management teams 73
critical incidents 55, 65, 71-74
critical patients 9, 10
CRT (capillary refill time) 95, 96*f*
cryotherapies 348
crystalloid solutions 123, 140
CT. *See* computed tomography

CTE (chronic traumatic encephalopathy) 225-226
cultural competence 20, 22-24
CUPS nomenclature 89, 89t
CVA (cerebrovascular accident). *See* stroke
cyanosis 84, 296-300

D

DBP (diastolic blood pressure) 97, 123, 304
DCAP-BTLS strategy 88-89
debridement 149
decerebrate 254
decorticate 254
deep vein thrombosis (DVT) 137-138, 141-142, 142f, 295-296
defibrillators. *See* automated external defibrillators (AEDs)
delayed-onset muscle soreness (DOMS) 355
delegation of tasks 18
dens 248, 248f
dental anatomy 219, 219f
dental injuries 242, 243-244t
dependability 18
depressed fractures 221
dermographism 160, 169, 169f
dexamethasone 377
dextrose solution 124, 125t, 129-130, 129t, 347
diabetes mellitus (DM) 344-348
    diagnostic accuracy for 346
    field assessment techniques 345
    immediate management techniques 346-347, 347f
    incidence and epidemiology 344
    risk factors for 344-345
    signs and symptoms of 345
    transport of patients for 348
diagnostic peritoneal lavage (DPL) 334
diaphoresis 144, 369
diastatic fractures 221
diastolic blood pressure (DBP) 97, 123, 304
diazepam 235
DIC (disseminated intravascular coagulation) 142-143, 358
differential diagnosis
    anaphylaxis and 164-171
    in emergency examinations 77-79, 92
    exertional collapse associated with sickle cell trait and 361-362
    exertional rhabdomyolysis and 358
    sudden cardiac arrest and 323
direct contact transmission 30
disability, in ABCDE assessment approach 84
diseases. *See* communicable diseases; infectious diseases; *specific diseases*
disinfectants 40-41t, 40-42
dislocations
    ankle 197-200, 198f, 199t
    elbow 191-193, 192-193f
    finger 193-194

hip 194, 195f
knee 195-197, 196-197f
mechanism of 184, 187
shoulder 187-191, 189-191f
temporomandibular joint 242
disseminated intravascular coagulation (DIC) 142-143, 358
distracting injuries 254
distributive shock 154-156, 155t
diversity. *See* cultural competence
diving headaches 230, 231
DM. *See* diabetes mellitus
documentation practices 24-25, 47-52, 70-71
DOMS (delayed-onset muscle soreness) 355
dorsalis pedis artery 183, 183f
dorsal root 251-252
DPL (diagnostic peritoneal lavage) 334
drawing up medications 117, 118, 118f
drop foot 209
droplet transmission 30-31
drug administration. *See* medication administration
Dunphy's sign 338
dura mater 219, 227
DVT. *See* deep vein thrombosis
dysphonia 244
dyspnea 96, 114t, 292, 294-300
dysrhythmias 156

E

EAPs. *See* emergency action plans
ear injuries 240-241
ECAST. *See* exertional collapse associated with sickle cell trait
ecchymosis 139, 145, 209, 221, 292
ECG. *See* electrocardiogram
echo strategy 70
ECPs (exposure control plans) 34, 43, 379-382
ectopic pregnancy 339-340
edema 222
EDs (emergency departments) 10, 13
effort thrombosis 137
EHRs (electronic health records) 46-47
EHS. *See* exertional heatstroke
EIA (exercise-induced asthma) 299-300
EIA (exercise-induced anaphylaxis) 166-167, 174, 175
Einthoven's triangle 306, 307f
elbow anatomy 191, 192f
elbow dislocation 191-193
    field assessment techniques 192-193
    immediate management techniques 193, 193f
    incidence and epidemiology 191
    risk factors for 192
    signs and symptoms of 192, 192f
electrical conduction system 306-307, 306-307f
electrocardiogram (ECG) 306, 307f, 310, 315-317, 316-317f
electronic health records (EHRs) 46-47
electronic medical records (EMRs) 47-48

electronic protected health information (ePHI) 46-47
embolisms 141, 232. *See also* pulmonary embolism (PE)
embolus 141
emergencies, defined 55
emergency action plans (EAPs) 54-75
    for anaphylaxis 174-177, 176f
    checklist for 67-68
    communication system in 68-71
    coordinator of 58-59
    core elements of 55, 57
    defined 55
    development and implementation 56-57, 56f
    emergency response team in 59
    EMS integration into 59-60
    equipment and supplies in 62-65
    evacuation procedures in 72
    evidence for best practices 74-75
    facility designation in 61-62, 61t
    incident reports and documentation 70-71
    for mass casualty and catastrophic incidents 71-72
    overview 54-55
    personnel training on 66, 68
    post-catastrophic injury plans 72-74
    post-critical incident plans 72-74
    practice sessions for 66
    psychological first aid in 73-74
    purpose of 55
    review of 62, 64-66
    for sudden cardiac arrest 321-322
    templates for 61
    transfer of care in 70
    transport issues in 60-61
    for trauma and medical emergencies 57
    venue-specific 56-57
emergency departments (EDs) 10, 13
emergency examinations 77-103
    chief complaint identification in 89-91, 90-91t
    equipment for 82
    focused assessment 91-93
    full-body exams 91-92, 92t
    initial assessment 77-78, 82-89
    injury scoring systems and 101-103, 102t
    monitoring critical patients 93-99
    overview 77-79, 78f, 100f
    reassessment in 100
    review of systems in 92-93, 93t
    scene size-up in 79-82
    standard precautions in 80
    transfer of care following 100-101, 101t
    triage and 80-82, 81t, 82f, 103
    vital signs and 80, 91, 93-99
emergency medical responders (EMRs) 9, 11-13
emergency medical services (EMS)
    activation of system 60
    break tabs used by 106

integration into emergency action plans 59-60

mass casualty incident training with 72

nomenclature for patient transport decisions 89, 89*t*

role of 8-10

scope of practice 9-13

emergency medical technicians (EMTs) 9-13

emergency medicine specialists 10, 13, 14

emergency physicians 10, 255-256

emergent patients 9, 10

emesis 159

emotional intelligence 23

empathy 19, 20

EMRs (electronic medical records) 47-48

EMRs (emergency medical responders) 9, 11-13

EMS. *See* emergency medical services

EMTs (emergency medical technicians) 9-13

enteral routes of administration 108, 109*t*

envenomations 169

environmental emergencies 365-377

    altitude-related 375-377, 376*t*

    cold-related 372-375, 372*f*, 373-374*t*

    heat-related 368-372, 369*t*, 370-371*f*

    lightning strikes 365-368, 366*t*

eosinophilic esophagitis 166

ePHI (electronic protected health information) 46-47

epidemiology 25, 54

epidural hematoma 226-227

epilepsy 233-235. *See also* seizures

epinephrine

    administration of 106, 117, 173

    for anaphylaxis 62, 120, 170, 172-174

    for cardiac emergencies 321

    characteristics of 119*t*

epinephrine auto-injectors

    administration of 117, 122

    for anaphylaxis 62, 111, 166, 167, 169, 173

    cost considerations 120

    training on use of 174

epistaxis 139

equipment removal 269-279

    advantages of 269-270

    face masks 270-271, 270-271*f*

    guidelines and recommendations 279

    helmets 271-273, 273*f*

    shoulder pads 273-279, 273-279*f*

ER. *See* exertional rhabdomyolysis

errors 16-18, 48, 108

erythrocytes 123, 330, 359, 361, 362

ethical practice 5, 7, 18, 24-25

evacuation procedures 72

examinations. *See* emergency examinations

exercise-induced asthma (EIA) 299-300

exercise-induced anaphylaxis (EIA) 166-167, 174, 175

exertional collapse associated with sickle cell trait (ECAST)

    assessment of patients with 361

    diagnostic accuracy for 370-371

    differential diagnosis and 361-362

    incidence and epidemiology 360-361

    management of 362

    pathophysiology of 361-362, 361*f*, 361*t*

exertional heatstroke (EHS) 368-372

    diagnostic accuracy for 370-371

    field assessment techniques 369, 370*f*

    immediate management techniques 371-372, 371*f*

    incidence and epidemiology 368, 369*t*

    medical consequences of 368

    signs and symptoms of 368-369

    transport of patients for 372

exertional hyponatremia 368

exertional rhabdomyolysis (ER) 353-359

    assessment of patients with 358

    clinical presentation of 355-357

    complications of 143, 357-358

    diagnostic accuracy for 370-371

    differential diagnosis and 358

    incidence and epidemiology 353-355, 354*f*

    management of 358, 359*f*

    pathophysiology of 355, 355*f*

    risk factors for 354, 355, 360, 362

exposure, in ABCDE assessment approach 84

exposure control plans (ECPs) 34, 43, 379-382

expressed consent 44-45

exsanguinating blood loss 86, 136

external bleeding 86, 138, 146-148, 147*f*

external oblique muscle 328, 329*f*

external pressure headaches 230

extracardiac causes of shock 156

eye anatomy 219, 219*f*

eye injuries 238-240, 239-240*f*

F

face mask removal 270-271, 270-271*f*

facial anatomy and physiology 217-219, 218-219*f*

facial injuries 237-245. *See also* head injuries

    corneal abrasion and foreign object in eye 238-239, 239*f*

    dental 242, 243-244*t*

    fractures 241-242, 241*f*

    hyphema 240, 240*f*

    laryngeal 242, 244-245

    overview 237-238

    retinal detachment 239-240

    temporomandibular joint dislocation 242

    tympanic membrane rupture 240-241

Facility Principles (BOC) 28

fallopian tubes 331, 331*f*, 339-340

false ribs 282

family. *See* parents and guardians

Family Educational Rights and Privacy Act of 1974 (FERPA) 47

fasciotomy 215

fatigue 18

FDEIA (food-dependent exercise-induced anaphylaxis) 167, 175, 177

febrile seizures 234

female reproductive system 331, 331*f*

femoral arteries 182-183, 183*f*

femoral nerve 181, 182*f*

femur fractures 205-207

    distal 206-207, 206*f*

    proximal 205-206, 205*f*

    risk factors for 207

    shaft (diaphyseal) 206

    signs and symptoms of 210

FERPA (Family Educational Rights and Privacy Act of 1974) 47

field (on-site) diagnosis 77

field triage 80-82. *See also* triage

finger dislocation 193-194

"flash," in needles 128, 128*f*

flat torso technique 277, 277*f*

flexible splints 200

floating ribs 282, 282*f*

flu virus. *See* influenza virus

focused assessment 91-93

fomite 30

food allergies 62, 160, 163, 165-166

food-dependent exercise-induced anaphylaxis (FDEIA) 167, 175, 177

foreign object in eye 238-239, 239*f*

fractures

    ankle 208-210, 212, 212*f*

    classification of 183-184, 185-187*t*

    Colles' 202-203, 203*f*

    facial 241-242, 241*f*

    femur 205-206*f*, 205-207, 210

    humeral 200-202, 201-202*f*

    lower-extremity 209-214, 212*f*

    pelvic 203-205, 204-205*f*

    rib 291-293

    skull 221

    tibia-fibula 207, 210

frostbite 372, 372*f*, 374, 374*t*

full-body exams 91-92, 92*t*

G

gallbladder 330

gastroenteritis 32*t*

general impression 80, 84-86

general seizures 234

germicides 40-41

gestational diabetes 344-345

Glasgow Coma Scale (GCS) 83, 86, 220, 220*t*, 222, 228

Glisson's capsule 329

gloves 36-38, 37*f*

glucagon 117, 120, 120*t*, 343-344, 346, 349-351

glucocorticoids 207

glucometry 345-346, 346*f*, 350

go bags 323

golden hour 77, 89

Good Samaritan laws 45
grief counseling 73
guardians. *See* parents and guardians
Guideline for Disinfection and Sterilization in Healthcare Facilities (CDC) 39
gurneys 57, 59

H
habitus 84
HACE (high-altitude cerebral edema) 375-377
HAIs (health care–associated infections) 31-32*t*, 31-33
hand hygiene 15, 28, 30, 34-35, 38
HAPE (high-altitude pulmonary edema) 375-377, 376*t*
hazardous material (HAZMAT) 41, 41*f*, 55
HCM (hypertrophic cardiomyopathy) 310-311, 310*f*
HCPs. *See* health care providers
head, anatomy and physiology of 217-219, 218-219*f*
headaches 228-231
    field assessment techniques 231
    immediate management techniques 231
    incidence and epidemiology 229-230, 229*f*
    primary vs. secondary 228-230
    risk factors for 230
    signs and symptoms of 230-231
head impact sensors 224
head injuries 220-237. *See also* facial injuries
    altered mental status 236, 236-237*t*
    chronic traumatic encephalopathy 225-226
    classification of 220
    concussion 221-225, 223-224*t*
    epidural hematoma 226-227
    headaches 228-231, 229*f*
    intracerebral contusion 226
    intracranial pressure 226
    scalp lacerations 220-221
    seizures 233-236, 235*t*
    skull fracture 221
    stroke 231-233, 232*f*, 233*t*
    subdural hematoma 227-228, 228*f*
    traumatic brain injuries 220-222, 225, 228-230, 238, 240
HEADS UP Concussion in Youth Sports Initiative 225
head-tilt–chin-lift maneuver 256-257, 256*f*
health care–associated infections (HAIs) 31-32*t*, 31-33
health care informatics 24-25
health care providers (HCPs). *See also* emergency examinations; ethical practice; legal responsibilities; medication administration; *specific providers*
    ACLS-trained 319-320
    in collaborative practice 5

communication by 4, 6
ensuring safety of 79-80
errors by 17-18
evolution of 3, 4
professional attributes of 18-19
rules and regulations for 7
screening tests for 29
therapeutic behaviors of 19-25
vaccine recommendations for 29, 29*t*
health care system 3-6, 15, 57
health care teams. *See* team-based health care
health informatics 47
Health Information Technology for Economic and Clinical Health (HITECH) Act of 2009 46-47
Health Insurance Portability and Accountability Act (HIPAA) of 1996 46, 47
health status indicators 23
heart
    abnormal rates and rhythms 306-308
    cardiac output 138, 139*f*, 304
    chambers, valves, and vessels of 304-305, 305*f*
    electrical conduction system of 306-307, 306-307*f*
    protection of 281, 285
heatstroke. *See* exertional heatstroke (EHS)
helmet removal 271-273, 273*f*
hemarthrosis 209
hematemesis 139, 145
hematochezia 145
hematomas 226-228, 228*f*
hematuria 331, 336, 337, 356
hemicrania continua 229
hemiparesis 234
hemodialysis 357
hemoglobin 346, 359
hemoglobinopathies 359
hemolysis 359
hemolytic anemia 359
hemopneumothorax 297, 298
hemoptysis 145, 244, 296-298
hemorrhage 136-152
    assessment of patients with 144-146
    cardiovascular responses to 138
    classes of 139-140, 140*t*
    complications with 137, 141-143
    defined 136
    direct pressure applied to 146-147, 147*f*
    emergency care for 146-152, 146*f*
    external bleeding 86, 138, 146-148, 147*f*
    internal bleeding 138-139, 144-146
    pathophysiology of 137-144
    physiologic responses to 140-141
    systemic responses to 143-144
    types of 138-139
    wound closure for 147-152, 149*f*
hemorrhagic shock 123, 137, 146, 155, 155*t*, 159
hemorrhagic strokes 232, 232*f*

hemostasis 140-141, 141*f*
hemostatic agents 147
hemothorax 297-299
    diagnostic accuracy for 298-299
    field assessment techniques 298-299
    immediate management techniques 299
    incidence and epidemiology 298
    indications and contraindications 299
    overview 297-298, 297*f*
    risk factors for 298
    signs and symptoms of 298, 298*f*
    transport of patients for 299
heparin 141-143, 143*t*
hepatitis B vaccine 29*t*, 43, 381
hepatitis B virus 32*t*, 38, 40
hepatitis C virus 32*t*, 38
hepatomegaly 333
high-altitude cerebral edema (HACE) 375-377
high-altitude headaches 230, 231
high-altitude pulmonary edema (HAPE) 375-377, 376*t*
high-concentration oxygen 87
HIPAA (Health Insurance Portability and Accountability Act) of 1996 46, 47
hip dislocation 194, 195*f*
hip fractures. *See* pelvic fractures
Hippocratic method 189, 190*f*
histamine 160
HITECH (Health Information Technology for Economic and Clinical Health) Act of 2009 46-47
HIV/AIDS 32*t*, 38, 40
hives 169
Homan's sign 142
honesty 18, 20
hosts for infectious diseases 28, 30
humeral fractures 200-202
    classification of 201-202, 201-202*f*
    field assessment techniques 201-202
    immediate management techniques 202
    incidence and epidemiology 200-201
    risk factors for 201
    signs and symptoms of 201, 201*f*
humerus, anatomy of 200, 200*f*
hyperbaric chambers 377
hypercapnia 84, 230
hypercoagulable conditions 137
hyperglycemia
    causes of 349
    defined 343
    management of 347-348, 347*f*, 350-351
    signs and symptoms of 345, 349
    transport of patients for 351
hyperkalemia 358
hypernatremia 234
hyperoxemia 114*t*, 115
hyperpnea 286
hypersensitivity reactions. *See also* anaphylaxis
    classification of 160-161, 161*t*, 164

defined 160
drug-induced 170
food-induced 166
urticaria and 169
hypertension 304, 305
hypertensive crisis 96-97, 97t
hypertrophic cardiomyopathy (HCM) 310-311, 310f
hyphema 240, 240f
hypoglycemia
causes of 348
defined 343
diagnostic accuracy for 350
field assessment techniques 349, 350f
management of 120, 129, 346-347, 350-351
risk factors for 349
seizures and 234
signs and symptoms of 345, 349
transport of patients for 351
hyponatremia 234, 368
hypoperfusion 84, 88, 94, 95, 136
hypotension 96, 97t, 144, 296, 304, 305
hypothermia 372-374, 373t
hypovolemic shock 143-144, 154-155, 155t, 335
hypoxemia 297, 321, 375
hypoxia
altitude-related 375
blood oxygen saturation and 97
cerebral 307
headache and 230
level of consciousness and 84
medical oxygen for 114t
pulmonary embolism and 296
respiratory assessment for 87

I

iatrogenic pneumothorax 298
ICHART documentation technique 48, 50t
ICP (intracranial pressure) 226
ICS (incident command system) 72
icterus 170
ICU (intensive care unit) 14
I-gel airway 290f, 291
iliocostalis thoracis muscle 328
immunity 32t
immunizations 29, 29t
immunoglobulin E antibody (IgE) 160-162, 166, 170
immunologic emergencies. *See* anaphylaxis; hypersensitivity reactions
implied consent 45
incident command system (ICS) 72
incident reports 70-71
index of suspicion 80
indirect contact transmission 30
infarction 232, 295, 359. *See also* myocardial infarction
infectious diseases 28-43. *See also* pathogens; *specific diseases*
defined 28
exposure control plans for 34, 43, 379-382
health care–associated 31-32t, 31-33

multidrug-resistant organisms 33-34, 33t
nosocomial 30, 31
prevention of 28, 29, 29t
standard precautions for 28, 34-43
transmission routes 29-31
treatment for 28
infiltration 129
influenza virus 28, 29t, 30
informed consent 20, 44
infraspinatus muscle 283, 284f
inhalers 111-113, 113f, 113t
initial assessment 82-89
ABCDE approach to 83-84, 84f, 172, 210, 254
of airway 87
of blood loss 86
of breathing 87
of circulation 87-88
of consciousness level 86-87
general impression from 84-86
goals of 82-83
of life-threatening conditions 85, 86
overview 77-78, 85f
of perfusion 88
of priority of patient care and transport 89, 89t
rapid trauma assessment 88-89
of spinal injuries 85-86
injection practices 38-39, 38f, 116-120
Injury Severity Score (ISS) 102-103, 102t
injury surveillance systems 25, 25t
inline stabilization 257-259, 258f
insect bites and stings 167-169, 168t
Institute of Medicine (IOM) 5
insulin 108, 117, 343-344, 347-350
integrity 18
intensive care unit (ICU) 14
intercostal muscles 282-283, 284f
internal bleeding 138-139, 144-146
internal oblique muscle 328, 329f
interpersonal communication 20-22
interpersonal distance 20, 20f
interprofessional communication 5, 6, 18, 69
interprofessional practice 4-6. *See also* team-based health care
interspinous ligaments 250f, 251
intervertebral discs 251, 251f
intracerebral contusion 226
intracranial pressure (ICP) 226
intramuscular administration 109t, 117, 120, 121, 173
intravenous (IV) administration 120-131
benefits of 121-122
catheters for 123-124, 123f, 127-129
changing IV bags 129
discontinuation of 131
established IV access point for 129-130, 130f
fluid selection for 123, 124, 124-125t, 129-130, 129t
indications for 120-123
overview 109t

saline lock setup for 126, 126f, 130, 130f
spiking the bag for 126, 126f
supplies for establishing access 123-124
tubing selection for 124, 126
unsuccessful attempts at 130-131
vein selection for 127, 127f, 128
venipuncture and 126-129, 128-129f
intravenous urography (IVU) 337
IOM (Institute of Medicine) 5
I PASS the BATON strategy 70
ipratropium bromide 116, 116t
irrigation of wounds 149
ischemia 201, 304, 309
ischemic strokes 232, 232f
islets of Langerhans 343-344
ISS (Injury Severity Score) 102-103, 102t
IV administration. *See* intravenous administration
IVU (intravenous urography) 337

J

jaundice 94, 170
jaw-thrust maneuver 256, 256f

K

Kehr's sign 145, 332, 334
Kendrick Extrication Device (K.E.D.) 265-266, 265f
ketonuria 347
kidney injuries 335-337
clinical prediction rules for 337
diagnostic accuracy for 337
field assessment techniques 336-337
grading system for 336
immediate management techniques 337
incidence and epidemiology 336
protection from 335-336, 335f
risk factors for 336
signs and symptoms of 336
transport of patients for 337
kidneys, structure and function of 330-331
kidney stones 337
King airway 291, 291f
King-Devick test 224
knee dislocation 195-197
field assessment techniques 196-197, 196f
immediate management techniques 197, 197f
incidence and epidemiology 195, 196f
risk factors for 195-196
signs and symptoms of 196
knee ligaments 195, 195f
knowledge-based mistakes 16
Korotkoff sounds 97
Kussmaul breathing 347

L

lactated Ringer's (LR) solution 124, 125t, 140, 159
laparotomy 334

lapses (errors) 16
laryngeal anatomy 219, 219*f*
laryngeal injuries 242, 244-245
laryngeal mask airway (LMA) 290-291, 290*f*
latent infections 29
latex allergy 62, 166
latissimus dorsi muscle 283, 284*f*, 328
Le Fort fractures 241, 241*f*
legal responsibilities 43-52
   confidentiality 23, 46-47, 69
   documentation of care 47-52
   Good Samaritan laws 45
   mandated reporting 45-46
   patient consent 20, 43-45
level of consciousness (LOC) 84, 86-87, 220, 334
levels of trauma centers 61, 61*t*, 103
licensure 9, 105
Lichtenberg figure 367
lifelong learning 19
ligamentum flavum 250*f*, 251
lightning strike injuries 365-368
   diagnostic accuracy for 367
   field assessment techniques 367
   immediate management techniques 367-368
   incidence and epidemiology 366
   medical consequences of 366
   methods and effects of 365, 366*t*
   signs and symptoms of 366
   transport of victims 367-368
linea alba 329, 329*f*
linear fractures 221
lipohemarthrosis 209
liver, structure and function of 329-330
liver injuries 332-335
   contraindications 335
   diagnostic accuracy for 334-335
   field assessment techniques 334-335
   grading system for 334
   immediate management techniques 335
   incidence and epidemiology 332, 333
   risk factors for 333
   signs and symptoms of 333
   transport of patients for 335
LMA (laryngeal mask airway) 290-291, 290*f*
LOC. *See* level of consciousness
log-roll technique 259, 262-265, 262*f*, 264*f*, 278, 278*f*
longissimus thoracis muscle 328
longitudinal ligaments 250-251, 250*f*
long QT syndrome 314, 314*f*
lower-extremity anatomy 181-183, 182-184*f*
lower-extremity fractures 209-214
   clinical decision rules for 211-212
   field assessment techniques 209-212
   immediate management techniques 212-214
   immobilization of 213
   sign and symptoms of 209, 210

transport of patients for 214
   types and sequencing 210-211
LR solution. *See* lactated Ringer's (LR) solution
"lub dub" sound of heart 305
lucid intervals 226-227
lumbar vertebra 248, 248-249*f*, 249
lungs, structure and function of 285-286, 285*f*
lymphadenopathy 142

M
magnetic resonance imaging (MRI) 212, 226, 376
Maisonneuve fracture 208, 209*f*
malocclusion 241, 242
mandated reporting 45-46
mandibular fractures 241, 242
Marfan syndrome 311-312, 311*f*
marriage and family therapists (MFTs) 15
mass casualty incidents (MCIs) 71-72, 80-81
maturity 19
maxillary fractures 241
McBurney's point 145, 331, 338, 338*f*
MDIs (metered-dose inhalers) 111-113, 113*f*, 113*t*
MDQ (medically disqualifying) injuries 53, 54, 75
MDROs (multidrug-resistant organisms) 33-34, 33*t*
mean arterial pressure (MAP) 123
mechanism of injury (MOI)
   ankle fractures 208
   Colles' fracture 202
   determination of 80
   elbow dislocation 191
   femur fractures 206
   finger dislocation 193
   general impression and 84
   hemorrhage assessment and 145
   knee dislocation 195
   laryngeal injuries 244
   liver and spleen injuries 333
   pelvic fractures 203, 204
   ring avulsion 215
   shoulder dislocation 187
   spinal injuries 252-253
   sternoclavicular joint injuries 293, 294
   testicular injuries 340
   tibia-fibula fractures 207
   triage and 103
median nerve 180, 180*f*
mediastinum 285, 285*f*, 298, 299
medical abbreviations 48, 49*t*
medical alert bracelets 108, 108*f*
medical devices 39-40, 39-40*t*, 42
medical directors 8, 9
medical ID mobile apps 108, 108*f*
medically disqualifying (MDQ) injuries 53, 54, 75
medical oversight 9, 105-106
medical specialties 10

medication administration 105-131. *See also* oxygen administration; *specific medications*
   allergic reactions to 160, 170-171
   aseptic technique and 110
   best practices for 107-108
   drawing up medications 117, 118, 118*f*
   emergency injections 116-120
   errors in 108
   intramuscular 109*t*, 117, 120, 121, 173
   intravenous 109*t*, 120-131, 123*f*, 126-130*f*
   metered-dose inhalers 111-113, 113*f*, 113*t*
   nebulized 112, 114-115, 114-115*t*, 114*f*
   oral 109*t*, 110
   routes of 108, 109*t*
   scope of practice and 105-106
   six rights of 107, 108
   subcutaneous 109*t*, 117, 117*f*, 119, 119*f*, 347
   sublingual 109*t*, 110-112, 112*f*
   for sudden cardiac arrest 320-321, 320*t*
medication storage 106, 108, 117
medulla oblongata 218, 218*f*
melena 145
memory, dependence on 17-18
meninges 219
menorrhagia 139
mesentery 328
metabolic emergencies 343-351
   anatomical structures in 343-344, 344*f*
   diabetes mellitus 344-348, 347*f*
   hyperglycemia 343, 345, 347-351, 347*f*
   hypoglycemia 120, 129, 234, 343, 345-351, 350*f*
metered-dose inhalers (MDIs) 111-113, 113*f*, 113*t*
methicillin 33*t*
methicillin/oxacillin-resistant *Staphylococcus aureus* (MRSA) 33*t*, 36
MFTs (marriage and family therapists) 15
microbes 28
microbicides 40, 41
migraines 229-231, 229*f*
Milch technique 189, 190*f*
minors. *See* children and adolescents
mistakes, defined 16
mitral valve 304-305, 305*f*
mittelschmerz 340
modified Trendelenburg position 335
MOF (multiple organ failure) 136, 153, 154
MOI. *See* mechanism of injury
mononucleosis 333
MRI (magnetic resonance imaging) 212, 226, 376

MRSA (methicillin/oxacillin-resistant *Staphylococcus aureus*) 33*t*, 36
multiculturalism. *See* cultural competence
multidrug-resistant organisms (MDROs) 33-34, 33*t*
multilumen airway 291, 291*f*
multiperson lift and slide 259-261, 260*f*, 273-274, 273-274*f*
multiple organ failure (MOF) 136, 153, 154
musculocutaneous nerve 180, 180*f*
musculoskeletal injuries 183-216. *See also* dislocations; fractures
    compartment syndrome and 192, 207, 209, 214-215
    immediate management for 214
    ring avulsion 215-216
    secondary survey for 188
    subluxations 184, 187
musculoskeletal system 179-184
    bones of 179-181
    ligaments of 179-180
    lower-extremity anatomy 181-183, 182-184*f*
    tendons of 180
    upper-extremity anatomy 180-181, 180-181*f*
myocardial infarction 156, 296, 309-310, 316
myocardial ischemia 309
myocarditis 311
myoclonic jerking 315, 318, 325
myoglobin 356, 357
myoglobinuria 354, 356, 357

N

NaCl (sodium chloride) 368
nail blanch test 95, 96*f*
naloxone 117, 120, 121*t*, 129, 130
nasal cannula 115*t*, 287, 288*f*
nasal fractures 241-242
nasopharyngeal airway (NPA) 115, 288-289, 289*f*, 289*t*
National Athletic Trainers' Association (NATA)
    ATs Care program from 74
    Code of Ethics 18, 24
    on dental trauma 242
    on exertional rhabdomyolysis 355
    on medication administration 106, 115, 122
    position statements on emergency response 57, 58*t*
    on sickle cell trait 359
    time-out system recommended by 65-66
National Center for Catastrophic Sport Injury Research (NCCSIR) 153, 360, 368
National Collegiate Athletic Association (NCAA) 54, 197, 206, 247, 359, 360
National Weather Service 367
nature of illness (NOI) 80

nebulized medication administration 112, 115-116, 116*f*, 116*t*
needlestick injuries 38-39
neglect, mandated reporting of 45-46
nephrectomy 336
nerve plexuses 251*f*, 252
nerves of upper and lower extremities 180-182, 180*f*, 182*f*
nervous system 251-252
neurogenic shock 155*t*, 156
New Severity Injury Score (NISS) 102-103
NEXUS criteria 254-256
nitroglycerin (NTG) 111, 111*t*, 320*t*, 321
NOI (nature of illness) 80
noninvasive blood pressure (NIBP) devices 97
non-rebreather masks 115, 115*t*, 287-288, 288*f*
nonverbal communication 21, 21*t*
normal saline (NS) 123-124, 124-125*t*, 149, 159, 220, 238
nosocomial infections 30, 31
notice of privacy practices 46
NPA. *See* nasopharyngeal airway
NSAIDs (nonsteroidal anti-inflammatory drugs)
    anaphylaxis and 171
    anticoagulant effects of 141, 142, 143*t*
    asthma and 300
    for pain management 169, 231, 292-293
NTG. *See* nitroglycerin
nucleus pulposus 251, 251*f*
numeric pain rating scale 99, 99*t*

O

oblique muscles 328, 329*f*
obstructed airway 87
obstructive shock 154, 156, 157*t*
obtundation 157
occlusion of blood flow 128, 129*f*
occult pneumothorax 299
occupational exposure 34, 43
Occupational Safety and Health Administration (OSHA)
    blood-borne pathogen standards from 43
    on medical-grade oxygen 287
    risk reduction guidelines from 31
    on standard precautions 34
    workplace safety standards from 55, 107
occupational therapists (OTs) 14
OIT (oral immunotherapy) 177
oliguria 157
on-site (field) diagnosis 77
OPA. *See* oropharyngeal airway
open-ended questions 21, 22, 90
open fractures 183-184
OPIM (other potentially infectious materials) 34, 43
OPQRST questions 90-91, 91*t*
oral administration 109*t*, 110

oral immunotherapy (OIT) 177
oral reports 69
oropharyngeal airway (OPA) 115, 288-290, 289*f*, 289*t*
orthopedic technologists, certified (OTCs) 15
OSHA. *See* Occupational Safety and Health Administration
osmotic demyelination syndrome 236
osteoporosis 203, 292
other potentially infectious materials (OPIM) 34, 43
OTs (occupational therapists) 14
ovarian cysts 339-340
ovaries 331, 331*f*
over-the-head technique 276, 276*f*
overtriage 103
oxygen administration
    delivery devices 115, 115*t*, 287-288, 288*f*, 318
    indications for 112, 114*t*, 115, 320*t*, 321
    maximization of delivery 319, 319*f*
    steps for 287
    tanks and cylinders for 114-115, 114*f*, 287

P

padded splints 200
Paget-Schroetter syndrome 137
pain, assessment of 90-91, 99, 99*t*
palliation 90
palpation 96, 97, 99, 332, 334
pancreas 343-344, 344*f*
paramedics 10-13
parenchyma 329, 330
parenteral contact 34
parenteral routes of administration 108, 109*t*
parents and guardians
    consent obtained from 44
    disclosure of medical conditions by 174
    professional boundaries with 22
    role in care process 8
participation indicators 23
participatory care 5
participatory decision-making process 8, 19
PASG (pneumatic antishock garment) 9
PAs (physician assistants) 14
pathogens. *See also* infectious diseases
    blood-borne 28, 36, 43, 107
    defined 28
    in health care settings 31, 31-32*t*
    multidrug-resistant 33, 33*t*
    respiratory 43
    standard precautions for 34-39, 42-43
    transmission routes for 29-31
patient care reports (PCRs) 48
patient-centered care 5, 6, 15, 57
patient presentation 80
patients. *See also* transport of patients
    communication with 4, 20-22
    consent obtained from 20, 43-45

(continued)

patients *(continued)*
 critical 9, 10
 documentation of care 24-25, 47-52
 emergent 9, 10
 primacy of 22
 refusal of care by 48, 50-52, 51*f*
 role in care process 8
 transfer of care 48, 70, 100-101, 101*t*
PCRs (patient care reports) 48
PE. *See* pulmonary embolism
peak flow meters 300, 302*f*
PEA (pulseless electric activity) 313, 319
pectoralis muscles 282, 284*f*
pectus excavatum 312
pediatric patients. *See* children and adolescents
pelvic fractures 203-205
 field assessment techniques 204-205, 204*f*
 immediate management techniques 205, 205*f*
 incidence and epidemiology 203
 risk factors for 203
 signs and symptoms of 204
pelvic girdle 203, 204*f. See also* abdominopelvic region
penetrating trauma 145
penicillin 171
percussion 332, 332*f*
percutaneous exposure incidents 38-39
percutaneous techniques 10, 110
perfusion
 capillary refill and 95, 96*f*
 defined 136
 determinants of 136, 137*f*
 hypoperfusion 84, 88, 94, 95, 136
 initial assessment of 88
 as physiological basis for shock 123
 reperfusion 154
 skin characteristics and 94-95, 95*f*
pericardium 285
peripheral nerve injury 358
peripheral nervous system (PNS) 251
peritoneum 328, 329
peroneal artery 182, 183*f*
peroneal nerves 182, 182*f*, 196, 206, 209
personal protective equipment (PPE) 30, 35-38, 37*f*, 42, 107
petechiae 139
PFA (psychological first aid) 73-74
pharmacists 14, 16, 106, 231
PHI (protected health information) 46-47
phonophobia 229, 230
photophobia 229, 238, 240
physical therapists (PTs) 15
physical urticaria 170
physician assistants (PAs) 14
physicians. *See* health care providers (HCPs)
pia mater 219, 226
PIOs (public information officers) 72, 73
platelet plugs 140-141, 141*f*
platinum 10 minutes 77, 89
pleural cavities 285, 285*f*

pneumatic antishock garment (PASG) 9
pneumonia 292, 293
pneumothorax 297-299
 diagnostic accuracy for 298-299
 field assessment techniques 298-299
 immediate management techniques 299
 incidence and epidemiology 298
 indications and contraindications 299
 overview 297-298, 297*f*
 risk factors for 298
 signs and symptoms of 298, 298*f*
 transport of patients for 299
PNS (peripheral nervous system) 251
pons 218, 218*f*
popliteal artery 182-183, 183*f*, 196-197, 206
positive feedback loops 141
positive-pressure ventilation 87
post-catastrophic injury plans 72-74
post-concussive syndrome 222
post-critical incident plans 72-74
post-event evaluations 73
post-phlebitic syndrome 142
post-traumatic stress disorder (PTSD) 73-74
PPE. *See* personal protective equipment
practice acts 7, 43, 105-106, 117
pregnancy, ectopic 339-340
pre-hospital care reports 48
premonitory symptoms 310
pre-shock 154
pressure dressings 146-147, 147*f*
pressure urticaria 169
primacy of patients 22
primary care 5-6, 13
primary exercise headaches 230
primary survey. *See* initial assessment
Privacy Rule (HIPAA) 46
professional attributes 18-19
professional boundaries 22-23
protected health information (PHI) 46-47
proteinuria 357
protocols 55, 57
proximal tibiofibular joint (PTFJ) 207
pruritus 163
psychiatrists 15
psychological first aid (PFA) 73-74
psychologists 15
PTSD (post-traumatic stress disorder) 73-74
PTs (physical therapists) 15
public crest 328, 328*f*
public information officers (PIOs) 72, 73
pulmonary circulation 304, 304*f*, 306
pulmonary embolism (PE) 295-297
 clinical prediction rules for 297
 as complication of hemorrhage 137
 as consequence of misdiagnoses 142
 defined 295
 diagnostic accuracy for 296-297
 field assessment techniques 296-297
 immediate management techniques 297

 incidence and epidemiology 295, 296*f*
 risk factors for 295-296
 signs and symptoms of 296
 transport of patients for 297
pulmonary valve 304, 305*f*
pulseless electric activity (PEA) 313, 319
pulse oximetry 97, 99, 99*f*, 286-287, 286*t*, 376
pulse points 181-183, 181*f*, 184*f*
pulse rate 87-88, 96
pulse rhythm 96
purpura 139
P wave 306, 307*f*
pyrogenic reaction 125*t*

Q
QRS wave complex 306, 307*f*
quick-release helmets 270-271, 271*f*
quick-release shoulder pads 279, 279*f*

R
radial artery 180, 181, 181*f*
radial nerve 180, 180*f*, 201
rapid trauma assessment 88-89
rectal thermometers 369, 370, 371*f*, 374
rectus abdominis muscle 282, 284*f*, 328, 329*f*
recumbence 165, 293, 295
red blood cells. *See* erythrocytes
refusal of care 48, 50-52, 51*f*
renal failure 357
reperfusion 154
reporting practices 45-46, 48, 69-71
reprocessing 39
reproductive system 331, 331*f*, 339-341
respect 18, 20-22, 24
respiratory arrest 115
respiratory assessment 87, 96, 286
respiratory distress 112, 115
respiratory failure 115
respiratory hygiene 42-43
responsibility, as professional attribute 18
responsiveness, assessment of 86-87
retinal detachment 239-240
retroglottic airway 291, 291*f*
retroperitoneum 328
return of spontaneous circulation (ROSC) 321
return to participation (RTP)
 concussion and 225
 criteria for 7
 exertional rhabdomyolysis and 358
 liver and spleen injuries and 334
 rib fracture and 293
 treatment options and 8
rewarming techniques 374-375
Reye's Syndrome 110*t*
rhabdomyolysis. *See* exertional rhabdomyolysis (ER)
rhinorrhea 160
rib fracture 291-293
 clinical prediction rules for 292
 diagnostic accuracy for 292

field assessment techniques 292
immediate management techniques 292-293
incidence and epidemiology 291-292
indications and contraindications 293
risk factors for 292
signs and symptoms of 292
transport of patients for 293
ribs, structure and function of 281-282, 282f
Riddell quick-release pin system 270, 271f
ring avulsion 215-216
risk management 27-28
ROSC (return of spontaneous circulation) 321
Rovsing's sign 338
RTP. *See* return to participation
rule-based mistakes 16

S

sacrum 248-250, 248f, 328, 328f
SAC (Standardized Assessment of Concussion) 224
SADS (sudden arrhythmic death syndrome) 314
SAMPLE questions 90, 90t, 92
SAM (structural aluminum malleable) splint 200, 202
SA (sinoatrial) node 306, 306f
SBAR communication tool 100-101, 101t
SBP. *See* systolic blood pressure
SCA. *See* sudden cardiac arrest
scalp lacerations 220-221
SCAT-5 (Sport Concussion Assessment Tool) 223-224, 230, 383-391
SCD. *See* sudden cardiac death
scene size-up 79-82
Schutt Twist Release Retainer 270-271, 271f
sciatic nerve 181-182, 182f
SC joint. *See* sternoclavicular (SC) joint
SC joint injury. *See* sternoclavicular (SC) joint injury
scoop stretchers 266-268, 267f
scope of practice 9-13, 105-106
screwdrivers for face mask removal 270, 270f
scrotum 331-332, 332f, 340-341
SC (sternoclavicular) ligament 282, 283f, 293
SCT. *See* sickle cell trait (SCT)
secondary injuries 253
second impact syndrome 222
Security Rule (HIPAA) 46, 47
seesaw breathing 96
Segond sign 209
seizures 233-236
    categorization of 234
    immediate management techniques 235-236
    incidence and epidemiology 234
    indications and contraindications 235
    participation in sports and 233-234
    procedures and protocols 235-236

risk factors for 234
    signs and symptoms of 234-235, 235t
selective serotonin reuptake inhibitors (SSRIs) 207
self-awareness 23
semilunar valves 304
sepsis (septic shock) 31t, 136, 143, 154-156, 155t
serial vitals 93, 94, 108
serratus muscles 283, 284f
7-strap system 268, 268f
sharps, defined 41
sharps disposal 38, 41-42, 42f
sharps injuries 38-39
shivering 373
shock 152-160. *See also* anaphylaxis
    assessment of patients with 156-158
    cardiogenic shock 154, 156, 156t, 304
    defined 152
    distributive 154-156, 155t
    emergency care for 158-160, 159f
    epidemiology of 152-153
    hemorrhagic 123, 137, 146, 155, 155t, 159
    hypovolemic 143-144, 154-155, 155t, 335
    medical consequences of 136
    neurogenic 155t, 156
    obstructive 154, 156, 157t
    pathophysiology of 153-156, 153f
    perfusion as physiological basis for 123
    risk factors for 152
    septic 31t, 136, 143, 154-156, 155t
    signs and symptoms 138, 157, 158
    stages of 154
    undifferentiated 156-160
shoulder dislocation 187-191
    field assessment techniques 189
    immediate management techniques 189-191, 190-191f
    incidence and epidemiology 187
    risk factors for 188-189
    signs and symptoms of 189, 189f
shoulder pad removal 273-279, 273-279f
shunting 138
sickle cell disease (anemia) 359
sickle cell trait (SCT) 358-362. *See also* exertional collapse associated with sickle cell trait (ECAST)
signs, defined 79
simple oxygen masks 115t, 287, 288f
simple triage and rapid treatment (START) strategy 81-82
sinoatrial (SA) node 306, 306f
sinus bradycardia 306, 308
sinus rhythm 306, 307, 313f
SIRS (systemic inflammatory response syndrome) 156
skeletal system. *See* musculoskeletal system
skin, assessment of 88, 94-95, 95f
skin adhesives 149-150, 149f
skull fracture 221
slips (errors) 16

SLPs (speech and language pathologists) 15
small-volume nebulizers (SVNs) 116, 116f, 116t
SMR. *See* spinal motion restriction
SOAPM documentation method 48, 50f
social workers 15
sodium chloride (NaCl) 368
solar urticaria 170
somnolence 225
Spaso technique 189-190
speech and language pathologists (SLPs) 15
Speed Clips 268
spermatic cord 331-332, 332f, 340, 341
spider bites 167-169, 168t
Spider-Strap system 268, 268f
spinal column 248-250f, 248-251, 253
spinal cord 251-253, 251f
spinal injuries 252-280
    airway management and 256-257, 256f
    cardiac arrest and 257
    cervical 85-86, 257-259, 258f
    emergency medical care for 254-256
    equipment removal for 269-279, 270-279f
    growth of 247
    immobilization for 85-86, 254-269
    mechanism of injury 252-253
    pathophysiology of 252-253
    signs and symptoms of 253
spinalis thoracis muscle 328
spinal motion restriction (SMR) 254-269
    Canadian C-Spine Rule for 254-256, 255f
    cervical 85-86, 257-259, 258f
    equipment for 266-268, 267f
    guidelines and recommendations 269
    NEXUS criteria for 254-256
    for prone patients 263-265, 264f
    for seated patients 265-266, 265f
    strapping techniques 268-269, 268f
    for supine patients 259-263, 260-262f
spine boards 266, 267f
spleen, structure and function of 330
spleen injuries 332-335
    clinical prediction rules for 335
    contraindications 335
    diagnostic accuracy for 332-334
    field assessment techniques 334-335
    grading system for 334
    immediate management techniques 335
    incidence and epidemiology 333
    risk factors for 333
    signs and symptoms of 333-334
    transport of patients for 335
splenectomy 330
splenomegaly 333
splints 199-200, 202, 203, 213
Sport Concussion Assessment Tool (SCAT-5) 223-224, 230, 383-391
sports-related injuries. *See also* emergency examinations; mechanism

(continued)

sports-related injuries *(continued)*
of injury (MOI); *specific types of injuries*
catastrophic 54-55, 72-74, 153
costs associated with 75
epidemiology of 25, 54
medically disqualifying 53, 54, 75
surveillance systems for 25, 25*t*
SSRIs (selective serotonin reuptake inhibitors) 207
Standardized Assessment of Concussion (SAC) 224
standardized procedures 16-17, 25
standard precautions 34-43
for biohazardous material 41, 41*f*
compliance with 28
for contaminated equipment or surfaces 39-41*t*, 39-42
defined 34
in emergency examinations 80
hand hygiene 15, 28, 30, 34-35, 38
injection practices 38-39, 38*f*
personal protective equipment 30, 35-38, 37*f*, 42, 107
respiratory hygiene and cough etiquette 42-43
for sharps disposal 41-42, 42*f*
Standards of Professional Practice (BOC) 18
Staphylococcus aureus 28, 33*t*
staples 150
START (simple triage and rapid treatment) strategy 81-82
sterilization 40-42, 40*t*
sternoclavicular (SC) joint 282, 283*f*, 285, 293, 294*f*
sternoclavicular (SC) joint injury 293-295
diagnostic accuracy for 295
field assessment techniques 294-295
immediate management techniques 295
incidence and epidemiology 293
indications and contraindications 295
risk factors for 293
signs and symptoms of 294
transport of patients for 295
sternoclavicular (SC) ligament 282, 283*f*, 293
sternocleidomastoid muscle 282, 284*f*
sternum 282, 282-283*f*
Stimson's hanging arm technique 189, 190*f*
straddle technique 259, 261, 261*f*, 274, 274*f*
strapping techniques 268-269, 268*f*
stress 18
stroke 231-233
comorbidities and 233
field assessment techniques 232-233, 233*t*
immediate management techniques 233
incidence and epidemiology 231-232
risk factors for 232

structural aluminum malleable (SAM) splint 200, 202
subclavian artery 180, 181*f*
subcutaneous emphysema 244
subcutaneous (SubQ) administration 109*t*, 117, 117*f*, 119, 119*f*, 347
subdural hematoma 227-228, 228*f*
sublingual administration 109*t*, 110-112, 112*f*
subluxations 184, 187
subperitoneum 328
sudden arrhythmic death syndrome (SADS) 314
sudden cardiac arrest (SCA) 318-325
chain of survival 318-321
clinical decision making for 323, 324*f*
emergency preparedness for 321-323
field assessment techniques 315
immediate management techniques 315, 318-321
incidence of 307
from lightning strikes 366
pharmacologic intervention for 320-321, 320*t*
spinal injuries and 257
survival following 325
treatable causes of 319
sudden cardiac death (SCD) 307-315
arrhythmic causes of 312-315
incidence and epidemiology 307
population differences in 308-309, 308*t*
prevention strategies 303, 323, 325
structural causes of 309-312, 309*t*
superbugs 33-34, 33*t*
supraglottic airway 115, 290-291, 290*f*
supraspinous ligaments 250*f*, 251
SURETY model 21, 21*t*
sutures 150-151, 151*f*
SVNs (small-volume nebulizers) 116, 116*f*, 116*t*
symptoms, defined 79
syncope 89, 165, 236, 310, 314-315
syndesmotic joint 197
systemic circulation 304, 304*f*, 306
systemic inflammatory response syndrome (SIRS) 156
systems review 92-93, 93*t*
systems thinking 15
systolic blood pressure (SBP) 97, 99, 123, 304

T
tachyarrhythmias 156
tachycardia
in pneumothorax and hemothorax 298, 299
pulmonary embolism and 296
shock and 138
ventricular 306, 308, 310, 312, 313*f*
tachypnea 144, 286, 298
talar dome 197
TBIs. *See* traumatic brain injuries (TBIs)
TB (tuberculosis) 29, 29*t*
team-based health care 3-25

advantages of 4, 5
breakdowns in 15-18
characteristics of 4-6
core competencies of 5
defined 3-4
effective practices in 18
errors in 16-18
examples of 3, 5
principles for 4
professional attributes in 18-19
in sports medicine setting 6-15, 6*f*
therapeutic behaviors in 19-25
telangiectasias 139
temporomandibular joint (TMJ) dislocation 242
tendons 180
tension headaches 229, 229*f*, 231
teres muscles 283, 284*f*
testicles, structure and function of 331-332, 332*f*
testicular injuries 340-342
clinical prediction rules for 342
diagnostic accuracy for 341
field assessment techniques 341-342
immediate management techniques 342
incidence and epidemiology 340-341
risk factors for 341
signs and symptoms of 341
transport of patients for 342
tetraplegia 252
therapeutic behaviors 19-25
closed- and open-ended questions 21-22, 90
confidentiality issues 23
cultural competence and 20, 22-24
defined 19
emotional intelligence 23
ethical practice and 24-25
interpersonal communication 20-22
interpersonal distance 20, 20*f*
nonverbal communication 21, 21*t*
professional boundaries and 22-23
touch, appropriateness of 22
therapeutic space 21, 21*t*
thermistor thermometers 369, 370, 374
thermotherapies 348
thoracentesis 299
thoracic outlet syndrome 137
thoracic vertebra 248, 248-249*f*
thorax 281-286
bones of 281-282, 282-283*f*
cavities of 285, 285*f*
ligaments of 282, 283*f*
muscles of 282-283, 284*f*
organs of 285-286, 285*f*
thorax injuries 286-299
airway maintenance for 288-292, 289-291*f*, 289*t*
pneumothorax and hemothorax 297-298*f*, 297-299
pulmonary embolism 137, 142, 295-297, 296*f*
respiratory assessment for 286

rib fracture 291-293
to sternoclavicular joint 293-295
supplemental oxygen for 286-288, 288*f*
thrombocytopenia 143
thrombosis 137, 141, 143, 232. *See also* deep vein thrombosis (DVT)
thrombus 141, 295
thunderclap headaches 231, 232
tibia-fibula fractures 207, 210
tibial arteries 182, 183, 183*f*, 209
tibial plafond 197
tilt technique 275, 275*f*
time-out system 65-66
time shortages 16
TMJ (temporomandibular joint) dislocation 242
torsion, testicular 340-342
touch, appropriateness of 22
tourniquets 127-129, 127*f*, 151-152, 151-152*f*
traction splints 213
traditional handhold method 257, 258*f*
trainers. *See* athletic trainers (ATs)
transfer of care 48, 70, 100-101, 101*t*
transmission routes 29-31
transport of patients
    altitude-related emergencies and 377
    anaphylaxis and 120, 169
    appendicitis and 339
    asthma and 301-302
    cold-related emergencies and 374-375
    concussion and 225
    diabetes and 348
    ectopic pregnancy and 340
    in emergency action plans 60-61
    EMS nomenclature for 89, 89*t*
    exertional heatstroke and 372
    hyperglycemia/hypoglycemia and 351
    kidney injuries and 337
    lightning strike injuries and 367-368
    liver and spleen injuries and 335
    lower-extremity fractures and 214
    ovarian cysts and 340
    pneumothorax/hemothorax and 299
    priority conditions 79
    pulmonary embolism and 297
    rib fracture and 293

sternoclavicular joint injury and 295
testicular injuries and 342
transverse abdominis muscle 328, 329*f*
trapezius muscles 283, 284*f*
trap squeeze method 257, 258*f*
trauma center levels 61, 61*t*, 103
traumatic brain injuries (TBIs) 220-222, 225, 228-230, 238, 240
traumatic events 55, 57, 73-74
triage 80-82, 81*t*, 82*f*, 103, 366
tricuspid valve 304, 305*f*
trigeminal autonomic cephalalgias 229
Triple Aim of health care system 5
tripod fractures 241
tripod position 96
true ribs 281-282
tuberculosis (TB) 29, 29*t*
tuning forks 212
turgor 95, 95*f*
tympanic membrane rupture 240-241
type I hypersensitivity reactions 160-161, 161*t*
type 1 diabetes 344, 347, 348
type 2 diabetes 344-345

U

ulnar artery 180, 181*f*
ulnar nerve 180, 180*f*
ultrasound 298-299, 334-335, 337, 338, 340, 341
uncompensated shock 154
undertriage 103
unsecured protected health information 46
upper-extremity anatomy 180-181, 180-181*f*
urgent care 13
urinary tract infection (UTI) 338
urticaria 160, 164, 169-170, 169*f*
U.S. Department of Health and Human Services 46
U.S. Food and Drug Administration (FDA) 39
uterus 331, 331*f*

V

vaccines 29, 29*t*
vacuum mattresses 267-268, 267*f*
vacuum splints 199, 202, 203, 213
Valsalva maneuver 310

vancomycin 33*t*
vascular spasm 140, 141*f*
vaso-occlusion 359
venipuncture 126-129, 128-129*f*
venous thromboembolism (VTE) 137, 143, 295
ventral root 251, 252
ventricular fibrillation (VF) 306-308, 310, 313-314*f*, 313-315
ventricular tachycardia (VT) 306, 308, 310, 312, 313*f*
verapamil 321
vesicular sounds 286
vials, drawing medication from 117, 118, 118*f*
violations 15, 22-23
viricides 40
vital signs 93-99
    baseline 91, 94, 122
    blood oxygen saturation 97, 99, 99*f*
    blood pressure 96-99, 97*t*, 123, 304, 305
    oral report on 69
    pain 90-91, 99, 99*t*
    perfusion 88, 94-95, 95-96*f*, 123
    pulse rate 87-88, 96
    respiration rate and quality 87, 96
    serial 93, 94, 108
    trends in 93-94
Volkmann's contracture 209
VT. *See* ventricular tachycardia (VT)
VTE (venous thromboembolism) 137, 143, 295

W

warfarin 141, 142, 143*t*
wheals 169
wheezing 300
willful neglect 46
wind chill 372, 372*f*
windlass tourniquets 151, 151*f*
within normal limits (WNL) 95
Wolff-Parkinson-White (WPW) syndrome 314
World Health Organization (WHO) 5, 173
wound closure 147-152, 149*f*
wrist fractures 202-203, 203*f*

Z

zygomatic fractures 241

Michelle A. Cleary, PhD, ATC, CSCS, is an associate professor in the athletic training program and an associate dean of graduate health science at Chapman University. Prior to joining Chapman in 2012, Cleary taught at Temple University, where she earned her doctorate, and at Florida International University and the 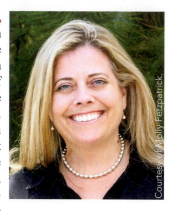 University of Hawaii. She is certified as an athletic trainer by the Board of Certification (BOC) and is certified as a strength and conditioning specialist by the National Strength and Conditioning Association. She is the chair of the Research and Grants Committee of the Far West Athletic Trainers' Association and is also a member of the American College of Sports Medicine. Cleary's primary research interests focus on heat-related illness and injury and other sport safety issues. In addition to numerous journal articles and book chapters, Cleary has written two national position statements for the National Athletic Trainers' Association (NATA). Her clinical experience includes time as an athletic trainer at the high school, NCAA Division I, and international/Olympic levels.

Courtesy of Molly Fetzpatrick.

Katie Walsh Flanagan, EdD, ATC, is a professor and director of the sports medicine and athletic training program in the department of health education and promotion at East Carolina University, where she has worked for more than 20 years, and is an athletic trainer certified by the Board of Certification (BOC). 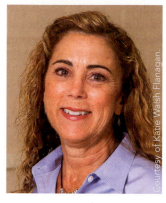 Walsh Flanagan previously worked as a lecturer and assistant athletic trainer at California State University, Fresno, and as the head athletic trainer for the Chicago Power, a men's professional soccer team. She has also assisted as an athletic trainer for various sports in international competitions, including the 1996 Summer Olympic Games and 1987 Pan American Games.

In 2012, Walsh Flanagan was elected to the North Carolina Athletic Trainers' Association Hall of Fame. The organization named her the North Carolina College/University Athletic Trainer of the Year in 2000 and 2006. She received the National Athletic Trainers' Association (NATA) Most Distinguished Athletic Trainer Award in 2010 and NATA's Service Award in 2006. In 2017, she was named a NATA board member as the director of District Three. She coauthored *Medical Conditions in the Athlete, Third Edition.*

Courtesy of Katie Walsh Flanagan.

CONTRIBUTORS AND EXTERNAL REVIEWERS

Contributors

Dewayne DuBose, PhD, ATC, LAT, NCPT
Assistant Professor
Health and Exercise Science/Athletic Training
Bethune-Cookman University

Dominique Francis DuBose, PhD, ATC, LAT
Adjunct Professor
Health Exercise Science
Bethune Cookman University

Adjunct Professor
Biology
Embry Riddle Aeronautical University

Kristan Erdmann, EdD, ATC, EMT
Assistant Professor
Applied Health Sciences
Murray State University

Eric J. Fuchs, DA, ATC, AEMT
Chair of the Department of Exercise and Sport Science
Professor
Athletic Training
Eastern Kentucky University

Priscilla Maghrabi, PhD, ATC
Assistant Professor
Applied Health Sciences
Murray State University

Laura Zdziarski-Horodyski, PhD, LAT, ATC
Clinical Outreach and Development Coordinator
University of Utah Health
University of Utah Orthopaedics

External Reviewers

Megan Colas, PhD, ATC, NREMT
Clinical Education Director, Athletic Training Program
Department of Health and Human Performance
Nova Southeastern University

Lindsey E. Eberman, PhD, LAT, ATC
Professor and Program Director
Doctorate in Athletic Training, Applied Medicine and Rehabilitation
Indiana State University

Eric J. Fuchs, DA, ATC, AEMT
Chair of the Department of Exercise and Sport Science
Professor of Athletic Training
Eastern Kentucky University

Kit Vreeland, EdD, MBA
Clinical Associate Professor
Department of Rehabilitation and Movement Science
University of Vermont

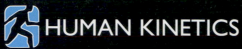
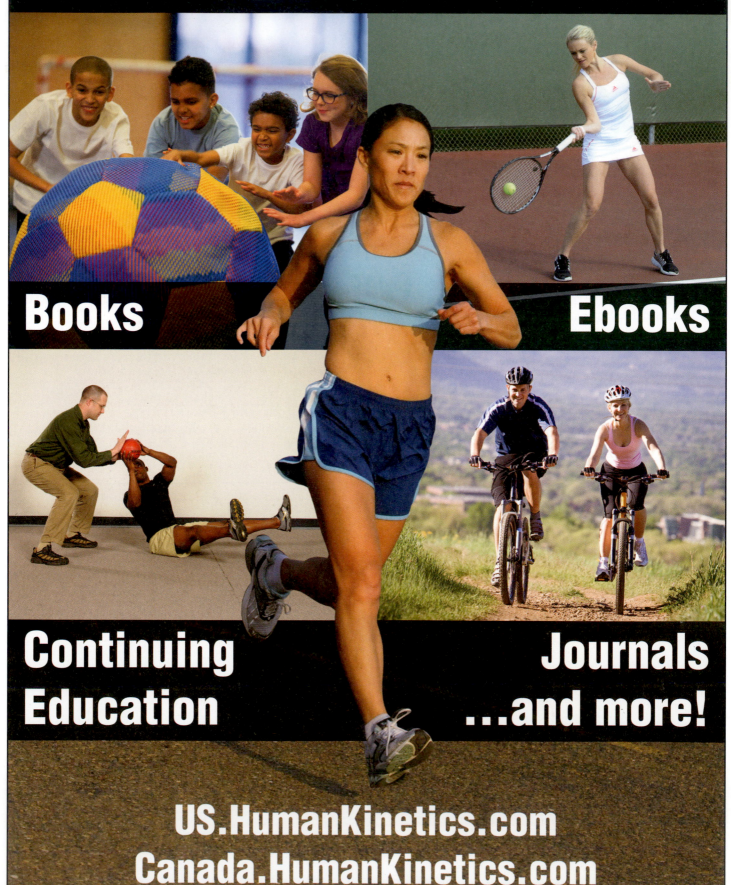